PHYSICAL DIAGNOSIS
The history and examination of the patient

PHYSICAL DIAGNOSIS
The history and examination of the patient

JOHN A. PRIOR, M.D.

Professor of Medicine,
The Ohio State University College of Medicine,
Columbus, Ohio

JACK S. SILBERSTEIN, M.D.

Clinical Professor of Medicine,
The Ohio State University College of Medicine,
Columbus, Ohio

JOHN M. STANG, M.D.

Assistant Professor of Medicine,
Director of Physical Diagnosis, Director of Coronary Care,
The Ohio State University College of Medicine,
Columbus, Ohio

SIXTH EDITION

with **492** illustrations

The C. V. Mosby Company

ST. LOUIS • TORONTO • LONDON   1981

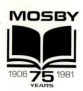

MOSBY

1906 **75** 1981
YEARS

A TRADITION OF PUBLISHING EXCELLENCE

Editor: John E. Lotz
Manuscript editor: Cheryl Zwick
Design: Jeanne Bush
Production: Debbie Wedemeier

SIXTH EDITION

The C.V. Mosby Company
11830 Westline Industrial Drive, St. Louis, Missouri 63141

Library of Congress Cataloging in Publication Data

Prior, John A.
  Physical diagnosis.

  Includes bibliographies and index.
  1. Physical diagnosis.   I. Silberstein,
Jack S.   II. Stang, John M.   III. Title.
[DNLM: 1. Diagnosis.   2. Medical history
taking.   QB 200 P958p]
RC76.P89   1981   616.07′54   81-38432
ISBN 0-8016-4054-7   AACR2

C/VH/VH 9 8 7 6 5 4 3 2 1   01/B/009

CONTRIBUTORS X

†NORMAN ALLEN, M.D.

Professor of Medicine (Neurology), The Ohio State University College of Medicine, Columbus, Ohio

JAMES H. CALDWELL, M.D.

Associate Professor of Medicine (Gastroenterology), The Ohio State University College of Medicine, Columbus, Ohio

RICHARD D. CARR, M.D.

Associate Professor of Medicine (Dermatology), The Ohio State University College of Medicine, Columbus, Ohio

HARRISON S. EVANS, M.D.

Professor and Chairman of Psychiatry, Loma Linda University College of Medicine, Loma Linda, California

WILLIAM H. HAVENER, M.D.

Professor and Chairman of Ophthalmology, The Ohio State University College of Medicine, Columbus, Ohio

ZEPH J.R. HOLLENBECK, M.D.

Professor of Obstetrics and Gynecology, The Ohio State University College of Medicine, Columbus, Ohio

ARTHUR G. JAMES, M.D.

Professor of Surgery, The Ohio State University College of Medicine, Columbus, Ohio

ERNEST L. MAZZAFERRI, M.D.

Professor and Chairman, Department of Medicine, University of Nevada, Reno, Nevada

ELIZABETH S. RUPPERT, M.D.

Professor of Pediatrics, Medical College of Ohio, Toledo, Ohio; formerly Professor of Pediatrics, The Ohio State University College of Medicine, Columbus, Ohio

WILLIAM H. SAUNDERS, M.D.

Professor and Chairman of Otolaryngology, The Ohio State University College of Medicine, Columbus, Ohio

†Deceased.

JOHN P. SMITH, M.D.

Clinical Associate Professor of Surgery (Neurology), The Ohio State University College of Medicine, Columbus, Ohio

RONALD L. WHISLER, M.D.

Associate Professor of Medicine, and Director, Division of Immunology, The Ohio State University College of Medicine, Columbus, Ohio

WIGBERT C. WIEDERHOLT, M.D.

Professor of Neurosciences, School of Medicine, University of California at San Diego, La Jolla, California; formerly Associate Professor of Medicine (Neurology), The Ohio State University College of Medicine, Columbus, Ohio

To our wives

HELEN P. and **HELEN S.**

for their devotion, encouragement, and understanding

PREFACE

In planning the sixth edition of this text we have emphasized our attempt to approach the subject from a physiologic standpoint. It is our philosophy that physical diagnosis should be meaningful and practical—not a mere mechanical process. The history and properly performed physical examination should afford the physician an insight as to whether various organs or organ systems are functioning normally or abnormally. At the same time they should provide insight into the patient as a unique and individual person. It is important to understand the physiologic mechanisms responsible for normal functions before we can accurately interpret the disturbed functions that result from disease. Just as animation adds life and interest to a picture, so does a physiologic approach add meaning and practicality to the physical examination.

With practice the physician can learn to identify the first and second heart sounds. However, only when the examiner understands the physiologic mechanisms responsible for the production of these sounds is he or she able to interpret alterations of their functions produced by various disease processes. One must understand why the second heart sound usually splits on inspiration and closes on expiration to diagnose conditions that result in abnormal splitting of this sound. To appreciate the significance of rales and rhonchi in the presence of pulmonary disease, the physician first must have a basic knowledge of respiratory function in the normal lung.

You will note that considerable space has been devoted to the development of the patient's history. It is our opinion that the little space devoted to the history in textbooks of physical diagnosis (none in some) is deplorable. Those of us who teach this course at The Ohio State University College of Medicine believe it *difficult to overemphasize* the importance of a *careful history* in the study of a patient. Therefore, one of our major objectives is to teach the student how to obtain an adequate history. When coupled with examination, the history will enable him to have a reasonably accurate impression of the possible causes of any given illness. It should serve not only as a guide for immediate care but also as an indication of the need for further diagnostic studies. It is well known that in some diseases significant physical findings are sparse or nonexistent. Thus far no substitute has been found for a good history.

A relatively detailed review of body systems has been included. This has been done with two purposes in mind. First, one of the problems confronting the medical student is the large number of clinical terms with which he must become familiar in a short time—terminology that is necessary in medicine for ease of communication. Knowledge of these meaningful terms is a fundamental part of the practice of medicine and an essential tool in the physician's daily work. This review of systems has been designed to serve as a glossary of commonly used medical terms and at the same time to explain the meaning of each term in language that a layman can understand. It is our responsibility to help the medical student become a physician. Second, an attempt has been made to explain the medical significance of the many terms to which the medical student is being introduced. An understanding of the significance of various conditions will thus serve as a guide for further questioning and will indicate body systems that may require particular attention.

Discussion of disease has been kept intentionally at a minimum because, first, we believe that a thorough concept of the normal is essential to the appreciation of the abnormal; therefore, the emphasis at this stage of the student's development should be on (1) the techniques of history-taking and physical examination and (2) the appreciation of the normal. Second, the mere volume of the material presented to the student today in textbooks of physical diagnosis, as well as in all other courses, is virtually overwhelming. Consequently, every effort has been made to maintain the utmost in simplicity and brevity.

Most textbooks of physical diagnosis contain a number of procedures, rarely used, that seldom serve any practical purpose, and it seems justifiable to leave them out of a modern text. This we have done wherever it seemed consistent with modern practice.

Physical diagnosis is not a static subject. As the result of new medical and surgical techniques in diagnosis, certain alterations in body functions assume increasing significance. For example, the growth of vascular surgery has made possible the repair of abdominal aortic aneurysms. As a consequence, such advances necessitate a more thorough consideration of examination techniques as applied to the abdomen. Tracings of heart sounds have resulted in a clearer understanding of the dynamics of production of these sounds. The chapter on the cardiovascular system has incorporated a number of heart sound tracings in order that the student may correlate the physical findings with the tracings. Also included is a more thorough evaluation and explanation of the pulse pressure curve, the understanding of which is absolutely essential to the physiologic interpretation of the various events in the cardiac cycle. Other additions to the current edition include evaluation of hearing from a clinical point of view and bedside tests for venous competency in the extremities. Various chapters, especially those dealing with the mental examination, cardiovascular system, abdomen, musculoskeletal system, and pediatric examination, have been revised considerably to ensure greater ease of understanding.

The use of personal names (eponyms) in medicine serves no purpose and contributes nothing to an understanding of the patient or his disease. As an example, the term "Stensen's duct" is absolutely meaningless until one has first learned that it is the parotid duct—the duct of the parotid salivary gland. This is a needless duplication of learning. Although we have great respect for the observations of the pioneers in medicine, we believe that it is much more important for the student to understand the fundamental principles and normal variations than it is to perpetuate a man's name, which serves no purpose in furthering the student's knowledge. Consequently, every effort has been made to use only *those terms that convey some meaning*. This is in accordance with the recommendations of *The Journal of the American Medical Association,* which has "long waged a fight against eponymic phrases generally in the medical vocabulary."* Therefore, eponyms have been eliminated whenever possible.

If, at the end of the course in physical diagnosis, the student has learned to extract from the patient an *organized, logical history* and to perform a *systematic examination, we believe that our goal has been achieved.* It should be the responsibility of his clinical teachers to instruct him in all the many findings of disease, thus helping him to build diagnostic skill on the fundamentals learned in physical diagnosis.

---

*Editorial: Meningitic breathing, J.A.M.A. **165:**1568, 1957; editorial: Confusion of tongues, J.A.M.A. **154:**1093, 1954.

We wish to thank the national office of the Arthritis Foundation for the slides in Chapter 19 reproduced from the Clinical Slide Collection on the Rheumatic Diseases, produced by the Arthritis Foundation, New York, 1972.

We are particularly pleased to have Dr. John M. Stang join us in editing this edition of *Physical Diagnosis: The History and Examination of the Patient.* In his usual energetic and well-organized fashion, Dr. Stang brings new and vital ideas to the teaching of physical diagnosis, and we are most happy that he will be assuming the major responsibility for the continuation of our textbook.

John A. Prior
Jack S. Silberstein

CONTENTS

PHYSICAL DIAGNOSIS

The history and examination of the patient

CHAPTER 1

INTRODUCTION

As a medical student you are the physician of tomorrow, and as such you need to understand that the physician is a medical detective. You will obtain information from any and every source possible to enable you to unravel the mystery of the patient's illness.

To solve the crime of murder or robbery the police detective asks many questions, often of many people, examines and photographs the premises (or body, as the case may be), and sends various items, such as blood, bullets, bits of paint, and fragments of clothing, to the crime laboratory for further study. Only after all possible data have been obtained is he in a position to identify the criminal with the greatest accuracy possible.

The physician in the same fashion is hunting for his criminal, the disease that makes the patient ill. After the witness (the patient) has told his story in his own way, the medical detective will ask many searching questions to elicit items of information that might otherwise be overlooked, or to more specifically characterize information already given. This may include interrogation of family and friends if the patient will not or cannot give a straight story. The body (of the patient) will be examined meticulously in every way possible by the physician, using all of his God-given senses. Other special investigative aids, such as the chemistry laboratory, x-ray films, and microscope, are called into the chase to add further clues to those that the physician has already uncovered by questioning and examining.

It is only after all the data have been assembled that the medical detective is in a position to begin his analysis. By clear thinking based on the information gathered, the physician is usually able to identify definitely the offending disease and to bring about the most effective remedy possible.

These are the methods that you, the medical detective of tomorrow, will use the rest of your days of practice in the never-ending search for the cause of the patient's illness. In this book you are being introduced to the *two most fundamental skills necessary for the medical investigation—interrogation and examination*. At first these procedures will be difficult for you, but with careful study and diligent practice they can be cultivated until you reach a high degree of proficiency. The development or lack of development of these skills differentiates the top-flight clinician from the mediocre.

CHAPTER 2

INTELLECTUAL PROCESS OF DIAGNOSIS

To obtain a good history requires considerable experience and a fundamental knowledge of medicine. A good case history taken by an experienced clinician is truly an invaluable component of the patient's record. Conversely, a poor history is useless, in fact, may be misleading, and is a detriment to the record. It is extremely difficult for the beginning student to take a history. His knowledge of medicine is naturally limited, and the mere task of eliciting a history is in itself complex. The student is all too acutely aware of his inadequacies in history-taking and requires thoughtful guidance and support as he learns to obtain an accurate medical history. Yet, as with other situations in life, the student must start, even though with faltering steps.

We wish to emphasize that eliciting the history is not a mere patient response to a stereotyped list of specific questions. Each item of information requires clarification and amplification. Furthermore, information must be carefully weighed as to its clinical significance and its possible relationship to the patient's complaints. These facts alone, in our opinion, make the computerized history inaccurate and untenable.

The verbal communication of information from patient to physician is the essential element of a good history. Each item of information requires interpretation that in turn may necessitate a further intelligently guided search for additional data to which the patient must respond as lucidly as possible. To obtain significant information from the patient, the physician must selectively guide him throughout the entire process, although to do so is extremely difficult because it requires a knowledge of the possible final outcome that the physician does not yet possess. The thoughtful and intelligent guidance of the patient is the hard part. In view of this dilemma just how does the beginning student take a history? He may employ four general steps in history-taking:

1. Write a brief, but accurate and comprehensive description of the patient's complaint. (This information is derived from the patient.)

2. List the various diagnoses suggested by the description. (This is a mental exercise on the part of the physician and does not involve participation by the patient.)
3. Ask the patient various questions that are designed to either confirm or exclude the tentative diagnoses. (This involves an interaction between the physician and his patient.)
4. Attempt to predict the positive physical and laboratory findings likely to result, on the basis of the information at hand. (This too is a mental exercise for the physician.)

The student should attempt to follow this step-wise analytic sequence. The expert clinician actually performs these same steps but at a more subconscious level rather than by consciously attempting to do so. The principal differences are that the clinician knows much more about the characteristics of many diseases than does the beginning student and has become skillful in developing the history by his previous experience.

Once having adopted the preceding four basic principles of history-taking, one may then consider the intellectual processes that are involved in establishing a diagnosis.

TAXONOMY OF INTELLECTUAL PROCESSES

The six progressively more complex levels of intellectual functioning are as follows: knowledge, comprehension, application, analysis, synthesis, and evaluation.

1. *Knowledge*. Knowledge is unedited factual information provided by the patient, and as such may not necessarily be accurate or precise. To serve a purpose in establishing a diagnosis facts are merely the foundation for other more complex thought processes.

2. *Comprehension*. Comprehension is understanding the facts as related by the patient to the physician. By means of further discussion the physician must affirm his comprehension of what the patient said. Misinterpreta-

tions of the history are so prevalent that two physicians frequently do not obtain exactly the same history from a given patient.

3. *Application*. Application entails an accurate and well-organized recording of the facts as related by the patient, which facilitates utilization of the knowledge as comprehended by the physician.

The preceding three steps can be performed by any reasonably educated person. The resultant product is a narrative account of an episode in the patient's life, which, if sufficiently accurate, may be of assistance to the physician. However, the next steps, analysis, synthesis, and evaluation, are progressively more complex and sophisticated intellectual processes. They are essential for the full utilization of the medical history in the solution of the patient's problem. It is only after the application of these higher intellectual processes to the history, as previously obtained, that it becomes the true medical history—one that serves as the foundation for accurate diagnosis and effective therapy.

4. *Analysis*. Analysis is sorting out or classification of the obtained data into related categories. The larger the number of abnormal components obtained in the history, the more diagnostic information available to the physician. It is the physician's difficult task to sort out, to weigh, and to differentiate minutiae from the more significant aspects of the narrative history. At this point it is prudent to consider everything that seems to be abnormal and to disregard those aspects that are clearly normal. Significant data must be placed into related categories.

5. *Synthesis*. Synthesis is reassembly of the many components obtained in the history into patterns of recognizable disease. This is much more difficult than analysis because it requires a knowledge of the disease that will best be described by the aggregate of the patient's symptoms. Because the human body is a complex

organism, many diseases are characterized by a mixture of many separate symptoms.

As the result of analysis and synthesis, one may then enumerate the diagnoses suggested by the patient's history (the differential diagnosis). The ability to accomplish this step is made possible by growing experience and further learning.

6. *Evaluation*. Most difficult and important of the intellectual processes is the final step applied to the history and ultimately to the most accurate diagnosis. Specific diagnoses become valid only if they pass the inspection of critical evaluation. This involves two basic steps previously mentioned: asking the patient questions that are designed to either confirm or exclude tentative diagnoses and predicting the likely physical and laboratory findings. As the result of evaluation, one decides whether the available information is compatible with the working diagnosis.

As mentioned previously, the lower levels (knowledge, comprehension, and application) are rather basic and within the capability of any reasonably well-educated individual. In the educational process learning at these lower levels is poorly retained because information tends to be disparate and unrelated rather than utilized as part of a composite unit. Although retention of large bodies of information is necessary in medicine, it clearly involves only the lower levels of thought. The higher levels of the taxonomy of intellectual processes (analysis, synthesis, and evaluation) involve a method of learning that compels information to make sense. Information that has been subjected to analysis, synthesis, and evaluation is apt to be retained for long periods of time, is easily refreshed, and is recaptured with accuracy. It becomes part of an integrated whole and, consequently, is far superior to simple knowledge. Alone, mere memorization of facts may actually defeat the higher intellectual processes of learning that are essential to the finest diagnostic and therapeutic care of the patient.

ESTABLISHING AND TESTING THE DIAGNOSIS

Basic skills and knowledge are mere tools used in the intelligent approach to evaluation and synthesis and ultimately in the solution of medical problems. A skilled clinician has the capability of selecting sometimes seemingly unrelated facts and perceiving their potential relationship. One must learn to deal with facts concerning medicine in accordance with basic scientific methods. It is not sufficient to merely suspect a relationship. The physician actually must establish and test this relationship, which is accomplished by developing a hypothesis (a tentative explanation of the relationship of various facts). The principal value of a hypothesis is that it serves as a guide to permit the recognition of additional pertinent facts. Thus, one must determine which facts are pertinent and which irrelevant. Unfortunately, pertinent facts are not always conspicuous and may require intensive search for their recognition.

The validity of a hypothesis is established by gathering and evaluating information that confirms or opposes the tentative diagnosis. This is the step in diagnosis that is most poorly performed by beginning students. Such a shortcoming is understandable because their experience and knowledge are limited at this point, and they therefore fail to search for relevant data.

When the hypothesis is confirmed, it is elevated to the status of a theory (definite diagnosis). A theory is a reasonably well-established concept that is of value because it permits prediction of as yet unknown future facts (appropriate treatment, response to treatment, and course of the disease).

SELECTED READING

Bloom, B. S., editor: Taxonomy of educational objectives: the classification of educational goals. Handbook I. Cognitive domain, New York, 1956, David McKay Co., Inc.

CHAPTER 3

MEDICAL HISTORY

The problem comes when the physician does not take the time for a careful history and analysis of the pain; then, unfulfilled at finding no cause, he looks for more tests to do or he operates.*

A patient consults his physician because of unpleasant or unusual subjective sensations (symptoms) that interfere with his comfort or productivity. Alterations in function or structure (signs) are produced by disease. Signs are the objective evidence of an illness that the physician detects by physical examination.

It is essential that the physician be familiar with the normal so that he can detect or determine which signs and symptoms are abnormal. Most patients consider all of their symptoms to be abnormal, which in turn gives them reason for concern. Other patients either minimize or fail to recognize important symptoms. For example, some patients with heat intolerance caused by thyrotoxicosis do not recognize this as abnormal, yet they open the windows in a cool room where others are comfortable. Similarly, some patients with obvious pallor, anemia, and shortness of breath fail to report the presence of blood in their stools because they interpret this as being from hemorrhoids rather than a possible carcinoma of the colon. One distinguishing feature of the physician is his ability to elicit symptoms, to accurately characterize them, then to establish a diagnosis and a prognosis, and to institute indicated therapy. What is really meant by a given symptom? The physician must be very clear in his understanding of each symptom so that he can accurately communicate his understanding to all persons associated with the patient's care. The *medical history* should be a chronologic record of the development of a patient's symptoms from the inception of his illness until the time he presents himself to the physician. It includes not only the history of the present illness but also all past illnesses, injuries, and operations, any of which may have an important bearing on the present illness.

An adequate history makes the physical examination more interesting and important and permits the physician to correlate the physical findings with the information previously acquired. Without the history, the physical examination is simply a routine mechanical procedure. The combined data obtained in the history and examination will serve as a guide for

---

*From Spiro, H. M.: Visceral viewpoints; pain and perfectionism—the physician and the "pain patient," N. Engl. J. Med. **294**(15):829, 1976.

additional diagnostic procedures. Finally, on the basis of all the information accumulated, the physician is enabled to make the most accurate diagnosis possible and thus is in a position to treat the patient's illness in the most intelligent and effective fashion. Accurate diagnosis is now and always will be the keystone of rational treatment.

There is no field of medicine in which history-taking is not essential. Since the history will be an integral part of the physician's study of his patients for the rest of his days, the art of history-taking should be cultivated to the highest possible degree.

ROLE OF THE STUDENT

In making the transition from the basic sciences to the clinical years the student must learn to complement his biologic knowledge with an understanding of the psychologic principles which enter into the physician-patient relationship. In the clinical setting the student is confronted with a situation entirely different from any he has previously encountered. For the first time he is charged with the responsibility of caring for human beings. He must learn to relate to people and to have a true understanding of their personalities, their strengths and weaknesses, as well as their medical problems.

The medical student is inexperienced in the art and science of dealing with patients and for all practical purposes is a layman. He usually feels quite insecure in his first patient experiences. However, he need not feel shy or embarrassed. The patient is seeking help, and the student can and does fulfill a very necessary role in the management of the patient. Because the student usually spends more time with the patient than any other member of the hospital staff, he has a great opportunity to develop a truly meaningful relationship with and insight into the patient. An alert, competent student takes advantage of this opportunity, with the result that in many instances his history and physical examination is the most comprehensive recorded on the chart. Most patients recognize the necessity for the educational experience of the student and thus do not resent his role in their management. On the other hand it is the obligation of the student to perform his role in a dignified, skillful, and professional manner.

For most students physical diagnosis is their first clinical experience on the hospital ward or in the clinic. It is in this setting that they are first exposed to a patient as well as to the various members of the hospital staff. Here, the students have an opportunity to observe the medical team in operation. Most important, each student has the privilege of interviewing and examining the patient and following the course of the patient's illness during hospitalization. In addition the student has the opportunity of hearing staff discussions and conferences regarding the diagnosis and management of the patient. The student can learn much about the hospital procedure by merely being observant at all times.

Just as a student's first exposure to the ward is a unique experience for him, so too is a patient's first stay in the hospital a novel event. Being admitted to the hospital requires a major adjustment for the patient. The entire hospital schedule and environment are vastly different from those which he experiences in his home and in the course of his daily life. The patient has little or no privacy in a hospital, he is separated from his family, the food is different, many new personnel are encountered, and the entire milieu seems strange. Superimposed on all of these inconveniences and oddities is his concern about his illness, financial matters, the welfare of his family, and many other personal details. Thus, it is important to utilize all the means necessary to make a patient feel secure and comfortable. Conscious striving to establish a good physician-patient relationship goes a long way toward accomplishing this goal.

It is important to observe how the patient

reacts to the medical and nursing staff, to the various procedures, to other patients on the ward, and to his family and visitors. The student should respect his patients and in turn command and deserve their respect. It is essential to be orderly, neat in appearance, mild in manner, but at the same time firm and secure. The student must pursue his work on the ward in a dignified, mature, and serious manner. He must be interested in all aspects of his patient and his care, be sensitive to his concerns and frustrations, and by all means be kind and gentle. With few exceptions patients of all economic and educational statuses will readily sense the compassionate and sincere feelings of a dedicated physician.

It is the physician's duty and moral obligation to observe and maintain the patient's right to privacy. Only those matters that directly relate to the patient's illness should be discussed with other qualified professional members of the hospital staff. Failure to preserve the patient's privacy is a serious breach of medical ethics.

Frequently the patient has visitors or members of his family at his bedside—a delicate situation and one that is often highly charged emotionally. History-taking and physical examination of the patient under these circumstances require considerable time if they are to be done properly. The student should inform both the patient and the visitors that the procedure will require an approximate period of time and ask the visitors if they will leave while the examination is being conducted. He should always be considerate and tactful in this situation. The history-taking and physical examination are strictly private affairs and should not be conducted before members of the family or other visitors.

The student should also be considerate of other personnel responsible for the patient's care. In order that his procedure does not conflict with meals, x-ray studies, or laboratory or other diagnostic tests, he should inform the charge nurse regarding the time he plans to examine the patient.

COMPUTERIZED MEDICAL HISTORY

In this age of mechanization and industrialization the computer has assumed a major role in scientific investigation and application. During the past few years there has been considerable research involving the use of computers in medical history-taking. Studies have shown that some medical-history data can be obtained from patients by various questionnaires based either on the paper-and-pencil medium or on data-processing equipment with the use of computer terminals. In regard to certain aspects of the history there is good correlation between the records derived from questionnaires and those obtained by physicians using the traditional methods of personal interview. In other areas of the medical history the correlation is not good and leaves much to be desired.

It is both possible and probable that in the future more refined techniques will be developed in this area, in which case computerized medical histories will become routine procedures. However, for the present it is advisable to retain the time-proved method of personal interview.

If one accepts the fact that in the near future the computer will become an integral factor in the physician's environment, he must then agree that it is essential to develop better-organized medical records. With this thought in mind Weed has conceived and developed the problem-oriented technique of recording medical data. Weed's method necessitates that each medical record have a complete list of all the patient's problems, including both clearly established diagnoses and all unexplained findings that are not clear manifestations of a specific diagnosis, such as abnormal symptoms or physical findings. This results in a dynamic, not static, list of problems on the patient's chart that can be challenged and altered as the situation demands. The problems may be charted as active or inactive, making it easier to recognize those of immediate importance.

In the utilization of Weed's method each problem is given a number, and all subsequent data in the patient's record, such as plan of therapy, progress notes, and orders, can be recorded under the title and numbered problem to which each properly belongs. The problem-oriented history absolutely necessitates thoroughness and completeness in the development of the problem list. As a result, the physician is compelled to think logically and intelligently about the patient's symptoms in order to arrive at an accurate diagnosis, which in turn is the basis for rational therapeutic decisions.

PHYSICIAN-PATIENT RELATIONSHIP

One of the most important factors in history-taking is that of establishing *rapport*, a relationship of mutual trust and respect, with the patient. The physician's approach to his patient will not only determine to a large degree the amount of information that the patient imparts, but, what is more important, may even affect the accuracy of these data. If the patient senses an attitude of sincerity, integrity, and warmth in his physician, he feels free to relate all matters pertaining to his health, regardless of how personal they may be. The patient will reveal his inner feelings only if he believes that the physician accepts him unconditionally. The physician must learn to conceal any moral judgments that he may have about the actions and attitudes of the patient and must learn more about the origins of his own feelings. The physician should be moral but not a moralist.

To know the details of a patient's history is not necessarily to understand him. To know how he has felt about the events in his life is to begin to appreciate the way life has looked to him. The effective communication of these feelings from the patient to the physician is the key to establishing an ideal physician-patient relationship. The term "feelings" is used to indicate the quality and intensity of emotional experience and is described positively as pleasure, joy, and pride, and negatively as fear, anxiety, anger, hopelessness, and rage.

In the practice of medicine it is essential that the physician understand the basic mechanisms of disease. However, it is just as essential that he understand the patient who is harboring the disease. Diseases are not abstract quantities; they are various abnormalities, physical and mental, that are part and parcel of human beings. There is no such entity as a disease without a patient. Thus the astute clinician not only recognizes the pathology but also observes and considers the patient's feelings and reactions to his disease.

There are many intangible but extremely important factors involved in establishing a good physician-patient relationship. These include general appearance of the examiner, a kind and considerate approach, professional attitude, and humility.

The physician who is negligent about his personal appearance, cleanliness, and mode of attire can hardly expect to command respect from his patient. The patient is likely to suspect, and often correctly so, that such a physician may be equally careless in his diagnosis and treatment. The ill patient is particularly sensitive to such attributes and will be reassured when approached by a neatly dressed, clean, well-mannered examiner.

Many people react differently when sick than when enjoying good health. They may be tense, anxious, apathetic, reticent, or argumentative, but behind these various facades is the common element of concern or fear.

One often hears the phrase, in both professional and lay circles, that "he or she has a low threshold for pain." Tolerance for pain or discomfort, although frequently related to the severity of disease, is also influenced by the emotional status of the patient. When people are fearful and insecure their pain may seem exaggerated or overwhelming. On the other hand, patients who are well adjusted and reasonably secure often tolerate the same disease with significantly less pain.

The patient's predicament must be kept in mind. He is sick. He does not know in what way or how seriously, and his ignorance enhances his fears. He is frightened for himself, his family, and their socioeconomic security. To make matters worse, he cannot usually see the relevance of the many details being inquired about by the physician. He will find reassurance and confidence in the physician who understands him and his problems and who is kind and gentle in both word and manner. Genuine kindness and sympathetic understanding come only from within. Fortunately, most medical students have more than a little compassion for their fellowmen; in fact, it is a powerful motivating factor in their selection of a career. It should not be necessary to point out that it is an attitude that may be fostered or stultified.

Professional attitude is difficult to define. Often it is such an integral part of one's personality that we may be inclined to say that some just have it and others never will attain it, but we hasten to add that it may be cultivated. Such an attitude includes many virtues that ideally should be developed to a high degree in the course of a physician's training. These include physical and mental maturity, poise, strength of character, gentleness, honesty, and many others. The sum of these characteristics constitutes the truly professional attitude so essential to successful physician-patient relationships.

Last but not least, the physician not only should feel but also should demonstrate humility in his relationship with the patient. There is no place in the care of the sick for arrogance, an attitude of superiority, or ultrasophistication. The patient, although he regards his physician as possessing superior skill and knowledge, prefers to think of him as a fellow human being whose life is dedicated to the welfare of humankind.

PRINCIPLES OF HISTORY-TAKING

The fundamental principles involved in history-taking are listening and questioning, observation, and integration.

Listening and questioning. To obtain a good history necessitates careful and attentive listening to the patient's story of his illness. Listening is an art in itself. If the patient is permitted to talk freely, he will often volunteer essential information that the examiner might not be able to elicit by more direct questioning. By listening carefully to the patient's story, the examiner often not only obtains factual information pertaining to his illness but also gains insight into the patient's personality and emotional status. Thus, history-taking should be a fascinating study in human nature as well as an analytic study of symptoms. After the patient has related in his own way the story of his illness, it will be necessary to ask more specific questions to elicit further information or to clarify the exact nature of his complaints.

Observation. Although we think of observation as being a part of the physical examination, nonetheless it is an inseparable and important part of the history-taking. Examination (by observation) actually begins when the patient enters the office and continues while the history is being obtained. During the time that the physician listens and asks questions, he should be observing many things: the general demeanor of the patient, reactions to questions, sense of physical as well as mental well-being, level of intelligence, socioeconomic status, alertness, and the patient's attitude toward his illness and the physician—all of which contribute to the sum of the physician's knowledge and understanding of his patient.

Integration. After the physician has obtained

information pertaining to the patient's illness from listening and asking questions and after he has observed the patient during the course of the history-taking, each item of information so obtained will have to be integrated and fitted into its proper place to formulate the most accurate impression of the patient's illness and his emotional reaction to it.

ELICITING SUFFICIENT INFORMATION FROM THE PATIENT

The establishment of a satisfactory relationship with one's patient is not a separate step or procedure. Instead, this rapport is developed throughout the process of the history-taking and the physical examination. At the same time it is essential to obtain sufficient accurate information to establish a diagnosis or at least a working hypothesis of the underlying disease.

After the amenities of introduction, the examiner usually initiates the interview by asking the patient what things are troubling him or what complaint caused him to seek medical attention. The patient is asked to describe his symptoms regarding their nature, location, date and mode of onset, frequency, duration, what accentuates or relieves them, and any associated symptoms.

Since the student doing physical diagnosis usually has little knowledge of clinical medicine, he may properly inquire, "How do I know what questions to ask my patient?" By following a history outline, the method of routine questioning can be learned rather quickly. At the beginning the student should be permitted to follow such an outline at the bedside of the patient. Although it may be embarrassing to the student at the onset to use this "crutch," it is an effective method to develop the basic procedure in obtaining the medical history. In the early stages of his development, the student will often neglect to inquire into many pertinent symptoms unless he utilizes such an outline. Although each history is an individual

experience and the questioning will be influenced by the nature of the patient's symptoms, still it is essential to follow some routine pattern of questioning to ensure coverage of all aspects of any given illness. After repeated use of this outline, the mechanics of history-taking become well developed. History-taking must be adjusted to each individual and his problem. The examiner who is poorly organized and literally at sea regarding the procedure of history-taking usually concludes with a disorganized and often conflicting history. Furthermore, the patient usually senses this state of confusion in the physician and considers him to be perplexed concerning the nature of his illness. However, the physician who appears certain of what he wants to know enhances the patient's confidence in him. History-taking becomes progressively easier as the physician grows in understanding symptoms of the diseases encountered in medical practice and the impact of emotions on the patient.

The method of questioning should be simple, the terminology must be that which the patient can readily understand, and the examiner should permit the patient to talk freely. If the patient is made to feel at ease and not hurried or interrupted unnecessarily, he will usually relate the pertinent details of his illness. Most patients quickly sense when the examiner is in a hurry to conclude the interview; consequently, they may fail to impart essential information.

In the process of obtaining a history, the physician may encounter a number of obstacles, the majority of which are not intentional on the part of the patient. Such obstacles include fear, mental cloudiness or incoherence, language barriers, and rambling and talkativeness. The perverse patient, who seemingly takes pleasure in making it difficult to extract each item of information, is another possible obstacle. Such obstacles are usually associated with his illness or are an integral part of his personality. Sometimes they may result from the physician's failure to establish a satisfactory relationship with his patient.

The fearful patient either has a sense of fear regarding physicians in general or is frightened concerning the seriousness of his illness. In either situation the physician can usually overcome this obstacle by employing a confident, skillful approach and a cheerful attitude during the interview. The patient's fear is not overcome by trite phrases such as, "You'll be all right" or "Everything is going to be okay," which often sound quite hollow to the anxious patient. An effective means of countering fear is through reassurance to the patient that the vast progress in medical science enables the physician to treat the majority of illnesses. However, the technique will differ in each case, depending on the willingness of the patient to discuss his fears.

The incoherent, irrational, or comatose patient constitutes a real problem. The physician is never more keenly aware of the importance of the medical history than when he is confronted with a critically ill patient who is unable to relate any information concerning his illness. Obviously, the history, if it is to be meaningful, must be obtained from a relative or friend who is familiar with the patient's illness. The situation becomes even more frustrating when neither relative nor friend is available to supply this information.

When there is a language barrier, it is necessary to secure the information through a member of the family or a friend who acts as an interpreter. The mentally retarded patient does not present as difficult a problem as one might think. The examiner must confine his questioning to simple phrases, using only terms that the patient can understand. If the line of questioning is above his level of comprehension, the patient usually feels embarrassed and may relate inaccurate information.

The best history is obtained when the proper relationship is established between the physician and his patient. The physician should be cheerful, neat in his attire, courteous, considerate of the patient, and modest in his attitude. In addition, he should be constantly observant of the various actions and reactions of his patient. The mechanics of history-taking can be perfected only by repetition and extensive clinical experience. The obstacles that may be encountered can usually be overcome by the skillful examiner.

CHAPTER 4

CHIEF COMPLAINT AND PRESENT ILLNESS

In the process of obtaining the medical history the physician obtains all necessary information regarding the patient's illness and at the same time establishes a growing, understanding relationship with the patient. Although the order of taking the history may vary slightly, the major categories include: (1) chief complaint—the symptom or symptoms that prompted the patient to consult his physician, (2) present illness, (3) past history, (4) family history, (5) review of body systems, and (6) social and personal history.

As a rule it is advisable to use the preceding format as a guide in obtaining the history. Although it is most important to obtain all necessary data in each of these categories, one often must deviate from the format because the patient's conversation may randomly drift into different areas. However, the student may keep written or mental notes and at the end of the interview can then assemble all information into a sequential, organized history.

BIOGRAPHIC DATA

Biographic information concerning the patient is essential and should include his full name, age, sex, race, occupation, nationality, marital status, and permanent home address. It is becoming increasingly important to have a record of the patient's federal identification number. The date of the initial and each succeeding interview must be included. Age, sex, and occupation may have a definite relationship to a medical problem. Different age groups are more susceptible to certain illnesses than others (obviously, cancer is much less likely in a 19-year-old girl than in a 55-year-old woman). Certain diseases have a sex and race predilection. Occupation may have great impact on the patient's health.

CHIEF COMPLAINT

The chief complaint should constitute in a few simple words the main reasons why the patient consulted his physician and should be stated as nearly as possible in the patient's own words. This is not the place for a dissertation on his illness. Instead, it should be a simple notation of the symptom or symptoms that are the most troublesome to the patient. The severity and duration of these symptoms are not included, since this material should be elaborated on in the history of the present illness.

The chief complaint should not include diagnostic terms or disease entities. Except for the very sophisticated, a patient never states that he is dyspneic or that he has edema of his extremities. Instead, he will say that he is short of breath or that he cannot get his breath and that he has swelling of his feet or swelling of his ankles. Some patients may say that they have "heart trouble." Although this is quite vague, "heart trouble" is a diagnosis, and there must have been some symptoms that led to this conclusion on the part of the patient. Although the patient's diagnosis of his own case may be correct, at times it is in gross error and may mislead the uninitiated. The student must not accept the diagnosis given by a patient, and similarly he should not accept unqualifiedly the diagnosis of previous physicians. It is essential that the student determine what are or were the symptoms that led to this diagnosis. As physicians we must never forget that it is our responsibility to arrive at the diagnosis, but this can be done with accuracy only after all available information has been obtained. Failure to obtain an accurate chief complaint may ultimately result in an incorrect diagnosis.

HISTORY OF PRESENT ILLNESS

The development of the patient's history is a painstaking task. It requires patience and perseverance on the part of the examiner, and a proper mode of interrogation is essential. The patient is gently and understandingly led to relate an unabridged and factual account of his illness, not tinged by what the physician thinks the circumstances should be or by the physician prematurely jumping to conclusions as to the nature of the patient's illness. The physician should phrase his questions so that the patient must provide the information rather than simply answer "yes" or "no." Some patients may be inclined to answer "yes" to almost every question, seemingly out of a desire to be agreeable; whereas others, more contrary, find it easier to answer "no" to virtually everything. Great care must be taken to avoid leading questions or to suggest answers. Some patients are quite suggestible and may even agree to statements of a forceful physician when they know such statements are not true. On the other hand, some physicians virtually put words into a patient's mouth with such statements as, "The only time you get this pain is when you are walking, isn't that right?" Instead, they should ask, "What brings on this pain?" so that the patient must proffer the information needed to qualify the factors precipitating the pain.

The history of the patient's present illness should be a well-organized, sequentially developed elaboration of his chief complaint or complaints. Taking this portion of the history entails a meticulous development of each symptom from its inception until the time the patient consults his physician.

Once a chief complaint has been determined, the examiner proceeds to elaborate on its various characteristics: (1) date of onset; (2) character of complaint; (3) mode of onset, course, and duration; (4) location; (5) relationship to other symptoms, bodily functions, and activities; (6) exacerbations and remissions; and (7) effect of treatment.

The majority of symptoms or complaints, with the exception of general symptoms, such as chills, fever, insomnia, fatigue, and weakness, will usually suggest the involvement of one of the body systems. For example, frequency of and burning during urination immediately suggest disease of the genitourinary system; whereas expectoration of blood, shortness of breath, or pain on inspiration indicates involvement of the cardiorespiratory system. On the other hand, certain symptoms may be related to several body systems. Although frequency of urination is often related to disease of the genitourinary system, it may also be a

symptom of diabetes mellitus, diabetes insipidus, or emotional tension. The student may
ask, "How can I develop such a symptom or in
what category do I place it for further evaluation?" The answer to this question lies in one
word—experience. With increasing clinical experience and accumulation of knowledge, the
physician learns to ask certain additional questions that assist him in pinpointing various
symptoms to specific body systems. For example, the more skilled physician knows through
previous experience that urinary frequency
along with increased thirst, increased desire for
food, and loss of weight suggest the possibility
of diabetes mellitus; however, urinary frequency, dribbling of urine, and urination during the night hours indicate involvement of the
lower urinary tract. The student and also the
experienced physician on many occasions must
inquire about each complaint with regard to
the body systems in which it might seem to
logically fall. Thus he will review all of the possible symptoms of the suspected body system
or systems during the course of recording the
history of the present illness. By doing so he
will promptly determine if frequent urination
is accompanied by dribbling, excessive urination at night, and hesitancy or whether it is associated with weight loss, excessive thirst, and
increased desire for food. This same procedure
applies to each of the patient's chief complaints.

Date of onset. Whenever possible, specific
dates relating to the onset of each symptom
should be included. This can best be done by
noting the actual date of onset or of variation of
each symptom. As an acceptable substitute, so
many days, weeks, or months before a specific
date of reference—usually the date of admission to the hospital or first consultation in the
office—may be used. Such vague terms as "last
Saturday" or "two weeks ago today" serve only
to confuse, are absolutely meaningless when

reviewing the record months or years later,
and are mentioned only to be deprecated.

Character of complaint. Each complaint
should be characterized as fully as possible. Often it is very difficult for the patient to describe
with accuracy the nature of the unpleasant sensation of which he complains. This is particularly true of pain or discomfort that is visceral
in origin. If the patient is having trouble describing the discomfort, unpleasant sensation,
or pain, frequently it is helpful if the examiner
provides descriptive terms. For example, pain
may be described in many ways, some of which
are burning, sharp, dull, aching, gnawing,
throbbing, shooting or lancinating, and viselike
or constricting. Likewise, pain should be further characterized as to severity—mild, moderate, severe, excruciating, or agonizing. At
the same time the physician should be observing the patient for confirmatory evidence of the
severity of the complaint while the patient describes it. The psychoneurotic patient may
claim that he has agonizing pain but may exhibit a general attitude of indifference or even
cheerfulness. In contrast, those with organic
discomfort usually have accompanying grimaces or gestures that indicate genuine distress.

Mode of onset, course, and duration. How
did each symptom first make its appearance?
Was the onset abrupt or gradual? In some illnesses the onset is so sudden that the patient
can relate the exact moment it began. In various chronic illnesses the onset may be so gradual that it is difficult to determine the exact
date of appearance of the various symptoms. In
such instances approximate dates are all that
one can hope for. What, if any, in the patient's
opinion were the precipitating factor or factors?
For example, certain digestive complaints may
be related to the ingestion of specific foods, a
backache may be associated with lifting a heavy
object, or a substernal pain may have occurred
while the patient was running for a bus. The

examiner next inquires into the course and duration of each symptom. Was the pain persistent or intermittent? How long did it last? Was the pain temporary, has it remained constant, or has it increased in severity?

Location. Where is the distress located? The examiner should insist on specific localization of pain or discomfort. Whenever possible, insist that the patient, with the use of one finger, point to the site of his discomfort. It is not sufficient to accept "pain in my chest" as a site of the distress. After all, the chest covers a large area and includes numerous structures, many of which may give rise to thoracic pain. Is the pain located beneath the sternum or just medial to the left nipple? Is the pain localized to one area, or does it radiate and extend to other regions? If radiating, describe the mode and extent of such radiation.

Relationship to other symptoms, bodily functions, and activities. What other symptoms accompany the patient's chief complaint or complaints? These will usually be enumerated when the examiner reviews the involved body system. However, it is important to point out that other symptoms, seemingly unrelated at the time, may be intimately associated with the chief complaint. For example, in a patient complaining of urinary frequency and pain on urination, a history of associated chills and fever immediately suggests an infection of the urinary tract. Is pain over the lower midabdomen affected by urination or bowel movement? Bodily functions often may either relieve or accentuate pain in various locations. Is pain in the region of the sternum precipitated or aggravated by walking or climbing stairs? Is the backache worse when the patient is reclining or walking? The relationship between symptoms and bodily activity often affords the examiner important diagnostic information.

Exacerbations and remissions. Very often, especially in chronic illnesses, there is a tendency for symptoms to undergo one or more exacerbations and remissions. Cycles of exacerbations and remissions characterize a number of diseases. When applicable to the present illness, these should be noted and dated in order to obtain a clearer concept of the course of the patient's disease.

Effect of treatment. In many instances, patients will have taken remedies on their own or on the advice of friends and family. Such measures may vary from proprietary medications to physical applications, such as heat, cold, and various appliances. The effect of such treatment, either beneficial or harmful, may be of importance and should be recorded as part of the history. In addition, the patient may have consulted other physicians and received various medications or applications. The patient's response to these measures is equally important and constitutes a pertinent segment of his history.

When the history is completed, it should give the physician in chronologic sequence a clear picture of the date and mode of onset of each symptom, its course and duration, precise location, character, exacerbations and remissions, what relieves or makes it worse, and any relationship to other symptoms, bodily functions, and activities. The history should have included a review of all possible symptoms referable to the body system or systems indicated.

When first seen, the patient may have any one of a thousand diseases, virtually everything known to medical science. The history, physical examination, and laboratory data eliminate various possibilities until only a few diagnoses remain as probabilities.

The history shown on p. 16 is the first obtained from a patient on the wards by a student early in his course in physical diagnosis. Although a very poor effort, it illustrates a number of mistakes frequently made by the novice

STUDENT HISTORY

When admitted?

This man is 67 years old and his chief complaints are that he has been having shortness of breath for seven years, and he has some swelling in his feet that has been coming on for the last ten days.

Qualifying statements should be under present illness

Implies he was short of breath before '69! If so, how did it begin? When? How much exertion?

The patient became so short of breath in 1969 that he could no longer work. He says that he has trouble in getting his breath out, which he says is due to his emphysema. He also has bronchitis that makes him cough and his asthma makes him wheeze. On a couple of occasions he has noticed some streaks of blood in the phlegm that he raises.

Diagnostic terms. Symptoms that indicate these diagnoses should be elicited.

Another conclusion based upon other symptoms

Indicates sputum. How much? Color? Odor?

He has a lot of trouble sleeping. He has paroxysmal nocturnal dyspnea that awakens him about every hour. He has to sit up and cough, and after he raises some phlegm he can breathe all right and go back to sleep. He has some swelling in his feet that he could not get rid of until he came into the hospital where they gave him some "water shots" that removed the swelling after a few days. Sometimes he has orthopnea when his feet are swollen.

How long had cough? Frequency? Severity? When worse?

When did this come on? First time? Day or night?

Does not support conclusion that he had paroxysmal nocturnal dyspnea

What led to this conclusion? How many pillows? How long?

His appetite is bad and he has lost weight and is very tired. Any little thing that he does wears him out. He has been in the hospital six times in the last four years for the same trouble.

Why? Pain? Not hungry? Nausea?

How much? Over what period? Best weight? Present?

Describe activities that produce this exhaustion. Onset? Duration? Getting worse?

What hospital? Dates? We may want chart or result of that hospital stay!

in obtaining and transcribing the history, as annotated in the margins.

The history of the same patient after reorganization into a sequential pattern and correction of the indicated mistakes is as follows:

#625434
C. D. _ _ _ _ _ _ _
22 Doe Street, Columbus, Ohio
AGE: 67   SEX: Male   COLOR: White
MARITAL: Single   NATIONALITY: American
OCCUPATION: Clothing salesman

C. D. was admitted to University Hospital for the seventh time on November 20, 1976. Chief complaints:
  1. Shortness of breath
  2. Swelling of feet
This man first noticed a sensation of being short of breath about 1954. Although it did not limit his activities, he noticed that more effort was required to do a given amount of physical exercise, and there was a sensation of not being able to "fully get his breath." At the same time he noted the onset of cough. Although this occurred only occasionally dur-

ing the day, it was troublesome on arising each morning, at which time he would cough intermittently for 15 to 30 minutes and would raise about two teaspoonfuls of thick, clear sputum.

Except for an occasional respiratory infection, at which time he had more cough and the production of yellow sputum, his cough, amount of sputum, and sensation of shortness of breath remained unchanged until 1969. At that time he noticed that his cough was rapidly becoming more frequent and that he had more thick sputum that was increasingly difficult to raise. At the same time his shortness of breath was now definitely limiting his physical activities. Although he could climb a flight of stairs, he would have to rest at the top in order to catch his breath. By the end of 1969 he had become so short of breath that he was no longer able to work.

In 1970 he first noticed that he was coughing at night, which disturbed his rest. Since 1971 he has been awakened frequently, as often as every hour, with a feeling of being smothered or choked up. He would have to sit up and cough; after raising some sputum he would be relieved and could go back to sleep. Also in 1971, he became aware of frequent wheezing, often relieved by coughing.

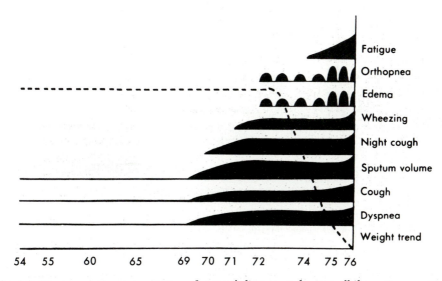

Fig. 4-1. Diagrammatic representation of patient's history, indicating all the major symptoms and their progress over a 22-year period. Although all the minor details cannot be illustrated, a clear picture of the development of the illness can be obtained by this technique.

Since 1972 he has had six bouts of swelling of his feet and ankles, accompanied by difficulty in lying flat in bed. He found that he could breathe better if he slept on two or three pillows. On each occasion he was admitted to this hospital, where he says he was given "water shots" that would remove the swelling in his feet. He could again sleep flat in bed.

Beginning in 1973 he became very short of breath while eating. As a consequence, he has been eating less and less and has lost approximately 48 pounds. Since 1974 he has experienced increasing fatigue.

On November 10, 1976 (10 days before his present admission to the hospital), he noticed that his feet were becoming swollen again, he was more short of breath, could not sleep unless propped up in bed, and was very tired and exhausted. At present, he is so short of breath that he can barely walk across the room. He states that he is coughing every few minutes and raises whitish or whitish yellow sputum. He is aware of considerable wheezing and is awakened almost every hour "filled with phlegm."

He smokes only three to five cigarettes per day; however, for over 40 years he smoked an average of two packages per day until 1975, at which time he reduced his smoking to the present level.

After the patient's history has been completed, it should be so logically developed and so thoroughly and sequentially organized that one could actually make a diagram of it, a diagram that would indicate the date and mode of onset, variations, and progression or disappearance of each symptom. Fig. 4-1 is a diagrammatic representation of the major features of the relatively long history just presented, which covers a span of 22 years.

The following is a history that was obtained from a patient who was subsequently shown to have cancer of the lung involving the left upper lobe. It is presented to show the use of the day of admission to the hospital as the date of reference.

#629041
R. L. _ _ _ _ _ _
222 East 32nd Ave., Columbus, Ohio
AGE: 57   SEX: Male   COLOR: White
MARITAL: Married   NATIONALITY: American
OCCUPATION: House painter
ADMITTED: 11-22-76

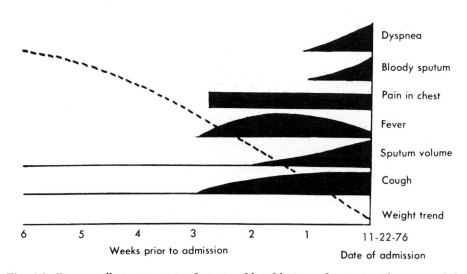

Fig. 4-2. Diagram illustrating major features of brief history of patient with cancer of the lung. The date of admission to the hospital is used as the date of reference.

R. L. was admitted complaining of:
1. Shortness of breath
2. Coughing up blood

Six weeks before admission the patient noticed the gradual onset of mild cough, present both day and night, that produced only very small amounts of white sputum. He thought that he had a "cold" and took some home remedies without benefit.

Three weeks before admission he noticed that his cough was becoming severe and more frequent. He would have paroxysms of cough that would sometimes last as long as 5 minutes, leaving him quite exhausted, but still producing only a small amount of thick sputum. At the same time he thought that he had some fever, since he would feel alternately hot and cold, especially in the afternoon and evening. Often he had sudden drenching sweats, although he denied that he had any night sweats. *About 2 days later* he developed pain in the upper chest anteriorly and laterally, which has persisted to the present time. It is present mainly as a dull ache of moderate severity, but he will have a more severe sharp pain in the same area that will cut off his breath if he coughs or breathes deeply. He has found that the pain is much worse if he lies on his right side, but it is relieved if he lies on the left.

About *2 weeks before admission* he noticed that his cough was even more frequent and more productive. The sputum was predominantly yellowish-white. *One week before admission* the sputum at times became frankly bloody. He said that sometimes it looked as if it was "all blood." At the same time he became aware of increasing shortness of breath. The sensations of fever and pain in the chest have improved during the past 3 to 4 days. At the present time he becomes short of breath if he does anything more than walk slowly about the room, and he is particularly short of breath after coughing.

Using this history as an example, the information presented can be reproduced in the form of a graph (Fig. 4-2).

In instances when the patient has been in the hospital one or more times or has been treated previously for his present illness, the name and location of such hospitals or physicians and the date of such admissions and treatments should be specifically recorded. This information ultimately may prove vital in assessing the present illness. Often seemingly unrelated illness in the past has an important bearing on the present study.

CHAPTER 5

PAST, FAMILY, SOCIAL, AND OCCUPATIONAL HISTORY AND SYSTEMS REVIEW

PAST HISTORY

A detailed review of the patient's past medical history may prove of inestimable value. A number of diseases are characterized by an acute phase that subsides, only to be followed by serious sequelae in later years. As an example, a history of rheumatic fever, recurrent tonsillitis, or scarlet fever in childhood may explain congestive heart failure occurring in later life, the result of rheumatic heart disease that originated in childhood. The past history should include a review of all past illnesses, surgical procedures, and injuries. All statements made by the patient regarding previous illnesses should be thoroughly evaluated and clarified. If the patient states that he had rheumatic fever in childhood, the examiner should not accept the patient's diagnosis, but instead he must make a thorough inquiry into the nature of the symptoms and the course of the disease.

Many physicians in recording this portion of the history are content to make a notation "the patient had the usual childhood diseases." After all, what is meant by this phrase—"usual childhood diseases"? Smallpox and diphtheria were common childhood illnesses 50 years ago, but immunization has resulted in effective control of these conditions. Each past illness should be specifically recorded, noting in particular its date of occurrence, significant complications, and sequelae.

Data concerning all past surgical procedures are an essential part of the case history. The dates of all operations, the hospitals in which they were performed, and the names of the surgeons should be recorded. In some instances this information may be essential in evaluating the patient's present illness. Frequently, patients who have been subjected to surgical procedures have little knowledge regarding the exact nature of or findings at the operation. The present examiner should either request a transcript of the patient's chart or contact the surgeon personally. Similar inquiry should be made regarding all major injuries.

FAMILY HISTORY

The family history is likewise an important part of every patient's record. Inquiry is directed toward the health status of the patient's family (mother, father, siblings, and children), their age if living, and, if deceased, the age at which they died and the cause of death. Hereditary and constitutional factors play an important role in the cause of certain diseases. These factors are recognized and accepted by all in some diseases, such as hemophilia and diabetes mellitus, whereas they are accepted with reservation in others, such as in some forms of cancer, hypertension, and arteriosclerosis. Nevertheless, there is sound basis for obtaining information in the family history relative to numerous diseases or disease processes, including diabetes mellitus, hypertension, cancer, blood dyscrasias (hemophilia, hemolytic jaundice), gout, obesity, allergic disorders, epilepsy, coronary artery disease, and mental illness.

After the physician has inquired into specific hereditary diseases, there are still many others that may be familial. The hereditary nature of the present illness may be revealed by asking, "Are there any other members of your family that have or have had a similar illness?" Frequently, this question will uncover evidence of a familial factor that will not be found in any other way.

SYSTEMS REVIEW

The systems review is a comprehensive account of all complaints referable to each body system, progressing in a logical manner from the head toward the feet. The purpose of this review is twofold: (1) a thorough evaluation of the past and present status of each body system and (2) a double check to prevent omission of significant data relative to the present illness that otherwise might be overlooked should this procedure be neglected. The importance of this portion of the patient's history cannot be too strongly emphasized. This review permits the examiner to group symptoms in a manner that helps him to arrive at a plausible diagnosis, often made possible by integration of apparently unrelated symptoms. For example, if a patient complains of epigastric pain, it may be the result of peptic ulcer, gastric malignancy, pancreatitis, biliary disease, or angina pectoris. By means of a careful review of systems, the physician can determine whether such pain is relieved by eating, precipitated by exertion, exaggerated by deep breathing, aggravated by fatty foods, or is unrelated to any other body processes.

It is our opinion that the absence as well as the presence of symptoms should be recorded in the review. Failure to follow this procedure may result in two grave errors: (1) important symptoms may be omitted because the examiner fails to inquire about them and (2) the case history is a permanent part of the patient's record and may in the future be reviewed by either the original examiner or other physicians, so if only the symptoms present are recorded, the person reviewing the chart may be in doubt regarding symptoms not listed.

Body weight. Information should include the patient's average, maximum, and least weight. If there has been an appreciable loss or gain in weight, the amount and time interval during which it occurred should be established. In the presence of a pronounced weight loss, the examiner must determine if this has occurred as part of the illness or because the patient has voluntarily reduced his caloric intake.

Skin, hair, and nails. The hair and nails are often referred to as appendages of the skin. Thus, these structures are grouped together and should be so considered in the system review. They are affected by both local and systemic diseases, and symptoms relative to these structures may provide diagnostic clues to the presence of disease in other body systems.

The physician should inquire about the texture of the skin, past or present dermatologic disease, excessive dryness or sweating, alteration of temperature, unusual discolorations or pigmentations, and itching (pruritus). Skin texture is influenced by metabolic disturbances, vitamin deficiencies, and other conditions. Excessive dryness or moistness of the skin may suggest the presence of hypothyroidism and hyperthyroidism, respectively. Profuse sweating is referred to as *diaphoresis* and may be attributed to psychogenic disorders or may accompany organic disease. The tense and apprehensive patient sweats profusely when under mental stress. This is often obvious during the physical examination.

Many of the dermatologic diseases, such as *acne, psoriasis,* and *seborrhea,* are recognized and known to the patient by their medical name. All dermatologic conditions and their therapeutic management should be recorded in the skin review.

In some instances patients will be aware of changes in their skin temperature. It is not unusual to have a patient complain of cold hands or feet or state that he is constantly cold when others in the same room are warm. In certain metabolic disorders the patient has legitimate reason to complain of feeling excessively cold or warm.

Itching may be local or generalized, may be associated with specific dermatologic diseases, and at times may be the result of systemic disease, such as obstructive jaundice. It is frequently encountered in patients with nervous disorders (neurodermatitis).

Symptoms referable to the hair include texture, baldness, itching of the scalp, and abnormal distribution. As in the skin, various diseases, both local and systemic, may affect the texture of the hair. The type or pattern of baldness is important. When it is hereditary in origin, it usually assumes a symmetric distribution, whereas in specific diseases affecting the scalp, baldness is either patchy or irregular in its outline.

Various factors relating to the nails should be recorded. These include texture, specific diseases, and biting of the nails. *Psoriasis, onychomycosis* (fungus infection of the nails), and other diseases may be responsible for various abnormalities of the nails. Nail biting is often indicative of nervous tension. This information may be helpful in evaluating the patient's emotional status.

Head. A review of symptoms referable to the head should include headache, vertigo, and trauma. Headache is a common but very difficult symptom to evaluate. To merely ask a patient whether or not he has headaches is inadequate. A more informative answer results from phrasing the question, "Do you have either unusually frequent or unusually severe headaches?" This question will cause the patient to consider his reply and not hastily answer in the affirmative. Most people occasionally experience headaches; however, the information sought is that concerning severe or frequent headaches and not the occasional mild headache.

Headaches are described as to their character, location, severity, circumstances under which they occur, and any associated symptoms. They are dull, throbbing or pounding, constricting or viselike, burning, and at times are described as sensations of pressure or weight over the cranium. In some instances the headache is confined to one side of the head and is referred to as *hemicrania*. Headaches are frontal, parietal, temporal, supraorbital, occipital, or generalized in location. The severity of a headache is described as mild, dull, moderate, severe, or excruciating. In some instances the headache is more pronounced or occurs exclusively at various times of the day or night. The headaches of frontal and sphenoidal sinusitis are commonly worse on arising in the morning because of the accumulation of secretions within the sinuses during the night. Headaches caused by increased intracranial pressure are diffuse, often intense, and frequently awaken the patient during the night. The headache of eyestrain is usually supraorbital or occipital and appears in the late afternoon or following prolonged use of the eyes as in reading or writing.

Associated symptoms often help to establish the cause of headache. In migraine the actual headache may be preceded by either a visual or an auditory disturbance, which is termed an *aura* and is often accompanied by nausea, vomiting, or both. In *labyrinthitis* (inflammation of the inner ear) the headache is frequently accompanied by nausea, dizziness, and tinnitus.

Mention of trauma to the head may have been omitted in reviewing the past history, and inquiry into this possibility should be made. It is important to determine if the head injury was accompanied by unconsciousness, the duration of coma, evidence of fracture, or if any other symptoms accompanied or followed such trauma to the head.

Vertigo is described as a sensation of dizziness, inability to maintain equilibrium, or both. It may be classified as *objective* vertigo (the room spins or reels about the patient) and *subjective* (the patient reels or spins with his environment remaining stationary). This is a symptom, not a disease and may be the result of numerous causes. The two most common causes are diseases of the cerebellum and diseases of the inner ear. It is essential to differentiate vertigo (true dizziness) from the sensation of *lightheadedness* or *faintness*, since the layman as well as some physicians confuse these terms.

Eyes. Symptoms related to the eyes include disturbances of vision, lacrimation, photophobia, itching, and pain within the eyeball or orbit. A history of visual disturbances should include details of blurring of vision, diplopia, fatigue with use of eyes, and "spots" in front of the eyes. *Blurred vision,* which is actually a decrease in visual acuity, may be the result of errors of refraction or ocular disease. If glasses are worn, the physician should determine to what extent the impaired vision is corrected. *Diplopia* is double vision (when the patient looks at a single object, two are seen) and is caused by imbalance of the extraocular muscles, resulting in the failure of both eyes to point directly at the same object. Undue fatigue following use of the eyes is commonly associated with refractive errors or muscular imbalance. "Spots" in front of the eyes are common and are usually not significant but occasionally may herald the onset of serious disease. *Lacrimation* (excessive watering) and *photophobia* (extreme sensitivity to light) are common symptoms associated with inflammation of or trauma to the eye. *Itching* is frequently suggestive of allergy. Evaluation of pain in the eyeball or within the orbit requires accurate description of the location and character of the pain, as well as determination of the presence of pain referred to other areas of the head.

Ears. Symptoms referable to the ears include deafness, pain, discharge, vertigo, and tinnitus. *Deafness* (partial or complete loss of hearing) should be evaluated as to degree, duration, whether of one or both ears, and the cause if known. Pain in or about the ear *(earache)* should be carefully analyzed, for it may result from disease in the ear or mastoid or may be referred from the mouth, teeth, throat, or paranasal sinuses. Its exact location, duration, mode of onset, and character should be determined.

Discharge may arise from the middle ear or the external auditory canal and is described as *serous* (clear, thin, and watery), *mucoid* (thick, clear, or white), *sanguineous* (bloody), or *purulent* (thick, yellow). The physician should inquire regarding previous infections of the ear, especially during childhood, mastoid infections, any surgical procedures such as *paracentesis* (surgical puncture for drainage) of the tympanic membrane, any of which may explain impaired hearing or persistent aural discharge.

Vertigo, which may accompany disturbances of the inner ear, has been previously described and its presence or absence should be verified. *Tinnitus* (a sensation of whistling or ringing in the ears) is entirely subjective. Tinnitus may be present in labyrinthitis, tumors of the eighth nerve, and cerebral arteriosclerosis.

Nose, nasopharynx, and paranasal sinuses. In reviewing the nose, nasopharynx. and paranasal sinuses, the examiner inquires about the presence of nasal discharge, obstruction, frequent colds, allergies, trauma, and sense of smell.

Nasal or *postnasal discharge*, depending on its color and consistency, is described as serous, mucoid, purulent, sanguineous, or mixtures thereof. The physician should determine the type and amount of secretion and the time of day or season of the year when it is most copious. When the discharge is frank blood, the condition is called *epistaxis*. In frontal and sphenoidal sinusitis, the discharge is often most copious in the morning on assuming the upright position. Some discharges (postnasal) run back into the nasopharynx, from which they are expectorated. Nasal infections may be accompanied by acute infections of the maxillary sinuses and, less frequently, of the frontal sinuses. When this complication occurs, the patient experiences pain over the infraorbital or supraorbital areas, respectively.

Obstruction is one of the most common complaints referable to the nose. Its duration, frequency, and degree should be determined, as well as the side involve, if unilateral. The physician should inquire whether the obstruction followed trauma to the nose.

A history of frequent colds is not uncommon, but when present, the physician should ascertain that the patient is actually experiencing "common colds" rather than recurrent sinusitis or nasal allergy (hay fever). Nasal allergies are accompanied by profuse serous drainage and some degree of obstruction. If nasal allergy is suspected, the season of year during which it occurs should be determined. The patient should be asked if he is aware of any disturbance of olfaction (sense of smell). If such is present, the duration should be determined.

Mouth and throat. Pertinent symptoms referable to the mouth and throat include pain, bleeding gums, soreness of mouth and tongue, dysphagia, changes in voice, and dental hygiene. The location, duration, and character of pain in the mouth and throat should be ascertained. In addition, if there is a history of frequent "sore throat," its frequency, severity, and such associated symptoms as arthritis or rash should be determined.

Bleeding gums and soreness of the mouth or tongue may be symptoms of local disease or manifestations of various systemic illnesses.

Status of the dental hygiene should include information regarding carious or abscessed teeth, dentures, and the character of oral care practiced by the patient.

Dysphagia (difficult swallowing) or *odynophagia* (painful swallowing) may be the result of disease of the pharynx, esophagus, or neuromuscular system. The physician should determine whether there is difficulty in swallowing only solids (usually indicating mechanical obstruction) or both liquids and solids (suggesting a disorder of esophageal motility). The location at which swallowed material seems to stick, the duration and rate of progress of the symptoms, and whether these symptoms are intermittent or continuous should be noted. If the difficulty is localized to the pharynx or cervical esophagus, special note of associated choking and coughing should be made.

Neck. Symptoms referable to the neck include pain, swelling, and limitation of movement. A history of injury in the neck may serve to explain the origin of various symptoms in this region. Pain is described as to its location, severity, character, and as to which movements of the neck either aggravate or alleviate it. Pain originating in the cervical spine often radiates to the shoulders, arms, and hands. Localized swelling in the neck may be the result of many causes. The mode of onset, the location of the swelling, the presence of tenderness or discharge, and finally the course of the pain should be ascertained. Enlargement of the anterior cervical lymph glands is a common occurrence in acute infections of the oropharynx and must be differentiated historically from a slowly enlarging chain of cervical lymph nodes, which may be caused by lymphoma. On the other hand, swelling in the anterior midline of the lower neck suggests the possibility of an enlarged thyroid gland or thyroid cyst.

Cardiorespiratory system. A thorough review of the cardiorespiratory system necessitates inquiry into dyspnea, orthopnea, paroxysmal nocturnal dyspnea, edema, cough, sputum, hemoptysis, pain, wheezing, palpitation, syncope, cyanosis, hypertension, hoarseness, and stridor.

Dyspnea (shortness of breath or difficulty in breathing) is usually a symptom of cardiac or pulmonary disorder but also may occur as the result of severe anemias, metabolic disorders, acidosis, and neuroses. Dyspnea should be differentiated from *sighing respiration,* which patients often falsely interpret as shortness of breath. The physician should determine the degree of dyspnea, its rate of progression, and whether it occurs on exertion, at rest, or both.

Orthopnea is the inability to breathe comfortably in the recumbent position. The patient obtains relief on elevating the upper portion of his body by the use of two or more pillows under his head or by sitting upright. It is often described as two-pillow or three-pillow orthopnea. It is usually a manifestation of congestive heart failure.

Paroxysmal nocturnal dyspnea is not to be confused with either dyspnea or orthopnea. It is defined as a sudden onset of severe dyspnea occurring in a patient sleeping in a recumbent position, relieved by the patient's assuming an upright or sitting position.

Edema is soft-tissue swelling that is the result of abnormal accumulation of fluid. It may occur in the lower extremities, sacral region, face, periorbital area, or may be generalized. A thorough history of edema regarding its location, conditions under which it occurs, and circumstances that may alleviate it is helpful in ascertaining its cause. Edema in the lower extremities, which is increased after standing and which decreases or disappears with bed rest, is usually cardiac in origin, although it may be caused by varicose veins. Periorbital edema, which is most pronounced upon arising in the morning, is often the result of renal disease and is frequently seen in acute and chronic glomerulonephritis. Edema in the lower extremities accompanied by scrotal edema and *ascites* (free fluid in the peritoneal cavity) may be the result of cardiac failure or cirrhosis of the liver. Generalized edema *(anasarca)* can occur in kidney disease and congestive heart failure. Unilateral edema in the extremities is usually caused by lymphatic or venous obstruction.

Cough, one of our most vital protective reflexes, is a symptom produced by inflammation, viscid secretions, or obstruction of the tracheobronchial system. Cough should be described as dry or productive of sputum. When the cough is productive, the sputum (the material expectorated as the result of the cough) should be further described as to its color, quantity, consistency, and any unusual odor. Purulent sputum is usually indicative of infection. A reddish or grossly bloody sputum should suggest a number of disease possibilities. In certain types of pneumonia, such as that caused by *Klebsiella,* the sputum is often very tenacious. In acute pulmonary edema the sputum may be either frothy white or pink as a result of blood in the secretions. Cough should be further characterized as *paroxysmal* (a prolonged episode of forceful cough), *hacking* (frequent brief periods of cough, usually not very severe), *explosive* (self-explanatory), and *brassy* (a harsh, dry cough that is often the result of extrinsic compression of the trachea or bronchus). Also, it should be determined if the cough occurs during the day, the night, or both, and if it is influenced by body position.

Hemoptysis is the expectoration of bloody sputum. The examiner should determine the color of the blood, the quantity, and whether or not it is pure or admixed with the sputum. (It may occur in clots.) An approximation of the amount of blood expectorated in any 24-hour period is quite important. Ordinarily, the coughing of blood is frightening and, as a result, the patient is inclined to exaggerate the quantity. Hemoptysis is frequently of serious significance and may occur in the course of pneumonia, tuberculosis, and cancer.

The presence of odor in the sputum is usually detected by the physician, but in some instances it can be noted by others who are present in the vicinity. The patient may or may not be aware of the odor of his sputum. Foul sputum is usually indicative of some putrefactive process in the respiratory tract, such as bronchiectasis or lung abscess.

Pain in the chest is a frequent complaint. Its significance as well as its probable cause frequently can be determined by a careful interrogation of the patient. First, the examiner should ascertain the exact location of the pain. Under what circumstances does the pain occur? What precipitates and relieves it? What is the nature and severity of the pain? In some instances the pain is brief and fleeting in duration, and in others it is persistent for minutes, hours, or days. Chest pain may be produced by respiration, eating, coughing, and physical exertion, or it may occur independently of any of

these mechanisms. Radiation of the pain to the shoulders, neck, arms, abdomen, or back should be ascertained. In order to clarify this symptom even further, several brief descriptions of various types of chest pain follow:

1. *Pleuritic pain* (the pain of pleurisy). Pleuritic pain is usually localized over the site of pleural irritation. Because there is a greater range of respiratory motion in the lower than in the upper thorax, most pleuritic pain is confined to the lung bases, especially anterolaterally. It is often severe and characteristically is aggravated by deep inspiration, coughing, or laughing.

2. *Precordial pain.* Precordial pain constitutes the most common type of chest pain causing the patient to seek medical advice. It is usually located to the left of the sternum, especially in the region of the cardiac apex. Such pain may be mild or moderate, is usually fleeting, stabbing, or sticking in character, and is unrelated to physical activity. Although it may occasionally radiate to other areas, it is usually localized. This type of pain tends to occur in the highly emotional or tense person and is rarely caused by organic heart disease. However, the patient with acute pericarditis may experience severe precordial pain.

3. *Substernal pain* or *oppression.* Substernal pain is of greater significance and usually indicates coronary artery disease. This pain may vary from mild to excruciating and from transient to persistent. It may be localized in any part of the sternum, from which it may radiate to the neck, mandibles, shoulders, down either or both arms, to the back or epigastrium; it may also extend over the entire anterior chest. It may be precipitated by physical exertion or emotional stimulation (*angina pectoris*) and is usually relieved rather promptly by rest. Similar pain occurring at rest is usually caused by *coronary thrombosis.* The patient often describes this pain as crushing or squeezing and frequently uses such phrases as "it feels as

though someone is standing on my chest" or "someone is squeezing me to death." Such descriptions are often volunteered by the patient, and they are so classic that the diagnosis may be obvious from the history alone.

4. *Heartburn*. A relatively common experience is that of heartburn. When persistent, it should be characterized, since many patients confuse it with other kinds of chest pain or fail to appreciate that it may not be a normal sensation. Substernal pain of burning quality, often with radiation to the neck and associated with pyrosis, regurgitation of gastric contents, and aggravation by increased abdominal pressure or the recumbent position, may signify important dysfunction of the lower esophageal sphincter. If associated with dysphagia or with other symptoms, heartburn should be fully investigated. The examiner should be aware that the esophagus is not accessible to physical diagnostic means and that a carefully taken history will be required to direct further study of the patient's symptoms.

Palpitation is a throbbing or pounding sensation experienced in the precordial region, which may be described by the patient as "my heart jumps" or "my heart flops around in my chest." Although it may result from unimportant disturbances of cardiac rhythm, such as premature systoles and paroxysmal tachycardia, it is usually associated with the tachycardia of excitement, exertion, and the toxic effects of coffee, alcohol, or tobacco. At times it may occur with important disturbances of rhythm in thyrotoxicosis and organic heart disease.

Cyanosis is a bluish or purplish discoloration of the mucous membranes, skin, and nail beds. Although usually an objective finding, occasionally it constitutes a major complaint of the patient. Cyanosis is caused by an increased percentage of reduced hemoglobin in the capillary blood.

Syncope is fainting or temporary loss of consciousness. This symptom may be of great significance in such conditions as complete heart block (Stokes-Adams syndrome) or aortic stenosis with temporary cardiac standstill, or it may be of little importance in other conditions such as emotional instability (simple fainting). Attacks of syncope were commonly observed in the armed services when a patient would faint at the very sight of a hypodermic needle long before he received the injection.

Stridor is a "crowing" sound heard primarily on inspiration. It is indicative of obstruction in the respiratory tract from the larynx through the major bronchi. It may be the result of numerous causes, including inflammation, foreign body, or neoplasm.

Wheezing is a peculiar whistling noise occurring during both inspiration and expiration, predominantly the latter. There is classically a musical quality to the sounds produced, which is often audible to others in the patient's vicinity. This symptom is caused by partial obstruction of the terminal bronchi and bronchioles, as seen in asthma or bronchitis.

Hypertension (high blood pressure) may result in serious cardiac disease. Strictly speaking, it is not a symptom but a sign observed by the examiner. Therefore the physician should ascertain if his patient has a history of hypertension, which may have been detected in previous examinations, and if so, how severe, its duration, what were the attendant symptoms, and what medication, if any, he has taken for this condition. It must be remembered that hypertension is not a disease but a result thereof and may be associated with other organic defects, such as kidney disease, adrenal tumors, thyrotoxicosis, and arteriosclerosis.

Gastrointestinal system. Since the gastrointestinal system is relatively inaccessible to the routine methods of physical examination, it is essential to elicit a detailed review of the various symptoms referable to this system. The gastrointestinal system is unique in three respects: (1) it is often involved in so-called functional disease syndromes wherein the patient has many symptoms and either a paucity or complete absence of physical findings; (2) organic lesions of this system may reach an advanced stage before physical findings become apparent; and (3) similar symptoms may result from diseases involving any of several organs in the abdomen, as well as more distant organ systems. For example, nausea and vomiting may occur not only in gastrointestinal disease but also in biliary and pancreatic diseases and in distant conditions, such as tumor or infection of the central nervous system. Thus, in these situations the significance of a comprehensive history should be obvious. Only by developing each system and correlating it with associated symptoms is it possible to obtain a clear picture of the whole disease.

Symptoms that are referable to the gastrointestinal system include character of the appetite, dysphagia, pyrosis, indigestion, food idiosyncrasies, nausea, emesis, hematemesis, flatulence, jaundice, abdominal pain or discomfort, change in bowel habits, diarrhea, constipation, character of stools, and hemorrhoids.

The character of the appetite may constitute an important diagnostic clue. *Anorexia* (poor appetite or a lack of desire for food) necessitates clarification. There is a distinct difference between lack of desire to eat and fear of eating because certain foods result in digestive disturbances. Loss of appetite indicates either organic disease of the gastrointestinal tract, mental depression, severe infections, or toxic states. On the other hand, good appetite is not synonymous with good eating habits. Some persons who are emotionally disturbed are constantly nibbling throughout the day (eating is an obsession), whereas others similarly affected may feel an actual revulsion for food.

Indigestion is an exceedingly vague term and is mentioned only because it is so widely used by both laymen and physicians, with a multitude of implications. It is apparent that the ex-

aminer must obtain a more accurate understanding of what his patient means by "indigestion."

Food idiosyncrasy is an actual intolerance to certain foods that produce unpleasant gastrointestinal symptoms. True food idiosyncrasy must be differentiated from the personal whims of the patient who will not eat certain foods simply because he does not like them. The fact that a patient dislikes cabbage does not imply that he has digestive intolerance to this food. However, if the ingestion of cabbage results in severe, colicky right upper quadrant pain, it then suggests that he may have biliary tract disease and actually cannot tolerate this food. Similarly, many patients avoid fat or fried food for different reasons. Some do it as part of a prudent diet, while others have various gastrointestinal symptoms after such a meal. While fat intolerance has been widely popularized as a symptom of biliary tract disease, it is equally common among those with normal digestive tracts.

Nausea and *vomiting* are obvious symptoms, requiring no further definition. Vomiting, which is also referred to as *emesis*, should be further characterized to include the nature and quantity of the vomitus and when the emesis occurs in relation to the previous meal. The vomiting of undigested food particles indicates that the food either is not retained for an appreciable length of time or that there is a high gastrointestinal obstruction that does not permit passage of the food into the small bowel. The color of the vomitus should be determined. The vomiting or regurgitation of blood is referred to as *hematemesis*. Fresh blood in the vomitus usually indicates a freely bleeding lesion, such as a ruptured esophageal varix or peptic ulcer. If blood has remained within the stomach for a sufficient period of time to undergo digestion, it will resemble grounds of coffee dispersed among the other digested food particles, the vomitus of which is referred to as *"coffee-ground emesis."* The quantity of blood or vomitus should be ascertained. Because it is a frightening experience, patients often exaggerate the amount of blood present.

Pyrosis is sour eructation or belching. This is a frequent complaint and may or may not be associated with organic disease. *Flatulence* is a sensation of fullness or gaseous distention in the abdomen and is often accompanied by the complaint of excessive belching and passage of flatus. Both pyrosis and flatulence are common in organic disease of the digestive tract, but their frequent association with *aerophagia* (air swallowing) and other functional disorders limits their diagnostic usefulness.

The complaint of *abdominal pain* requires a thorough history of onset, location, character, severity, associated symptoms, and what relieves or exaggerates it. After the mode of onset has been ascertained, exact determination of the location and radiation of pain is vital in establishing an accurate diagnosis. The next step is to determine the character of the pain and its subsequent course. Abdominal pain is described as dull, sharp, burning, gnawing, stabbing, cramping, aching, or colicky. *Colic* is a unique type of distress characterized by a gradual onset and increasing in crescendo fashion until it reaches the peak of its severity. Then it slowly subsides until the patient is either completely free of discomfort or largely so. Since pain is purely subjective, patients often find it difficult to express the exact nature of the discomfort that they are experiencing.

Jaundice (icterus) is a diffuse yellow pigmentation of the body and is caused by hepatic disease, biliary tract obstruction, or excessive destruction of red blood cells *(hemolysis)*. If the patient has had jaundice, the physician must then determine under what circumstances it occurred and what the accompanying symptoms were. Was the jaundice accompanied by pain, chills, and fever; and were there other similar cases in the home or neighborhood at the same time? In obstruction of the biliary tract, the stools will be light gray or clay colored *(acholic)* because of the absence of bile pigments, and the urine will be reddish brown or brown *(cola)* because of the excretion of the excess bile pigments in the urine.

An often neglected aspect of the history is that relating to the patient's bowel habits. All too frequently the statement is made that the bowel habits are normal, or that the patient has diarrhea or constipation, without further description. A history of *diarrhea* (abnormally frequent and/or loose stools) necessitates inquiry as to color, consistency, odor, and number. The presence of blood, pus, mucus, undigested food, and oil or fat should be noted. Acute infectious diarrheas may be accompanied by chills, fever, and prostration. In chronic diarrheas special attention also should be given to weight loss, abdominal pain, and relation to nature and timing of food intake.

While chronic *constipation* over many years without ill health does not usually cause concern, the onset of constipation in a patient with previously normal bowel habits may be the first clue to an obstructing cancer of the colon. On the other hand, alternating constipation and diarrhea, or the frequent passage of small, hard, dry stools ("rabbit-pellet" or scybalous stools) is more likely to be found in the irritable bowel syndrome, one of several functional digestive disorders. Finally, it should be appreciated that a single daily bowel movement is neither required for good health nor the only normal habit, since many normal people have two or three stools daily while others move their bowels only once every two or three days.

The patient should be asked to describe his stool as to color, consistency, and conformation. The normal stool is brown in color. Significant alterations are often associated with certain diseases *Clay-colored* (light gray) stools indicate an absence of bile pigment. Black or tarry stools *(melena)* are the result of digested blood and indicate upper gastrointestinal bleeding. Bright blood in the stool or on the toilet tissue usually indicates bleeding from the anus, rectum, or colon. The exact site of the bleeding can usually be determined only by other diagnostic procedures.

Hemorrhoids are quite prevalent, and the patient is usually aware of this defect. They may be accompanied by bleeding or pruritus, or both. Although bleeding is a common complication of hemorrhoids, the physician must keep firmly in mind that rectal bleeding may arise anywhere in the lower bowel and may be indicative of serious disease.

Genitourinary system. Symptoms referable to the urinary tract include frequency, nocturia, urgency, hesitancy, oliguria, hematuria, pyuria, renal colic, dysuria, dark urine, edema, and dribbling or incontinence.

Frequency of urination may be attended with large volumes of urine *(polyuria)* or small quantities passed at frequent intervals. Frequency may occur in primary diseases of the urinary tract or may result from diabetes mellitus, diabetes insipidus, or emotional tension. The patient with diabetes mellitus usually presents a triad of symptoms characterized by polyuria, *polydipsia* (increased thirst), and *polyphagia* (increased ingestion or desire for food). In any case the examiner should record the approximate number of times the patient urinates during a 24-hour period and the quantity of urine voided if it seems to be excessive.

Nocturia (urination at night) is usually indicative of urinary tract disease. Again the examiner should record the number of times his patient urinates at night and make a reasonable estimate of the amount voided.

Urgency, which may be constant or intermittent, is an intense desire to urinate. It is often accompanied by frequency. Urgency is usually the result of prostatic disease or infection of the bladder.

Hesitancy refers to difficulty in starting the urinary stream. There is the desire to urinate, but on reaching the lavatory the patient must wait before the stream is released. This may occur in nervous or tense persons but is commonly secondary to prostatic disease.

Oliguria (decrease in urinary output) is caused by a decrease in urinary production such as occurs in acute glomerulonephritis and other renal diseases.

Dysuria refers to pain, burning, or discomfort in the urethra that accompanies the flow of urine. It is indicative of disease in the kidneys, bladder, or urethra.

Dribbling (passage of a frequently interrupted small urinary stream with little or no force) usually indicates a urethral stricture, prostatic obstruction, or certain neurologic disorders.

Hematuria is blood in the urine. The site of bleeding may be at any point along the urinary tract. Bright blood that is passed at the onset of urination is the result of a urethral lesion. Terminal hematuria or bleeding that occurs at the end of urination usually indicates disease in the trigone of the urinary bladder or in the prostatic urethra. When bleeding is present throughout urination, it may arise from the kidneys, ureters, or bladder. Hematuria may or may not be accompanied by pain, depending on the site and nature of the disease process. For example, a cancer of the urinary bladder may cause intermittent, painless hematuria; whereas a benign process, such as hemorrhagic cystitis, may result in profuse hematuria accompanied by discomfort in the suprapubic region, as well as dysuria.

Pyuria (pus in the urine) is usually manifested to the patient as cloudy urine. Pyuria may be caused by infection at any point along the urinary tract. On the other hand, cloudy urine is not necessarily caused by pyuria. In alkaline urine, phosphates may produce a cloudy appearance.

Edema, as previously mentioned, may occur in renal as well as other diseases. When caused by renal disease, the edema may be localized in the hands and periorbital region, or it may be generalized. Such edema is commonly present in acute and subacute glomerulonephritis, nephrosis, and other less frequent diseases of the kidneys.

Incontinence (lack of control of the bladder) may be the result of infections, mechanical impairment of function, and neurologic disorders.

Pain referable to the urinary system may be mild, moderate, or severe and may be dull, sharp, or colicky. In typical renal colic, the result of a stone in the ureter, the pain is severe, originates in the costovertebral angle on either side, and radiates toward the groin, testis, or vulva on the respective side. Suprapubic pain may occur in cystitis or simply in an overdistended urinary bladder. In prostatic disease the patient may experience dull pain over the lumbosacral spine and also in the perineal region.

Venereal disease. An important part of every patient's history is the venereal disease review. Patients are often sensitive regarding this issue, and the examiner must be tactful in his questioning. In the majority of patients a correct answer will be obtained by asking, "Have you ever had syphilis, gonorrhea, or any other venereal disease?" To some patients such terms are meaningless, and the physician must either inquire about certain symptoms of these diseases, such as "Have you ever had a sore on your penis?" or he must resort to terminology in a vernacular familiar to the patient. In many instances the physician will have to use rather crude terms such as "clap" (which means gonorrhea to many patients), "hair cut" (which is often used to indicate a chancre on the penis), or "bad blood" (another equivalent for syphilis). Inquiry by means of common name and symptoms should be made for each of the venereal diseases. When a history of venereal disease is obtained, the date of the infection, the type and quantity of treatment administered, and any follow-up data should be recorded.

Menstrual and obstetric history. A thorough appraisal of the menstrual and obstetric history is essential for every female patient. The menstrual history should include date of last normal period, interval between periods, duration and amount of flow (the latter expressed in terms of the number of pads or tampons used in a 24-hour period), and age of onset *(menarche)*. The physician should inquire concerning the presence or absence of dysmenorrhea, metrorrhagia, menorrhagia, postcoital bleeding, vaginal discharge, and dyspareunia. Additional pertinent data should include information regarding tension, swelling and soreness of the breasts, and details concerning the *climacteric* ("change of life" or cessation of the menses).

Dysmenorrhea (painful or difficult menstruation) is described by patients as menstrual "cramps." It is pertinent to inquire as to the time relationship between dysmenorrhea and actual menstruation. In some patients pain occurs for several days prior to menstruation, whereas in others it appears coincident with the flow or even several days after the onset of menstrual bleeding.

Metrorrhagia is either frank bleeding or spotting of blood that occurs in the interim between menstrual periods. This symptom is often of grave significance and necessitates thorough study. *Menorrhagia* is excessive bleeding or actual hemorrhaging at the time of menstruation and is often manifested by the passing of large clots of blood. This symptom may be either functional or organic in origin. *Postcoital bleeding* (that which follows sexual intercourse) may be important and should be carefully investigated.

Vaginal discharge (frequently called *leukorrhea*) is a common complaint. The term leukorrhea implies that the discharge is white, but in many instances it is actually yellow, brown, or red. The color, amount, and time of occurrence of the discharge in relation to the menstrual cycle should be recorded. Many women experience a minimal white or pale yellow discharge following menstruation, and as a rule this is of little or no significance. On the other hand, a thick, persistent, profuse white, yellow, or bloody discharge may indicate a severe infection or malignancy of the cervix, uterus, or vagina. Further, it should be noted whether the discharge is accompanied by irritation or itching.

Dyspareunia refers to pain or discomfort in either the vagina or pelvis that accompanies sexual intercourse. Although it may be functional, it is usually organic in origin.

Premenstrual tension is manifest by emotional tension, apprehension, extreme nervousness, a state of depression, and other similar symptoms. Many women experience bloating of the abdomen and soreness of the breasts for several days prior to the menstrual flow.

In those patients in whom the *climacteric (menopause)* has occurred, the history should include the date of cessation of the menses, associated symptoms, and any treatment.

The obstetric history should include the number of pregnancies, the number of deliveries, and any significant complications. The number of pregnancies, for convenience, is referred to as *gravida* and the number of deliveries as *para*. For example, if a patient has had six pregnancies resulting in six deliveries, it is recorded as gravida 6, para 6. If, on the other hand, she has had six pregnancies and five deliveries with one spontaneous abortion, it is recorded as gravida 6, para 5, and abortion 1. When an abortion has occurred, the examiner should record the cause, if known, the duration of gestation, and determine whether the abortion was spontaneous or induced.

Nervous system. Evaluation of complaints referable to the nervous system is often difficult. Frequently it is necessary for the exam-

iner to clarify the patient's statements. For example, many patients complain of "nervousness." This term is quite vague, and its connotation is variable. To some, "nervousness" means anxiety or apprehension; to others, it designates tremors or even convulsions. When such a term is used, the physician should ask, "What do you mean by nervousness?" or "In what way do your nerves bother you?" Thus clarification of nervous symptoms is essential to an understanding of the basic illness and whether they are physiologic or pathologic in origin.

Inquiry should be made to determine the character of a patient's interpersonal relationships—how he has gotten along with his family, friends, associates, and in school or at work. Also, the physician should determine if the patient has had any "nervous breakdowns" or any condition in which he has been "out of his mind," "too nervous to work or do anything," under the care of a psychiatrist, or in a mental hospital. In most instances, information concerning changes in the patient's behavior, memory, or judgment must be obtained from relatives or friends. Attention to the family and past history may contribute to an understanding of the present complaints referable to the nervous system.

Inquiry should be made into the following important symptoms: convulsions, vertigo, sensory disturbances, pain, paresthesia, and paralysis and paresis.

Convulsions (commonly called "fits," "spells," or "falling out") are of great medical importance. They are *tonic* (a sustained muscular contraction), *clonic* (intermittent muscular contractions), localized, or generalized. Convulsions are usually sudden in onset and may be preceded by an aura (an auditory or visual sensation). Biting of the tongue and incontinence of urine and feces may be present. It should also be determined if the seizure is followed by stupor or sleep. Loss of consciousness may accompany the seizure, which may be followed by *amnesia* (absence of memory) for the entire episode. Convulsive seizures are the result of organic brain disease.

Vertigo (dizziness), headache, and tinnitus have been previously described.

Sensory disturbances include pain and paresthesia (anesthesia, hypesthesia, and hyperesthesia).

Pain is a subjective experience and must be evaluated not in terms of the patient's statement of severity but in terms of the extent to which it has interfered with his activities. One should determine the time incidence of the pain and any precipitating factors, such as relationship to movements. The location of the pain should be determined as precisely as possible, and the examiner should ascertain if it has shifted to other areas. Has the pain in the involved areas become more or less severe?

Paresthesia is an abnormal or perverted sensation, such as numbness, tingling, burning, or formication. It includes *hypesthesia*, which is a decrease in tactile sensation, *anesthesia*, which is a loss of sensation, and *hyperesthesia*, which is an excessive sensitivity of the skin or special senses. These alterations in sensation indicate abnormality of the peripheral nerves, sensory nerve roots, spinothalamic tract, or thalamus. *Formication* is the sensation of insects crawling on the skin.

Evaluation of the *motor components* of the nervous system should include inquiry for *paralysis* (loss of motor function) and *paresis* (weakness or incomplete paralysis). *Ataxia*, which is the result of a loss of muscular coordination, is a staggering or reeling gait. It is the result of lesions in the spinal cord or brain.

Musculoskeletal system. A review of the musculoskeletal system should include inquiry for muscular pain; swelling, pain, deformity, or disability of any joint; lameness; weakness; and symptoms of impaired circulation in the extremities. Also, the physician should inquire

for symptoms referable to the back and vertebral column.

If the patient has any complaints referable to his extremities, it is important to determine whether the discomfort is actually located in the joint proper or in the muscles and tendons. Often the patient assumes that any pain in the extremities is caused by arthritis. A review of joint symptoms should determine whether the pain is localized or migratory, aggravated or alleviated by movement, and accompanied by swelling, redness, and tenderness. In patients with symptoms suggestive of arthritis, it should be ascertained if there are associated constitutional symptoms such as fever, chills, and sore throat. Many patients experiencing joint pain will have tried such home remedies as local heat, aspirin, and other medications, and the effects of these measures should be noted.

Weakness of an extremity or a muscle group may be a presenting symptom of neurologic or primary muscle diseases such as poliomyelitis, polyneuritis, myasthenia gravis, and primary muscular dystrophy and muscular atrophy.

Peripheral vascular diseases are frequently encountered, and a careful history will often suggest the proper diagnosis. Pertinent symptoms of these conditions include coldness and numbness in the extremities, cyanosis or other types of discoloration, leg cramps, intermittent claudication, ulceration, and trophic changes in the digits and nails. The term *leg cramps* usually refers to cramping pain in the calf muscles, which may occur in the sitting, standing, or reclining position. *Intermittent claudication* is severe cramping in the calf muscles, precipitated by walking and relieved by rest. It is caused by arterial insufficiency, which may be the result of arteriosclerosis or thromboangiitis obliterans. Discoloration may vary from purple to red or white, depending on whether there is venous impairment, arterial insufficiency, or both. The term *trophic changes* refers to atrophy of the digits, nails, or both. This condition may progress to *gangrene* (necrosis). Also, the physician should inquire for the presence of varicose veins and phlebitis.

SOCIAL HISTORY

It is generally conceded that functional diseases are extremely common and constitute a large portion of the physician's practice. In addition, the course of organic disease is influenced considerably by the patient's emotional reaction to his disease and to his environment as a whole. Therefore, it is of paramount importance to inquire into the patient's social history in order (1) to determine his state of social adjustment and (2) to interpret any organic disease in light of his emotional tendencies. Questioning is directed, therefore, into the patient's personal habits, emotional adjustments, sex life, business life, personality factors, and recreation habits. This type of inquiry requires a great deal of tact and is both learned and perfected by repeated experience in interrogating patients. For example, many patients are unwilling to volunteer information concerning their sex habits. This and other data can be obtained, however, by establishing good rapport with the patient and by convincing him that such information is pertinent in arriving at a correct diagnosis.

The patient's emotional adjustment, sex habits, and business life are usually closely related and can be approached by a general method of inquiry. How does the patient adjust to his job, his friends, his business associates, and people in general? Is he temperamental, moody, depressed, euphoric, or cheerful? Is he mature or juvenile in his approach to everyday problems and his relations with people? Has he had any pathologic (perverted) sexual experiences, and if so, what is his reaction to them? A detailed survey of the social history will enable the physician to arrive at a more adequate understanding of his patient.

Habits

Personal habits include those relating to smoking, alcoholic beverages, sleeping, eating, recreation, and the use of narcotics or sedatives. Does the patient use tobacco and, if so, to what extent and in what form? Does he imbibe alcohol and, if so, to what extent? Does he drink coffee or tea to excess, and does he eat a balanced diet? Does he obtain sufficient rest at night? Does his schedule include some recreational program other than his routine work? Does he use narcotics, sedatives, or other types of medication, and to what extent?

Marital history

This review includes data concerning the health of the mate, sexual adjustment, the number of children and their physical status, and the general social adjustment within the family. Are the patient and his or her mate happily married, or is there constant turmoil, disagreement, and lack of adjustment? Are there congenial relationships between the parents and the children? If there is any sexual maladjustment, on what basis does it occur? An informative family history may be helpful in evaluating the patient's personality pattern.

OCCUPATIONAL HISTORY

It is recognized that certain occupations are associated with definite health hazards. These include exposure to certain irritating agents, contact with various domestic and wild animals, exposure to certain climatic and environmental conditions, and finally the physical and mental pressures of occupations that sooner or later take their toll on certain persons. Thus, the occupational history should include a record of all past and present types of work, the conditions of work, and specific details regarding exposure to various metals, gases, chemicals, fumes, dust, and radioactive materials.

A few specific instances of occupational diseases are pneumoconiosis (fibrosis of the lung caused by the inhalation of mineral dust), which may be encountered in foundry and pottery workers, miners, stonecutters, and grinders; lead poisoning, which may be acquired by painters, storage battery workers, and smelters; arsenic poisoning, which may be found in fruit-tree sprayers and those engaged in certain chemical industries; brucellosis, which may be found in veterinarians and slaughterhouse workers. In this modern atomic age, persons exposed to radioactive isotopes are prone to the development of blood dyscrasias.

CHAPTER 6

MENTAL STATUS

VALUE OF MENTAL EXAMINATION

The mental examination is a part of the total evaluation of the patient and can make a valuable contribution to the understanding of the patient and his illness. Because of its value and importance the physician needs to acquire competence in its conduct just as he would in any other examination procedure, such as the cardiac, pelvic, or neurologic examination. When it is omitted, the evaluation of the patient must be considered incomplete. The following are some of the more important contributions of the mental examination.

Identification of patient's personality. There is a high correlation between personality or life style and certain diseases or clinical syndromes. For example, migraine headache and ulcerative colitis are seen typically in people having a rigid, compulsive personality. Alcoholism and its sequelae are found typically in those with a moody or cyclothymic personality. These illnesses must be treated within the context of the patient's personality. A basic medical dictum is that one should treat the patient and not the disease. This is only possible when the physician knows and understands the patient's personality through the mental examination. The crucial importance of personality style in disease is emphasized by Rapaport, who points out that "All behavior is characteristic of the behaving personality."[1]

Identification of mental illness. One of the major goals of the mental examination is to ascertain whether or not the patient has troubled thoughts, disturbed emotional states, or mental conflict. Their presence might indicate an existing mental illness, and their identification may bring understanding to otherwise seemingly inexplicable somatic phenomena. It should be remembered that thoughts and feelings do not exist in isolation. Headache, backache, abdominal distress, or chest pain may be, and often are, the distant physiologic effects of a central emotional disturbance. This complex interaction of mind and emotion with the body is the concern of that field of medical science called psychosomatic medicine. A very high percentage of patients who consult their doctors for various complaints and disabilities have no organic disease but instead are suffering from a psychosomatic disorder.

Identification of somatic disease. The interrelation of mind and body is a two-way street, the mind influencing the body and the body, the mind. All parts of the body are represented directly or indirectly at the mental level, and changes in the body are therefore reflected consciously or unconsciously at the mental level. The mind can be viewed as a sensitive monitor of all that goes on in the body. It is not uncommon for different pathologic somatic states to be manifested first in the patient's mental life—in the patient's feelings and thoughts. For example, alteration in mood (depression or elation) is not infrequently associated with malignancy or metabolic disorders. Such mood changes may be the first sign of the disease. Impaired concentration, memory, or judgment may herald the presence of a brain tumor, brain infection, intoxication, or cerebral arteriosclerosis.

Value for the nonpsychiatric physician. Although it is perhaps obvious, it nevertheless should be emphasized that mental examination is a tool to be used by the nonpsychiatric as well as by the psychiatric physician. The nonpsychiatric physician in fact sees and screens many more patients with emotional and psychologic problems than the psychiatrist. He is able to help and treat many of these without psychiatric referral if their problems are properly understood and recognized through the mental examination. Therefore, it is important that he appreciate the value of the mental examination and acquire skill in its conduct. The purpose of this chapter is to assist the student in acquiring competence in this area.

THE INTERVIEW

The mental examination is carried out within the framework of the interview. In turn, the interview can be broken down into three basic steps: (1) obtaining the history of the problem, which compares with the medical history; (2) eliciting the patient's past history, including family history, and developmental, educational, medical, vocational and marital history; and (3) performing the mental examination itself.

Although these three procedures, of necessity, must be discussed separately, in practice one blends with another. For example, while the patient is discussing his problem or discussing his life experience, the physician is making observations and arriving at impressions. In other words, the physician is examining while taking the history. The way the patient tells his story, the things he chooses to tell or to omit, his life experiences, and his reactions to them all contribute to the data of the mental examination as well as to the clinical history. Furthermore, the story that the patient tells serves to guide the examiner in his subsequent mental examination, determining in part what areas of mental functioning will be explored and tested.

There are also ancillary techniques that can be used in the mental evaluation of the patient; however, they are not used routinely and ordinarily are administered by a specially trained person, the clinical psychologist. For example, in some instances special psychologic tests, such as the Rorschach test, the Wechsler-Belleview test, or the TAT, are used because they are often helpful in revealing information about the patient's mental functioning that might not be apparent in the mental examination itself. Also, on some occasions hypnotic techniques and drugs (narcoanalysis) are used, but they are highly specialized procedures and should be employed only by qualified specialists.

Importance. Interviewing is one of the most important techniques a physician can use in the evaluation of his patient. In spite of its great importance and value it is often sadly neglected, and many physicians never trouble themselves to become knowledgeable and skillful in its use. But it is through the interview that the physician learns about the patient's problem, becomes acquainted with the patient, and makes observations about the patient.

Nature. In essence the interview is a procedure that consists of two (or more) people sitting and talking together. It is a discussion or conversation, with one of the participants, because of his professional training, providing leadership and guidance. This leadership and guidance can prevent the interview from wandering aimlessly and can make it a productive and meaningful experience for both the patient and the physician.

Because the successful mental examination is dependent on the participation of the patient and on the information he provides, the atmosphere of the interview and the relationship that is established are of fundamental importance. If the patient is comfortable, if he can sense that the physician is interested and concerned, then he will feel more freedom to tell his story and to discuss his personal problems.

An interview is not carried out through the use of a questionnaire or through a bombardment of probing questions. Rather, the ideal interview is one in which, after a good relationship has been established, the patient is able to talk freely about things that are important to him—his conflicts, his problems, and the ways in which he is feeling badly. The interviewer's primary task is to provide the right atmosphere, to be a good listener, and to ask only those questions that help the patient to tell his story. A good interviewer can be compared with a skilled obstetrician who, in assisting with the delivery of a baby, lets natural forces play the dominant role and interferes only when there are obstructions that need to be removed.

Setting. A satisfactory and productive interview requires a special setting. As previously pointed out, one of the first considerations is to make the patient comfortable and help him feel at ease. An interview cannot be carried out with the physician standing impatiently by the patient's bed or trying to talk to the patient in a ward with other patients nearby and with ward personnel coming and going. An interview must be conducted in privacy, in a room in which the patient can feel that what he says is confidential and will not be overheard. Interruptions, such as incoming phone calls, should be kept to a minimum. The general atmosphere should be calm and unhurried. The interviewer should present a relaxed manner—professional but not stiff or formal. He should manifest appropriate warmth, be flexible, and apply the light touch when it is indicated. Consideration should be given to the lighting of the room and the seating arrangement. If possible, the room should be softly lighted, and the patient should not have to stare into a bright light or an unshaded window. Sometimes the patient is more at ease if the interviewer does not sit behind a desk but occupies a chair similar to the patient's in a conversational arrangement. However, on some occasions a desk between the interviewer and the patient provides a sense of security for the patient. The seating arrangement in general is not crucial, but the interviewer's attitude and manner are very important. The interviewer should not feel hurried, and should convey to the patient the idea that there is a reasonable period of time set aside for him to tell his story; if the story cannot be told in the allotted time, other interviews can be arranged. The interviewer should avoid being preoccupied and should be alert to the patient, giving the patient his undivided attention. Taking notes usually does not interfere with the natural flow of the story; however, when note-taking interferes with the interviewing process, or if a patient becomes apprehensive or suspicious of the note-taking, it should be avoided.

EMOTIONAL PROBLEMS IN INTERVIEWS

The purpose of all examination procedures is to gather clinical data and information. However, in contrast to most other diagnostic procedures the interview (history-taking) can be seriously blocked or interfered with by emotional factors on the part of the patient or the doctor. This is because of the peculiar nature of the interview and the mental examination. It deals with private and highly subjective material, which is difficult for all parties to deal with freely, openly, and honestly. Since the interview can be distorted by conscious and unconscious factors on the part of either the patient and physician, they therefore deserve our consideration at this point.

Problems of the patient. The physician must understand that an interview normally is an anxiety-provoking experience. Two basic factors underlie this anxiety. One is that the interview and mental examination tend to be self-revealing. The very purpose of the examination is to uncover and identify that which is normally hidden or denied. So every interview is to some extent a minor tug of war between patient and physician, the one defending himself against undue exposure and self-revelation and the other trying to get data that can help him to know and understand his patient better so that he in turn can be more helpful.

The second reason for the patient's anxiety is the way the physician is frequently perceived because of an unconscious mental process called *transference*. Transference is the unconscious displacement of affect or feeling associated with a significant person in the patient's past onto the physician. It is responsible for the physician's frequently being perceived in an authoritative, power-laden role, similar to the power and authority of parent to child. It should be emphasized that the physician assumes this role without the patient's conscious awareness. Transference interferes with the physician's being perceived as a basically kindly, neutral, helping scientist. Instead the patient tends to perceive the physician as judgmental, critical, and punitive. Transference only enhances the normal reluctance to self-revelation and openness.

The patient's anxieties lead to what is called *resistance*, a way of defending himself against anxiety. It is resistance that blocks, distorts,

and interferes wth the interview. In order to conduct an interview successfully the physician must be sensitive to the patient's anxiety and his resistance, both of which must be dealt with and overcome if the interview is to be successful.

Anxiety and resistance are evident in such behavioral responses as flushing, perspiration, dry mouth, trembling, going "blank," and blocking. Some patients deal with anxiety by a certain bravado, by cracking jokes, or by dominating and taking over the interview. Other patients may be critical and verbally attack the physician, as if an offense is the best defense. Other patients may withdraw and become suspicious and distrustful. These responses require calm, wise, unhurried leadership along with respect for the patient's limitations in talking about certain topics. Not pushing the patient but giving him time along with reassurance and encouragement are often enough to overcome his anxiety and resistance.

In every interview distortions, omissions, memory lapses, or exaggerations are observed. These too are evidences of resistance. The physician should be slow to point them out and tactful when he does. Very often, as the patient becomes more comfortable he corrects them himself.

Problems of the physician.[2,3] Interviewing is not a one-way street. The physician can also have emotional blocks and attitudes that interfere in the process. Just as it is ordinarily more comfortable for the patient to undergo a physical examination than to be interviewed, so in general it is more comfortable for the physician to conduct a physical examination than an interview.

By training, physicians are accustomed to being active and doing things. They examine, cut, inject, ask direct questions, and give orders. An interview is a free-flowing, unstructured, interpersonal process, in which neither party assumes a dominating or controlling role.

A good interview is a mutual process. His role in the interview may not be a comfortable one for the physician because he may not feel he is in charge.

Furthermore, an interview that is personal to the patient is also, to some extent, personal to the physician. What he asks the patient or what the patient reveals, directly or indirectly, frequently touches the physician's life, such as in discussions about sex, infidelity, love, hate, etc. Thus, the physician may omit certain areas or he may probe unduly into other areas because of his own conscious and unconscious conflicts, curiosities, and interests. There are very few physicians who are adept at taking good sexual histories, not only because of a lack of skill, but also because most physicians are not comfortable in discussing this aspect of life and behavior.

Besides blatant conflicts and anxieties that interfere with the interview, the physician may carry to the interview certain attitudes, prejudices, and biases that are equally interfering. In the emotional and psychologic field the physician must continue to be an objective scientist and must avoid being judgmental, condemning, or nonaccepting. To provide the physician with the material he needs to know, the patient must feel unconditionally accepted, respected, and liked as a decent human being.

Hawthorne[4] has provided a model of the sensitive, inquiring physician to which all students should give serious consideration.

He deemed it essential, it would seem, to know the man, before attempting to do him good. Whenever there is a heart and an intellect, the diseases of the physical frame are tinged with the peculiarities of these. In Arthur Dimmesdale, thought and imagination were so active, and sensibility so intense, that the bodily infirmity would be likely to have its ground work there. So Roger Chillingworth—the man of skill, the kind and friendly physician—strove to go deep into his patient's bosom, delving among his principles, prying into his recollections, and probing everything with a cautious touch, like a treasure seeker in a dark cavern. Few secrets can escape an investigator who has opportunity and license to undertake such a quest, and skill to follow it up. A man burdened with a secret should especially avoid the intimacy of his physician. If the latter possess native sagacity, and a nameless something more,—let us call it intuition; if he show no intrusive egotism, nor disagreeably prominent characteristics of his own; if he have the power, which must be born with him, to bring his mind into such affinity with his patients, that this last shall unawares have spoken what he imagines himself only to have thought; if such revelations by received without tumult, and acknowledged not so often by an uttered sympathy as by silence, an articulate breath, and here and there a word, to indicate that all is understood; if to these qualifications of a confidant be joined the advantages afforded by his recognized character as a physician,—then, at some inevitable moment, will the soul of the sufferer be dissolved, and flow forth in a dark, but transparent stream, bringing all its mystery into the daylight.

CONDUCTING THE INTERVIEW

Beginning. Often the most difficult and awkward time in the interview is at the very beginning when the examiner is trying to establish the relationship from which he can project his study of the patient. Probably one of the most important factors in initiating the interview is that the examiner himself feel comfortable and be relatively free from anxiety. If the physician remembers several basic things, he can approach the interview and the examination with considerably more confidence and poise. First, most patients welcome the opportunity to have someone to talk to. It is often a source of considerable relief for patients to have someone who is willing to take time to listen and to hear them out. A common complaint on the part of many patients is that their physician does not take time to talk to them. Second, the examiner need not feel that he must or should learn everything about his patient or understand his patient completely in one interview. Not infrequently, repeated interviews are necessary for a patient's problem to be well understood. Third, if the examiner approaches each patient with an appropriate sense of humility, not needing or desiring to impress the patient with what he knows or what he can do, but only wanting to understand the patient's problem and, if possible, to be more helpful to the patient, then the examiner is better able to start the interview in a more natural and relaxed manner.

Discussion of a problem. At the start of the interview the examiner must necessarily take the initiative. He should introduce himself and have the patient identify himself and provide certain basic information, such as his age, marital status, spouse's name, children's names and ages, address, telephone number, and occupation. A brief period of informal small talk at the beginning is quite appropriate to help the patient relax and feel more comfortable. From this point the examiner then moves to the main content of the interview.

An important part of the interview is concerned with the story of the patient's problem. A carefully detailed account of the beginning and course of the problem is the single most valuable source of information in the total study of the patient. Probably more errors in diagnosis and treatment result from an inadequate or faulty history of the patient's illness than from any other single cause. There is no stereotyped routine that the physician can use, but there are guidelines for him to follow, which can be helpful if they are employed with imagination.

Physician's initiation of discussion. To initiate the discussion, the interviewer can use any number of phrases such as, "Tell me about your problem; what is it that is troubling you?" "In what way have you been feeling bad?" "Tell me about your symptoms." "What problem made your physician feel you should see me (or be admitted to the hospital)?"

Permitting patient to tell his story. Once the patient has started to talk, he should, as much as possible, be permitted to tell his own story in his own words and in his own way. The interviewer should avoid unnecessary interruptions since his primary task is to listen attentively and quietly and to extract meaning from what the patient is saying. It requires adequate time to obtain a good history and the patient needs to be heard out. If, in telling the story, the patient becomes emotionally stirred and weeps, usually it is best to remain quiet and not make any comment other than a word of reassurance indicating that the interviewer understands and that such an emotional display is quite acceptable.

Guiding discussion. Being a good listener, however, does not mean that the interview should be permitted to wander aimlessly on irrelevant topics. The interviewer has the responsibility of guiding the patient's discussion and of clarifying points through discreet questioning. The main problem in providing guidance and structure for the interview is to avoid overstructuring that prevents the patient from telling his own story and instead causes him to relate what he feels the interviewer wants him to say. The patient is sensitively tuned in to what he feels are the interviewer's major interests and thoughts (expectations), and in his desire to cooperate he provides information that he believes the interviewer is searching for rather than providing freely and spontaneously what he has actually experienced.

Overstructuring the interview can be avoided by nondirective and open-ended questions and responses. For example, a point can be clarified or the patient can be encouraged to continue talking by such responses as: "Could you tell me more about that?" "I am not sure I understand; could you elaborate a little more on that point?" "What do you mean?" "What was it you felt?" "What was your reaction to that?" The physician should, for the most part, avoid questions that put words in the patient's mouth.

Nature of problem and etiologic factors. It is important to know when and how the problem started. In some patients the physician finds that the problem has existed for many years or has been virtually lifelong, in contrast to a problem of more recent origin. It is characteristic of certain illnesses, such as anxiety reactions and vascular crises, to have a sudden and dramatic onset. Other illnesses, such as depressions and various somatic diseases, tend to begin more slowly and follow a more progressive course. Questions useful in gathering data in this area are: "Has the illness or problem been constant, has it fluctuated in intensity, or has it been marked by periods of well-being?" "Have symptoms of a similar nature ever been experienced before, and if so, when and in what way?"

A problem is understood through its relationship to etiologic factors. As a rule, emotional and psychologic problems represent a reaction to something that has happened in the individual's life situation. Therefore, the interviewer should inquire into the various areas of the patient's life—vocational, social, and family situations—to see if there have been any significant changes. Depressed states are frequently precipitated by adverse life experiences such as losses or disappointments. Anxiety reactions frequently occur as the result of provocative situations that have aroused impulses (angry or sexual) that have consciously or unconsciously frightened the patient. Life crises of a great variety can arouse feelings and conflicts beyond the individual's capacity to handle them. Some of the common crises of life occur during the adolescence of the patient's children, when they are growing up and leaving home; at the time of retirement; when there is lack of success at work; during sickness in the home; or when a spouse has been unfaithful. Therefore, no significant event in the individual's life can be overlooked or considered insignificant in precipitating emotional conflict leading to the patient's illness.

Discussion of history. A review of the patient's past history constitutes another major area to be covered in the interview. The discussion of the present problem provides a basis for an understanding of the patient's illness, but is does not provide significant information about the patient as a person—what his life experiences have been, how he has adapted, or what his style of living has been.

Knowledge of the patient's personality and life style gives an indication of basic strengths and weaknesses and is of diagnostic and prognostic value. For example, a patient was referred for evaluation because her physician thought a conversion reaction might explain the distress and the disability that she was experiencing in her right upper extremity. A careful clinical history indicated that she probably had an underlying organic illness involving her nervous system.—namely, multiple sclerosis—that had caused both sensory impairment and ataxia of the right hand and arm. The knowledge that the patient probably had this illness did not preclude the possibility of a superimposed and complicating conversion reaction; however, an assessment of her basic attitudes and life patterns made it improbable. The assessment showed her as a conscientious, serious-minded, compulsive person, to whom self-control had always been important. Until the onset of her present illness she had enjoyed good health and had demonstrated no evidence of emotional difficulty. In other words, her life adjustment and personality pattern did not suggest a person who would react to crises or conflicts with a conversionlike pattern. Rather, her personality pattern suggested an intensified need to control the malfunctioning part of her body. Of course, this need to control the malfunction could lead to concern, anxiety, increased tension, and preoccupation with the involved part and thereby could lead to added distress.

The following abstract will serve to illustrate further the importance of the past history in providing an understanding of the person and his basic personality pattern. A married woman had been subjected to various diagnostic and therapeutic measures because of symptoms referable to her heart, characterized chiefly by episodes of tachycardia, weakness, and marked anxiety. Physical studies failed to reveal anything basically wrong; therefore, it was evident that she did have an emotional problem—an anxiety neurosis. This conclusion, however, did not provide any basis for understanding why she had the emotional problem or what could be done about it.

An evaluation of her life experiences and of her personality pattern did provide, in much greater depth, an understanding of her illness. It was found that she was the only child of rigid and strict parents who placed a high premium on the home being quiet and orderly. They discouraged any expression of anger or healthy assertiveness. As a consequence she developed a personality pattern characterized by compliance, agreeableness, and denial of angry feelings. Throughout her life she had never been consciously aware of being angry. Yet she now found herself in a life situation—an adult, married, and the mother of several active and normally boisterous children—for which her personality pattern was not adequate. Her life situation could not help but arouse feelings of frustration and irritability because it really demanded assertive, positive, and aggressive action. It would have been healthy for her on occasion to "blow up," to "let off steam," and to exert firm discipline. But such behavior would have been in conflict with her training and past experiences. Her personality pattern would not permit it. Consequently, for her to be helped required not only a recognition that her illness was emotional in nature but also an under-standing of her personality pattern and how it needed to be modified through psychotherapeutic measures so that she could be more expressive of her feelings and thereby relieve inner tensions.

The major areas of the person's life that should be investigated are (1) *his family*, (2) *his developmental and medical history*, and (3) *his school, social, and vocational history*. When and how each of these areas will be explored depends somewhat on the circumstances and natural flow of the interview. However, it is important that each of these areas be covered.

Family history. Because a patient's life begins with his family and since it is from this source that he acquires both his constitutional endowments and early training, it is understandable that a careful review of one's family and family experiences is of basic importance.

The mental interview, like the traditional medical interview, is concerned with the medical history of the family: illnesses, deaths, ages and causes of death, and so on. But the mental interview is especially concerned with what the home was like and what kind of interpersonal relationships existed in the home. Was there an atmosphere of security and peacefulness or of turmoil, tension, anxiety, and insecurity? The patient can be drawn into a discussion of his family and family life by such phrases as, "Tell me about your family and your home life." "What was your father like?" "Describe your mother to me." "Could you tell me something about your brothers and sisters?" "How did you see the relationship between the various members of your family?"

The patient should be requested to give a brief characterization of his parents and siblings, telling what they were like, describing their attitudes, what he believed they felt toward him, and how he in turn felt toward them. It is important to learn about the family's religious, social, educational, vocational, and sexual attitudes. The family's situation in the community, such as its economic status and group identification (ethnic and religious), should be explored. Such family experiences as a broken home, chronic illness, alcoholism, quarreling, threats and intimidations, and attitudes of rejection and disapproval or of love and acceptance are all of basic importance in the understanding of the person and his illness.

Developmental and medical history. The patient should be requested to give as much information as he can (either from recall or from hearsay) about his early life experiences, including birth, nursing, weaning, toilet training, and adolescence. The medical history should include all significant illnesses, accidents, operations, and previous psychiatric problems, the circumstances surrounding them, and the patient's emotional reaction to them—namely, how the patient felt about these experiences and what they meant to him.

School, social, and vocational history. A review of these areas tells the examiner much about the patient's basic capacities, emotional maturity, and aspirations. Educational goals and achievements are indicative of the patient's motivations and his intellectual capacities. The patient's social history concerns all of his interpersonal relationships, family, friends, schoolmates, teachers, fellow workers, and others. This area can be investigated by such questions as: "Tell me how you feel you have gotten along with people." "Was it easy for you to make friends in school?" "Who has to take the first step in making friends?" "How do you get along at work? Do you feel comfortable around your superiors? Are your co-workers friendly?"

Consideration of the patient's vocational experiences is often most informative. The positions the patient has held, his effectiveness as a worker, his ability to assume leadership and responsibility, his work stability, and his capacity to get along with others, all tell a great deal about his life adjustment and basic abilities.

Inquiry into habitual patterns of behavior.

A review of the past history tells one a great deal about the patient. However, to clarify further what kind of person the patient is, one should inquire into some of his enduring attitudes and reaction patterns that serve as the basis for what is known as the patient's personality.

After having talked about school, work, and relationships, it is quite easy and natural to inquire into how the patient envisions himself and how he reacts in various life situations. The subject can be introduced by such questions as, "Could you tell me what kind of person you feel you are? By this I mean are you serious minded and highly conscientious? Or are you carefree and nothing bothers you, so to speak?" "When doing something, do you have to do it perfectly?" "Are you a stickler for details?" "Do you worry and fret about things?" "Do you get blue and discouraged easily?" "Have you thought of yourself as being a moody person or are you more even tempered?" "Do you meet emergencies well?" "Does the thought of a fight or argument upset you?" "Do you avoid quarrels or do you enjoy a good scrap?" "What is your reaction to seeing an accident or seeing some one sick or injured?"

The patient's response to such questions enables the examiner to arrive at some tentative impressions about his personal characteristics. The compulsive person is serious minded, conscientious, and great for details. The hysterical personality is often light hearted, carefree, and emotionally labile. The moody personality is readily discouraged and easily gets into "black moods." The anxious and insecure person avoids arguments, fights, or emergencies whenever possible.

DATA FROM THE CLINICAL HISTORY

Before proceeding with the mental examination let us review the information that the clinical history has already provided. The data obtained from the clinical history will guide one in the examination procedure itself, for it will suggest those areas of behavior and mental functioning that need to be explored.

The clinical history provides clues about the nature of the patient's illness, which the mental examination can help to prove or to disprove. It will indicate the nature of the precipitating factors and in turn suggest the patient's points of vulnerability and weakness. If precipitating factors cannot be clearly identified, one is forced to consider that the illness is possibly of endogenous origin or that it is primarily a physical problem. The historical study also enables the examiner to learn something about the patient's major identifications, basic attitudes, and personality pattern. The examiner has begun to become acquainted with his patient as a person, and this is a valuable frame of reference for the diagnosis of his problem and for the estimation of the prognosis and planning the course of treatment.

MENTAL EXAMINATION

In performing the mental examination, one explores and studies in detail those areas of behavior and mental function that the clinical history has indicated might be disturbed. As previously pointed out, the history reveals clues about the nature of the patient's illness, which the examination can help to prove or disprove.

The mental examination is dependent on the art of *observation* and *questioning,* just as the clinical history is dependent primarily on the art of intelligent *listening.* The data of the mental examination are derived from (1) *observation* of the patient, noting his behavior, appearance, manner and attitude, expression, speech, and motor activity; (2) *assessment* of the patient's intellectual function, considering such things as intelligence, clarity of thought, insight and judgment, and ideational content; and (3) *evaluation* of the emotional state.

Observation

Observation is fundamental in all examinational procedures, both physical and mental, and is essential in all scientific studies. Being a good observer is basic to being both a good clinician and a good scientist. Observation can be carried out in many ways: by observing the patient and his behavior, by carrying out special tests and observing their results, and by using special instruments, such as the fluoroscope, the x-ray machine, or even the microscope.

Observation derives its great importance in psychiatry from the fact that one is viewing behavior that has significance and meaning. First, behavior can be a form of nonverbal communication. Behavior is in many respects an attempt, consciously or unconsciously, to convey a message or to leave an impression. We are all reminded of the old adage: "Actions speak louder than words." Very often a patient's behavior is far more informative than the data that he can or is willing to relate verbally.

Second, behavior is a reflection of the integration of the total person, both physiologically and psychologically. Disturbances in this integration, no matter at what level, may be reflected in the patient's behavior. For example, rigidity of facial expression, a slight tremor, a shuffling gait, or slowed movements are behavioral changes that indicate underlying organic disease of the nervous system. Likewise, tension, flushing, a furtive glance, or mannerisms are behavioral signs that indicate underlying disturbances in the patient's emotional and psychologic integration.

One must always keep in mind that overt behavior should not be taken at face value alone but rather should be considered in depth. The overt or manifest behavior may be a disguise for or a reaction to underlying tendencies, feelings, and conflicts. For example, a person who acts "brash" and "cocky" in reality may feel dreadfully inferior and insecure and is only "covering up." Or a person may act quite "sweet" and ingratiating but in reality and underneath this facade may be quite hostile and aggressive.

The beginner needs assistance in learning

what he should notice or look for in appreciating the significance of what he has observed. The following are some of the things that the examiner should notice.

Patient's response. Is the patient alert, readily accessible, and appropriate? Or is he preoccupied and hard to make contact with? Does he seem confused and disoriented? Patients with organic brain disease are likely to demonstrate confusion or disorientation. The schizophrenic patient may be withdrawn, preoccupied, and inaccessible. Retarded or slowed responses are quite characteristic of the severely depressed patient, while in contrast the manic individual is hyperalert and hyperactive.

Patient's grooming. How is the patient dressed? Is he neatly dressed and well groomed? Is his grooming appropriate? There is a correlation between a patient's dress and appearance and his personality or illness. The compulsive patient's grooming reflects his careful, meticulous approach to life. Ostentation and seductiveness in dress are characteristic of the hysterical, narcissistic individual. Schizophrenic patients or those with schizoid personality often display an odd choice of clothing, colors, and style. A disheveled, unkempt appearance is more in keeping with the psychotic or organically deteriorated patient. The beard, long hair, blue jeans, sneakers, and other unconventionalities in grooming are the hallmark of the rebellious adolescent. There is also the grooming, in both the male and female, suggestive of disturbances in sex role identification—namely, overt or covert homosexual attitudes.

Patient's manner and appearance. How does the patient present himself? Is he friendly and cooperative, negative or sullen, angry or suspicious? Some patients are dramatic, affected, or highly ingratiating. Is there flirtatiousness, the quick smile, or sly wink? The anxious patient may display flushing, tension, and dryness of the mouth. Is he perspiring?

Are his nails bitten? Does he show other nervous habits or mannerisms?

The patient's physique, posture, and facial expression can tell a great deal about his personality and mental state. For example, we think of the obese person as being "jolly" and good natured, whereas a muscular, athletic build suggests rigidity and aggressiveness. Slumping posture is associated with the depressed and the discouraged individual, the lordotic posture with the confident and arrogant personality. The facial expression as well as the look of the eye can reveal sadness and depression. A patient's expression can also suggest hope and confidence, skepticism or apprehension, strength or weakness, passivity or independence, determination or stubbornness, or shrewdness or cunning.

Speech and motor activity. How does the patient speak and express himself? What is the tone of his voice? Is his speech calm, assured, and deliberate, or does he talk rapidly and under pressure? Is there a need to impress or to intellectualize? Is his verbal production slowed or blocked? Is his conversation coherent and easy to follow, or is it rambling, circumstantial, and disconnected? Does he use neologisms? Is there echolalia? In patients with organic disease of the nervous system, one might observe perseveration, slurring, dysarthria, or aphasia.

Along with observation of speech, which is a form of expression or motor activity, one should notice the patient's overall motor pattern. Is he tense and ill at ease, restless or agitated, retarded or blocked, hyperactive or relaxed and well poised? Are there any conspicuous mannerisms, tics, or involuntary movements?

Assessment of intellectual function

The most important part of the mental examination is concerned with the patient's thinking—what he thinks and how he thinks.

Because this part of the examination can be especially threatening to the patient, it needs to be carried out with considerable tactfulness and consideration for the patient. Much information about the patient's thought content and thinking processes will have already been obtained during the interview, at which time he discussed his illness and life history. Therefore, inquiry into specific areas and functions of the patient's mental life should be made only when there are special indications and when the preceding interview has not provided the desired information. For example, if a patient is obviously intelligent, alert, and well educated, it would be insulting to ask him if he knows the day of the week, the day of the month, or the month of the year. The interview, with its discussion of events in the patient's life and the dates when such events occurred, no doubt has already answered such questions. It is only when the examiner has observed deficiencies and disturbed functions that he will want to move in closer and make a more detailed study through special inquiry and special tests.

Orientation, memory, and concentration. The patient's behavior and the information that he has provided during the interview will have already afforded clues regarding his mental status in these areas. If the patient is alert, relates well to his surroundings, and speaks knowledgeably of his problem and life situation, with no evidence of forgetfulness or confusion, there is probably no question concerning these functions. However, when one has reason to question the patient's memory or orientation, then the examiner should tactfully inquire into these functions. One might ask, for example, "Have you observed that it has been harder for you to remember recently than it used to be?" Can you tell me how long you have been in the hospital?" "Do you remember my name (the examiner)?" "What is the date today?" "Where are you now?" "Can you tell me your name?" Frequently in cases of senility and cerebral ar-

teriosclerosis, the memory is more impaired for recent than for remote events. The patient might very well recall when and where he was born but be unable to recall what he ate for breakfast, what happened yesterday, or who visited him last night.

The patient's memory and ability to concentrate can be tested further by asking him to repeat a series of digits or to perform the serial seven test. A normal person should be able to repeat six digits forward or should be able to reverse four digits. In giving the patient the digits, either to be repeated or reversed, they should be chosen at random and should not represent any historical date or be given in numerical sequence. Also, they should be given at a uniform rate of one per second. The examiner can say, "If you do not mind, I would like to give you a few simple tests to see how well you can do them. Repeat for me 641, now 6528, 31859, 529746, 6273981." If the patient fails at one level, an alternative series can be provided to see if the patient has not been blocked by anxiety. Likewise, the patient can be asked to reverse 25, 295, 8526, 92518, 471952.

The serial seven test is carried out by requesting the patient to successively subtract 7 from 100, 7 from the previous answer, and so on until the series of subtraction has been completed. The speed and accuracy of the patient's performance are an indication of his mental efficiency, memory, and ability to concentrate. Deteriorated patients may become confused, lose the thought entirely, or make gross errors. It should be remembered that anxiety can interfere with performance in both repeating digits or in doing the serial seven test.

Insight and judgment. A person might be quite intact in his more gross mental functions, such as intelligence, memory, or power of concentration, but at the same time be quite deficient in the capacity to understand himself or his problem or to direct his life with judgment and wisdom. Insight is the capacity for self-observation or self-reflection, to have some degree of awareness or of understanding of one's problem, or to recognize that one has a problem for which he needs help. Insight is relative, depending on degrees of understanding and self-awareness. The extremely sick person, such as the paranoid individual who must blame his environment, the chronic alcoholic who must deny his problem, or the obese person who cannot recognize his deep insecurities, lacks insight. He is unable (and unwilling) to recognize that he has a personal problem, that he has conflicts, and that he needs help.

Some patients may recognize that they are ill and are in need of help but may be lacking in any insightful understanding of the nature of the illness. Still other patients, who are troubled and disturbed, may have a keen awareness of the nature of their conflict and its causes. The patient's insight can be tested by such questions as, "Do you think emotional factors or tension and worry could be causing your symptoms?" "Do you think you have primary physical disease or do you think your trouble could be of nervous origin?" "When you feel people are critical of you or are talking about you, do you think this is really so, or do you think such feelings could be the result of your anxiety and sensations of guilt or insecurity?"

Judgment reflects the capacity to foresee the future, to act and plan wisely, and to profit by experience. The patient's life history, the decisions he has made, his attitudes, his plans and purposes are all an index of his judgment. Of course, patients who have in the past exercised excellent judgment may under the onslaught of illness (organic or functional psychoses) suddenly show gross defects in this area, becoming impulsive and erratic. Although insight and judgment are subtle indices of mental health and intellectual integrity, they are important and should be carefully noted and observed.

Intelligence. Every mental examination should include some consideration of the patient's intelligence—namely, his basic capacities and endowments. There are special tests available for arriving at the patient's IQ, but in most instances the use of such tests is not necessary. The patient's experiences, his achievements, both educational and vocational, his vocabulary and general fund of information, and his interests all serve as a good basis for estimating his intelligence—whether he is dull, average, or superior.

The patient's capacity for humor and wit, his ability to see the funny side of things, his readiness to accept a new point of view or a different interpretation, will indicate his level of intelligence, healthy mindedness and mental flexibility. Rigidity, arbitrary thinking, and sticking pedantically to details are indicative of impaired mental agility and of restricted mental functioning.

The quality of the patient's thinking, the maturity of his concepts, or the concreteness of his thinking usually can be quite accurately estimated by his responses and by his evident comprehension and interpretation of his life experiences. As a rule, the examiner does not subject the patient to definitions and interpretations in order to test his ability to conceptualize or to abstract meaning. But if such testing is thought to be necessary, he can, for example, be asked to tell the difference between laziness and idleness, poverty and misery, character and reputation, evolution and revolution. This provides some idea of the maturity of his concepts. Likewise to test his ability to abstract, he can be asked the meaning of such proverbs as (1) people who live in glass houses shouldn't throw stones; (2) a bird in the hand is worth two in the bush; (3) when the cat's away, the mice will play; or (4) don't cry over spilled milk. Patients who have brain damage, who are schizophrenic, or who are feebleminded may have difficulty or find it impossible to define the above terms or abstract the subtle meaning implicit in the proverbs.

Thought processes and associations. Normally a person's thoughts are logically related, are coherently expressed, and are easily followed and understood. But in patients whose emotional conflicts are intense and overwhelming, the integration of thought processes may be seriously impaired. Ideas may no longer be expressed in a relevant and coherent fashion. What the patient says may be difficult or impossible to follow. What he says may not have any meaning. Some very sick patients may talk freely but the words tumble out in an unrelated, hodge-podge fashion, without inner direction or organization. The verbal productions and thought processes are rambling and tangential. Words may be selected on the basis of their sounds and not on the basis of their meaning. This is referred to as "clang" association. Still other associations are determined by unconscious guarding, leading to evasiveness and circumstantiality. The patient in such instances is endeavoring to hide rather than reveal what he means or is thinking. Therefore, it is important to observe the patient's clarity of thought and expression, for this is indicative of his capacity to organize his thinking and to integrate conflicting tendencies.

Mental content. Up until now in our consideration of intellectual function, we have been considering processes such as remembering, reflecting, making judgments, conceptualizing, abstracting, and the organizing thoughts. We are now concerned with what the patient is thinking, what is in his mind, what are his dominant and pervasive ideas, attitudes, and beliefs; in other words, with what he is preoccupied.

Traditionally, the psychiatric examination has been particularly concerned with the presence of delusions, phobias, obsessions, or hallucinations. It is important to determine whether such things are present. But as the mental examination is broadened in its application to include evaluation of all patients and not just strictly "psychiatric patients," one must be sensitive to other content that is highly significant and must not be preoccupied only with those grosser evidences of illness and disturbed function.

A patient who primarily presents medical symptomatology, such as fatigue and exhaustion, may be harboring highly significant thoughts and ideas that are not delusional or otherwise strictly "psychiatric." If the patient is encouraged to talk about what he is thinking or encouraged to talk about his life situation, he might very well begin to express thoughts and attitudes that had never been revealed previously and that are clinically significant. For example, following an accident at work, a 36-year-old woman, the mother of six children, continued to be disabled with headaches, dizziness, forgetfulness, and emotional lability. It was thought that a cerebral concussion, at least in part, explained these symptoms. However, it was found in the mental examination that she had had a "lifetime" of worry and insecurity, that she was constantly worried about current financial security, and that she had attitudes of resentment and bitterness. She then revealed the following meaningful content: "Things bother me. I have been meaner since the accident. I am more hateful. If people just talk to me, it bothers me. And my husband! Poor guy! I am like a tiger. I can't give him a civil answer anymore, and I am sexually cold. I cannot stand to look at a baby. If we can only rear the children we have, then I will be happy."

Such meaningful content as expressions of bias, prejudice, worry, resentment toward members of one's own family or toward others, guilt, and anxiety is present in many ostensibly medically sick patients; but unless it is searched for it will never be uncovered or identified. Heretofore the search for such mental content was not considered an important part of the evaluation of the patient, nor was it given a place of primary importance in the mental examination. Consequently, we must now realize that the search for such content is an important part of the mental examination, just as the mental examination is an important part of the total physical examination of every patient.

The exploration of mental content is a highly sensitive and delicate procedure and requires great tact. The examiner probes into the patient's thinking by following up the leads that are provided by the information that the patient has already related. "You say that you feel you have not been treated fairly. Can you tell me a little more about it?" "Do you feel you have been discriminated against?" Do you feel uncomfortable in crowds?" "Do you ever feel people are watching you or talking about you?" "Do you think people make slighting remarks about you? What do you think they are saying?" "Do you feel your life is in danger?" "Have you felt there might be a plot to get you?"

Other delusions, such as delusions of guilt and unworthiness, are equally important to identify. Frequently, the patient is not as defensive in talking about these as in talking about paranoid delusions. If it is suspected that the patient feels troubled and self-critical, the examiner again follows up whenever possible the statement that the patient has given. "You say you feel discouraged? How discouraged?" "Do you feel you have done something wrong? How strongly do you feel about this?" "You have indicated you feel you are no good. What do you mean? What do you feel you have done that is so bad? Are you convinced these ideas you have about yourself are true?"

Hallucinations may occur in any of the sensory modalities, but they are most common in the auditory sphere. Visual hallucinations are most frequently seen in toxic states. A patient who is hallucinating may be preoccupied, his attention may be hard to get or to maintain, and he may be manneristic or smile to himself. In some instances, a highly disturbed patient may actively converse with the hallucinated voice, oblivious and unresponsive to his sur-

roundings or to others. When it is suspected that the patient is hallucinating, one again tries to make tactful inquiry. "Would you mind telling me what is on your mind? At times you seem preoccupied. Are there thoughts that dominate your mind? Are they just thoughts or do you actually experience something such as noise, a sound, or even a voice? You say there are voices that speak to you. Can you tell me what they say? Do you recognize the voices? Do they tell you what to do? What do they tell you to do?" Similar questions could be used regarding hallucinatory experiences in other modalities.

Illusions are distortions of actual perceptual experiences in contrast to hallucinations, which are perceptual experiences of internal rather than external origins. Usually illusions appear in confused states and are often of toxic origin. Noises or sounds are misinterpreted, are mistaken for the cry of a child or the voice or call of someone.

Phobias and obsessions are not uncommon mental phenomena and are more typical of neurotic disorders. A *phobia* is a fear of an external situation or object determined by internal conflicts and attitudes. All phobias may have a substance of justification but for the most part represent an excessive or irrational fear. Most patients are quite willing to talk about their fears. The main thing is not to forget to inquire into such experiences. The patient can be asked such questions as, "Are there things that you are especially afraid of or that you avoid?" "Are you afraid of the dark, of high places, of flying, of crowds, or of small or restricted areas?" "How do you feel in an elevator?" "Are there any animals that you especially fear or dread, such as snakes, dogs, horses, or cats?"

Phobias can exist for almost any situation or experience of life. The type of phobia is suggestive of the kind of internal conflict the patient has. Fear of high places suggests a conflict over ambitious strivings; a fear of animals suggests sexual conflict, expecially fear of snakes; fear of crowds or closed places suggests a conflict over dependency. There also can be phobias regarding disease or illness: cancerophobia, syphilophobia, cardiophobia, and so on. These usually reflect internal conflict over certain impulses with associated guilt and fear of retribution.

An *obsession* is the repeated and involuntary appearance of an objectionable thought or idea into consciousness—thoughts or ideas that are associated with carrying out some kind of antisocial act. The thought of cursing, blasphemy, shouting an obscene word, striking or killing someone, or putting disgusting objects into the mouth is typical of obsessional thinking. Frequently associated with obsessional thinking is compulsive behavior, a forced behavior to forestall or to undo any actions associated with obsessive thinking. For example, a person who is preoccupied with destructive thoughts will be ritualistically and meticulously careful in carrying out certain acts. If there is a fear of contamination of the food, a mother may check every ingredient three times or carefully wash the dishes a certain number of times before using them. Other common compulsions are checking the door several times to see if it is locked, checking the gas stove repeatedly to see if it is turned off, or checking a sleeping child a certain number of times to be sure he is all right and is not smothered.

The patient in whom such ideation is suspected can be questioned about disturbing thoughts or feelings. "Are you troubled by unpleasant or annoying thoughts or urges?" "Do you ever have the thought that you may say or do something contrary to your wishes, such as striking someone or an object or shouting a forbidden word?"

Occasionally patients may have strange or unreal feelings. This can apply to both external objects and to oneself. When objects seem strange, different, or unreal, this is referred to as *estrangement,* or feelings of unreality. When the self appears strange or unreal, this is referred to as *depersonalization.* In patients who are highly anxious or insecure, such feelings or experiences should be investigated. "Have things seemed strange, different, distant, or unfamiliar to you?" "At times do things seem unreal?" "Do you feel changed in any way?" "Do you feel as if you were 'walking in a dream'?"

Evaluation of emotion

The evaluation of the patients's emotional life is concerned with the patient's feelings—how he feels about things, the meaning that things have for him, and what he is interested in. Emotion, mood, and affect are terms that refer to one's feelings and feeling responses, and they are used interchangeably, although they are technically different.

All during the interview and the examination the examiner is formulating an impression of the patient's emotional state. His behavior, what he says, and how he expresses himself will indicate how he feels about things. In most instances the patient's emotional life will not be tested separately but will be investigated along with discussion of his problem and conflicts. It is important to remember that the mental examination is not a compartmentalized procedure. Thoughts, feelings, and actions are parts of an integrated whole. The examination involves a consideration of many different details and features simultaneously.

Nevertheless, to describe a procedure it is necessary to discuss separately different aspects of the total procedure. This is the only way techniques and procedures can be taught. It is the examiner's responsibility to synthesize and organize his knowledge and techniques so that the examination is carried out smoothly and effectively.

The following are some of the questions that the examiner should ask himself and endeavor to answer by means of his examination: Is the patient emotionally depressed? Is his mood elated or pathologically "high"? Is there evidence that the patient is anxious, apprehensive, or fearful? Are the patient's feelings appropriate, consonant with his ideas or his life situation? Some of these questions will be answered by observation. Where it is indicated, the examiner will inquire into these areas of the patient's emotional life. The following are some suggestions regarding technique and procedure.

Emotional depression. When the patient's behavior or symptoms suggest a depressed state, the examiner can delve more deeply by saying, "Tell me a little more about the way you have been feeling." "You have spoken about being discouraged. How discouraged have you felt?" "Has life been less enjoyable?" "Do you have less zest for living?" "Do things seem harder, more of an effort, or less worthwhile?" "Do you feel tired and worn out?" "Is it hard to get up in the morning?" "What time of the day do you feel worse, in the morning or evening?" "How is your appetite?" "Have you lost weight? How much?" "Has your sexual drive been less?" "Do you feel at times that you cannot carry on or that you do not want to go on?" "Have you ever wished you would go to sleep and not wake up?" "Has the thought ever entered your mind that you would just as soon end it all?" "Do you worry?" "Do you feel guilty about anything?" "Do you feel you are no good?"

Emotional elation. A patient who is emotionally "high" or elated is unusually animated, hyperalert, hyperactive, and hypertalkative. This mood can be investigated by such questions as, "Are you feeling quite well?" "Do you think you are feeling more optimistic and confident than usual?" "Does the future seem unusually bright?" "Have you noticed that you have more than your usual amount of drive and energy?" "Do you require less sleep than usual?"

Anxiousness. Anxiety is an affect or emotion that is usually quite evident in the patient's behavior and that colors his thoughts. However, frequently such feelings need to be explored more fully. This can be done by asking the patient about his tendencies to worry, to feel apprehensive, his feelings of discomfort, racing of the heart, shortness of breath, or fear of disease.

Appropriateness of affect. The appropriateness of the patient's feeling is often quite evident in his behavior and in what he says. Inappropriateness of mood can range from being maudlin and sentimental, shallow and mercurial, impulsive and erratic to unfeeling and indifferent. In discussing serious or tragic events, the person's mood would be expected to be sober and concerned. When discussing humorous experiences he should be able to laugh and be amused. In certain illnesses and in certain personalities, one finds the mood to be "out of step" with the patient's ideas or life situation. A patient may discuss his father's death or a tragedy and instead of feeling sad may feel indifferent or even laugh. Some individuals lack a normally warm, tender feeling; instead they are cold, distant, and aloof. Still others display emotional responses that are inappropriately excitable, giddy, or superficial.

Emotional lability. In evaluating the patient's emotional state, one also should take into consideration the stability of the patient's feelings. Most people are able to manage or control their feelings. However, in some illnesses a person's feelings may overflow in different directions—weeping or laughter—on the slightest provocation and in some cases without any provocation. There are those who weep or become teary-eyed with the discussion of a relatively minor life incident and in the next moment are full of laughter or jocularity over an equally trivial life situation. In organic disease involving the cerebral structures, emotional lability, characterized by swings from crying to laughter and back to crying, is quite common.

DIAGNOSTIC FORMULATION

Following the mental examination the examiner should be in the position to have certain opinions about the patient and his mental status, which can be referred to as a diagnostic formulation. This formulation should include a clear picture of the patient's life situation, including its stresses and pressures, which could serve as precipitating factors in the illness. This part of the formulation is called the *situational diagnosis*.

The second part of the formulation, which is called the *personality diagnosis*, identifies what kind of person the patient is. It has been emphasized before that the person the physician treats is as important as the disease. Therefore, in caring for a patient one should be sure he knows what kind of person the patient is, since this will provide certain guidelines in understanding and managing him.

The last part of the formulation, which is the *clinical diagnosis*, labels the kind of emotional reaction the physician believes the patient has. One should be acquainted with the standard nomenclature of mental and emotional disorders as well as with the different types of personality. The clinician should strive to be able to label psychologic reaction as accurately as he would other kinds of illness.

REFERENCES

1. Rapaport, D.: The structure of psychoanalytic theory, Psychol. Issues **2**(2):43, 1960.
2. Werner, A., and Schneider, J. M.: Teaching medical students interactional skills, N. Engl. J. Med. **290**(22):1232, 1974.
3. Ward, N. G., and Stein, L.: Reducing emotional distance: A new method to teach interviewing skills, J. Med. Educ. **50**:605-613, 1975.
4. Hawthorne, Nathaniel: The scarlet letter.

SELECTED READINGS

Garrett, A.: Interviewing: its principles and methods, New York, 1942, Family Service Association of America.
Menninger, K. A.: A manual for psychiatric case study, ed. 2, New York, 1962, Grune & Stratton, Inc.
Stevenson, I.: The psychiatric examination, Boston, 1969, Little, Brown & Co.
Sullivan, H. S.: The psychiatric interview, New York, 1970, W. W. Norton & Co., Inc.

CHAPTER 7

GENERAL INSPECTION

General inspection is a series of accurate and meaningful observations. It involves the use of at least four of one's special senses—namely, sight, hearing, touch, and to a lesser extent smell. In addition, it involves integration of the information detected by these sensory mechanisms. The application of general inspection is an art unto itself, difficult to describe and usually perfected through years of experience. The ability to make a "snap diagnosis," although described as intuitive, usually stems from the physician's ability to correlate his current observations with previous experiences in similar medical problems. Cerebration is an integral component of careful observation. When abnormal traits or findings are observed, the wheels begin to spin, and the astute clinician attempts to channel these findings into a specific diagnosis or syndrome. In essence, careful observation is a highly developed art that requires time and experience to perfect but can be acquired and developed by all who aspire to attain this goal.

The first step in every physical examination is the general inspection of the patient. This includes a general survey of the patient's mental status, posture, body movements, gait, speech, breath odor, state of nutrition, stature, temperature, and skin. Examination of the skin is discussed in detail in Chapter 8, and appraisal of the mental status is reviewed in Chapter 6. To satisfactorily inspect the patient necessitates above all that the examiner be alert and observant. Small yet pertinent details may escape the attention of the casual, hasty, and careless physician. The patient should always be examined in the presence of good lighting conditions. Although daylight is preferable, good artificial light will suffice in most instances.

Actually, general inspection begins while the physician establishes his introduction to the patient and takes the medical history. The physician should be constantly alert to any unusual personality traits as well as conspicuous physical abnormalities. For example, slow speech; dull, expressionless puffy face; sparse eyebrows; thick lips; and waxy pallor of the skin are indicative of myxedema (thyroid insufficiency). This type of "armchair diagnosis" is applicable to a number of other diseases. We do not necessarily stress the significance of snap diagnoses, but it is essential to appreciate the importance of keen, alert observation in arriving at the correct diagnosis.

The experienced examiner learns to observe

body movements, emotional reactions, and general demeanor when the patient is preoccupied and least suspicious that he is being carefully evaluated. Malingerers and hysterical patients often try consciously or subconsciously to mimic disease conditions, especially when they are aware that the physician is closely observing them. For example, a true malingerer complaining of a backache may be unable to bend forward when asked to do so. The same patient, however, may stoop with ease to pick up a coin that the physician has intentionally dropped on the floor.

In recent years an increased understanding of a variety of genetic disorders has led to widespread recognition of certain characteristic appearances that are diagnostic of such disorders (for example, Marfan's, Hurler's, and Down's syndromes).

PREPARATION OF PATIENT AND TECHNIQUES OF EXAMINATION

The patient should be made as comfortable as possible during the examination. When possible, the examining table should be situated so that the examiner has access to both sides of the patient. When one side of the examining table is placed against a wall, it is difficult for the physician to conduct a satisfactory examination without inconvenience to the patient and to himself. An ideal arrangement is to have the table located in the center of the examining room.

The patient should be properly draped and prepared for the examination. He or she should disrobe to whatever extent is necessary. In most instances it is advisable to have the patient completely undress and wear an examining gown. A practical gown is one that can be tied in the back. This type is suitable for either sex and can be adjusted as necessary to expose those areas to be examined. For example, when examining the breasts, the physician may lower the top portion of the gown for a few minutes without exposing the remainder of the body. *It is to be emphasized that failure to expose the area to be examined will often result in inadequate findings that may lead to an erroneous diagnosis.*

Some patients, especially women, resent exposure even in the presence of their physician. Therefore, the examiner should explain the necessity for disrobing. When the reasons are tactfully explained, there is usually no resentment on the part of the patient. The physician, on the other hand, should be careful not to embarrass the patient by unnecessary exposure or tactless remarks. A competent nurse can be of great assistance in preparing the patient as well as in providing legal protection for the male physician while he is examining the female patient.

The examination should be conducted with gentleness, dignity, and consideration. If the physician is unduly hasty or rough, there may be a loss of the rapport established during the history-taking. On the other hand, rapport may often be enhanced by conversation during the examination, especially when directed to some aspects of the patient's complaints. This is an effective way of demonstrating the physician's continued interest in the patient and his problem. A tactfully performed and well-executed examination is reassuring to the patient. It serves to cement or enhance the relationship established during the course of the history-taking.

POSTURE

The patient's position or posture may reveal significant information. The patient whose spine is fixed and whose neck is so rigid that he must rotate his entire trunk to view an object not directly in front of him is suspected of having arthritis. Persons with congestive heart failure often sit in a chair the entire night rather than experience the marked difficulty in breathing that occurs when they attempt to recline. Patients with carcinoma of the body or tail of the pancreas often complain of pain over the lower thoracic spine when they are in a supine position. They frequently obtain relief by assuming an upright or sitting posture. In patients with meningitis or tetanus the back may be severely arched and the head is in extreme extension. Thus, the position of the patient at the time of the examination may suggest certain disease possibilities. A history of assuming certain positions to obtain relief from pain also may be of diagnostic importance.

BODY MOVEMENTS

Body movements are classified as voluntary and involuntary. Voluntary movements are associated with normal routine body activity and require no further discussion. Involuntary movements are usually abnormal and may occur in patients in either conscious or comatose states.

Among the more frequently observed involuntary movements are the *tics*. These are habit spasms and usually involve the muscles of the eyes, face, and neck. They generally occur in tense or emotional persons. The eyes may be rolled about, the eyelids may constantly twitch, or there may be twitching at the corner of the mouth. The patient may rhythmically jerk his head to one side.

Convulsive movements are a series of violent involuntary muscle contractions. These may be either *clonic* or *tonic* in character. Tonic convulsions are sustained contractions, whereas clonic ones are characterized by intermittent contraction and relaxation. Convulsions may be unilateral or generalized and may occur in both the comatose and the conscious patient. They occur in a variety of disease states, such as epilepsy, uremia, drug poisoning, and tetanus. In chorea (St. Vitus' dance) there are purposeless, awkward movements, usually involving the arms and legs but occasionally involving other parts of the body.

Tremors are trembling movements that are the result of various causes, such as fatigue, alcoholic intoxication, certain drugs, thyrotoxicosis, multiple sclerosis, parkinsonism, hysteria, and nervous tension.

A flapping tremor (*asterixis*) can frequently be seen in the presence of hepatic coma. This is best seen in the hands, although it may occur in the feet or tongue. With the arms outstretched on the bed, the wrists dorsiflexed, and the fingers spread apart there occur episodes of rapid alternating flexion and extension movements at the patient's wrists and the metacarpophalangeal joints.

GAIT

The manner in which a patient walks is often of diagnostic value. There are a number of abnormal gaits, many of which are either typical or suggestive of certain diseases.

In *parkinsonism* the patient walks with his body held rigid and with his trunk and head bent forward. He takes short, mincing steps, and his arms do not swing as he walks. He may suddenly run forward (*propulsion*) or backward (*retropulsion*) and is unable to stop this sudden change of pace unless he can grasp some object at hand. This type of gait is so typical that a specific diagnosis can be made on inspection alone.

Diseases of the cerebellum, brain, and cerebellar tracts are often accompanied by an *ataxic* gait, resembling alcoholic intoxication, in which the patient staggers or reels.

In diseases involving the posterior column of the spinal cord the patient may have a *slapping* gait. This is commonly seen in *tabes dorsalis* because of a loss of the sense of position. The patient walks on a broad base with his feet wide apart, raises his legs high, and then slaps his feet on the ground. These persons usually fix their eyes on the ground when walking to observe where they are going and to place their feet. Consequently they usually manage well in the light but walk with great difficulty in the dark.

Patients who have *hemiplegia* drag the affected leg around in a semicircle. They also hold the ipsilateral arm rigidly against the chest wall.

In *multiple sclerosis* the patient walks with jerking incoordinated movements, referred to as a *spastic* gait. The *scissors* gait of spastic paraplegia is characterized by walking with the thighs close together, because of the rigidity of the adductor muscles.

SPEECH

The character of a patient's voice and the manner of his speech may be of considerable diagnostic aid. Involvement of the larynx by inflammation, tuberculosis, or malignancy may result in hoarseness. In cerebral vascular accidents the speech is often thick and the words are enunciated with considerable difficulty. In paralysis of the recurrent laryngeal nerve the voice is weak and loses its normal resonating quality.

One may encounter three different basic speech defects: aphonia, aphasia, and anarthria. *Aphonia* is loss of the voice. In *motor aphasia* the patient usually understands what the examiner says but is unable to repeat words or speak spontaneously. If asked to identify a given object, the patient cannot express his answer in speech. For example, if shown a pencil and asked what the object is, he is unable to answer "pencil." On the other hand, if the examiner asks, "Is this a knife?" the patient will usually signify "no." "Is this a flashlight?" He will again signify "no." If the examiner asks, "Is this a pencil?" the patient will signify "yes." *Anarthria*, on the other hand, implies the inability to articulate distinctly.

Certain defects in speech are suggestive of specific neurologic diseases. These may be detected during ordinary conversation and at times only during the repetition of test phrases. In *paresis* the speech is slurred, and the patient has great difficulty in pronouncing certain consonants. Paretics pronounce "Methodist Episcopal" as "Messodis Epistobal," and they also slur other test phrases such as "Massachusetts General Hospital" or "round the rugged rock the ragged rascal ran." In multiple sclerosis the speech is *scanning* and is characterized by rhythmically recurrent pauses. There are still other speech disturbances in such conditions as delirium tremens, parkinsonism, and chorea.

BREATH ODORS

An offensive breath odor is commonly associated with poor oral hygiene, dental caries, and various infections in the oral cavity. Putrefactive diseases of the lungs, such as abscess and bronchiectasis, are also accompanied by a fetid breath.

In certain diseases or metabolic disorders accompanied by acidosis, such as diabetes mellitus, one can detect acetone on the breath; this is a sweet fruity odor. In the presence of uremia the breath may reek with an odor of ammonia. In hepatic coma the breath at times has a musty odor *(fetor hepaticus)* thought to be caused by the presence of methyl mercaptan. Although alcohol on the breath usually indicates that the patient has been imbibing, it is mandatory to rule out trauma and ingestion of drugs containing alcohol before arriving at a diagnosis of alcoholic intoxication.

NUTRITION

As part of every physical examination the physician should record the patient's weight, height, temperature, pulse, and respiratory rate. The state of a patient's nutrition is usually obvious. Although affected by many factors, including electrolytes and vitamins, a patient's state of nutrition is usually evaluated in terms of being overweight or underweight.

Overweight or obesity may be either *exoge-*

nous or *endogenous* in origin. The most common cause for obesity is excessive caloric intake (Fig. 7-1, *A*). Although many fat people insist they do not overeat, they nevertheless ingest sufficient food to maintain or augment their already obese status. In exogenous obesity, caused by overeating, the fat distribution is usually generalized. Certain endocrine diseases, such as Fröhlich's and Cushing's syndromes (Fig. 7-1, *B*), are characterized by en-

dogenous obesity. In these conditions the fat distribution is localized in certain regions of predilection, usually the girdle area, and is often accompanied by abnormalities in sexual characteristics.

Edema (the accumulation of fluid in subcutaneous tissues) must be differentiated from obesity. Edema occurs in the presence of congestive heart failure, nephritis, and numerous other conditions. In edema the tissues *pit*

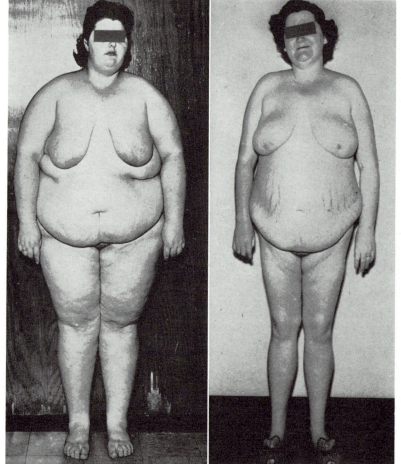

Fig. 7-1. A, Exogenous obesity; generalized fat distribution. **B,** Cushing's syndrome; girdle obesity. Note normal arms and legs.

(indent) when pressed with the finger. This phenomenon is not present in obesity.

Underweight may vary in degree from mild to severe, and severe underweight is referred to as *cachexia*. A slender patient is not necessarily ill. The examiner should evaluate the patient's present weight in terms of his average weight; that is, has the patient always been slender or has he lost weight? Patients exhibiting mental depression may have marked weight loss on the basis of anorexia associated with worry. People may lose weight as the result of voluntarily decreased caloric intake or because of various wasting diseases, such as pulmonary tuberculosis, malignancy, and hyperthyroidism.

STATURE

"Stature" here refers to height and body build. Excessively tall people are referred to as

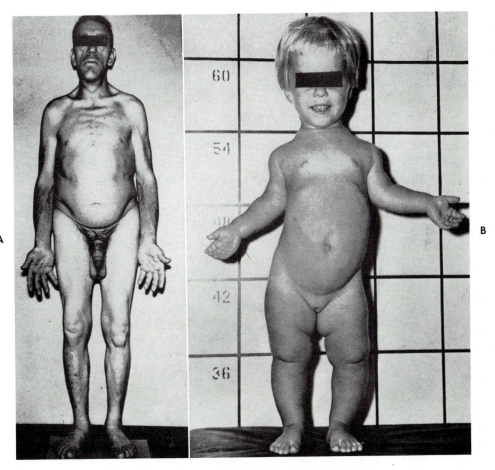

Fig. 7-2. A, Acromegaly. **B,** Achondroplastic dwarf.

giants, and those whose height is decidedly below normal are called *dwarfs.* There are, however, many normal persons who are either very short or very tall. Height and body configuration are governed to a great extent by hereditary background. If the parents are both small, it is not unusual that their children also will be small.

Gigantism is of two essential types, both of which are caused by hypersecretion of the anterior pituitary growth hormone. If this overactivity of the anterior lobe begins before the bony epiphyses fuse (for which gonadal hormones are essential), there results an individual of abnormally large stature with absent or retarded sexual development. If, on the other hand, the anterior lobe becomes overactive following union of the epiphyses, *acromegaly* results (Fig. 7-2, *A*). Acromegaly is characterized by enlargement of the head, a prominent jaw, a huge nose, and massive hands and feet.

Dwarfs are usually classified as *midgets* or *achondroplastic dwarfs.* Midgets are merely very small people who are perfectly proportioned in all respects. Achondroplastic dwarfs have short curved legs and arms, but their body and head are of normal size (Fig. 7-2, *B*). *Cretins,* another type of dwarf, are characterized by arrested physical and mental development as a result of congenital lack of thyroid secretions. The cretin is usually stocky and overweight and has a broad, flat nose. The features are coarse, with thick lips, eyes set wide apart, protruding tongue, and pale skin. The hands are stubby and the muscle tone is poor.

TEMPERATURE

The patient's temperature should be recorded as part of every physical examination. In the United States the Fahrenheit scale is still commonly used, but the centigrade system is increasingly employed. As a rule, the temperature is taken orally and normally should not exceed 98.6° F. In children, patients who are confined to oxygen tents, and those unable to cooperate, the temperature is taken rectally and is normally a degree higher than the oral temperature. On rare occasions the temperature is taken by placing the thermometer in the axilla; normal axillary temperatures are about a degree below below those taken orally. The temperature should be taken, whenever possible, under basal conditions, preferably before eating, drinking, or smoking.

It should be remembered that the so-called normal temperature of 98.6° F. is only an average. Although in the majority of persons the normal oral temperature does not exceed 98.6° F., there are some whose normal temperature is 97° F. and still others in whom it is 99° to 99.6° F.

Temperatures normally vary during any 24-hour period, being lowest in the early hours of the morning and highest in the late afternoon. This variation may range from 0.5 to 2°.

Subnormal temperatures are important when they occur in shock, congestive heart failure, or excessive exposure to cold.

Fever is an increase in temperature above 98.6° F. taken orally. "This patient has a temperature." is often heard. Obviously this is incorrect, because all living beings have a body temperature. The correct statement is, "This patient has 1 or 2 or more degrees of fever." Fever is primarily the result of tissue injury and occurs in many conditions: infections, malignancies, injuries, cerebral vascular accidents, and hemorrhage into various serous body cavities. Fever is usually of three types: continuous, intermittent, and remittent.

In *continuous fever* the temperature remains consistently elevated throughout the patient's illness, although it varies or fluctuates during any 24-hour period (Fig. 7-3). Continuous temperature elevation is commonly seen in typhoid fever.

In *intermittent fever* the temperature is elevated at some time during each day but falls to

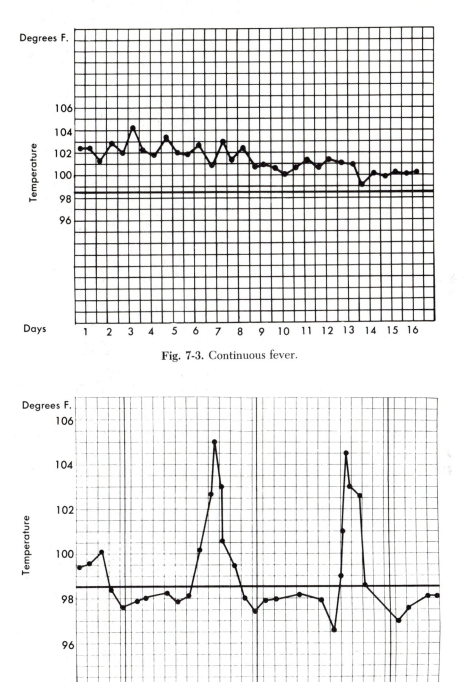

Fig. 7-3. Continuous fever.

Fig. 7-4. Intermittent fever.

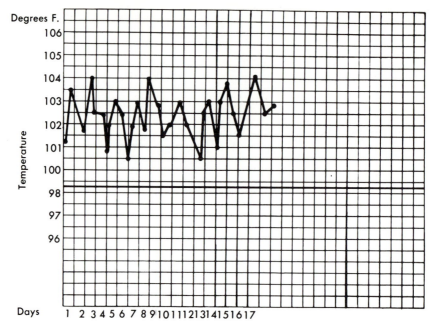

Fig. 7-5. Remittent fever.

normal or subnormal levels during the same 24-hour period (Fig. 7-4). Intermittent fever commonly occurs in infection.

Remittent fever is characterized by continuous temperature elevations with marked rise and fall, but never to a normal level (Fig. 7-5). This differs from continuous fever, in which there is only slight variation in the daily temperature.

A *relapsing fever* is one in which short febrile periods are interspersed by one or more days of normal temperature. This type of fever may be seen in Hodgkin's disease.

Fevers resolve or disappear by either *lysis* or *crisis*. Those that gradually recede to normal over a period of days are said to resolve by lysis. Those that abruptly fall to normal in less than 36 hours do so by crisis.

Diaphoresis (sweating) may occur in many diseases as well as in the very nervous patient. Sweats occurring during sleep (night sweats) may be present in the course of many illnesses associated with profound weakness and exhaustion. Profuse sweating accompanied by a sensation of excessive body heat even in cold weather is quite common in hyperthyroidism. In the majority of infectious diseases sweating accompanies fever.

Chills and rigors (shivering) occur with many of the infectious diseases. With the onset of a chill the patient usually becomes pale, cyanotic, apprehensive, and his skin is cold. This is followed by an elevation of temperature, then a rapid fall in temperature often accompanied by profuse diaphoresis.

SELECTED READINGS

Brain, Sir W. R.: In Walton, J.N., editor: Diseases of the nervous system, ed. 8, London, 1977, Oxford University Press.

Grinker, R. R., and Sahs, A. L.: Neurology, Springfield, Ill., 1966, Charles C Thomas, Publisher.

Harrison, T. R.: In Wintrobe, M. M., editor: Principles of

internal medicine, ed. 7, New York, 1974, McGraw-Hill Book Co.

MacBryde, C. M., and Blacklow, R. S.: Signs and symptoms, ed. 5, Philadelphia, 1970, J. B. Lippincott Co.

Merritt, H. H.: Textbook of neurology, ed. 6, Philadelphia, 1979, Lea & Febiger.

Tepperman, J.: Metabolic and endocrine physiology, ed 3, Chicago, 1973, Year Book Medical Publishers.

Turner, C. D., and Bagnara, J.: General endocrinology, Philadelphia, 1976, W. B. Saunders Co.

Villee, D. B.: Human endocrinology, Philadelphia, 1975, W. B. Saunders Co.

CHAPTER 8

SKIN

The skin has been called the "mirror" of an individual's health, since disease of any of the other organ systems is often reflected in it. It may be compared to a "window" in physical diagnosis, because a major part of the physical examination takes place at this translucent interface between the individual and his environment. Thus, inspection involves visual changes on or immediately beneath the skin; palpation requires superficial or deep feeling of the skin surface; and even in percussion and auscultation the skin acts as a sounding board between the examiner and the underlying organs.

STRUCTURE AND FUNCTION

Before proceeding to the techniques and findings, normal and abnormal, involved in the physical examination of the skin, a brief review of the structure and function of this organ system will help in better understanding the significance of such findings. The skin is composed of three layers (Fig. 8-1), whose functions may be outlined as follows:

I. Epidermis
   A. Keratinocytes → stratum corneum
      Barrier function—prevention of ingress of microorganisms, particulate matter, chem- icals, ultraviolet irradiation; prevention of egress of water, electrolytes
      Heat regulation—conduction, radiation, convection
   B. Melanocytes → melanin
      Barrier function—prevention of ingress of ultraviolet irradiation
   C. Epidermal appendages
      Eccrine sweat glands—heat regulation by evaporation
      Hair, nails, sebaceous and apocrine glands—semivestigial
II. Dermis
   Barrier function—protection from physical trauma
   Neurologic function—contains sensory nerve endings
   Depot function—water and electrolyte storage
III. Subcutis
   Depot function—fat storage
   Heat regulation—insulation

The epidermis forms the multilayered, stratified, squamous, epithelial, outer sheath of the body. It is composed of two cell populations: the keratinocytes and the melanocytes. As they migrate outward toward the skin surface, the keratinocytes form the stratum corneum, which is most important as a protective barrier of the

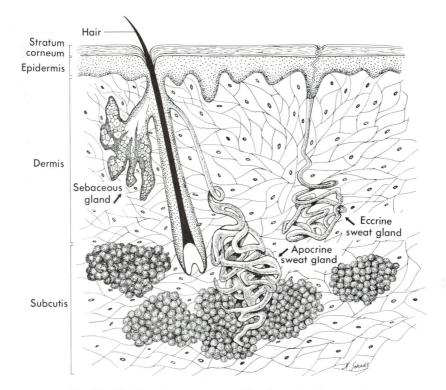

Fig. 8-1. The histologic anatomy of the skin and its appendages.

skin. The melanocytes produce melanin pigment, which acts as the body's principal protection against ultraviolet radiation.

Extending into the underlying dermis from the epidermis are the epidermal appendages: hair, nails, sebaceous glands, apocrine glands, and eccrine sweat glands. These keratinocytic structures serve specialized functions. If the epidermis is destroyed, they can act as centers of epidermal regeneration. Hairs are threads of hard keratin that are projected outward from epithelial bulbs in the dermis. Of their several important functions in lower animals, only the least significant function of ornamentation remains in humans. Similarly, nails serve no important function in humans. The sebaceous glands and the apocrine glands are usually attached to the hair shafts. The sebaceous glands

produce sebum, which has a lubricating effect on the horny stratum corneum. The female breasts contain specialized apocrine glands and have obvious practical and esthetic importance, but apocrine glands serve no other useful purpose. On the other hand, eccrine sweat glands are of great functional importance to humans, since the evaporative dissipation of heat that occurs with sweating allows humans to remain homeothermic when exposed to high environmental temperatures. Although the other skin appendages have become semivestigial in humans, the unique and vital eccrine glands more than compensate for these losses.

The dermis structurally holds the epidermis in place and contains the vasculature and peripheral nervous system of the skin. In addition to its function in protecting the body from gross physical trauma, it serves as the body's largest readily available storage compartment for water and electrolytes.

The subcutis (subcutaneous fatty layer) beneath the dermis is the principal area of fat storage for the body, is an important temperature insulator, and is a hammock for the skin, allowing it to move over the inner body core.

TECHNIQUE OF EXAMINATION

Although examination of the skin is quite simple, all too often it is performed inadequately. Its easy accessability and the lack of need for specialized tools of examination should in no way detract from the importance of the skin in the overall physical evaluation. All too often the examiner lacks sufficient expertise to decide whether a finding in the skin of a patient suggests internal disease, represents a purely cutaneous disorder, or is a variant of normal. Only careful, repeated examinations of the integuments of many patients under the supervision of teachers possessing a thorough knowledge of the cutaneous organ system can correct this deficit.

Although the skin is commonly surveyed as each part of the body is examined, a brief, careful survey of the entire integument at the very beginning of the general physical examination has obvious advantages. Thus, the skin is considered by the examiner as a separate and important organ system. Differences between various parts of the body surface are seen, and hints of abnormalities in other organ systems can be noted so that great care can be taken in looking for further suggestions of altered structure and function in these areas as the general evaluation proceeds. Since visual examination is most important, adequate lighting is essential in the evaluation of the skin. Superficial and deep palpation and the noting of odors emanating from the skin surface are of less importance.

If the need for further specialized proce-dures is indicated by the preliminary examination, bacterial and fungal smears and cultures, skin biopsies, patch and intradermal tests, Wood's lamp examination for the presence of fungi, and testing for normal and abnormal functioning of the skin (for example, sweating) are easily accomplished, since the skin is the most easily accessible organ of the body.

Nomenclature

Although dermatologic nomenclature has amused and irritated physicians for years, it is no more complex or irrational than the rest of the specialized language used in medicine. We are frustrated by what we do not understand, and many physicians simply never learn to use the terms that allow for brief, intelligent communication of information on the state of the skin. Like "rales" or "clonus," the following terms must be learned for professional description of physical findings (Fig. 8-2).

Cutaneous abnormalities are divided into primary and secondary lesions. Primary lesions are those that appear as the immediate result of some causative factor. Macules, papules, plaques, nodules, tumors, cysts, wheals, vesicles, bullae, and pustules are all primary lesions. A *macule* is a flat circumscribed area of color change in the skin less than 1 cm. in diameter; for example, a freckle or flat nevus. A *papule* is a solid elevation of the skin less than 1 cm. in diameter; for example, a wart. A *plaque* or *patch* may be either macular or papular, but is larger than 1 cm. in diameter; for example, vitiligo or mongolian spot. A *nodule* is a solid mass less than 1 cm. in diameter, extending deeper into the dermis than does a papule; for example, a dermatofibroma. A *tumor* is a solid mass in the skin that is larger than 1 cm. in diameter; for example, a cavernous hemangioma. The term is also used for all new growths and for any localized swelling. A *cyst* is an encapsulated, fluid-filled mass in the dermis or subcutis; for example, an epidermoid cyst. A *wheal* is a papule or plaque resulting from the acute extravasation of serum into the dermis; for example, urticaria. A *vesicle* is a fluid-filled elevation in the skin less than 1 cm. in diameter, caused by the focal accumulation of serum or blood within or just beneath the epidermis; for example, smallpox and chickenpox. A *bulla* is like a vesicle, but larger; for example, a second degree burn. *Pustules* are like vesicles and bullae, but contain pus, as seen in acne.

Secondary lesions never appear originally but result from alterations in the underlying primary lesions. Scales, crusts, fissures, erosions, ulcers, and scars are secondary lesions. *Scales* are flakes of skin, as seen in psoriasis. A *crust* is dried exudate on the skin, as seen in impetigo. *Fissures* are cracks in the skin, as

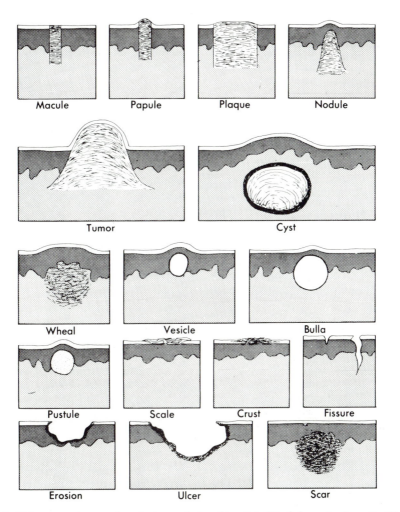

Fig. 8-2. Primary and secondary lesions of the skin. (Modified from Becker, S. W., and Obermayer, M. E.: Modern dermatology and syphilogy, ed. 2, Philadelphia, 1947, J. B. Lippincott Co.)

seen in chapping. An *erosion* is a loss of the superficial epidermis that does not extend into the dermis, as seen in superficial scratches or syphilitic chancres. If the entire epidermis is destroyed, an *ulcer* is present, as seen in stasis ulcer of varicose veins. When an injury extending into the dermis heals with the production of excess collagen, a *scar* results, as seen after vaccination.

Inspection

Inspection is the most important part of the examination of the skin. Color and shape are noted.

Obviously, skin color varies greatly from person to person and even from area to area on the same person. If possible, by use of photographs or findings from earlier examinations, the previous skin pigmentation should be ascertained so that the present coloring can be evaluated more precisely. Usually, an area of increased or decreased pigmentation in skin that is otherwise normally pigmented signifies some abnormality; for example, postinflammatory hyperpigmentation or vitiligo.

The normally occurring skin pigments are malanin, hemoglobin, and carotenoids. Diffuse or localized melanin hyperpigmentation can be seen in such conditions as Addison's hypoadrenocorticism, hyperthyroidism, pregnancy, hemochromatosis, and, most commonly, after exposure to sunlight. Melanin pigment is lacking in albinism (diffuse) and vitiligo (patchy). Erythema of the skin results from increased amounts of oxygenated blood in the dermal vasculature, such as might occur with fever or sunburn. Increases in deoxygenated blood hemoglobin result in a bluish tint to the skin (cyanosis) in such conditions as congestive heart failure, pneumonia, and congenital heart disease with right-to-left shunts. Localized red or purple changes result from vascular neoplasms, birthmarks, and hemorrhage into the skin (petechiae and ecchymoses). Pallor results if the

hemoglobin content of the blood is decreased, as in anemia or shock.

Changes in the color of the skin may result from the deposition of pigments normally not found in significant quantities in the skin. Thus, the yellow or even greenish hue of jaundice results from increases in tissue bilirubin in the skin and sclerae. Carotenemia also results in yellowing of the skin, but, unlike jaundice, the sclerae are not involved. This pigment change is caused by increased amounts of carotenoids in the skin and results from myxedema, diabetes, or ingestion of excess amount of foods containing these pigments, principally carrots. Carotenemia is occasionally present during pregnancy. Certain metal salts, such as silver, gold, and bismuth, when administered over prolonged periods as medications, may be deposited in the skin and cause a greyish discoloration. Foreign bodies, such as carbon-containing particles, can also cause localized pigmentation of the skin; for example, tattoos.

Palpation

Generally, palpation of the skin is used to confirm and amplify the findings observed on inspection. Inspection and palpation are inseparably interrelated, and the examiner often uses them synchronously. Such findings as temperature, moisture, texture, elasticity, and presence of edema in the skin are detected by palpation.

Although the skin temperature is a poor gauge of the temperature of the inner body core, it may reflect a maladjustment in the thermoregulatory mechanism of the body. Thus, if a febrile person's skin is warm and dry, one knows that sweat evaporation is not cooling the body and that the patient's temperature is probably rising. On the other hand, if the skin is warm and wet, then the sweating is probably acting to reduce the temperature. Skin temperature depends on the amount of blood circulating through the dermis. Thus, localized hyperthermia indicates localized increased blood flow, as noted in localized burn or furuncle. Generalized skin hyperthermia suggests increased blood flow in the entire integument; for example generalized sunburn and hyperthyroidism. Localized reduced blood flow results in coolness of that area; for example, peripheral arteriosclerosis and Raynaud's phenomenon. Generalized cutaneous hypothermia signifies a generalized reduction of skin blood flow; for example, shock.

Sweating results from autonomic discharge arising from stimulation of either the central nervous system or the peripheral nervous system. Various combinations of skin moisture and temperature findings can be evaluated on the basis of the previously described physiologic principles. Thus, cool wet hands indicate vasoconstriction and adrenergic sweating—a combination often resulting from autonomic nervous system stimulation caused by anxiety.

"Skin texture" refers to the quality and character of its surface. Is it rough and dry as it may become in hypothyroidism, the postmenopausal state, or "winter itch?" Is it velvety smooth, as in hyperthyroidism?

Loss of elasticity of the skin refers to its inability to return promptly to its normal position when stretched or pulled. This occurs most commonly in such areas of chronic actinic damage as the backs of the hands and the face. Increased elasticity of the skin and joints occurs in the Ehler-Danlos syndrome (cutis hyperelastica). Laxness or laxity of the skin refers to sagging or looseness of the integument and is seen following rapid weight loss and in the aged as the result of a lifetime of gravitational pull on the loose tissues of the face, buttocks, and other areas of the body.

Since the skin is a large depot for body water and electrolytes, much can be learned about the state of total body hydration by careful palpation. Thus, if the skin is loose, wrinkled, and lax in areas not previously subjected to chronic sun damage, this suggests dehydration of the entire body. On the other hand, excess body water may also be stored in the skin and may be manifested by pitting edema, wherein firm pressure against the fluid-filled area results in an indentation in the skin.

EPIDERMAL APPENDAGES

The normal distribution of hair over the body is well known. After puberty, distinct male and female hair patterns evolve. A decided variation in the pattern toward that of the opposite sex suggests the presence of an endocrinologic problem; for example, a masculinizing ovarian tumor. Greying or whitening of the hair *(canities)* is a common sign of senescence, but also may occur prematurely on an hereditary basis or from birth in albinos. Although hair may be dry and brittle in hypothyroidism, such changes more often are caused by physical or chemical injury resulting from efforts to change its color or shape in order to enhance its appearance. In hyperthyroidism the hair has a fine texture. In hypopituitarism there is a general decrease in body hair. Focal hair loss can be caused by such conditions as alopecia areata, fungus infection, secondary syphilis, and pulling of the hair as a manifestation of some psychiatric problem.

Hyperfunction of the sebaceous glands is manifested by oiliness of the skin and is most pronounced over the face and scalp, where these glands are most numerous. This hyperfunction results from androgenic stimulation and is quite common in both sexes at adolescence. On the other hand, in an adult woman or preadolescent child sudden increase in facial and scalp oiliness, with or without acne, suggests a virilizing hormonal imbalance.

While examining the fingernails and toenails, several points should be kept in mind. The visible nail plate is a dead sheet of hard keratin generated from the nail matrix. Thus, many of the changes seen in the nails reflect matrix damage by local or systemic abnormalities that occurred days, weeks, or even months earlier. Since nails grow approximately 0.1 mm. each day, one can calculate roughly when the injury to the matrix occurred. Although certain nail abnormalities may reflect systemic disease, practically none is specific. Thus, transverse furrows seen in nails (Beau's lines) may reflect earlier temporary matrix growth arrests as the result of a variety of systemic diseases, but more commonly they are the result of direct injury to the matrix, such as overzealous manicuring. Since the nail plates are transparent, changes in the underlying dermal vasculature can be seen with ease; consequently, the changes of cyanosis and anemia are especially obvious in the nail beds. Ridging, hypertrophy, subungual separation, and other changes may be seen with local trauma, dermatologic conditions with matrix or nail bed involvement (for example, psoriasis, local bacterial or fungal infection), and ischemic disease of the extremity. Hippocratic nails, in which the nails become curved like a watchglass, are associated with bulbous clubbing and enlargement of the fingertips and are seen most commonly in chronic lung disease and congenital heart disease. Although the nails may be dry and brittle in hypothyroidism and may separate prematurely in hyperthyroidism, these changes are not specific enough to be helpful in diagnosing thyroid disease.

In conclusion, careful examination of the skin may be of vital diagnostic importance. All deviations from normal should be noted and recorded, and often these will lend genuine assistance in arriving at the correct diagnosis of the patient's illness.

SELECTED READINGS

Fitzpatrick, T. B., and others: Dermatology in general medicine, ed. 2, New York, 1979, McGraw-Hill Book Co.

Montagna, W.: The structure and function of the skin, ed. 3, New York, 1974, Academic Press, Inc.

Rook, A., Wilkinson, D. S., and Ebling, F. J. G.: Textbook of dermatology, ed. 2, Philadelphia, 1972, J. B. Lippincott Co.

CHAPTER 9

HEAD, FACE, AND NECK

A detailed examination of the head, face, and neck involves a number of specialized examinations, such as those of the eyes, ears, nose, mouth, skin, and cranial nerves, which are beyond the scope of this chapter but are discussed in detail elsewhere in this text. However, careful inspection and palpation of the head and neck, a natural extension of the initial general inspection of the patient, is an important source of diagnostic information sometimes overlooked by the casual observer. For example, certain systemic disorders, such as acromegaly or Graves' disease, are accompanied by changes in the head and neck that are so characteristic as to be diagnostic of the disorder. More often, careful inspection and palpation may disclose subtle changes in the head and neck that reflect the presence of a systemic disorder. Hence, this chapter will be concerned primarily with the techniques of inspecting and palpating the head, face, and neck, with special emphasis on disorders readily recognized by these simple maneuvers.

CRANIUM

The size and shape of the cranium vary considerably from patient to patient. Although the normal skull is generally round, examination will demonstrate that the frontal areas are prominent anteriorly and the parietal areas posteriorly. A ridge representing the sagittal suture is often felt running anteroposteriorly, and a definite prominence is often noted over the extreme posterior aspect of the occiput. The mastoids are bony prominences behind each ear. Variations within the normal range can best be appreciated by the inspection and palpation of the skulls of many normal people.

The skull is palpated by using the palmar aspect of the fingertips, beginning at the front and proceeding systematically to the occiput. A gentle rotary motion is most satisfactory. Since small lesions may be missed, especially if the hair is thick, it is well to inquire if the patient is aware of any lumps, tenderness, or depressions in his skull.

Certain deformities of the skull result from congenital malformations. *Microcephaly* is a congenitally small skull resulting from failure of the brain to develop normally in size and function. The result, a skull much smaller than normal, is always accompanied by severe mental retardation. In contrast, *craniosynostosis (oxycephaly* or *steeple skull),* which results from premature union of the cranial sutures that leads to grotesque malformations of the calvarium, is not ordinarily accompanied by mental retardation. For example, in this disorder the skull of an otherwise normal child may be quite long in its anteroposterior axis, narrow in width, and pointed at the vertex. A *meningocele,* which is a congenital outpouching of the meninges that occurs in the midline of the occiput or vertex, may be accompanied by serious neurologic sequelae.

An abnormally large head *(macrocephalus)* may occur with several conditions:

1. *Hydrocephalus* is an enlarged infantile skull caused by increased intracranial pressure, which in turn results from an abnormal accumulation of cerebrospinal fluid within the ventricles of the brain. This is most commonly the result of an obstruction of the internal circulation of the cerebrospinal fluid. The ventricles distend with fluid and enlarge the calvarium before the sutures are closed, leading to marked enlargement of the skull with widely separated suture lines. In contrast, the bones of the face, which are normal in size, appear small compared to the enlarged calvarium. Pressure atrophy of the brain, with resultant mental retardation, occurs with this condition. Hydrocephalus usually becomes apparent early in life, occasionally being obvious at birth.

2. *Osteitis deformans (Paget's disease* of bone) may cause enlargement and deformity of the skull. This disease of unknown cause, which most often affects men over age 45, is characterized by excessive and abnormal remodeling of bone. Although usually localized to one or several regions of the skeleton, it occasionally may become widespread when it primarily involves the axial skeleton and long bones of the lower extremities. It results in painful thickening and bowing of the long bones, especially the femurs and tibias. With more extensive disease the skull is involved, and the entire cranium enlarges, particularly in the frontal region. The face, which usually remains normal, may appear small in contrast to the enlarged skull. The patient may note that his hat size is enlarging and usually complains of severe headaches. Bony overgrowth of the skull may result in compression of the brain and cranial nerves, leading to deafness and other serious neurologic impairments.

3. *Acromegaly* is a disorder resulting from chronic hypersecretion of growth hormone in the adult, characterized by striking deformities of the skull (Fig. 9-1). Excessive secretion of growth hormone leads to a proliferation of bone, connective tissue, and muscle that is particularly apparent in the skull, hands, and feet. Perhaps the most striking clinical abnormality in acromegaly is the typical facial appearance that results from a combination of bony and soft tissue overgrowth. Striking as these changes are, however, patients ordinarily do not complain about their facial appearance, since the alterations occur very slowly over many years and are usually attributed by the patient to advancing age. The skin, which characteristically becomes coarse, leathery, thickened, and oily, develops deep folds (Fig. 9-1) and widened pores (Fig. 9-2). The mandible frequently grows in length and thickness, causing the "lantern jaw" and overbite *(prognathism)* so characteristic of acromegaly (Fig. 9-3). As the mandible enlarges, the teeth become abnormally separated (Fig. 9-2), and the patient notices malocclusion. Soft tissue growth is particularly apparent in the tongue, which may become very enlarged *(macroglossia),* as depicted in Fig. 9-4. The frontal, nasal, and malar bones and the paranasal sinuses overgrow, giving the patient the typical appearance of acromegaly characterized by a prominent forehead and large nose. On occasion, one part of the skull may enlarge disproportionately and cause asymmetry of the face. In addition to these changes, the hands and feet become enlarged and thickened, causing the patient to notice an increase in glove and shoe size. Careful inspection of the head and face can lead to early rec-

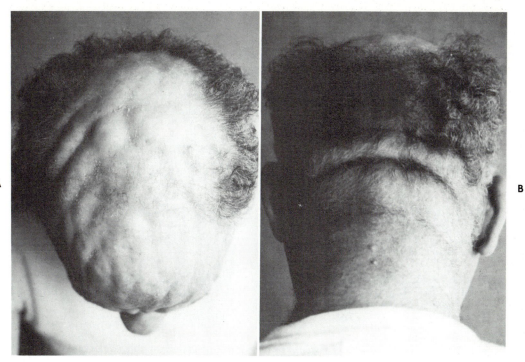

A   B

Fig. 9-1. Acromegaly. Marked thickening of the skin is apparent on the scalp and posterior neck.

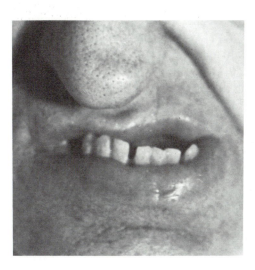

Fig. 9-2. Acromegaly. Notice the enlarged skin pores and separation of the lower teeth.

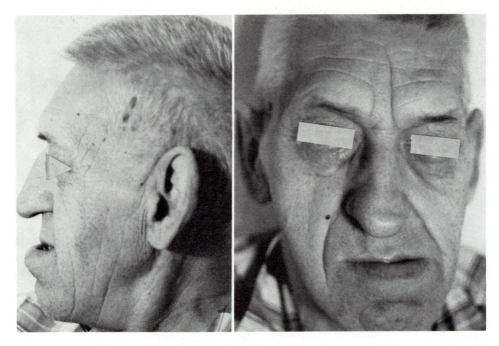

Fig. 9-3. Acromegaly. Notice the coarse facial features, prominent forehead, large nose, and large jaw with prognathism. (Reproduced with permission from Mazzaferri, E. L.: Endocrinology case studies, ed. 2, Flushing, N.Y., 1975, Medical Examination Publishing Co., Inc.)

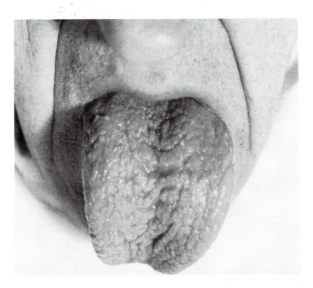

Fig. 9-4. Acromegaly. A large tongue (macroglossia) is characteristic of this disorder.

ognition of this disorder, which may result in a gratifying reversal of the soft tissue changes if the underlying cause, a pituitary tumor, is appropriately treated.

• • •

There are other conditions accompanied by characteristic deformities of the head. Congenital syphilis may be manifested by prominent bilateral "frontal bosses." Vitamin D deficiency (*rickets*) causes enlargement of the frontal and parietal prominences, producing a somewhat square head.

Tumors of the skull, such as osteomas, cysts, or metastatic nodules, may be seen or palpated by the careful examiner. In cases of trauma one might palpate an indentation or depression resulting from a fracture of the skull. Percussion of the skull rarely is useful; however, auscultation may disclose valuable information. Cranial bruits may be the only clue of an angioma in the proximity of the meninges or an arteriovenous fistula of the cerebral vessels. Occasionally cranial bruits can be heard over some intracranial tumors and vascular malformations.

Changes in the fontanels are discussed in Chapter 20.

HAIR AND SCALP

The character and color of the hair should be noted. Hair may be fine or coarse, dry or oily, and occasionally is quite brittle. In modern practice it may be difficult to evaluate accurately either the normal color or character of hair, especially among women. Dyes, bleaches, and rinses not only change the color but frequently make hair much coarser, drier, and more brittle. Often it is necessary to specifically inquire into these characteristics. The scalp should be inspected as well as palpated. *Seborrhea* (dandruff) is frequently observed. Lice, although frequent in the past, are seldom found today, as a result of improved hygiene.

Alopecia, a thinning of the hair or actual baldness, is the result of injury or death of the hair follicles. Although a number of conditions may cause loss of scalp hair, the most common is *hereditary alopecia*. Perhaps as many as half of all normal adult males are destined to have some degree of baldness, either prematurely or later in life. Hereditary male baldness usually begins with a generalized thinning of the hair associated with recession of the anterior hairline, particularly in the area of the temples. It is always symmetrical in distribution, in contrast to other forms of alopecia, which may be patchy or irregular. Although hereditary factors influence the appearance of baldness, endocrine factors, particularly male sex hormones, also play a role in the pathogenesis of alopecia. Baldness is usually associated with normal secretion of male hormones. For instance, eunuchs (men with hypogonadism) do not develop the normal male temporal hairline recession and usually do not become bald. Similarly, although normal women may develop some degree of generalized alopecia of the scalp, balding in a female should be regarded with suspicion. In fact, it should be considered as a possible indicator of virilization if it occurs principally at the temples or on the top of the head in a woman.

Other forms of alopecia are toxic or symptomatic alopecia and alopecia areata. *Toxic or symptomatic alopecia* is a rapid and sometimes total loss of hair that follows prolonged, exhaustive illnesses or severe emotional upsets. As a rule there will be regrowth of hair on recovery from the illness. Presently, the most common cause of sudden hair loss among hospital patients is the side effect of drugs used for palliation of malignant tumors and leukemia. *Alopecia areata* refers to the patchy loss of hair that may involve the scalp and at times even the beard. The areas involved are usually completely devoid of hair. On occasion, the baldness is total (alopecia totalis) involving not only the scalp but almost every hair follicle on the body. In severe instances, the nails show pitting, ridging, and increased friability; rarely they are shed. This type of baldness, the cause of which is not known, may be temporary or permanent.

Occasionally in the course of secondary syphilis there is a patchy alopecia that is "moth-eaten" in appearance and is readily observed about the periphery of the scalp.

In hypothyroidism (myxedema) the hair is commonly coarse, dry, and brittle. It is similarly affected in the cretin (congenital thyroid deficiency). In hyperthyroidism the hair is fine and soft.

Sebaceous cysts (wens) are frequently found in the scalp as smooth round nodules attached to the overlying skin. They are the result of occlusion of the duct of a sebaceous gland.

FACE

General appearance (facies). Certain individuals possess a gifted ability to look at another's face and, almost instinctively, sense a great deal of information. The physician who works at developing this attribute is richly rewarded. He is said to understand his patients. He responds quickly to changes in their emotions, and he can frequently make an instantaneous diagnosis because he recalls without conscious effort a set of associated findings.

Edema. It is often difficult for the examiner to detect small amounts of facial edema. In fact, minor degrees may be detectable only by the patient or by those quite familiar with his personal appearance. It may manifest itself mainly by puffiness of the eyelids. Edema appears earlier in the eyelids than in the rest of the face because the loose subcutaneous tissue

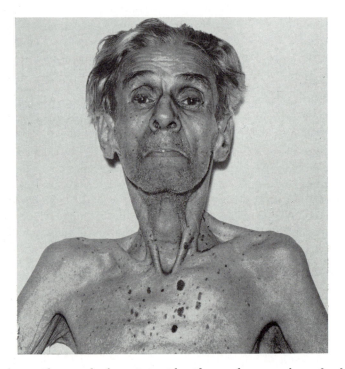

Fig. 9-5. Cachexia. Photograph of a patient with widespread cancer taken a few hours before his death. Notice the sunken eyes, drooping eyelids, and temporal muscle atrophy.

of the lids permits accumulation of fluid. As it becomes more advanced, it involves the entire face. Edema of the face may be the result of a variety of causes, including kidney disease and congestive heart failure. It may also be the result of obstruction to the superior vena cava, usually by a mediastinal malignancy. Superior vena cava obstruction is accompanied by cyanosis and dilated neck veins.

Cachexia. Many severe or prolonged illnesses will cause profound changes in the facial appearance (Fig. 9-5). With prolonged and severe sepsis, severe diarrhea, starvation, and malignant disease there will develop a relatively characteristic facial appearance that has been known for generations as the *cachectic* or *Hippocratic facies*—sharp nose, sunken eyes, drooping eyelids, hollow temples and cheeks, and dry, roughened skin.

Myxedema. This condition is the result of longstanding thyroid hormone deficiency. With this disorder the entire face is puffy and the patient often has the appearance and attitude of an individual just having been awakened from sleep (Fig. 9-6). The eyelids are edematous and tend to droop *(blepharoptosis)*, the lips and tongue are thickened, the speech is slow and sometimes slurred, and the skin is coarse and dry with a waxy, yellow pallor. Spasm of the orbicularis oculi muscle may rarely occur, in which case the patient is unable to open his eyes after closing the lids tightly. Patients with thyroid hormone deficiency move, speak, and think slowly, and, as a consequence, may be mistakenly thought mentally dull. However, replacement therapy with thyroid hormone reverses these changes completely.

Cretinism. This syndrome results from thyroid hormone deficiency during fetal development and is characterized by retardation of mental and physical growth. The distinctive features of cretinism, while usually present at birth, are often subtle, and, unfortunately, in many instances go unrecognized until late in the first year of life. An infant affected by this syndrome may or may not have a goiter. The cretin's face is typically dull, has a somewhat yellow appearance, and is characterized by a flattened nose. The thick lips, grossly enlarged tongue that often protrudes from the mouth, edematous eyelids, wrinkled forehead, and listless attitude complete the general appearance of apathy and mental retardation characteristic of these infants. In addition, the hair is dry, coarse and brittle, the frontal suture is widened, and the anterior fontanelle is enlarged. The child characteristically experiences difficulty in feeding, has a protuberant abdomen, and is constipated. The cretin has a reasonable expectation of normal physical and mental development if adequate treatment with thyroid hormone is begun within the first few months of life. However, tardy recognition remains the most important reason for therapeutic failure. When this occurs, the cretin is severely re-

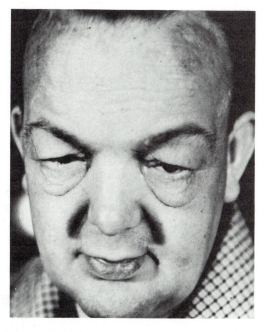

Fig. 9-6. Myxedema. Notice the periorbital edema, blepharoptosis, and facial puffiness.

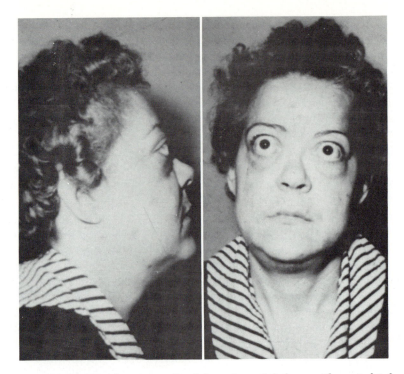

Fig. 9-7. Graves' disease. This patient has bilateral exophthalmos with periorbital edema. Notice the visible sclera above and below the cornea.

tarded mentally and remains short-statured throughout life. Hence, early recognition of this syndrome if of utmost importance.

Thyrotoxicosis. The syndrome of thyrotoxicosis is caused by an excess of thyroid hormone and is characterized by an alert, startled, flushed appearance. The skin is warm, moist, and smooth and the hair thin, silky, and fragile. Thyrotoxic patients speak rapidly and have abrupt body movements. They blink infrequently and have retraction of the upper eyelids, resulting in exposure of the white conjunctiva above the cornea. "Lid lag," in which the upper eyelid lags well behind the globe is easily demonstrated during downward rotation of the eyeball. These features tend to give the thyrotoxic individual a general appearance of great anxiety. One form of thyrotoxicosis,

caused by *Graves' disease*, is also characterized by protrusion of one or both eyes (*exophthalmos* or *proptosis*). This is often associated with conjunctival and periorbital edema and extraocular muscle dysfunction (Fig. 9-7). A characteristic sign of proptosis caused by Graves' disease is exposure of white conjunctiva both above and below the limbus of the cornea.

Acromegaly. Acromegaly not only causes enlargement of the head but also characteristic changes in the face, as described previously.

Cushing's syndrome. Cushing's syndrome, caused by an excess in circulating plasma cortisol concentration, often in turn caused by hyperfunction of the adrenal glands, has a typical facies characterized by a rounded facial appearance "moon face," plethora, acne, hirsutism, and thin skin with telangiectases (Fig. 9-8). Al-

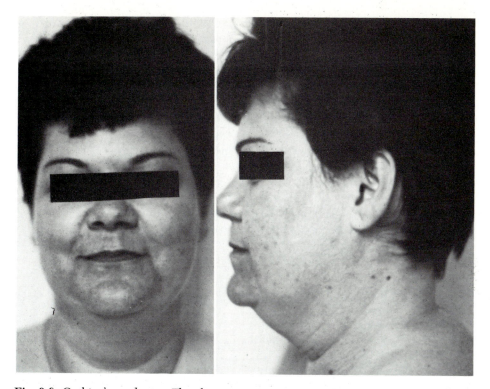

Fig. 9-8. Cushing's syndrome. The characteristic appearance of this syndrome is the round "moon" face with prominent jowls, preauricular fat, and hyperpigmentation. In the lateral view the deposition of fat (or *buffalo hump*) in the low posterior cervical area, which is characteristic of this disorder, is seen. (Reproduced with permission from Mazzaferri, E. L.: Endocrinology case studies, ed. 2, Flushing, N.Y., 1975, Medical Examination Publishing Co., Inc.)

though to the casual observer these patients may merely appear to be obese, careful inspection often discloses signs of Cushing's syndrome. The distribution of facial fat in patients with this syndrome tends to be preauricular, which obscures vision of the ears when the examiner places himself directly in front of the patient. In addition the ruddy complexion, telangiectases, hyperpigmentation, and hirsutism tend to be seen more often in the patient with Cushing's syndrome than in the obese individual.

Paralysis of facial (seventh) nerve. In paralysis of the seventh nerve the eye cannot be closed on the affected side of the face, and there is loss of the normal nasolabial fold. The changes are most obvious when the patient attempts to smile or show his teeth, since he cannot elevate the corner of his mouth on the affected side. When he tries to whistle, air escapes from the paralyzed side. It should be emphasized that if the lesion is in the brain (*central* to the nucleus of the facial nerve) the patient will retain the ability to wrinkle his forehead on the affected side, although all of the other paralytic phenomena will be present.

If the lesion is in the *nucleus* or *peripheral* to it, the forehead on the affected side cannot be wrinkled.

Scleroderma. Scleroderma is a systemic disease characterized by a tightening and atrophy of the skin, which becomes bound to underlying structures. It particularly involves the hands, feet, extremities, and face. When the face is involved, the skin becomes taut and glistening and the nose appears pinched. As the process becomes more severe, the mouth is drawn, often baring the teeth, and there may be difficulty in closing the eyes and wrinkling the forehead—the face becomes expressionless. A diffuse increase in pigmentation with spotty areas of depigmentation also occurs. In addition, telangiectases are usually present, which may involve skin and mucous membranes of the mouth and lips.

Acne, telangiectatic lesions, and vascular nevi. Acne, telangiectatic lesions, and vascular nevi (birthmarks) may be observed on the face as well as elsewhere on the body. Occasionally, lesions that appear to be acne or certain vascular lesions are important diagnostic clues to systemic disease. *Encephalotrigeminal angiomatosis* (Sturge-Weber-Dimitri disease) is characterized by a unilateral port wine facial nevus ordinarily confined to the distribution of the first, and occasionally to other divisions of the trigeminal nerve. This is associated with a capillary hemangioma of the ipsilateral cerebral cortex, often leading to seizures and other neurologic sequelae. *Tuberous sclerosis* is a congenital disease characterized by tumors of the brain, skin, and viscera and *adenoma sebaceum*, which consists of firm, small tubercles located over the bridge of the nose and the cheeks and sometimes the rest of the head. These lesions develop near the end of the first decade, around the time of puberty, and may be mistaken for acne. *Ataxia telangiectasia* is a congenital disease characterized by telangiectasis of the face and eyes associated with atro-

phy of the cerebellar cortex. Near the age of four, telangiectases appear on the bulbar conjunctiva, spreading eventually to the malar surfaces of the face in a butterfly distribution, and to the ears, palate, and along the neck. A variety of neurologic signs, including severe ataxia, accompany this disorder. *Hereditary hemorrhagic telangiectasia* is an inherited disorder of blood vessels, characterized by telangiectases of the skin and mucous membranes that is associated with nose bleeds and gastrointestinal hemorrhage. In this disorder the areas around the mouth, lips, and tongue ordinarily are involved with telangiectases, which may be florid

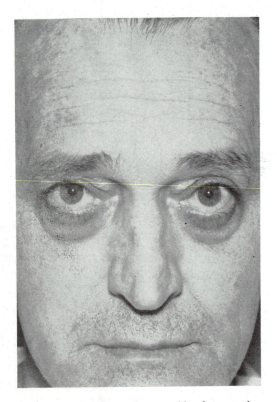

Fig. 9-9. Xanthelasma. Plaques of lipid material are present in the medial aspects of each upper lid. These lesions are yellowish to orange in color and are usually irregular in outline and elevated.

and easily identified, or, as in the case with young adults, subtle and easily overlooked.

Xanthelasma. Xanthelasma are circumscribed collections of lipid material in the eyelids, which are occasionally associated with hypercholesterolemia or diabetes but which may occur without any associated disease. Xanthelasma may be flat but are often elevated, and vary in size from 1 mm. to 2 cm. In the eyelids, they tend to occur first near the intercanthus (Fig. 9-9).

Color and pigmentation. Examples of color and pigmentation changes are vitiligo, mask of pregnancy, jaundice, carotenemia, cyanosis, lupus erythematosus, polycythemia, pallor, and melanin.

Vitiligo. Vitiligo, which is the absence of pigmentation of the skin, is most obvious in those races that are heavily pigmented, but even in the white race it usually can be seen with ease. The areas so affected will not tan upon exposure to the sun. Although this condition most commonly occurs in patches, large areas may be entirely devoid of pigment.

Mask of pregnancy (chloasma gravidarum). Chloasma gravidarum is a yellowish brown pigmentation that tends to occur rather symmetrically on the forehead, cheeks, and neck of some women during pregnancy. It is probably the result of the hormonal changes that occur during pregnancy, since the pigmentation disappears soon after delivery. In recent years it is seen, most frequently in those women who have taken birth control pills.

Jaundice (icterus). In jaundice mild degrees of yellow pigmentation may not be detectable on the skin but can be found by careful scrutiny of the sclerae, the underside of the tongue, and the posterior portion of the hard palate. More pronounced jaundice will be seen as a definite yellowish cast in the skin of the face as well as in the sclerae. It should be emphasized that jaundice, obvious in daylight, may not be visible in artificial light.

Carotenemia. Carotenemia, which may result from excessive ingestion of carrots or be secondary to increased levels of body carotene in diseases such as hypothyroidism and nephrosis, should not be confused with jaundice. This pigment localizes in certain layers of skin but, in contrast to jaundice, does not appear in the sclera or mucous membranes.

Cyanosis. Cyanosis is a bluish cast to the skin that is mostly readily seen on the tip of the nose, lips, cheeks, ears, oral mucosa, tongue, and the nail beds. Cyanosis is usually caused by an increased amount of unoxygenated hemoglobin in the circulating blood, which may be the result of a wide variety of causes, some of which are pneumonia, heart failure, congenital heart disease, and severe chronic pulmonary disease. It should be noted that our ability to estimate visually the degree of cyanosis is very poor, and moderate cyanosis may be present before it can be detected with certainty.

Systemic lupus erythematosus. Lupus erythematosus is a systemic disease that in about half the cases is accompanied by a typical facial rash with a butterfly distribution over the malar skin surfaces and bridge of the nose. This may only be a blush and swelling or may develop into a scaly, erythematous, macular papular rash. More serious lesions associated with scaling, follicular plugging, telangiectases, hyperpigmentation, and hypopigmentation (vitiligo) occur and are often called "discoid" lupus erythematosus.

Polycythemia. Polycythemia is a condition in which there is an abnormal increase in the number of red blood cells. It may be the result of a primary excessive production of red blood cells and hemoglobin by the bone marrow *(polycythemia rubra vera)*, or it may be secondary to reduced oxygen saturation of the blood. The cheeks, ears, lips, and nose have a dusky red hue that sometimes is sufficiently bluish to be confused with cyanosis. However, in polycythemia there is usually enough reddish cast to the skin to differentiate it from true cyanosis.

Pallor. Pallor (paleness of the skin) occurs in many prolonged illnesses, in persons who remain continuously indoors, with the more marked degrees of anemia, and frequently in elderly patients. It may also be caused by hemorrhage, shock, and malnutrition.

Melanin. Melanin pigmentation in the skin varies greatly depending on the density of melanin granules in the epidermis. Genetic and racial influences are obviously important considerations in evaluating the pigmentation. In *albinism* there is an inability to form melanin. If melanin is deposited in the dermis rather than in the epidermis, a grayish blue color results, as seen in Mongolian blue spots or blue nevi.

Increased melanin pigmentation is associated with *Addison's disease*, pituitary tumors, hyperthyroidism, estrogen therapy, *neurofibromatosis* (café au lait spots), *polyostotic fibrous dysplasia, porphyria, hemochromatosis*, trauma from heat and light, chronic inflammation, *acanthosis nigricans*, vitamin deficiencies, and various medications. Clinically, perhaps one of the most important causes of hyperpigmentation is Addison's disease, the result of long-standing idiopathic adrenocortical insufficiency. Other causes of chronic adrenocortical insufficiency, such as tuberculosis, also produce hyperpigmentation of the skin. Adrenal insufficiency results in abnormally high secretion of the pituitary hormones, adrenocorticotropin and melanocyte-stimulating hormone, resulting in an intense hyperpigmentation of the skin

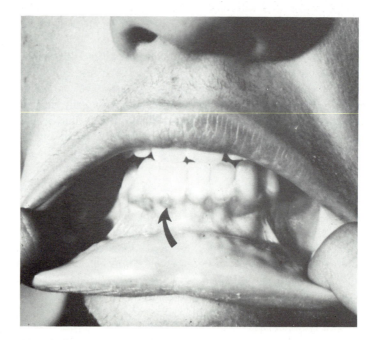

Fig. 9-10. Addison's disease. Hyperpigmentation of the alveolar ridge mucosa, which is readily apparent in this patient, is in most instances diagnostic of Addison's disease. (Courtesy Mazzaferri, E. L.: Endocrinology: a review of clinical endocrinology, ed. 2, Flushing, N.Y., 1980, Medical Examination Publishing Co., Inc.)

and mucous membranes. The patient's face appears deeply suntanned; however, in areas normally unexposed to sunlight, such as the areola and genitalia, hyperpigmentation is also intense. The diagnosis is also particularly suspect when nevi become intensely pigmented and when freckles are seen behind the ears. Hyperpigmentation of the alveolar ridge mucous membranes, depicted in Fig. 9-10, and pigmentation under the tongue are diagnostic of Addison's disease when the patient has cutaneous hyperpigmentation.

Hirsutism. Two basic types of hair occur on the human body: (1) *lanugo,* or *vellus hair,* which is soft, usually unpigmented, and rarely longer than several millimeters, and (2) *terminal hair,* which is coarser, pigmented, and continues to grow. Hair follicles occur all over the human body except for the palms of the hands, soles of the feet, and terminal portions of the penis and clitoris. In certain areas, such as the scalp, eyebrows, and eyelashes, terminal hair growth is present in all humans with few exceptions, regardless of age or sex. However, in other body areas, such as the face, pubis, axilla, chest, and abdomen, the degree of hair growth is dependent on the presence of male hormones (androgens). The conversion of hair in the axillae and pubic area at puberty to coarse, terminal, mature hair occurs under the influence of androgen secreted by the adrenal glands and awakening gonads. In contrast, facial, chest, abdominal, and sacral hair require exposure to male levels of androgens for conversion to terminal hair. Thus only the degree of hormone-dependent hair growth distinguishes the male from the female pattern. In women, hirsutism generally means the excessive growth of hormone-dependent hair. This is to be distinguished from *hypertrichosis,* which generally refers to excessive growth of hair on the extremities, head, and back that is primarily genetically determined, although it may be influenced by male hormones.

Ordinarily, in the male, terminal facial hair appears at the time of puberty and over several years develops into a full facial beard, covering the cheeks, upper lip, chin, and upper neck. In most men the rate of facial hair growth approximates 0.5 mm. per day. However, in both men and women, there is a substantial racial, genetic, and ethnic influence on hormone-dependent hair. For example, Mediterranean people tend to be more hirsute than Scandinavians, Caucasians more hirsute than Blacks, and Blacks more hirsute than Japanese, American Indians, or Eskimos. A localized loss of facial hair growth in the male may be the result of certain skin disorders or may be of uncertain cause. However, if the entire beard fails to grow or slows perceptibly in its rate of growth after puberty, this may be a signal of hypogonadism, hypopituitarism, or an abnormal source of female hormones, such as an adrenal carcinoma.

Most normal women have a light growth of lanugo hair on the face. Some women become unnecessarily alarmed when they suddenly discover it when looking in the mirror with a tangential light source, but they only require reassurance from the physician. Although terminal facial hair growth may be the sign of a serious endocrine disorder in a woman, most often it is the result of ethnic, racial, or hereditary factors. It is in this group of women that the most difficult problems in differential diagnosis arise (Fig. 9-11). In patients with hereditary hirsutism terminal facial hair appears at puberty and continues to increase until the early twenties. It also may become slightly more apparent during pregnancy and at the time of menopause. However, a documented abrupt change or any marked increase in facial hair growth after age 25 should be regarded as highly indicative of an underlying endocrine disorder. Diseases of the ovary, such as androgen-secreting tumors and polycystic ovaries (Stein-Leventhal syndrome); disorders of the

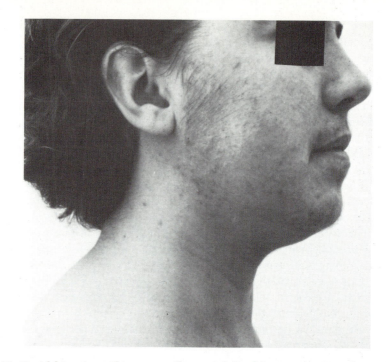

Fig. 9-11. Facial hirsutism. This patient first noted facial hair at age 18 and was found to have an adrenal carcinoma. (Courtesy Mazzaferri, E. L.: Endocrinology case studies, ed. 2, Flushing, N.Y., 1975, Medical Examination Publishing Co., Inc.)

adrenal gland, such as benign adenomas, adrenocortical cancer, or hyperplasia; and certain drugs, such as androgens, birth control pills, and phenytoin, all may cause hirsutism. Some patients with these disorders may have virilization that, in addition to hirsutism, is characterized by temporal balding, a loss of female secondary sex characteristics, enlarging muscle mass, and a deepening voice. The most diagnostic sign of virilization is an enlarging clitoris.

Thus perhaps the most difficult aspect of inspection of the face is the evaluation of facial hair because of the wide range of normal patterns in both men and women. This difficulty is best overcome by obtaining a complete history and carefully examining the genitalia, breasts, and other areas of the body covered with hormone-dependent hair.

MOVEMENTS OF THE HEAD

Abnormal positions of the head are usually quite obvious. Fixation or limitation of range of motion can be determined by the following:

1. Active motion of the patient's head as a result of his own voluntary effort
2. Passive movement, in which instance the head is moved in all directions by the examiner

When the examiner moves the patient's head, caution should be taken not to exert force. This is especially true if there has been an injury to the neck, under which circumstances the cervical spinal cord is particularly susceptible to serious, permanent injury.

In the normal patient, the head can be flexed anteriorly until the chin rests on the sternum. The inability to do so suggests: (1) central nervous system disease with irritation of the meninges, such as meningitis or encephalitis, (2) inflammation of muscles of the neck, or (3) mechanical limitation of motion, such as seen in arthritis of the cervical spine. Normally the head can be rotated 90 degrees to each side. Lateral motion may be limited as the result of arthritis of the spine or inflammation of the neck muscles.

The head may be tilted to the side as the result of shortening of the sternomastoid muscle. This condition is known as *torticollis* (wryneck). Although this is usually a congenital defect, it may be caused by inflammation of the muscles.

A not uncommon observation in elderly people is the constant rhythmic tremor of the head caused by cerebral arteriosclerosis and its attendant degenerative changes in the brain.

Bounding (a slight up-and-down movement) of the head that is synchronous with the pulsation of the heart may be noted in patients with aortic regurgitation as the result of the widened pulse pressure. This cardiac defect is usually the result of syphilis or rheumatic fever.

Habit spasm or *tic* is a sudden movement of the head, usually to the side, and often accompanied by facial grimaces. Tic is not the result of organic nervous disease but instead is a nervous habit reflecting emotional tension. It often becomes worse at times of stress.

NECK

Techniques of examination. Examination of the neck is conducted primarily by inspection, palpation, and auscultation. A careful examination of the neck, in addition to revealing local cervical disease, may give valuable diagnostic clues to: (1) systemic diseases with manifestations in the neck, (2) neoplasms of distant organs metastatic to the neck, and (3) infections or tumors of the oral pharynx and nasopharynx that have extended to the neck. Many important anatomic structures reside primarily in or pass through the neck, making it a veritable storehouse of normal and pathologic physical findings. Satisfactory examination is based on a sound knowledge of the anatomy of the neck. Because it is a relatively complex structure, which is readily accessible to the palpating fingertips, the neck may serve as a source of valuable diagnostic information; or its examination may lead to considerable confusion, depending on the skill with which it is examined. First, the general techniques utilized in the examination of the neck will be explored, followed by a detailed discussion of the systematic examination of various structures.

Inspection. Inspection of the neck should be done with the patient seated in a chair or standing directly in front of the examiner. An oblique light, such as an examination lamp, placed directly above and slightly in front of the patient's shoulder with its beam directed toward the opposite shoulder, offers a good source of contrast lighting to the neck, throwing subtle neck structures into stark contrast. The neck is first inspected for evidence of asymmetry, limitation of motion, abnormal pulsations, and enlargement of the thyroid and lymph glands. Inspection is facilitated by moderate extension and deviation of the head to the side opposite that which is being observed. With this technique, in the nonobese patient, the examiner should be able to easily identify the sternocleidomastoid muscles, jugular veins, thyroid cartilage, trachea, clavicle, and pulsations of the carotid and subclavian arteries. (Examination of neck vein pulsations is discussed in detail in Chapter 14.) Additionally, lymphadenopathy, thyroid enlargement, neck masses, and vascular dilatation or pulsation are made readily apparent by these simple maneuvers in contrast to their obscurity when the head is in the usual position and the light is improper. With the head tilted straight back, the patient is asked to swallow. This maneuver sometimes permits visualization of the normal thyroid as it moves upward with swallowing, and almost always reveals an enlarged thyroid gland. The examiner should inspect the neck for scars, such as those resulting from previous thyroidectomy or tracheotomy. Finally, the patient should protrude his tongue while the examiner looks for abnormal upward movements of midline cervical masses or abnormal skin adhesions in the neck.

Palpation. Palpation of the neck should be done with the patient seated in a chair while the physician examines the neck from both behind and in front of the patient. Certain structures are more readily apparent when palpated from behind the patient, while others are felt more easily when the examiner is positioned in front of the patient. Indeed, small neck masses, such as a supraclavicular lymph node or small thyroid nodule, are sometimes best palpated while the patient is supine because the neck structures are thrust slightly cephalad and anterior in this position. By placing one hand over the occiput, the physician can move the patient's head into any desired position while palpation is conducted with the other hand. The palmar surfaces of the fingertips are used primarily. A gentle, slow, to-and-fro or rotary motion is especially helpful in detecting and evaluating the characteristics of any palpable lymph node. Deep, firm palpation may force nodes into surrounding structures so that they cannot be detected.

As in any area of the body, but perhaps even more importantly in the neck because of the proximity and number of structures, a systematic approach to examination is essential. As a rule, first, with the patient's neck relaxed and the patient looking directly forward, the occiput, posterior neck, and posterior triangle are palpated for lymph nodes and masses. Then, with the head tilted slightly toward the side being examined (Fig. 9-12), the lateral neck is palpated. This is followed by palpation of the anterior cervical triangle, searching for carotid artery pulsation, enlargement of the lymph

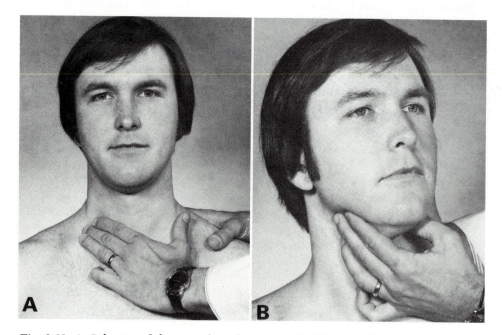

Fig. 9-12. A, Palpation of the supraclavicular region. **B,** Palpation of the anterior cervical triangle, which includes careful study of the underside of the jaw.

nodes, and tumors. The underside of the jaw is examined for induration, masses, and lymphadenopathy. The parotid, salivary glands, and preauricular lymph nodes are palpated (Fig. 9-13). The anterior midline of the neck is palpated for tumors, cysts, and tracheal position; and, finally, the thyroid is examined.

Auscultation. Auscultation of the neck with the bell of the stethoscope is an important part of the examination. Both carotid arteries should be carefully auscultated along their entire course in the neck, up to the angle of the mandible. During auscultation of the carotid arteries, the head should be straight forward and only gentle pressure should be applied to the stethoscope, since rotation of the head or heavy pressure on the stethoscope may cause factitial bruits. Bruits heard over the carotid arteries may indicate partial obstruction caused by an atheromatous plaque, tumor, or vascular abnormality. Since heart murmurs may be transmitted to the neck, a carotid bruit must be distinguished from an abnormal heart sound. This is best done by "inching" the stethoscope from the anterior chest to the neck, while listening for a heart murmur that might be transmitted to the carotid arteries. Auscultation should also be carried out over the carotid bifurcation and over the course of the innominate and subclavian arteries. Occasionally, a low-pitched hum (venous hum) can be heard in the area of the supraclavicular fossa. Although ordinarily not of particular significance, a continuous venous hum, particularly in the right supraclavicular fossa, may be heard in patients with diffuse toxic goiter. Additionally, a systolic bruit is usually heard directly over the thyroid gland in patients with diffuse toxic goiter.

Cervical lymph nodes. Cervical lymphadenopathy may be the result of: (1) infections or neoplasms of the oral pharynx or nasopharynx, which have extended to the neck; (2) systemic diseases such as Hodgkin's disease, leukemia, and metastatic cancer; (3) infections such as measles and infectious mononucleosis; or (4) drugs such as phenytoin. By far the most frequent cause of enlarged cervical lymph nodes is infection of the mouth or oral pharynx.

When there is significant enlargement of the lymph nodes, they should be described as to: (1) exact location, (2) size, (3) presence or absence of tenderness, (4) consistency, (5) presence or absence of visible or palpable surrounding inflammation, and (6) whether they are freely movable, adherent to the deeper structures, or matted together. A careful description of the lymph nodes will often give valuable clues as to the general type of disease process causing the lymphadenopathy.

In Fig. 9-14, the superficial lymph nodes of the neck are schematically depicted. Each group of lymph nodes must be examined in a systematic fashion so that none are omitted

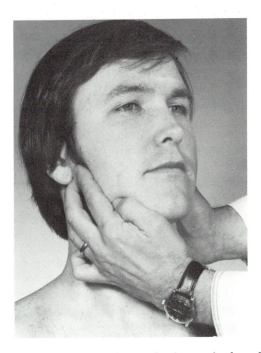

Fig. 9-13. Palpation of parotid salivary glands and preauricular lymph nodes.

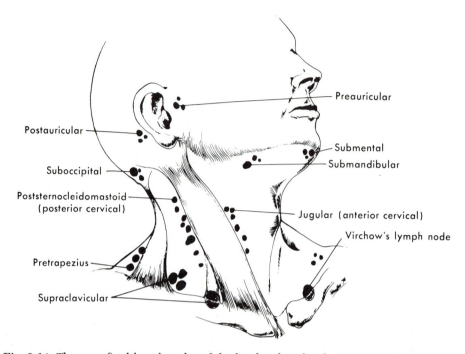

Preauricular

Postauricular

Submental

Submandibular

Suboccipital

Poststernocleidomastoid
(posterior cervical)

Jugular (anterior cervical)

Virchow's lymph node

Pretrapezius

Supraclavicular

Fig. 9-14. The superficial lymph nodes of the head and neck. There are nine major groups of superficial lymph nodes that should be carefully palpated in a systematic fashion during examination of the head and neck. In addition a careful search for a sentinel lymph node (Virchow's node) should be made in the left supraclavicular area, particularly in patients suspected of having a neoplasm.

during palpation of the neck. When an enlarged lymph node is found, the region drained by the lymph gland must be carefully searched for a primary lesion. Anterior cervical lymphadenopathy can be caused by lesions of the anterior third of the scalp, the facial structures, and the thyroid gland. Lymphadenopathy in the posterior cervical triangle can be caused by local disease of the posterior two thirds of the scalp and the thyroid. Preauricular lymphadenopathy may be the result of local scalp lesions, infections of the external auditory canal, and inflammatory or neoplastic processes involving the forehead and upper facial structures. Submental and submandibular lymph node enlargement may result from inflammatory or

neoplastic disorders involving the tongue, floor of the mouth, and oropharynx. Enlargement of a single lymph node in the left supraclavicular group, classically referred to as a *sentinel node* (Virchow's node), has been described as a sign of carcinomatous metastasis from a primary lesion in the upper abdomen. However, Virchow's node is probably more common today as a result of neoplastic disease metastatic from the left lung. In contrast, enlargement of the right supraclavicular lymph node may occur with neoplasms arising in the right lung and left lower pulmonary lobe. Often, a sentinel node is so deep in the neck that it escapes casual examination. The examiner must carefully explore the region behind the muscle head.

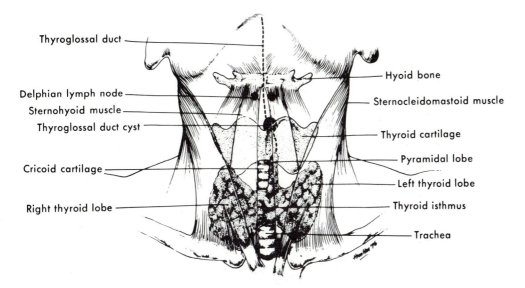

Fig. 9-15. Location of the normal thyroid. In the adult the thyroid weighs from 10 to 25 gm. Normally the right lobe is 5 cm. in length, and the left lobe is 4.5 cm. The greatest width of each lateral lobe is about 3 cm., and the normal gland varies from 1 to 2 cm. in thickness. Notice the relationship of the isthmus to the cricoid cartilage, the position of the pyramidal lobe, and thyroglossal duct cyst. Note also that the thyroid is deep to sternocleidomastoid and sternohyoid muscles, thus requiring flexion of the neck anteriorly during physical examination to facilitate palpation of the gland.

Also, a forceful Valsalva maneuver or coughing may move a sentinel node upward momentarily so that it is easily palpated.

Acute localized inflammation of the mouth and throat produces enlargement of the lymph nodes in the anterior cervical triangle, predominantly in the angle between the sternocleidomastoid muscle and the jaw. These nodes are tender, firm, and freely movable, and, as a rule, there is relatively little evidence of surrounding inflammation. Chronic inflammatory changes that accompany fungus infections or tuberculosis produce an enlargement of the lymph nodes, especially in the anterior cervical triangle. However, these nodes tend to be firm, but not hard, large, and multiple. They are often associated with surrounding inflammatory reaction that causes the nodes to become matted together and adherent to adjacent structures. Occasionally, there may be draining sinuses associated with chronic lymphadenopathy, particularly when involved with *Actinomyces bovis*. With this infection the draining sinuses exude pus that contains sulfur granules that are 1 to 2 mm. in diameter. Lymph nodes involved by metastatic cancer are ordinarily "stony" hard, variable in size, nontender, and not fixed to the surrounding tissues until late in the disease. Hodgkin's disease is often characterized by cervical lymph node enlargement that, on occasion, is the only manifestation of the disease. The nodes, which frequently have been present for months, tend to be nontender, nonsuppurative, and discrete. The cervical lymph node enlargement with Hodgkin's disease is ordinarily much greater than with acute adenitis. *Delphian nodes* are lymph nodes in the midline of the thyrohyoid membrane (Fig. 9-15). Usually, they enlarge only in patients with thyroid carcinoma and subacute thyroiditis.

Salivary glands. Unless enlarged and firmer than normal, the *parotid* gland is not palpable. It lies anterior to the ear, beginning superiorly at the zygoma, extending downward and increasing in size until it is approximately 1 inch in width directly anterior to the external auditory canal. There is a slender continuation or "tail" of the gland that runs posteriorly under the ear for approximately 0.5 inch. Enlargement of the parotid salivary gland produces a relatively characteristic picture of swelling anterior to the ear, bounded above by the zygomatic process and extending downward below and posterior to the ear. Enlargement of the tail of the gland tends to displace the lobe of the ear laterally. The parotid duct can be seen on the buccal mucosa as a small nipplelike structure opposite the second upper molar, in the center of which is the minute orifice that appears slightly redder than the rest of the structure.

The normal *submandibular* gland is usually palpable, but because it is soft in consistency and rather poorly outlined, it can be felt only with difficulty and frequently cannot be detected by the inexperienced examiner. When enlarged or indurated, it can be felt quite readily. It is slightly movable, approximately 1.5 cm. in diameter, essentially circular in outline, and located just below the jaw, 1 to 2 cm. anterior to the angle of the mandibles. The pinhead-sized orifices of the submandibular glands may be seen on the floor of the mouth at each side of the frenulum of the tongue. The *sublingual* glands, which normally are not palpable, lie within the anterior curvature of the mandible. They empty through a number of invisible openings along a ridge lateral to the orifices of the submandibular salivary glands.

By far the most common cause of enlargement of the salivary glands in children is *mumps (epidemic parotitis).* There is usually diffuse swelling of the parotid salivary gland, and occasionally the submandibular glands are involved as well. There is usually considerable tenderness on palpation and discomfort on chewing.

A much less frequent cause of enlargement of the parotid gland is acute *suppurative parotitis*, which may occur in the course of the chronic wasting diseases or following serious operations, especially in older patients. The involved gland is acutely inflamed, red, and diffusely swollen.

The parotid gland also may be enlarged as a result of tumor. The most common is the *mixed tumor*, which is usually benign but may become malignant.

A *calculus* (stone) in the parotid duct may cause swelling of the parotid gland, and a calculus in the duct of the submandibular salivary gland may produce swelling of that structure. Frequently the patient will notice that the swelling is most prominent while eating.

Bilateral, firm, nontender parotid enlargement may occur in a number of other circumstances. For example, patients with lymphoma, chronic alcoholism, sarcoidosis, and diabetes mellitus and individuals who chronically ingest starch may all develop parotid enlargement.

Lateral neck tumors. *Branchial cysts* result from anomalous involution of the branchial clefts. The tumor, which usually appears in adult life, not in childhood, forms a soft, cystic swelling in the anterolateral neck. Typically, the mass is just anterior but deep to the upper one third of the sternocleidomastoid muscle. The cystic tumor is soft to palpation except when intercurrent infection causes it to become hard and tender. Fluid aspirated from a branchial cyst appears to be pus, but microscopically contains cholesterol crystals, which is diagnostic of branchial cyst. A *carotid body tumor* arising from chromaffin tissue within the carotid body is seen as a mass near the bifurcation of the common carotid. Because it may not pulsate, may feel cystic, and appears in middle life, it may be confused with a branchial cyst. A carotid body tumor, which is usually somewhat fusiform with the long axis parallel to the carotid artery, can usually be identified by its lateral mobility and restricted vertical movement. Ipsilateral pupillary dilatation may occur with this tumor, which is an important diagnostic sign. Pressure on the tumor may cause slowing of the pulse. A *hygroma* is a large, multiloculated, cystic mass in the neck, which is composed of occluded lymphatics that are present from childhood. The mass usually is in the upper third of the anterior cervical triangle but may extend down the neck and under the jaw. The distinguishing feature of this lesion is its translucence, which is easily demonstrated by placing a bright light directly on the mass in a darkened room. A *pharyngeal pouch* is a cystic mass that may appear in the lateral neck, usually on the left side, during eating or drinking. The patient ordinarily complains of regurgitation of food during eating or when lying on the side. A *laryngocele* is a laryngeal diverticulum that occurs in the lateral thyrohyoid membrane. This causes intermittent swelling of the neck, often observed while blowing the nose, coughing, or blowing on musical instruments.

Blood vessels. Abnormally forceful pulsations may be seen in the carotid arteries of patients with thyrotoxicosis or aortic regurgitation and occasionally in those with hypertension. An aneurysm of the carotid artery will produce an expansile pulsation that is synchronous with the heartbeat. Careful palpation will show that this enlargement expands in all directions with each pulse wave. Palpation over the carotid arteries in elderly patients should be performed gently. Occasionally as the result of elongation of the aorta and buckling of the carotid artery, pulsation may be felt above the right clavicle. This condition is seen especially in older patients with hypertension and arteriosclerosis. It may be erroneously diagnosed as an aneurysm of the carotid artery.

Auscultation over the carotid arteries may reveal bruits that indicate stenosis of major arteries in the neck. These changes are usually caused by atherosclerosis and may produce serious brain damage. Most significant is the high-pitched bruit heard over the bifurcation of the carotid artery. It usually indicates a stenosis of the internal carotid artery that is remediable by surgery. The low-pitched murmurs heard over the base of the neck are commonly caused by atherosclerosis of the subclavian artery.

Carotid arteritis is a poorly described disorder characterized by pain in the side of the neck, which is intensified by swallowing and associated with exquisite tenderness of the carotid artery to palpation. The carotid bulb may seem dilated and its pulsations exaggerated. Gentle digital compression of the carotid causes the pain to spread to distal branches of the artery in the ear, temple, and jaw. The disease is self-limited in most instances. However, it must be sharply distinguished from *temporal arteritis* (cranial giant cell arteritis), a disorder that only occurs past middle life and is characterized by an abrupt onset of severe pain, usually in one temple but sometimes in the occipital area, face, jaw, or lateral neck. This may be associated with exquisite hyperesthesia of the scalp and face, which causes combing the hair or touching the scalp to be painful. The temporal artery may be tender, thickened, or nodular, a condition that is virtually diagnostic of this disorder. Conversely, the vessel may become occluded and can be pulseless and impalpable. Temporal arteritis may lead to visual impairment and sudden blindness when the blood supply of the retina is affected. Thus·it is extremely important to carefully palpate the temporal arteries in elderly patients complaining of headache or facial pain.

The *jugular veins* are ordinarily not distended when the patient is in a sitting position, although filling of these veins will be seen as he reclines. When there is distention of these veins in the upright position, it usually indicates congestive heart failure. On the other hand, it may be the result of any obstruction to the return flow of blood from the head and neck into the thorax, such as constrictive pericarditis, tumor of the mediastinum, or obstruction of the superior vena cava.

Trachea. First, the trachea is palpated for evidence of deviation. The trachea is probably best palpated just above the suprasternal notch. The trachea may be displaced laterally by an aortic aneurysm, a mediastinal tumor, or a unilateral thyroid enlargement. In similar fashion, a large amount of fluid or air in the pleural space will push the trachea and other mediastinal structures toward the opposite side. If there are pleural adhesions, fibrosis within the lungs or atelectasis, there may be displacement of the trachea toward the affected side. Second, the trachea is palpated for evidence of *tracheal tug*. This is most easily detected by having the patient tilt his head backward, which tightens the trachea. Gently, but firmly, the trachea is grasped between the thumb and fingers just below the cricoid cartilage, and gentle pressure is exerted upward against the inferior margin of this cartilage. A definite downward pull synchronous with the cardiac pulsation will be felt if a tracheal tug is present. Tracheal tug is usually the result of an aneurysm in the arch of the aorta. Care must be taken to differentiate tracheal tug from forceful pulsation of the carotid arteries.

Thyroid gland. An understanding of the development and anatomy of the thyroid is nec-

essary for the diagnosis of thyroid disorders. The thyroid is derived from the embryonic pharynx, where it first appears as an outpouching of the foregut. During fetal development, the thyroid migrates caudally, losing its pharyngeal connection by the fifth gestational week and reaching its proper position in the neck by the tenth week of gestation. Fully developed, the thyroid contains two *lateral lobes* connected by a median band of thyroid tissue, termed the *isthmus,* that lies at the level of the second and third tracheal rings. Normally, the right lobe is larger than the left by about 25%, and the thyroid gland itself is slightly larger in women than in men. In about one third of normal individuals, a thyroidal remnant of the connection between the thyroid and embryonic pharynx, the *pyramidal lobe*, extends upward from the isthmus, lying slightly to the left of the midline (Fig. 9-15). Although normally the embryonic connection between the thyroid pyramidal lobe and pharynx obliterates, a remnant may persist as the *thyroglossal duct*. In this case, the thyroglossal duct may extend from the *foramen cecum* of the tongue, the site of embryonic origin of the thyroid to the pyramidal lobe of the thyroid. In other instances, the duct may partially obliterate, resulting in a *thyroglossal cyst*. Anatomic alterations of the thyroid are usually associated with disturbances of function, making the bedside evaluation of this gland extremely important in the diagnosis of thyroid disorders.

Inspection. With the patient seated in a good crosslight carefully inspect the neck, particularly the lower half. Although the thyroid gland is not usually visible in this position, a relatively small goiter or thyroid nodule often may be readily seen during careful inspection (Fig. 9-16). As noted elsewhere, the patient is then asked to tilt his head straight back, which renders the enlarged thyroid more easily seen. Next, the patient is asked to swallow. Normally, the thyroid ascends during swallowing, and any mass or enlargement that moves upward is likely to be within or adherent to the thyroid. If the patient is obese or has a short neck, it is extremely important to tilt his head back before he swallows.

Auscultation. Listen carefully with the bell of the stethoscope directly over the thyroid, particularly if the gland is enlarged or contains a nodule. A systolic bruit heard over the thyroid is almost diagnostic of diffuse toxic goiter. This physical finding, caused by increased blood flow to the thyroid, also may rarely be heard over thyroid tumors. A continuous venous hum in the supraclavicular areas (particularly on the right), also caused by increased blood flow to the thyroid, is another good sign of diffuse toxic goiter.

Palpation. Seat the patient in a chair and stand behind him. He must be relaxed and comfortable with his chin lowered and the back of his head resting against your body. Place your fingers anteriorly with their tips over the patient's thyroid, and the thumbs resting on the patient's posterior neck (Fig. 9-17). Throughout the examination, repeatedly ask the patient to swallow to facilitate identification and delineation of the gland. Identify the cricoid cartilage, an easily located landmark in the midline of the neck just below the laryngeal cartilage, and find the superior border of the isthmus just inferiorly (Fig. 9-15). Thyroid tissue is almost always within 1 cm. of the cricoid cartilage. With the fingertips of both hands

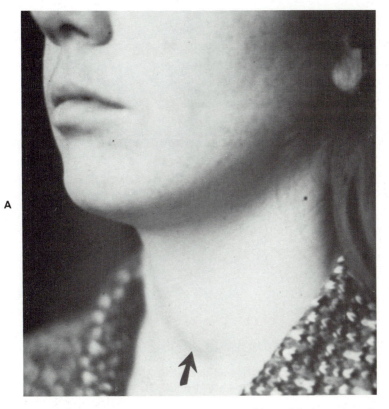

Fig. 9-16. A, Thyroid nodule. A thyroid nodule is readily visible (arrow) in this patient's neck when inspected with tangential light.

Continued.

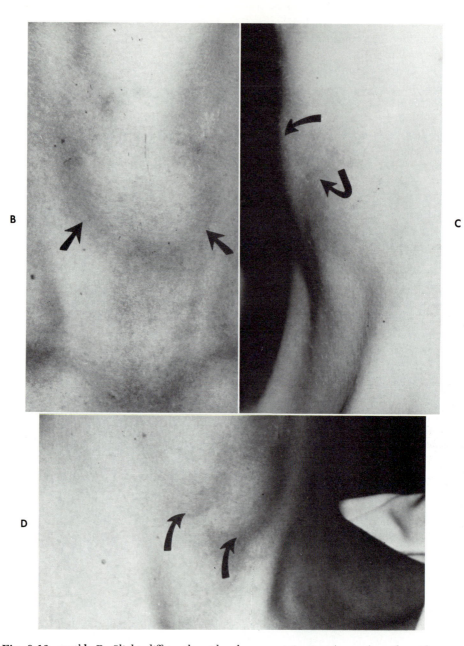

Fig. 9-16, cont'd. B, Slight diffuse thyroid enlargement is seen (arrows) easily with cross lighting from the, **B,** anterior position and, **C,** left and, **D,** right lateral positions.

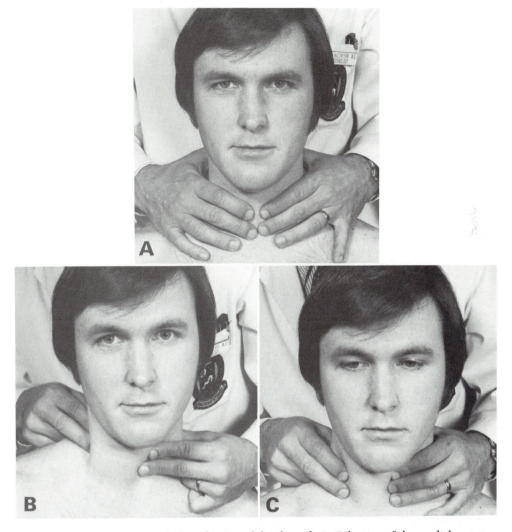

Fig. 9-17. Posterior approach for palpation of the thyroid. **A,** Palpation of the medial aspect of the gland, including the isthmus. **B,** Palpation of the lateral edge of the right lobe. **C,** Palpation of the body of the right lobe. Notice the position of the examiner's fingers in relation to the sternocleidomastoid muscle and the cricoid cartilage as well as the relaxed position of the patient's head.

resting on either side of the trachea (Fig. 9-17, A), ask the patient to swallow. This gives a general impression of the overall size and configuration of the isthmus and medial aspects of the lateral lobes. Then, to examine the right lobe and isthmus, tilt the patient's head to the right, being careful to keep his chin down. Place the fingertips of the right hand behind the patient's right sternocleidomastoid muscle, while the fingertips of the left hand gently displace the trachea to the right (Fig. 9-17, B). Ask the patient to swallow while evaluating the extreme right lateral border of the gland. Next, repeat this maneuver while placing the fingertips of the right hand anterior to the right sternocleidomastoid muscle, retracting it slightly posteriorly (Fig. 9-17, C). This permits evaluation of the main body of the lateral lobe. Next examine the left lobe in a similar fashion.

One may also palpate the thyroid while standing in front of the patient (Fig. 9-18). An anterior approach is preferred by some examiners, but generally, it seems to be less satisfactory for beginners. However, both approaches should be perfected since subtle abnormalities of the thyroid are sometimes detected only after examinations from both positions. To examine the left lobe place your left thumb against the right side of the thyroid cartilage and exert lateral pressure to the left. Place your right thumb along the medial margin of the sternocleidomastoid muscle, and your index and middle fingers along its lateral aspect. This enables you to palpate the underlying thyroid gland with the thumb and fingers around the belly of the muscle. The right lobe is examined in a similar fashion, using the right thumb to displace the larynx to the right and

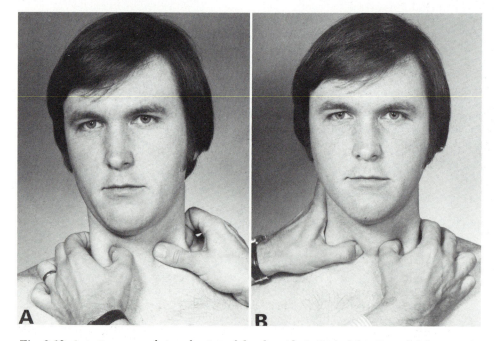

Fig. 9-18. Anterior approach to palpation of the thyroid. **A,** Right lobe. **B,** Left lobe. Notice the position of the patient's head, displacement of the larynx toward the side being examined, and the examiner's exploring fingers that virtually encircle the ipsilateral sternocleidomastoid muscle.

the left hand to examine the right lobe of the thyroid.

The examiner should feel as much of the thyroid gland as possible. The size, configuration, consistency, presence, and number of abnormal nodules should be carefully recorded. The size is usually evaluated in comparison to a normal gland, a popular method being to estimate the weight of the thyroid in grams. The normal thyroid gland weighs less than 25 g. and can be estimated roughly as consisting of a right and left lobe weighing 10 g. each and an isthmus weighing approximately 5 g. Thus, if the right lobe is estimated at three times normal size (30 gm.) and the left lobe and isthmus are normal (15 g.), the estimated overall weight is about 45 g. Such a gross estimate is useful to determine from time to time whether the size of the thyroid gland is changing.

Diffuse goiter. The thyroid may become diffusely enlarged in a number of disorders, such as diffuse toxic goiter (Graves' disease), iodine deficiency, chronic lymphocytic thyroiditis (Hashimoto's thyroiditis), use of antithyroid drugs, and certain congenital forms of goiter. In most instances the gland is smooth or slightly irregular (particularly with thyroiditis), of moderate consistency, and moves upward freely with swallowing. The right lobe is often larger than the left even in the diffusely enlarged gland. Multinodular goiter, an enlarged thyroid containing multiple nodules (Fig. 9-19), may be associated with thyrotoxicosis (multinodular toxic goiter), thyroiditis, and neoplasms. Ordinarily, the nodules are more firm than the surrounding thyroid parenchyma. The thyroid gland may or may not move upward freely with swallowing. Restriction of gland

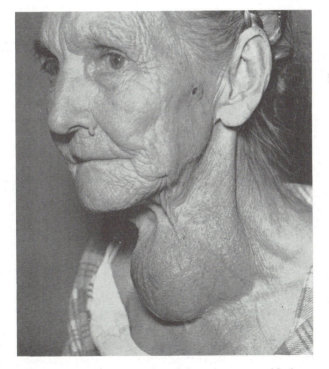

Fig. 9-19. A large, nontoxic, multinodular goiter in an elderly patient.

movements strongly suggests a neoplasm. Frequently, an isolated thyroid nodule is palpated within an otherwise normal thyroid gland. Such nodules, which may be cysts, benign or malignant tumors, areas of hemorrhage, or thyroiditis, vary considerably in consistency, size, and configuration. A tender nodule suggests subacute thyroiditis or recent hemorrhage into an adenoma or carcinoma. Any thyroid enlargement or nodule should prompt a careful search for surrounding lymphadenopathy, including palpation for midline Delphian nodes that enlarge with thyroid cancer or subacute thyroiditis.

Tracheal deformity can be caused by goiter. Indeed, in rare instances the trachea can be almost completely obstructed by massive thyroid enlargement. More commonly, however, slight thyroid enlargement causes displacement of the trachea, which, although creating symptoms in the patient, is difficult or impossible to recognize by physical examination alone.

Substernal goiter. Although on occasion, as in the examination of obese individuals, the normal thyroid cannot be palpated, the absence of palpable thyroid tissue should raise the suspicion of either hypothyroidism or an ectopic thyroid gland. Ectopically located thyroid is most commonly retrosternal (substernal or intrathoracic goiter). Although in most instances the upper border of a retrosternal goiter can be palpated during swallowing, rarely, it cannot be felt. A retrosternal goiter may produce dullness to percussion over the upper sternum, venous distention in the neck, and hoarseness. Another maneuver that may disclose signs of a retrosternal goiter is to hold the patient's arms vertically, high above his head for a few minutes. In this position, a goiter which is obstructing the thoracic outlet will cause congestion and venous distention in the head and neck, along with dyspnea and cyanosis of the face.

Other midline neck masses. The pyramidal lobe of the thyroid may normally extend to the top of the laryngeal cartilage. It can be identified as a soft, elongated structure, slightly to the left of the midline, which moves upward with swallowing. A thyroglossal cyst, which may appear at any time in life, is a firm or resilient mass that can be located in several areas in the neck. Above the hyoid bone it is a midline structure that may be difficult to distinguish from a sublingual dermoid cyst. Between the hyoid bone and thyroid cartilage, the cyst is midline; at the level of the thyroid cartilage, it deviates from the midline, usually to the left (Fig. 9-15). A thyroglossal cyst is perhaps best identified by its upward movement when the tongue is protruded. A thyroglossal fistula may result from rupture of an inflamed cyst. A dermoid cyst may occur in the midline of the neck in the area of the suprasternal notch. It does not move upward with swallowing. In patients with Cushing's syndrome, a soft, nontender mass of fat may form in the suprasternal notch. Because of its resemblance to the skin fold of a cow, it is referred to as a *dewlap*. Rarely, a pulsatile *aortic aneurysm* is present in the suprasternal notch. However, more commonly, such a pulsatile mass is an enlarged and tortuous aorta or innominate artery without an aneurysm.

SELECTED READINGS

Beeson, P. B., and McDermott, W., editors: Textbook of medicine, ed. 15, Philadelphia, 1979, W. B. Saunders Co.

Kuiper, D. H., and Papp, J. P.: Supraclavicular adenopathy demonstrated by the Valsalva maneuver, N. Engl. J. Med. **280:**1007, 1969.

Mazzaferri, E. L.: Endocrinology case studies, ed. 2, Flushing, N.Y., 1980, Medical Examination Publishing Co., Inc.

Werner, S. C., and Ingbar, S. H.: The thyroid: a fundamental and clinical text, ed. 4, New York, 1978, Harper & Row, Publishers, Inc.

CHAPTER 10

EYES

EXTERNAL EXAMINATION

Visual acuity. *The most rewarding single test of ocular function is the evaluation of visual acuity.* Reduced acuity will betray the presence of a great variety of diseases as well as the need for refractive correction. Determination of visual acuity should be a part of every complete physical examination.

Distant acuity is measured with a letter chart (Fig. 10-1) placed 20 feet from the patient. Acuity is expressed as a fraction; the numerator represents the distance to the chart and the denominator the distance at which a normal eye can read the line. Thus 20/30 means the patient is 20 feet away and can read the line that a normal eye should read at 30 feet. By 20/200 is meant that he can read only the largest letter, ordinarily legible to the normal eye at 200 feet. Less visual acuity than this may be recorded as *hand movements (H. M.)* or *light perception (L. P.).* An eye is not termed blind unless it cannot even perceive light.

Acuity is measured in one eye at a time. The other eye should be occluded with an opaque card. Always be on the alert for failure to cover the eye completely or for head turning, which permits the patient to peek around the card. Such "cheating" may be an involuntary attempt

to see with the only good eye, or it may be a deliberate fraud. *Never* allow a patient to cover his eye with his fingers, because he may see between them. Glasses should be worn if the patient customarily uses them for distance. Reading glasses will often blur distant vision.

Always coax the patient with apparently reduced visual acuity to try to read another line. Surprisingly often, he can! Illiterate patients may say they "can't see it" rather than admit their ignorance. Number charts answer this problem, since practically everyone can count money. Charts composed of "E" letters of various sizes and positions are useful for children who simply indicate the direction the E is pointing. An intelligent $3^{1}/_{2}$- or 4-year-old child can usually cooperate enough to permit accurate measurement of acuity.

Measurement of near vision is relatively unimportant as a routine procedure except in patients complaining specifically of reading difficulty or in persons over 40 years of age. With increasing age, the lenses become more inflexible, resulting in loss of accommodation for near vision and interfering with reading. This condition is known as *presbyopia.* Most patients who cannot read newspaper print at 1 foot while using their own reading glasses will

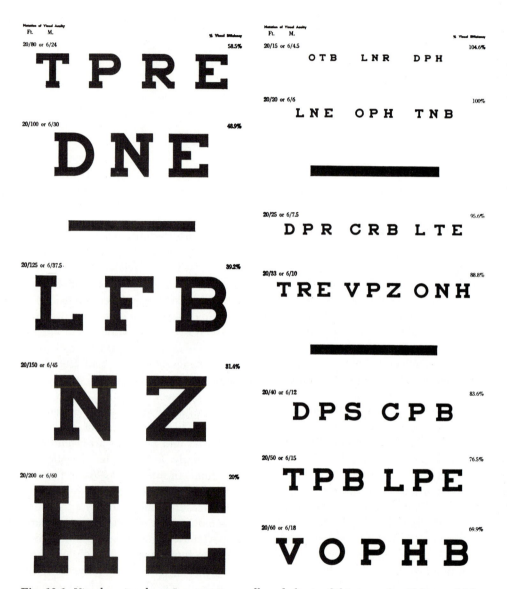

Fig. 10-1. Visual acuity chart. Inexpensive cardboard charts of this type should be available for use during a complete physical examination.

benefit from an ophthalmologic examination and refraction.

Lids. Lid examination has three objectives:

1. To ascertain the adequacy of protection of the eyes
2. To seek signs that betray systemic disease
3. To detect local disease

Do the lids close completely? This question should be answered for all patients and particularly for those with abnormally prominent eyes or facial paralysis. Potentially serious damage may be sustained through drying of eyes when lids do not close properly, as in unconsciousness caused by trauma or anesthesia, serious systemic disease, or if lid defects are present (Fig. 10-2).

Systemic disease (for example, nephrosis, heart failure, allergy, or thyroid deficiency) may be suspected in the presence of lid edema, provided purely local inflammation and the slight bulging of lid skin commonly caused by aging are excluded. *Ptosis* (drooping of the up-per lid) may be an early sign of involvement of the third nerve by any cause. Congenital defects rank high among causes of ptosis.

Infections of glands of the lid margin are quite common (Fig. 10-3). A *hordeolum* (sty) is a localized infection of the small glands about the eyelashes. A *chalazion* is an infection or retention cyst of the meibomian (sebaceous) glands, which lie within the tarsal plates and open on the posterior portion of the lid margins. Crusting of the lashes, often with very fine scales adherent to the lid margin, is an easily observed sign of lid infection.

Faults in position include outward rolling of the lids (*ectropion*) and inrolling (*entropion*). The lashes normally project away from the eye. Should they be misdirected backward, as in entropion, considerable corneal irritation may be produced.

Gentle palpation of the lids may be done by sliding the examining finger across the closed lid surface. In this way any masses (such as a

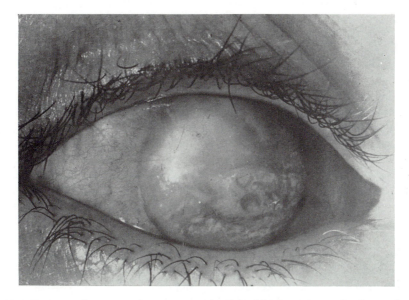

Fig. 10-2. Exposure damage to the cornea results if the lids do not properly close. Adequacy of closure of the lids should be checked during the physical examination.

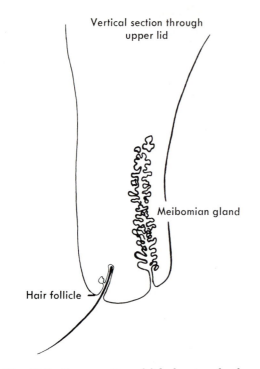

Fig. 10-3. Cross section of lid showing the large meibomian gland situated posteriorly and the smaller glands at the anterior edge.

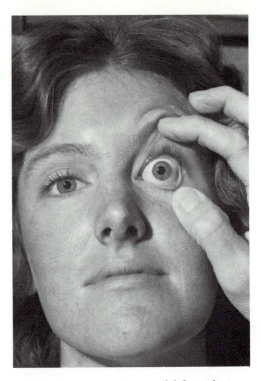

Fig. 10-4. Proper separation of lids without any pressure on the eye.

chalazion) within the lid may be felt between the finger and the eyeball and are often recognized more readily than by observation.

Great care must be taken in examining an injured eye. *Never* press over the eye when trying to separate the lids, since this may destroy the eye. Always limit manipulations to the portion of the lids overlying the bony orbital rims. The upper eyelid may be elevated by pressing upward over the brow, and the lower lid is retracted by pulling down the skin overlying the cheek bone (Fig. 10-4). This must never be forgotten when trying to open an injured eye for inspection. If at any time during examination of an injured eye it is ascertained that the eye has been penetrated (obvious laceration, prolapsed iris, protruding vitreous,

and so on), the examination should be stopped immediately to avoid the possibility of further damage through unwise manipulation.

Lacrimal apparatus. Tears are produced by the lacrimal gland, which is situated in the upper lateral orbit. A portion of this gland can often be seen beneath the retracted upper lid when the patient looks down and must not be mistaken for a tumor. Tears are carried to the lacrimal sac through the lacrimal puncta, which are situated on a tiny elevation on the nasal side of both upper and lower lids. If the lower lid margin does not touch the eye (as in ectropion), tears cannot enter the punctum, and *epiphora* (pathologic tearing) will result. The lacrimal sac is a small pouch situated in the lacrimal fossa. Should passage of tears via the na-

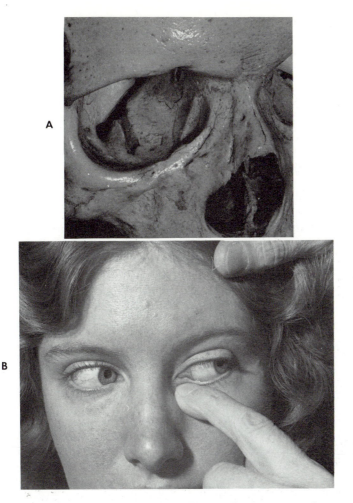

Fig. 10-5. A, The lacrimal fossa is situated *inside* the orbital rim. **B,** When examining the lacrimal sac for regurgitation of infected material, the examiner must direct pressure into the orbit, not on the nose.

solacrimal duct to the nose be obstructed, finger pressure on the lacrimal sac (Fig. 10-5) will cause regurgitation of fluid through the punctum. The finger must be applied *inside* the lower inner orbital rim, not on the side of the nose as is often erroneously done. After pressing on the sac, move the finger inferiorly so as to pull down the lower lid. This facilitates observation of any mucopurulent fluid expressed from the punctum.

Conjunctiva. The conjunctiva is divided into two portions, palpebral and bulbar. *Palpebral conjunctiva* lines the posterior lid surface. *Bulbar conjunctiva* covers the eye up to the *limbus* (junction of cornea and sclera). Conjunctiva is normally quite transparent, and the white color of the eye is caused by the underlying white sclera.

The bulbar conjunctiva is readily examined by separating the lids widely and by having the patient look up, down, and to each side. Many small blood vessels are normally visible in the conjunctiva and underlying structures. Dilation of these vessels is responsible for the various patterns of redness characteristic of many eye diseases. Both vessels and nerves penetrate the sclera at several points about 0.5 cm. above the limbus. At these scleral penetrations, particularly in dark-complexioned persons, uveal pigment often proliferates. These tiny black dots often resemble foreign bodies, as many an unwary beginner has learned to his sorrow. A small fleshy elevation known as the caruncle is situated in the nasal corner of the conjunctiva. Fine hairs and tiny yellowish spots (sebaceous glands) are normally seen in the caruncle and become more prominent with age. Lateral to the caruncle is a flat fold, the plica semilunaris.

The palpebral conjunctiva overlies fleshy tissue and therefore appears much redder than the bulbar conjunctiva. Vertical yellowish striations may be conspicuous in the portion of palpebral conjunctiva overlying the tarsal plates. These striations are the underlying meibomian glands. In response to irritation, virus infection, and particularly allergy, the lymph follicles of the palpebral conjunctiva enlarge, causing a finely nodular appearance that is best seen from the side with flashlight illumination in a semidarkened room.

The palpebral conjunctiva cannot be seen until the lids are everted. The lower lid is easily everted by sliding downward the skin overlying the lower orbital rim (Fig. 10-6). More of the conjunctiva will be exposed if the patient simultaneously looks upward.

Adequate inspection of the upper tarsal conjunctiva requires eversion of the upper lid. One of the common sites where foreign bodies lodge is on the inner surface of the upper tarsal plate, where they are particularly irritating to the cornea. Everting the lids is the simplest approach to removal of foreign bodies.

Five simple steps are required to evert the upper lid.

1. The patient must look down. This relaxes the levator muscle, which is attached to the upper border of the tarsal plate. When the patient looks up, the tarsal plate is retracted into the orbit, a position from which eversion is impossible.

2. The patient must not squeeze the lids shut. Such contraction of the orbicularis muscle effectively blocks eversion attempts. To ensure relaxation and avoid squeezing, reassure the patient, move slowly, and do not hurt him.

3. Hold the upper eyelashes. Grasping them is facilitated by lifting the upper lid, thereby causing the lashes to protrude straight forward. *Do not pull* on the lashes; this only causes the patient to squeeze his lids. Eversion is *not* accomplished by pulling the lashes upward or using them to roll the lid over a stick. In fact,

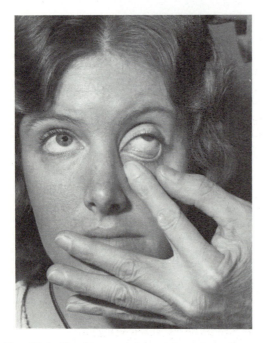

Fig. 10-6. The lower conjunctival sac is easily examined by pulling down the lower lid while the patient looks upward.

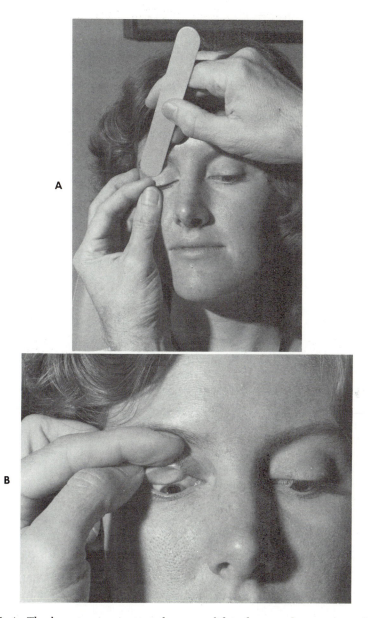

Fig. 10-7. A, The key step in everting the upper lid is downward pressure applied 1 cm. above the lid margin. **B,** The everted lid.

pulling gently down and forward simplifies the subsequent procedure.

4. Push down on the upper tarsal border with a small stick, such as an applicator or tongue blade (Fig. 10-7). The upper tarsal plate extends 12 mm. above the lid margin; therefore, pressure must be applied at least 1 cm. above the edge of the lid margin. You will find that this simple maneuver of pushing down the upper tarsal border is the key to easy lid eversion. *Do not push in against the eye.*

5. As soon as the lid is everted, appose the fingers holding the lashes to the brow, and the lid thus may be held securely in eversion during inspection of the conjunctival surface.

Because the upper lid is normally concave toward the eye, eversion causes a vertical fold to appear, usually in the nasal portion of the lid. This fold should not be misinterpreted as a mass.

To restore the everted upper lid to normal position, remove your hand completely from the patient. If he is still looking down, the lid remains everted. Take hold of the lashes and pull gently forward. Ask the patient to look up, and simultaneously move the lashes down into normal position.

Almost all medical students are much too rough during examination of the eyes. All manipulations, including eversion of the lid, must be performed far more gently than palpation of the abdomen or movement of the extremities. Move slowly, gently, and carefully, and you will retain the patient's confidence.

Cornea. Good vision requires a perfectly smooth and transparent cornea, which is normally invisible except for reflection from its surface. Two of the most common abnormalities of the cornea are *abrasions* and *opacities*. Oblique, moving illumination with a small flashlight is particularly effective in demonstrating corneal abnormalities (Fig. 10-8). Superficial irregularities are best detected by noting the defects appearing in the light reflec-

tions of the normal surface (Fig. 10-9). Occasionally a defect casts shadows on the iris, which may be more readily visible than the corneal lesion producing the shadow. Abrasions of the cornea are often almost invisible except when stained with fluorescein. This staining technique simply requires touching a sterile fluorescein paper to the lower conjunctival sac. Sufficient fluorescein will readily dissolve in the tears and is spread on the cornea by spontaneous blinking. Abrasions will be stained a brilliant yellow-green color. Oblique illumination and movement of the light will also help to differentiate corneal opacities, surface debris, deposits in the anterior chamber, and cataract. If the anterior chamber is abnormally shallow, oblique illumination will cast a characteristic crescent-shaped shadow on the far side of the anteriorly displaced iris (Fig. 10-10). Recognition of a shallow anterior chamber is important because it predisposes the eye to glaucoma and may contraindicate the use of dilating drops. Furthermore, shallowness of the chamber is caused by a number of serious disorders (for example, leaking corneal wound, inflammatory block of aqueous flow, and swollen lens).

Corneal sensitivity (fifth nerve) is tested by touching a wisp of cotton to the center of the cornea and noting the brisk lid closure. This lid closure is a normal and important protective reflex. Approach the eye from the side so that the patient cannot see the cotton, since he might blink from fear. Do not touch the lashes, for a touch will also cause blinking. Because of the great individual variation in corneal sensitivity, comparison of the corneal reflexes of the two eyes with each other is the best standard of reference (unless the patient has bilateral fifth nerve loss).

Pupil. Normal pupils are perfectly round and equal in size and constrict visibly to light and during accommodation. The *direct reaction to light* refers to constriction of the pupil receiv-

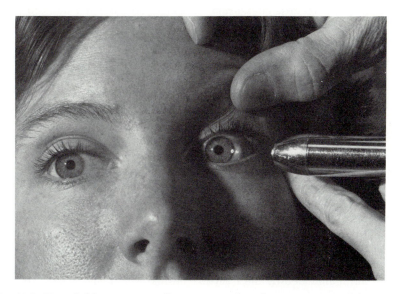

Fig. 10-8. Use of oblique moving illumination is best for examination of the cornea.

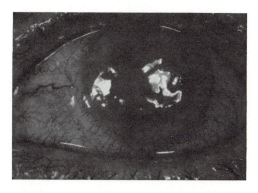

Fig. 10-9. Irregular reflections from a damaged corneal surface as seen by oblique illumination.

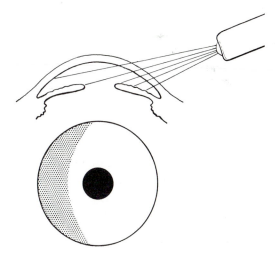

Fig. 10-10. Crescent-shaped shadow typical of shallow anterior chamber illuminated obliquely.

ing increased illumination. Constriction of the opposite pupil (even though no light increase strikes this opposite eye) is termed *consensual pupil reaction*. Either optic nerve may transmit the afferent part of the pupillary reflex. Efferent pupilloconstriction stimuli are distributed evenly to both eyes via ciliary nerves. Thus in monocular blindness, as with a severed or diseased optic nerve, the affected eye will have no direct pupil response but will react consensually to stimulation of the opposite eye. Stimulation of the blind eye, however, will not cause consensual reaction of the opposite normal eye. The "swinging flashlight" test is of great value in detecting defects in the afferent pupillary pathway. Simply alternate the flashlight from one eye to the other. If both afferent pathways are normal, the pupils will remain constant in size. If one side is defective, that pupil will dilate when illuminated by the flashlight (because the normal side is no longer illuminated and therefore both pupils dilate). A positive swinging flashlight test denotes neural disease—it does not result from opacities of the media, such as cataract.

The reaction to accommodation is best tested by holding one fingertip about 4 inches from the eye being tested. Request the patient to look alternately at the fingertip and at the far wall directly beyond the finger. This will greatly simplify observing the pupil, since the eye will not move. If the pupil reacts to light, it ordinarily may be assumed that reaction to accommodation will be present. Do not check the light reflex with a flashlight by approaching the patient from straight ahead, since the patient will accommodate on the light source as on any other object. You should bring the light in from the side (which also is the best position for inspection of the eye). Failure to react to light with preservation of convergence (Argyll Robertson pupil) is very characteristic of central nervous system syphilis. Careful check of the accommodation response is mandatory if

light response is absent. Absence of the light reflex should not be diagnosed unless the examination has been done in a darkened room with a bright light source.

Pupils are normally smaller in infancy and old age. Five percent of normal people will have a noticeable difference of pupil size *(anisocoria)*, but this finding should be regarded with great suspicion, since it may be caused by many types of central nervous system disease. Enlargement of the pupil *(mydriasis)* may be caused by ocular injury (recent or old), acute glaucoma, systemic poisoning by parasympatholytic drugs, and local use of dilating drops. Constriction of the pupil *(miosis)* is seen in iris inflammation, in glaucoma patients treated with pilocarpine, as an effect of morphine, and physiologically in sleep.

Irregularity of pupil contour is invariably abnormal, occurring in iritis, syphilis of the central nervous system, trauma, and congenital defects.

Intraocular pressure. By indentation of the eye with the examining fingers, a crude estimate of intraocular pressure may be made. Pressure measurement is important because elevated intraocular pressure, known as *glaucoma*, causes slow death of nerve fibers and is responsible for 12% of blindness in the United States. The determination of intraocular pressure by finger tension is a rather crude test that will detect only gross pressure alterations. Greater accuracy requires the use of a tonometer (Fig. 10-11). Early detection of lesser increases in pressure also requires use of tonometer. Routine tonometry at 5-year intervals is highly desirable in all patients over 40 years of age.

For tonometry the eyes are anesthetized by instillation of 1 drop of 0.5% proparacaine. Anesthesia is adequate in 1 minute. It is well to instill an additional drop in apprehensive patients and wait another minute to be absolutely certain of good anesthesia. During the waiting

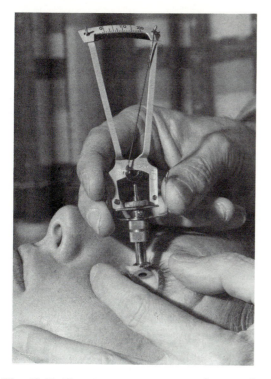

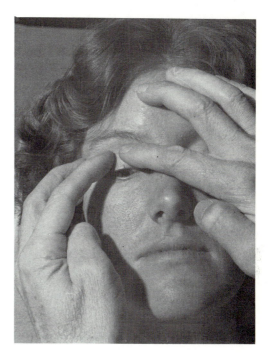

Fig. 10-11. Tonometer measurement of intraocular tension. This should be performed routinely in persons over 40 years of age because chronic simple glaucoma exists in 2% of patients in this age group.

Fig. 10-12. Finger tension technique. This is a gross screening procedure effective in determining only rather large increases or decreases in pressure.

period tonometer accuracy should be checked on the metal test block, on which the scale reading must be exactly zero. The indicator must swing freely without sticking.

In a reclining position the patient looks exactly vertically. He must hold his eyes steady and avoid squeezing his lids. The examiner gently separates the patient's lids, with his thumb and forefinger applied to the upper and lower orbital rims. If pressure is exerted into the orbit, a falsely high reading will register. The sterile tonometer footplate is placed perpendicularly on the center of the cornea. Tilting or eccentric positions readily produce erroneous readings. The tonometer is held by its

metal sleeve, which slides freely up and down on the lower portion of the tonometer. The sleeve serves simply to balance the tonometer and should be held in midposition, neither lifting nor pressing down the tonometer. The instrument is calibrated to measure intraocular pressure when its own weight rests on the cornea.

Tonometer scale readings are transposed to millimeters of mercury with the aid of the table supplied with each tonometer. Pressure of 25 mm. Hg or higher indicates thorough ocular evaluation by the specialized tests used to evaluate patients with glaucoma.

Tonometry is contraindicated in the pres-

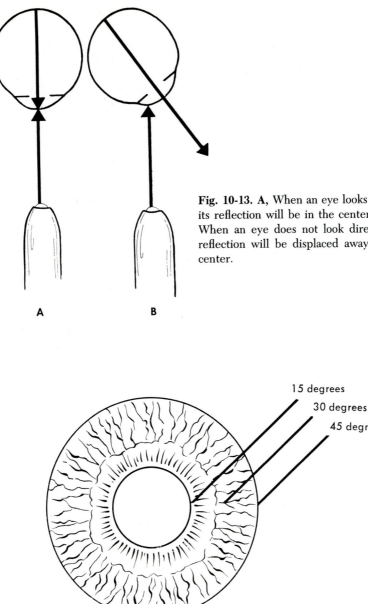

A   **B**

Fig. 10-13. **A,** When an eye looks directly at a light, its reflection will be in the center of the cornea. **B,** When an eye does not look directly at a light, its reflection will be displaced away from the corneal center.

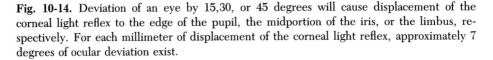

15 degrees
30 degrees
45 degrees

1 mm. = 7 degrees

Fig. 10-14. Deviation of an eye by 15,30, or 45 degrees will cause displacement of the corneal light reflex to the edge of the pupil, the midportion of the iris, or the limbus, respectively. For each millimeter of displacement of the corneal light reflex, approximately 7 degrees of ocular deviation exist.

ence of superficial ocular infection, corneal edema, or corneal exposure damage.

The technique of finger pressure (Fig. 10-12) is best explained by first describing what it is *not*. You are *not* balloting the eye in the orbit as a liver in an ascitic abdomen. You are *not* measuring orbital compressibility as you investigate for thyrotropic exophthalmos caused by increased orbital tissue volume. You *are* indenting the eye and feeling for the rebound of the sclera as your finger withdraws.

The most reliable estimates of intraocular pressure are obtained by pressure on the sclera and not on the cornea, which gives a false impression of abnormal firmness. If the patient simply closes his eyes, Bell's phenomenon will turn his cornea upward to an unpredictable degree. It is best to have him look down, and then palpate the sclera through the upper lid. One finger alone *cannot* distinguish between globe indentation and displacement of the entire eye into the orbital fat. Thus, because of orbital compressibility, even a glass eye may seem soft to one finger. You *must use two fingers*, preferably the forefingers of both hands. Gentle alternating pressure is applied to the upper sclera. The advancing finger holds the whole eye in position against the orbital fat and is not used to interpret softness. The rebound

of the depressed sclera against the *withdrawing* finger is the most reliable criterion of intraocular pressure.

Extraocular muscles. Straightness of the eyes is most easily demonstrated by observing the reflection of a light on the cornea (Figs. 10-13 and 10-14). The flashlight should be held directly in front of the examiner's eyes, and the patient's gaze should be directed at the light. Normally the light reflection is symmetrically situated in the two pupils. An asymmetric light reflex will readily betray a deviating eye.

Many young children have a bilateral skin fold (epicanthus) curving down from the nasal end of their upper lid. This partially conceals the eyes, especially when in looking to the side one eye is turned toward the nose. Epicanthus is commonly mistaken for crossing of the eyes. The corneal light reflex is a quick and reasonably accurate way to differentiate epicanthus and crossed eyes. Fig. 10-15 shows a child with both epicanthus and crossed eyes. Note the light reflex is centered in the left cornea but is displaced to the temporal side of the right cornea.

A paralyzed extraocular muscle may be one cause of ocular deviation. Muscle paralyses are best detected by moving the eyes into the six cardinal positions of gaze (Fig. 10-16). These cardinal positions are chosen because the muscle designated is paralyzed if the eye will not turn to a given position (Table 10-1). Be sure to carry the fixation point well out to the extremes of gaze since this will exaggerate a defect, thereby permitting easy recognition.

When looking far to the side, some eyes will develop a rhythmic twitching motion (end-positional nystagmus). The quick portion of end-positional nystagmus is always in the direction of gaze and is followed by a slow drift back. This differentiates end-positional nystagmus (a benign condition) from pathologic nystagmus (in which the quick component is always in the

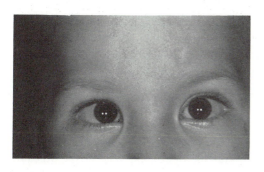

Fig. 10-15. Epicanthus and strabismus may coexist. Recognition of an eccentric corneal light reflex will establish the presence of strabismus.

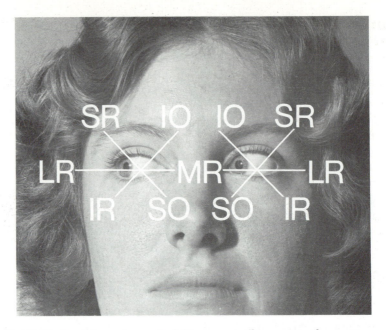

Fig. 10-16. Cardinal positions of gaze. Inability to move the eye into the positions specified indicates paralysis of the corresponding extraocular muscle.

Table 10-1. Cardinal positions of gaze*

Position to which eye will not turn	Paretic muscle
Straight nasal	Medial rectus (third nerve)
Up and nasal	Inferior oblique (third nerve)
Down and nasal	Superior oblique (fourth nerve)
Straight temporal	Lateral rectus (sixth nerve)
Up and temporal	Superior rectus (third nerve)
Down and temporal	Inferior rectus (third nerve)

*Note that straight up and down are *not* cardinal positions of gaze.

same direction, regardless of the direction of gaze).

The complaint of diplopia should initiate careful investigation of muscle function. The *cover test* is a more delicate method than simple observation to determine whether the eyes are straight and will detect deviations of less than 5 degrees. While the patient looks with both eyes at a specific fixation point (such as the flashlight), one eye is covered by a card or other type of occluder. Watch the uncovered eye. If this eye moves to fix on the light, it was not straight before the other eye was covered. If the uncovered eye does not move, then it was straight. Repeat the test for the other eye. Normally, both eyes should be perfectly straight by this test.

The *alternate cover test* shifts occlusion back

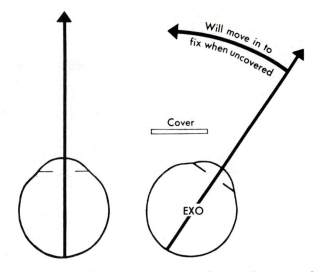

Cover

Will move in to fix when uncovered

EXO

Fig. 10-17. Exophoria causes an eye to diverge when covered.

and forth from one eye to the other as the patient looks at the fixation light. Watch the eye that is just being uncovered. As shown in Fig. 10-17, an eye may turn out while covered. When occlusion is shifted to the other eye, a corrective inward movement will straighten the eye just uncovered. Simultaneously, the newly covered eye will turn out by the same amount, since the angular relationship of the two eyes with each other remains unchanged. Movement of less than 5 degrees (estimated or measured by a prism) is normal in this test, since this much deviation may result from blocking binocular fusion reflexes.

Orbit. The position of the eye in its bony socket may be altered by tumor, inflammation, trauma, thyroid disease, or developmental defect. Forward displacement is termed *exophthalmos;* backward displacement is called *enophthalmos*. Although abnormal prominence of the eye is recognizable by inspection, the false impression of exophthalmos may be produced by widely open lids and the impression of enophthalmos by a drooping upper lid.

Measurement of exophthalmos may be done by placing a millimeter ruler so that it extends straight forward from the lateral orbital rim. If the examiner sights the corneal apex over the ruler from a lateral position he will obtain a rough measurement of the distance the cornea protrudes anteriorly from the lateral orbital rim. Normal measurements rarely exceed 18 mm. The examiner must guard against errors of parallax in this determination. More accurate measurements may be made with an exophthalmometer (Fig. 10-18).

Orbital compressibility is estimated by pressing firmly on the eye through closed lids. Normally the eye may be displaced almost 0.5 cm. into the orbital fat. Increased resistance to compression results from abnormal tissue (inflammatory infiltrate or tumor) within the orbit. Sometimes a tumor mass may be palpated by introducing the little finger between the orbital rim and the eye.

The orbital rims may be displaced by fracture. Do not mistake the occasionally palpable infraorbital and supraorbital notches for frac-

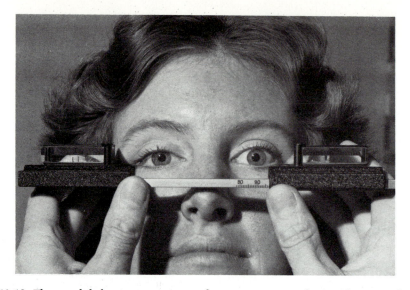

Fig. 10-18. The exophthalmometer measures the anteroposterior distance between the corneal apex and the lateral orbital rim.

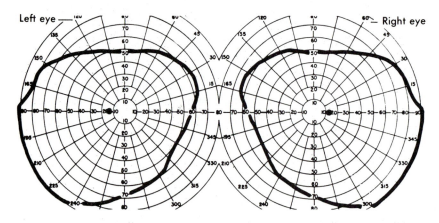

Fig. 10-19. Normal visual fields. The extent of the field in each direction is indicated in degrees.

tures. These contours are best investigated by passing a finger about the orbital edge.

Visual fields. A crude estimate of the function of the visual pathways may be obtained by confrontation testing of the peripheral extent of the field of vision. With one eye covered, the patient must look steadily straight ahead at a specific fixation point, not at the test object approaching from the periphery. A small object, such as a pencil, should be used rather than a gross object, such as the hand. This object is placed beyond the limits of the field of vision and advanced centripetally until seen. Normally a patient should see about 60 degrees na-

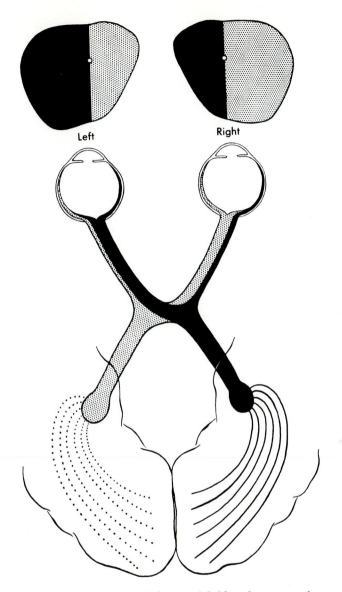

Fig. 10-20. Representation of the visual field in the optic pathways.

salward, 50 degrees upward, 90 degrees temporally, and 70 degrees downward as measured from the anteroposterior axis of the eye (Fig. 10-19). At least eight equally spaced meridians should be tested for each eye.

The confrontation method will fail to detect early evidence of damage to the visual pathways; hence, it is unsatisfactory for clinical use (unless, of course, a large defect is clearly demonstrated with confrontation testing).

Quantitative measurement of the visual field is a much more accurate and certain method of detecting, evaluating, and following visual pathway damage. Measurement of the visual

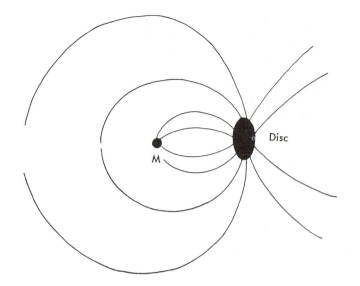

Fig. 10-21. Distribution of nerve fibers within the retina. Note that fibers radiate from the optic disc throughout the retina. Defects at the macula *(M)* will result in a central blind spot.

field should be included in the complete neurologic examination and in the evaluation of many eye complaints (for example, unexplained visual acuity loss uncorrectable with glasses, possible malingering or hysteria, and ocular aches or headaches of undetermined cause).

A brief review of the anatomy of the visual pathway (Fig. 10-20) is appropriate. Since nerves from both eyes intermingle behind the chiasm, lesions posterior to the chiasm will impair the opposite half of the visual field of both eyes. Lesions at the chiasm may cause a wide variety of defects, usually involving both eyes. Midline chiasm damage (as from pituitary tumor) damages the crossing fibers from the nasal retina and classically causes bitemporal field loss. Naturally, damage to one optic nerve will affect only the field of the involved eye.

The anatomy of the nerve fiber layer of the retina (Fig. 10-21) will determine the pattern of field defects caused by retinal disease. Macular defects cause a central blind spot. Edema

of the optic disc enlarges the blind spot. Localized damage to a group of nerve fibers (as by injury, infection, or glaucoma) will cause a sector of blindness corresponding to the involved area of retina.

Malingering and hysteria cause variable, bizarre, and nonphysiologic defects of the visual field. The most common functional defect is marked constriction, so that the patient may claim to see nothing beyond 10 degrees from the fixation point. That he actually does see peripheral to this is clear from his behavior, for he does not bump into chairs and other objects as does the diseased patient who actually cannot see peripherally.

USE OF THE OPHTHALMOSCOPE

Thorough physical examination should always include careful study of the details of the posterior eye (fundus) with an ophthalmoscope. In addition to the detection of ocular disease, this procedure will often permit the diagnosis

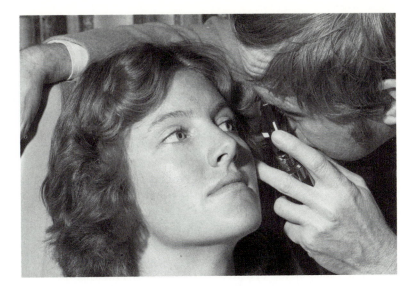

Fig. 10-22. Proper position for ophthalmoscopic examination. The ophthalmoscope is most effective if brought very close to the patient.

of serious systemic disorders. Since a careful study of the retina, vessels, and nerve is so often important to the diagnosis of both local and systemic disease, it is highly desirable to dilate the pupils. This will permit a much more adequate examination of the fundus.

Successful ophthalmoscopic examination requires cooperation from the patient. He must hold his eyes still. This is facilitated by pointing out a distant object at which you wish him to look (or pretend to look if your head interferes). If he is seated and you are standing, the optimal direction of gaze is about 20 degrees upward and temporally (Fig. 10-22). A darkened room is necessary for proper examination. Dilatation of the pupil with 10% phenylephrine hydrochloride greatly simplifies the examination. Glasses need not be worn by examiner or patient unless a high degree of astigmatism is present. Examiner and patient should keep both eyes open.

The ophthalmoscope is held in the exam-

iner's right hand before his right eye during examination of the patient's right eye. It is held in the left hand and before the left eye to examine the patient's left eye. The index finger rests on the lens wheel to permit focusing during observation. The head of the ophthalmoscope should be braced firmly against the physician's brow or nose with the viewing aperture positioned exactly in front of his eye. This relative position of the ophthalmoscope and physician will not be changed during any part of the examination. The beginning student should place the ophthalmoscope in this position and turn his head about in various directions as he looks through the aperture in order to emphasize the great importance of firm fixation of the ophthalmoscope against his head. Failure to do this will result in misalignment of the eye and viewing aperture, with consequent loss of the fundus view.

A number of more or less useless apertures and colored filters are incorporated in most ophthalmoscopes. The small, round, white light is best for almost all purposes. The light is used at maximum brightness unless this is not tolerated by the patient. It is probably easiest to start with the ophthalmoscope lens set at zero (unless the examiner has a significant spherical refractive error that can be corrected by the ophthalmoscopic lens). Red (minus) numbers focus farther away; black (plus) numbers focus nearer.

Looking through the aperture of the ophthalmoscope, which is held firmly against his head, the examiner should approach to within 1 foot of the patient and direct the light into his pupil. A uniform red glow (the red reflex) will now be seen to fill the pupil of normal eyes. Opacities in the clear portions of the eye will appear as black defects within the red reflex. Absence of the red reflex indicates that some abnormality is blocking transmission of light through the eye or that the ophthalmoscope is not properly positioned.

Always keeping the red reflex in sight, the physician should approach the patient's eye until his forehead touches the patient. Loss of the red reflex during the approach means the light is not directed into the pupil and is best corrected by backing away until the red reflex is again located. Another possible cause for loss of the light reflex is blinking by the patient. If this is annoying, the free hand may be rested on the patient's head and the thumb gently used to elevate the upper lid. To prevent bumping the patient's nose with the ophthalmoscope, the handle should be directed down and slightly away from the patient, a position achieved by slight tilting of the examiner's head.

In contact with the patient's forehead, the examiner should now perceive some fundus detail such as a vessel, pigment, or the optic disc. Whatever detail is first encountered should be brought into sharp focus by rotating the lens wheel as necessary. Because the patient's eye is only 1 inch away, the examiner will reflexly converge and accommodate. Since the amount of this accommodation may be variable, it interferes with focusing and causes the picture to blur and clear in annoying fashion. This is easily avoided if the examiner pretends he is looking through the patient's head at some far distant landscape. Focusing should be done with the lens wheel, not by the examiner's accommodation.

In systematic examination of the fundus the examiner should first locate the optic disc. If the ophthalmoscope light is directed into the eye from a position about 15 degrees temporal to the straight-ahead gaze of the patient, the optic disc will be the first detail seen (Fig. 10-23). If not located immediately, the disc may be found by following down the vessel bifurcations, just as following down the branches of a tree will lead to the trunk.

When the ophthalmoscope light is moved from one part of the retina to another, the beginner will often lose the fundus view completely. This is because the light has been moved so that it no longer enters the pupil. To understand this problem and its correction refer to Fig. 10-24, which illustrates the beam of light passing between ophthalmoscope and retina. To change the area of retina illuminated requires movement of the ophthalmoscope in the opposite direction so that *rotation of the light beam is centered at the pupil.*

Dazzling light reflections from the corneal surface may be quite annoying, especially during examination of the posterior pole of the eye. These reflections may be avoided by moving the ophthalmoscope very slightly to one side or the other.

When ophthalmoscopy or external ocular examination must be performed on an uncooperative child, some type of restraint becomes necessary. (Distraction with lollipops is better but will not always work.) "Mummying" by wrapping the child snugly in a sheet is the usual method of holding him quiet. A quicker, simpler, and more effective way of simulta-

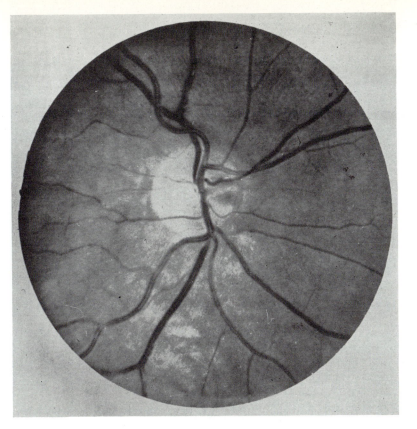

Fig. 10-23. Normal retinal details.

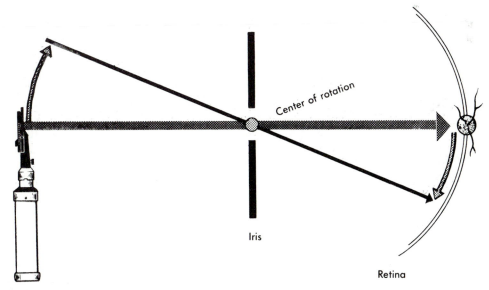

Center of rotation

Iris

Retina

Ophthalmoscope

Fig. 10-24. To look at another part of the retina requires movement of the ophthalmoscope so that the rotation of the beam of light will be centered at the pupil.

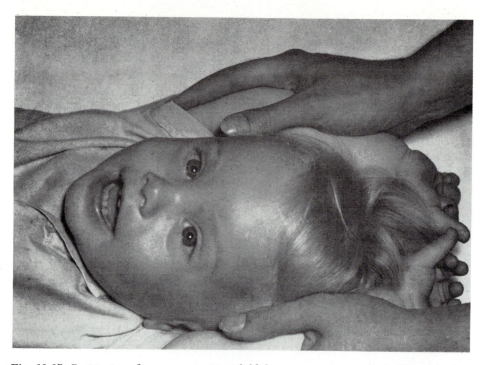

Fig. 10-25. Positioning of an uncooperative child for eye examination by holding his arms firmly against his head.

neous immobilization of head and arms is to lay the child on a cot, take hold of both his elbows, and press his arms firmly against his ears (Fig. 10-25). The parent can easily be instructed to hold the child in this way during examination. If the child moves his body and legs enough to disturb the eye examination, the parent can lean gently on the child's body by standing beside him.

Examination of the ocular fundus

A definite routine should be followed in examination of the fundus, beginning with the optic disc.

Optic disc. The optic disc is the most conspicuous feature of the fundus, and the following details should be noted:

1. Size. Normal discs appear of a uniform size, which is readily recognized with little ex-

perience. High myopic refractive errors magnify the disc; hyperopic errors minify it. For example, after cataract extraction the disc looks very small. Fundus distances are conveniently estimated in terms of disc diameters (DD). Thus a lesion slightly larger than the disc and situated in the upper fundus may be described as being 1 × 2 DD in size and 3 DD away from the disc at 1:30 o'clock (Fig. 10-26). The disc is approximately 1.5 mm. in diameter. All fundus details appear magnified 15 times because of the focusing effect of the cornea and lens.

2. Shape. The disc is normally round or vertically oval. Gross irregularities in shape and size should not be interpreted as being part of the disc but are ordinarily caused by adjacent disease.

3. Color. The healthy disc is a creamy pink

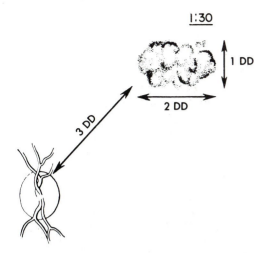

Fig. 10-26. Method of giving position and dimensions of a lesion in terms of disc diameters.

color. This is caused by a rich capillary network, the larger vessels of which are normally just visible. The center of the disc may be grayish if a deep physiologic cup exposes the lamina cribrosa. Infants have very gray discs that may easily be misconstrued as atrophic.

4. Physiologic depression. Most discs have a small depression just temporal of center. This may be quite large but *never* extends completely to the disc margin. It may be deep enough to permit a clear view of the fine fenestrations of the lamina cribrosa.

5. Margins. Ordinarily the disc outline is more or less regular, frequently with scattered pigment overlying the margins. Normally it is possible to focus clearly on these physiologic irregularities of the edges, indicating absence of edema or inflammation. Dense pigment deposits are often situated about the disc margin. As a normal variant, a grayish crescent of sclera is frequently visible immediately adjacent to the disc.

Vessels. The central retinal artery and vein appear in the depths of the disc. Bifurcations are variable and may occur deep in the disc or not until the vessel reaches the retina. Each large vessel should in turn be carefully observed along its whole length, from disc to periphery.

1. *Arteries* usually are about 25% narrower than veins. (Absolute size varies with the number of branches, and it is easily understood that if two veins drain an area fed by one artery, the artery will be the largest vessel.) A narrow band of light, the *arteriolar light reflex*, is reflected from the center of an artery. Arteries and veins may cross and entwine each other in any fashion, but *normal arteries do not indent* or displace veins. Arteriovenous crossings should be sought out and evaluated for the presence of such abnormal indentations, which are characteristic of arteriolar sclerosis.

2. *Veins* are darker in color than arteries and do not have a prominent light reflex. At the proximal end of the vein, overlying the disc, there is usually visible a slight pulsation (*spontaneous venous pulsation*) synchronous with the arterial pulse. This is caused by the forcing of venous blood out of the eye with each arterial systole. External pressure on the eye with a finger during ophthalmoscopic examination will produce venous collapse or pulsation (only at the disc end of the vein) in all normal eyes.

Macula. The macula is an area about 1 DD in size and situated 2 DD temporal to the disc. It is avascular, not even capillaries being present in its center, and is nourished by the choroid. The minute glistening spot of reflected light seen in the center of the macula represents a pinpoint depression, the *fovea centralis.* Delicate vessels run toward the fovea from all directions. Fine pigment granularity is normally seen in the macula as well as in the periphery of the retina.

If difficulty is encountered in finding the macula, instruct the patient to look directly at the ophthalmoscope light. This will place the macula in the center of the examiner's field of vision. This area deserves careful inspection, since it is the region of the retina with the highest visual acuity.

Periphery. Although the retina adjacent to the disc may be seen by aiming the ophthalmoscope beam in different directions, it is necessary to enlist the patient's aid to see the extreme periphery. Instruct the patient to look upward as the ophthalmoscope beam is directed upward, to the left as the beam is directed to the left, to the right as the beam is directed to the right, and downward as the beam is directed downward. In this manner the entire periphery of the retina can be visualized.

Normal variations. Various types of fundi exist normally.

1. Tesselated fundi are those that are fairly darkly pigmented except for prominent, crisscrossing, linear, light-orange streaks, which represent choroidal vessels.
2. Albinoid fundi are quite light in color, showing clearly the reddish choroidal vessels lying on the gray-white scleral background.
3. Negroid fundi are uniformly quite dark.
4. Most fundi are fairly uniform in coloration and of a finely granular texture with oc-

casionally visible choroidal vessels. The peripheral retina is usually lighter than the central portion.

Light reflexes. Light reflexes are glistening, movable reflections from undulations in the smooth retinal surface. They characteristically parallel the vessels and often encircle the macula. Light reflexes are more prominent in young persons than in older persons.

Media. On completion of the fundus examination, the more anterior portion of the eye may be examined by turning to higher plus (black) lenses. In sequence, this will focus on the posterior vitreous, anterior vitreous, and lens, which appear perfectly transparent and invisible in the the normal eye. Usually a +15 or +20 lens will be needed to see the iris and cornea at this close distance. About fourfold magnification of the iris results.

INTERPRETATION OF OPHTHALMOSCOPIC FINDINGS

When the mechanical difficulties of ophthalmoscopy have been mastered through practice, the problem of interpretation of the clinical ob-

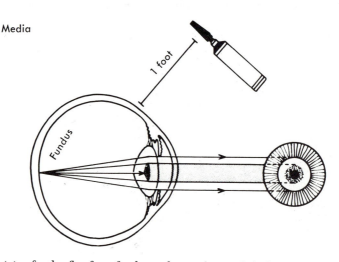

Fig. 10-27. Origin of red reflex from fundus and typical central shadow produced by nuclear cataract in the lens. (From Havener, W. H.: Synopsis of ophthalmology, ed. 5, St. Louis, 1979, The C. V. Mosby Co.)

servations will arise. The practical experience of seeing a variety of lesions under clinical supervision is indispensable; nevertheless, description of the more common ocular abnormalities will be helpful to the beginner.

Ophthalmoscopic observation of the eye from a distance of about 6 inches normally causes the pupil to glow with a reddish light (*red reflex*). This light is composed of reflections from sclera, choroid, retina, optic nerve, and the blood vessels within these structures. Originating from the back of the eye, the red reflex will be interrupted by any opacities of the media if they are located on the path of the emerging light rays. The method of formation of the typical central shadow so characteristic of a nuclear cataract is illustrated in Fig. 10-27. Even the smallest cataract, corneal scar, or vitreous opacity will produce a corresponding shadow in the red reflex. Vitreous hemorrhage or dense cataract may destroy the red reflex completely. A brilliant, uniform red reflex rules out most of the serious defects of the axial portion of the cornea, aqueous, lens, and vitreous. Observation of the red reflex is not only helpful in aligning the ophthalmoscope properly before the patient's eye but also provides immediate information as to the health of the transparent portions of the eye.

Abnormalities of the optic disc

Ophthalmoscopic study of the optic nerve requires evaluation of its size, shape, color, physiologic depression (or abnormal elevation) and margins. Three of the most important diagnoses that can be made from observation of the optic disc are optic atrophy, papilledema, and glaucoma. *Optic atrophy* indicates partial or complete death of the optic nerve. Optic atrophy is significant not only because it destroys sight but also because it may result from serious diseases of the central nervous system. *Papilledema* is particularly important because it is a sign of increased intracranial pressure and may be the first easily recognizable and definite indication of a brain tumor or hematoma. *Glaucoma*, an abnormal increase in intraocular pressure, is the most common *preventable* cause of blindness in the United States.

The color of the disc may be useful in the diagnosis of these three serious conditions. The healthy pink color of the disc is caused by the presence of its normal blood supply. On careful inspection, perhaps a dozen very tiny vessels can be distinguished on the disc surface (Fig. 10-28, A). These tiny vessels do not pass from the disc to the retina but remain on the disc alone. The disc vessels do not originate from or drain into the central artery and vein, but rep-

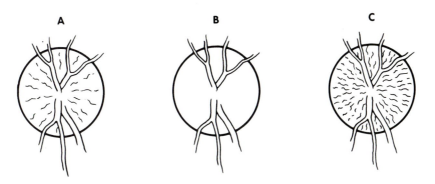

Fig. 10-28. Disc capillaries: **A**, normal; **B**, optic atrophy; **C**, papilledema.

resent an entirely separate circulation. Hence, the vascular status of the disc is independent from that of the retina.

Optic atrophy. Death of the fibers of the optic nerve results in a secondary disappearance of the tiny disc vessels. This is ophthalmoscopically recognizable as pallor or whiteness of the disc (Fig. 10-28, *B*). Because of the wide range of normal variation, the diagnosis of optic atrophy should not be made until the disc capillaries are completely absent from at least a sector of the disc. Comparison of the two discs with each other is often helpful in assessing the significance of a normally variable feature such as disc color. Ordinarily the two discs are quite similar in appearance.

The pallor of optic atrophy is either diffuse throughout the area of the disc or may involve only a sector of the disc. Sector involvement extends uniformly from center to edge of the disc. Optic atrophy does *not* cause pallor limited to a small portion of the center of the disc or to a crescent-shaped rim on the outside edge

of the disc. Marked whiteness in these areas is commonly seen as a normal variant and represents a prominent physiologic depression or a developmental temporal crescent, respectively. The appearance of a temporal crescent of a sclera is illustrated in Fig. 10-29. Such a disc is often misinterpreted as a round disc with temporal pallor. Actually, it is a perfectly normal vertically oval disc. As a normal developmental variant, the various pigmented layers of the retina and choroid often stop a short distance from the disc, leaving a space of uncovered white sclera. As illustrated, this white sclera is ordinarily somewhat crescent shaped, and usually lies just temporal to the disc. Sector optic atrophy must extend from center to edge of the disc (the anatomic distribution of the nerve fibers) and cannot exist as a crescent peripheral to the normal disc.

Papilledema. The venous drainage of the disc is to a plexus surrounding the optic nerve and within its meningeal sheaths. Increased intracranial pressure may be transmitted anteri-

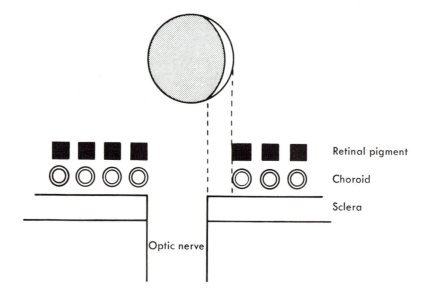

Retinal pigment

Choroid

Sclera

Optic nerve

Fig. 10-29. Normal scleral crescent in cross section (bottom) and ophthalmoscopic view (top).

orly within the meningeal sheaths of the optic nerves and may compress these veins, thereby impeding the venous drainage of the optic disc (Fig. 10-30). Such venous stasis of the disc is called papilledema. The ophthalmoscopic characteristics of papilledema are easily remembered by considering the sequelae of increased venous pressure. Most importantly, the tiny vessels of the disc become dilated and tortuous, are more readily visible, and therefore appear more numerous. This is the cause of the hyperemic disc (Fig. 10-28 *C*) and is the earliest definite sign of papilledema. Conversely, pallor of the disc excludes papilledema, even if it is slightly or definitely elevated with blurred margins. This is a most helpful point in the differential diagnosis of papilledema. Dilated capillaries leak their contents—fluid, blood, and protein. Fluid leak causes elevation of the disc, which may spread very slightly beyond the disc margin, causing its edges to become indistinct. The circumference of the edematous disc reflects light more conspicuously than usual. Such increased reflections are characteristically found at the edge of any area of retinal edema. Diapedesis of red cells from the dilated disc

capillaries causes small linear hemorrhages in the nerve fiber layer of the retina immediately adjacent to the disc (not further away than one or two disc diameters). Other causes of linear retinal hemorrhages are *not* confined to the area near the disc. Protein leakage may cause small gray deposits, also directly adjacent to the disc. To remember the appearance of papilledema, simply imagine the consequences of stasis of the disc capillaries.

Glaucoma. Disc color may also be altered by glaucomatous optic atrophy. Regardless of the cause of optic atrophy, pallor of the disc is characteristic of advanced disease. The diagnostic feature of glaucomatous optic atrophy is the so-called *glaucomatous cup*. The increased pressure of glaucoma seems literally to push the optic disc out of the eye. Depending on the stage of the disease, the disc surface may gently slope back from the disc edge or may abruptly drop back into a deep excavation (Fig. 10-31). In either case, the abnormal contour begins at the edge of the disc, without leaving a rim of normal disc tissue in the disc periphery. The backward displacement of the disc surface is often best recognized by observing

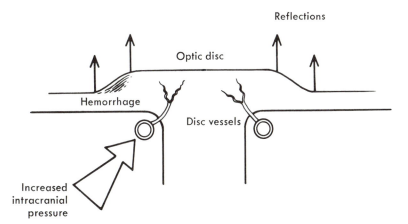

Fig. 10-30. Papilledema, caused by compression of disc capillary drainage, results in disc elevation, linear hemorrhages, and the circular reflections of edema.

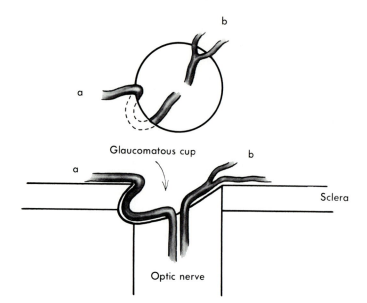

Fig. 10-31. Disappearance of retinal vessels into glaucomatous cup (no rim of normal tissue along disc edge).

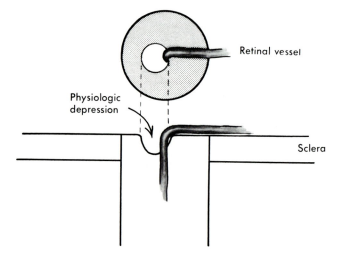

Fig. 10-32. Physiologic depression. It is important to note that, in contrast to glaucomatous cupping, a physiologic depression is entirely surrounded by a rim of normal tissue.

the course of a retinal vessel. In advanced glaucomatous cupping a retinal vessel may disappear abruptly from sight at the disc edge, only to reappear in the depths of the atrophic excavation as indicated by vessels a in Fig. 10-31. Glaucomatous atrophy often affects the two eyes unequally (in the early stages of the disease) and commonly various portions of the circumference of a glaucomatous disc are more deeply cupped than others. Usually the temporal side of the disc is more severely affected. In early glaucomatous atrophy the slight posterior sloping of the disc may be difficult to recognize, as shown with retinal vessel b in Fig. 10-31.

The student should be aware that the progress of disease only gradually changes the appearance of the optic disc from normal to that of optic atrophy, papilledema, or glaucomatous cupping. Very early ophthalmoscopic diagnosis may be impossible, but with time the characteristic features of each disease become progressively more evident. Since these diseases cause serious and permanent damage, the alert physician seeks to recognize such abnormalities as early as possible. Conversely, however, he does not wish to misdiagnose a normal anatomic variant as evidence of disease, since this causes the patient needless worry and expense.

Physiologic depression. The normal physiologic depression can easily be differentiated from a glaucomatous cup because of the presence of a rim of normal tissue in the disc periphery. The physiologic depression is within the disc and never extends to the disc edge (Fig. 10-32). The retinal vessels commonly drop abruptly over the edge of the physiologic depression—this is normal. The center of the physiologic depression may be very pale. Such central pallor does *not* indicate optic atrophy. The prominence of the physiologic depression varies greatly between patients. It may be very conspicuous or entirely absent.

The relationship of size between the cup and the disc is called the cup-disc (C/D) ratio. This is measured across the horizontal diameter of

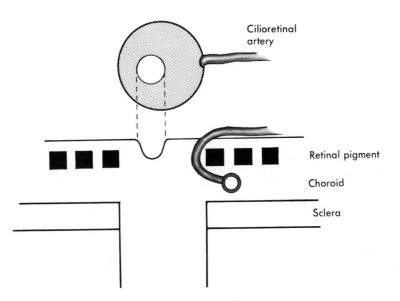

Fig. 10-33. Cilioretinal artery.

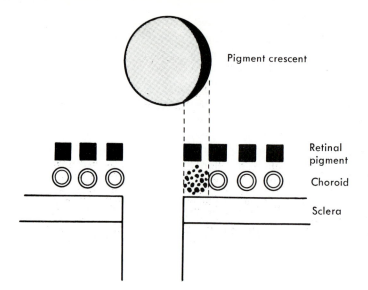

Fig. 10-34. Normal *pigment* crescent in cross section (bottom) and ophthalmoscopic view (top).

the disc and is expressed as a decimal. A C/D ratio of 0.4 means the cup occupies $^4/_{10}$ of the horizontal diameter of the disc. Normally, a physiologic cup does not exceed 0.4, and the two physiologic cups do not differ by more than 0.2. You should suspect the possibility of glaucoma if the C/D ratio is 0.5 or larger or if the two discs differ by more than 0.2.

Cilioretinal artery. Cilioretinal arteries occur on the temporal side of the disc in about 20% of patients. Although these vessels feed the retina, they do not originate from the central retinal artery but arise from the ciliary circulation (Fig. 10-33). Appearing abruptly at the disc edge, cilioretinal vessels simulate the disappearing vessels at the edge of a glaucomatous cup. The important differentiation between this common normal variant and the serious blinding disease is made by the presence of the normal disc tissue central to a cilioretinal vessel and its absence in a glaucomatous cup.

Temporal crescent. Description of the disc cannot be complete without reference to the developmental pigment crescents that so commonly lie just temporal to the disc (Fig. 10-34). Such pigment crescents are of varying width and prominence. They represent normal variants and are not to be misconstrued as disease. Although the pigmented scars of disease may somewhat resemble developmental pigment crescents, scars are much more irregular in shape and rarely conform smoothly to the disc edge.

Hemorrhage

Hemorrhage is one of the most conspicuous and significant fundus abnormalities recognizable with the ophthalmoscope. The typical red or dark appearance of a hemorrhage is obvious proof of disease, even to an inexperienced observer. The type and distribution of hemorrhages offer important clues to the diagnosis of both systemic and ocular diseases. Useful evaluation of fundus hemorrhages requires their exact localization. Fig. 10-35 is a diagrammatic cross section of the fundus. Note that two en-

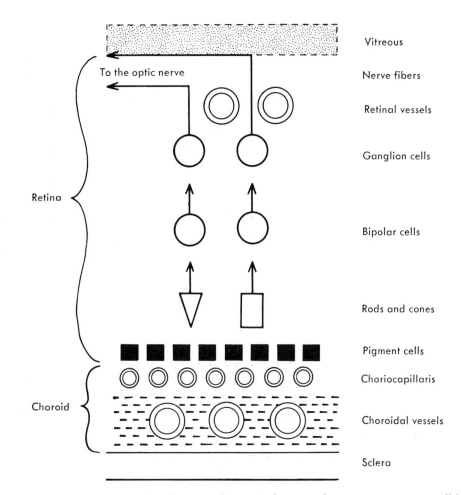

Vitreous

Nerve fibers

Retinal vessels

Ganglion cells

Bipolar cells

Rods and cones

Pigment cells

Choriocapillaris

Choroidal vessels

Sclera

To the optic nerve

Retina

Choroid

Fig. 10-35. Cross section of fundus. In subsequent drawings the various structures will be symbolized as shown here.

tirely separate circulatory networks exist: choroidal and retinal. The retinal vessels lie within the retina and tend to be near the vitreous side of the retina. The choroidal vessels nourish the outer layers of the retina by diffusion but do not physically extend into the retina.

Hemorrhages tend to form in well-defined potential spaces within the fundus (Fig. 10-36). Since the retina has a relatively compact structure, intraretinal hemorrhages are fairly small. Deep intraretinal hemorrhages are confined within the retinal substance and appear as irregularly rounded red spots. Small, rounded hemorrhages are commonly found in diabetes. Intraretinal hemorrhages in the nerve fiber layer are shaped into linear patterns by the anatomic distribution of the nerve fibers. As shown in Fig. 10-37, the nerve fibers run more or less radially toward the disc, hence the linear hemorrhages in the nerve fiber layer have a comparable orientation to the disc. Linear hemorrhages are commonly found in hyperten-

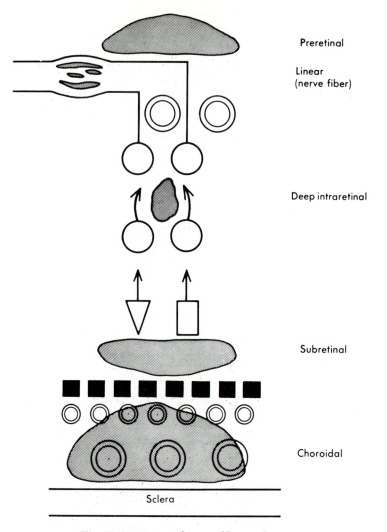

Fig. 10-36. Nomenclature of hemorrhages.

sion. Although both types of intraretinal hemorrhage are small, large numbers of such small hemorrhages may coalesce to form large red areas. To identify the type of hemorrhage, seek out the individual small components, which may be more readily separated from the red mass at the edges of a hemorrhagic area.

Hemorrhages that are superficial or deep to the retina may dissect into large potential spaces, hence are characteristically very much larger than individual intraretinal hemorrhages. These include preretinal, subretinal, and choroidal hemorrhages. Preretinal hemorrhages are most common in blood dyscrasias and subarachnoid hemorrhage. Subretinal and choroidal hemorrhages are found in chorioretinitis and senile macular degeneration.

Differentiation between these three types of

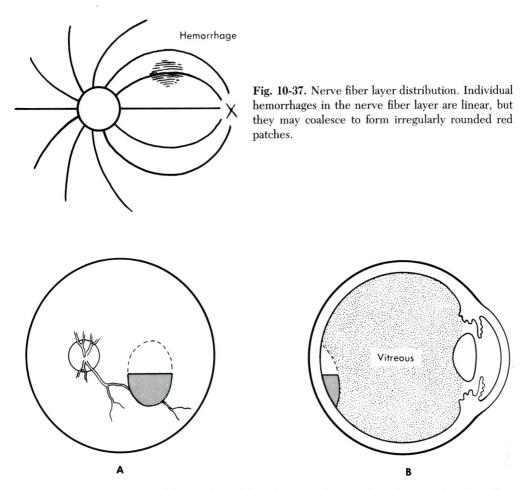

Hemorrhage

Fig. 10-37. Nerve fiber layer distribution. Individual hemorrhages in the nerve fiber layer are linear, but they may coalesce to form irregularly rounded red patches.

Vitreous

A

B

Fig. 10-38. A, Preretinal hemorrhage. Note that top of hemorrhage is a gravity-oriented straight line; hemorrhage conceals retinal vessel. **B,** Preretinal hemorrhage, confined between retina and healthy well-formed vitreous body.

large fundus hemorrhages is made on the basis of relationship to retinal vessels and the color of the hemorrhage. Obviously a preretinal hemorrhage will lie anterior to the retinal vessels and will conceal them from ophthalmoscopic view, whereas the retinal vessels are clearly visible in front of subretinal and choroidal hemorrhages. Preretinal hemorrhages frequently show a clearly defined horizontal line (gravity oriented) separating the dependent red cells from supernatant plasma (Fig. 10-38, *A*). Preretinal hemorrhages are confined between the retina and vitreous (Fig. 10-38, *B*) and are differentiated from vitreous hemorrhages, which extend into the vitreous substance.

The color of a fundus hemorrhage is modified by its relationship to the retinal pigment epithelium. As expected, preretinal and subre-

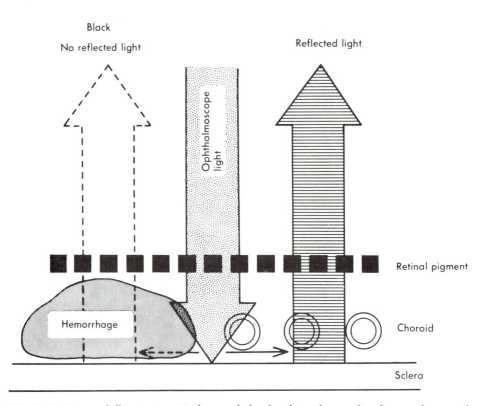

Fig. 10-39. Proximal illumination. To detect a light-absorbing abnormality deep to the retinal pigment layer, direct the ophthalmoscope light *beside* the lesion, not *on* it.

tinal hemorrhages will appear red. Choroidal hemorrhages, being deep to the retinal pigment layer, usually appear slate gray or black. This color is determined by the density of the retinal pigment.

Ophthalmoscopic light striking the choroid will scatter sideways through the tissue (Fig. 10-39). Normally, a substantial amount of this light reflects back from the sclera and is seen as the typical luminous red fundus background. If such scattered light encounters a hemorrhage, it will be absorbed and the examiner will see a nonluminous (black) area corresponding to the choroidal hemorrhage. Note that ophthalmoscopic evaluation of a choroidal lesion (deep to the retinal pigment layer) is greatly enhanced by directing the ophthalmo-

scope light adjacent to the lesions (*not* directly on it), as indicated by the beam of light in the center of Fig. 10-39. Such proximal illumination will permit easy recognition of a pigmented choroidal lesion (hemorrhage, hyperpigmentation, melanoma). Similarly, atrophic areas within the choroid will appear as light-colored defects by proximal illumination. Direct illumination of a choroidal lesion will often show nothing except the overlying retinal pigment layer, which may appear almost normal.

Hemorrhage scattered within the vitreous cavity tends to disperse and absorb light (Fig. 10-40). For this reason, the ophthalmoscopist will not see a red reflex in an eye with extensive vitreous hemorrhage but rather will perceive only darkness. The beginner might ex-

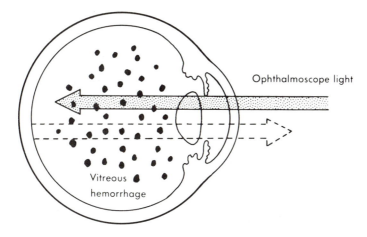

Ophthalmoscope light

Vitreous
hemorrhage

Fig. 10-40. Vitreous hemorrhage absorbs light, causing loss of the normal red reflex.

Table 10-2. Localization of hemorrhage

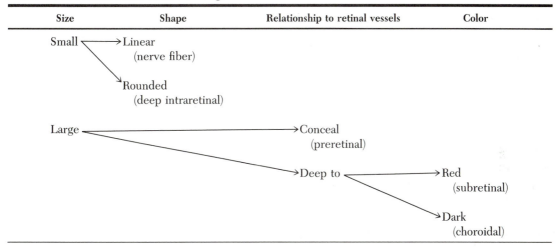

Size	Shape	Relationship to retinal vessels	Color
Small →	Linear (nerve fiber)		
	Rounded (deep intraretinal)		
Large		Conceal (preretinal)	
		Deep to →	Red (subretinal)
			Dark (choroidal)

pect vitreous hemorrhage to make the red reflex more red. This does not occur. Vitreous hemorrhage may result from injury or can develop spontaneously from diseases that damage intraocular blood vessels. Advanced diabetic retinopathy is a relatively common cause of vitreous hemorrhage. Vitreous hemorrhage may also result from purely ocular disease, such as tears of the retina.

Localization of hemorrhage. The accurate localization of hemorrhage as to its depth within the fundus (Fig. 10-36) can be presented as a series of simple steps. By the consecutive evaluation of size, shape, relationship to retinal vessels, and color, one can establish the location of a fundus hemorrhage. As indicated in Table 10-2, one first determines *size* of the hemorrhage. Small hemorrhages are evaluated as to *shape*. Hemorrhages that are linear lie in the nerve fiber layer; those that are rounded lie in the deeper retina. Large hemorrhages are evaluated as to *relationship to retinal vessels*. The hemorrhage that conceals the vessel is preretinal. When the large hemorrhage is deep to the retinal vessels, evaluate its *color*. If red, it is subretinal; if dark, it is choroidal.

Precise ophthalmoscopic information is required for this localization sequence. "Small" is defined as about the diameter of a retinal vessel near its disc origin. "Large" is any size exceeding this. Avoid the trap of misinterpreting an area containing *many small* hemorrhages as being *one large* hemorrhage. Relationship to vessels is not a conspicuous finding, but is easily observed when specifically sought. The color of a choroidal hemorrhage depends on the density of the retinal pigment epithelium—it may be almost black in a brunette or simply a shade of red in a blonde. To evaluate color, use as a color standard the blood in a retinal vein. A subretinal hemorrhage will be the same color as the venous blood, whereas hemorrhage beneath the pigment epithelium will be variably darker, depending on the pigment density.

Etiologic diagnosis is the purpose of localization of hemorrhages. To oversimplify, spontaneous bleeding originating from choroidal vessels is of degenerative or inflammatory cause; from retinal vessels, of systemic cause; from disc vessels, of neurologic cause. Choroidal vessel bleeding causes choroidal or subretinal hemorrhages. Retinal vessel bleeding causes deep intraretinal, nerve fiber layer, and preretinal hemorrhages. Disc vessel bleeding causes nerve fiber layer hemorrhages located within a disc diameter of the optic disc (*not* far away) and preretinal hemorrhages (usually near the disc, although the space between retina and vitreous is sufficiently loose to permit some migration of the blood).

Other red abnormalities

Not all red abnormalities in the fundus are hemorrhages. Microaneurysms and neovascularization are common changes characteristically found in diabetes and venous occlusion. In diabetes the distribution of the microaneurysms is relatively diffuse, though somewhat concentrated about the posterior pole (near the macula) of the eye. In venous occlusion, the microaneurysms are confined to the tributary area drained by the faulty vein.

Microaneurysms. Tiny, discrete red dots are of great diagnostic significance to the ophthalmoscopist. These dots are usually in the size range of 30 to 90 μ. Since the average large vessel leaving the disc is about 100 μ in diameter, the characteristic microaneurysm will be recognized as a red dot smaller than the caliber of a large vessel (Fig. 10-41, *A*). Close observation of a microaneurysm will reveal its edges to be smooth and discrete, as would be expected in an aneurysmal dilation of a tiny vessel (Fig. 10-41, *B*). Since microaneurysms originate from capillaries, which are too small to see with the ophthalmoscope, they appear as tiny isolated red dots with no obvious vascular connections. Very small hemorrhages may be distinguished from microaneurysms by their irregular and slightly blurred edges. In the absence of recognizable venous disease, even a few microaneurysms suggest the strong possibility of diabetes.

Neovascularization. Compact patches of new-formed blood vessels may simulate retinal hemorrhages, but are readily differentiated by recognition of the individual vessels. These abnormal new vessels are characteristically tortuous, narrow, and numerous. One reason for neovascularization is to bypass a site of venous occlusion (Fig. 10-42).

Spontaneous patches of neovascularization of similar appearance, except that they bear no relationship to an occluded vein, occur in dia-

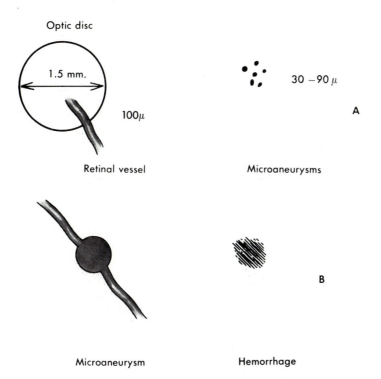

Fig. 10-41. **A,** Size relationships of microaneurysms and disc. **B,** Differentiation between microaneurysm with its sharp margins and a small hemorrhage that has irregular and blurred edges.

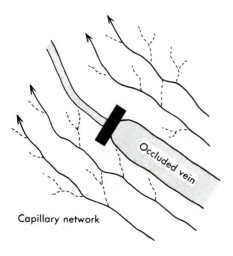

Fig. 10-42. Neovascularization to bypass site of venous occlusion. (From Havener, W. H.: Synopsis of ophthalmology, ed. 5, St. Louis, 1979, The C. V. Mosby Co.)

betic retinopathy. *Retinitis proliferans* is the name applied to the extensive growth of new vessels and accompanying connective tissue on the inner surface of the retina that may occur in diabetes. Diabetic retinopathy is now the most common cause of blindness (15%).

Retinal vessels

Observation of the retinal vessels may permit diagnosis of severe hypertension, arteriosclerosis, blood dyscrasia, and a variety of inflammatory, toxic, and degenerative changes. Study of the vessels should include evaluation of their caliber (particularly at arteriovenous crossings) and color (determined by the transparency of the vessel wall, the vascular light reflex, and any abnormal perivascular sheathing). Vessel abnormalities are usually unevenly distributed; hence, study of the retina requires orderly scanning of all the retinal vessels. Otherwise, diagnostically valuable changes in one vessel branch may be overlooked. A good method is to follow each large vessel from the disc to the periphery, returning to the disc to locate and follow out the next vessel in clockwise sequence.

Caliber. No figure can be given for the standard diameter of retinal arterioles and veins, since their size varies inversely with the number of branches. The best guide as to proper size of the vessels is the relationship of the vessel diameters to the disc diameter, as perceived by experience. In general, if an arteriole and a vein supply the same tributary area, the arteriole will probably be from two thirds to three fourths the width of the vein.

Fig. 10-43 illustrates a hypothetical retinal arteriole and vein with identical branching and tributary area. All arteriolar branches are smaller than the corresponding venous branches. However, arteriole *a* is larger than vein *b* because it supplies a larger tributary area. Note that when an arteriole is occluded (as by an embolus in arteriole *c*) the distal vessel segment is abnormally narrow, whereas occlusion of a vein (at the arteriovenous crossing

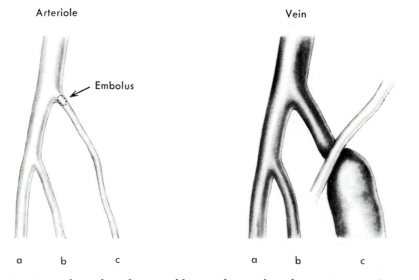

Arteriole

Embolus

Vein

a   b   c   a   b   c

Fig. 10-43. Size relationship of comparable retinal arteriole and vein. See text. (From Havener, W. H.: Synopsis of ophthalmology, ed. 5, St. Louis, 1979, The C. V. Mosby Co.)

of vein *c*) causes dilation of the distal segment.

Increase in vessel diameter is caused by diseases that cause more blood to circulate within the eye or that impede its exit from the eye. Examples of such diseases are polycythemia, carotid cavernous fistula, or venous occlusion. Decrease in vessel diameter results from functional constriction of the vessel walls, reduced inflow of blood to the eye, or retinal atrophy. Typical causes are severe hypertension, occlusion of the central retinal artery, or retinitis pigmentosa. These conditions primarily reduce the arteriolar caliber, the venous diameter often being virtually unchanged.

A localized apparent narrowing (called "nicking") of the vein is commonly seen at the arteriovenous crossings in arteriosclerosis and hypertension. This apparent narrowing is caused by partial concealment of the underlying vein by the abnormally opaque wall of the overlying diseased arteriole (Fig. 10-44). (Normally, the vessel walls are almost completely transparent.)

Although the caliber of the retinal vessels uniformly decreases toward the periphery as the branches become more numerous, such a relationship is not characteristic of the choroidal vessels. Depending somewhat unpredictably on nearness to vortex vein exits and ciliary artery entry, the choroidal vessels are extremely variable in size. No systemic or ocular abnormality can be diagnosed on the basis of caliber of choroidal vessels.

Color. Oxygenated arteriolar blood is a brighter red color than the reduced hemoglobin of the veins. Normally the ophthalmoscopist sees only the blood column of the retinal

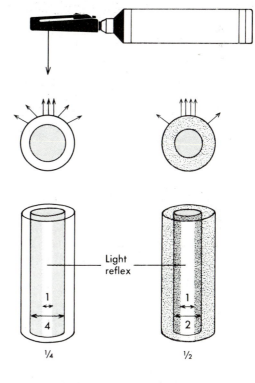

Fig. 10-45. Relationship of arteriolar light reflex and width of blood column in normal and arteriolar sclerotic vessels. (From Havener, W. H.: Synopsis of ophthalmology, ed. 5, St. Louis, 1979, The C. V. Mosby Co.)

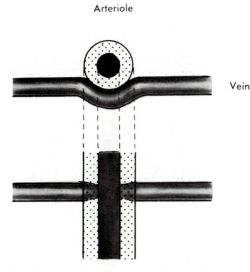

Fig. 10-44. Arteriosclerotic "nicking" of vein at arteriovenous crossing.

vessels, their walls being transparent. In arteriolar sclerosis the vessel wall becomes thicker and partially opaque (Fig. 10-45). With progressively increasing severity of arteriolar sclerosis the retinal arterioles change from red through orange, reddish gray, and finally dirty gray. Critical evaluation will reveal that part of the impression of the "color" of a vessel is caused by the width of its light reflex. The light reflex, a reflection from the vessel wall, is related to the transparency and reflectiveness of the vessel wall. Normally, the arteriolar light reflex is about one fourth the width of the blood column (Fig. 10-45). One of the early and definite signs of arteriolar sclerosis is widening of the arteriolar light reflex to one third or more of the width of the blood column, which is itself reduced in caliber.

"Sheathing" is the term applied to gray deposits surrounding a vessel wall. Sheathing may discolor the entire vessel thickness or may be more conspicuous as parallel white streaks running on each side of the vessel. Sheathing is usually the result of cellular infiltration of the perivascular spaces. Causes include leukemia, perivasculitis associated with retinal inflammations, occlusion of either arteriole or vein, and multiple sclerosis.

Light-colored retinal changes

A considerable variety of grayish or whitish changes may occur in the retina. These include exudates (soft and hard), drusen, chorioretinitis, myelinated fibers, edema, and reflections.

Exudates. Dense, grayish, localized retinal infiltrates are termed "exudates." They are of two types: "soft" and "hard." This improbable nomenclature, unverifiable by palpation, nevertheless is useful since it identifies two distinct types of retinal abnormality. Soft exudates are arteriolar microinfarctions (Fig. 10-46, A), whereas hard exudates occur in areas of stasis such as may accompany venous microinfarction (Fig. 10-46, B).

Soft exudates are somewhat fuzzy and indistinct gray patches. As would be expected from their origin as arteriolar microinfarctions, soft exudates may appear quite rapidly. Rarely are they numerous. They gradually are absorbed and disappear, leaving no visible scar.

Hard exudates are usually numerous, relatively discrete, with distinct edges and smooth, solid-appearing surfaces. They are rather small but may partially coalesce to form larger, irregular infiltrates. Characteristically, hard exudates form roughly circular patterns surrounding the venous microinfarction. Tiny hemorrhages, dilated vessels, or microaneurysms are commonly recognizable within the circle of hard exudates. Histologically, hard exudates are intraretinal lipoid deposits. These lipoid deposits develop slowly during the course of retinal disease.

Another pattern characteristic of hard exudates is the *star*, or fan, distribution, which is

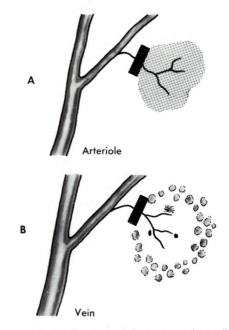

Fig. 10-46. Mechanism of formation of, **A,** "soft" and, **B,** "hard" exudates.

determined by the anatomy of the macula. The outer molecular layer of the retina slopes radially away from the fovea (Fig. 10-47). This anatomic pattern results in the typical radial distribution of hard exudates in the macula.

Exudates are conspicuous abnormalities that alert the ophthalmoscopist to search more closely for other features of diagnostic significance. The exudates themselves are of absolutely no help in making an etiologic diagnosis. Exudates may occur in many systemic diseases, including diabetes, hypertension, and collagen disorders. Also, they are found in many types of inflammatory or degenerative disease of the retina.

Drusen. Commonly seen in the eyes of older people, drusen are benign degenerative hyaline deposits on the elastic membrane between retina and choroid (Fig. 10-48). They appear as small, rounded, grayish or yellowish spots, almost always symmetrically located in the two eyes. In different individuals, drusen may be concentrated in the macula, in some sector of the periphery, or may be scattered diffusely throughout the fundus. Drusen are frequently mistaken for hard exudates. The distinction between these two lesions is important, since the presence of exudates indicates definite systemic or ocular disease demanding further investigation. The resemblance between these two entities is so close that the individual lesions may be almost identical in ophthalmoscopic appearance. The best differentiating feature is the pattern formation of hard exudates. Hard exudates frequently form circular or linear patterns, whereas drusen are haphazardly distributed. Drusen do not signify systemic disease, nor do they interfere with vision. However, senile macular degeneration is more likely to occur in patients with extensive macular drusen. Macular exudates ordinarily produce extensive loss of central vision.

Chorioretinitis. Acute focal inflammation of choroid and retina causes localized infiltration of inflammatory cells, the ophthalmoscopic appearance of which is very similar to that of a soft exudate. Accurate differentiation is usually possible on the basis of associated changes. An encircling halo of retinal edema invariably surrounds acute chorioretinitis, but is not often prominent around exudates. Hemorrhages are often found within or immediately adjacent to a focus of chorioretinitis. Since hemorrhages and exudates also often coexist, this feature would seem to be of little diagnostic value.

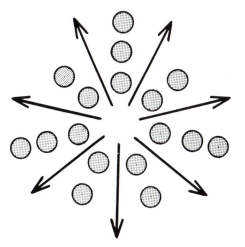

Fig. 10-47. Radial anatomic configuration at macula, illustrating formation of "star" pattern of exudates.

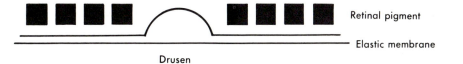

Drusen

Retinal pigment

Elastic membrane

Fig. 10-48. Drusen formation that results from localized disruption of pigment layer.

However, the hemorrhages of chorioretinitis are typically choroidal as well as subretinal, whereas those associated with exudates are retinal. (An exception to this is macular degeneration, which sometimes produces choroidal hemorrhages and retinal exudates.) Because they are covered by the retinal pigment layer, choroidal hemorrhages are much darker than the typically bright red retinal hemorrhages; hence, ophthalmoscopic differentiation is easy.

Acute chorioretinitis is usually localized to a relatively small area, whereas the conditions causing soft exudates commonly produce recognizable abnormalities throughout much of the retina, bilaterally. Chorioretinitis has a tendency to recur at a nearby site; therefore, the atrophic and pigmented scars of old chorioretinitis will often be found adjacent to an acute chorioretinitis. Soft exudates do not cause pigmentary disturbances. With time, chorioretinitis subsides, leaving a scar within which the retina and choroid are partially destroyed. The pigment has aggregated into irregular clumps that often line the edge of the lesion, more or less gray scar tissue is deposited, and the sclera may be partly visible. No edema or hemorrhage is found in a completely inactive scar.

Myelinated fibers. Normally the nerve fiber layer of the retina is unmyelinated. In about 0.5% of patients a small sector of the nerve fiber layer is myelinated. This appears as a light-gray patch, usually but not always adjoining the disc margin. Within the patch the individual myelinated axons are confluent and cannot be differentiated. The peripheral edges of a myelin patch will often appear frayed, resembling a feather's edge. This is because the myelin sheaths are of unequal length, a few extending beyond the others. Obviously, myelin sheaths will run in the same direction as the nerve fiber axons—radially away from the disc (Fig. 10-49). Any lesion oriented in another direction cannot be a myelinated fiber.

Myelinated fibers remain unchanged throughout adult life and do not cause pathologic conditions such as edema or hemorrhage. Recognition of myelinated fibers is primarily important to avoid confusion with inflammation, exudates, or papilledema. Perhaps the most common serious mistake is to misinter-

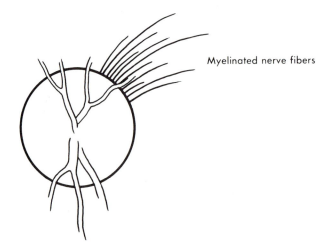

Myelinated nerve fibers

Fig. 10-49. Myelinated nerve fibers in ophthalmoscopic view.

pret myelinated fibers adjacent to the disc as representing papilledema. This differential diagnosis is easily made since the disc area is abnormally hyperemic in papilledema and abnormally pale with myelinated fibers.

Edema. An edematous retina is less transparent than normal and consequently will appear gray. The density of this discoloration varies with the amount of edema, ranging from obvious change to an inconspicuous delicate haze recognizable only by comparison with the opposite normal eye. The surface of an edematous retina shows more glistening reflections than normal, although in a young person very similar reflections are physiologic. Reflections are particularly well defined at the edge of an area of edema.

Edema is present only around recent or continuing lesions and is therefore a sign of active disease. Furthermore, edema is confined to the diseased portion of the retina. In papilledema or optic neuritis, edema will be confined to the region near the disc. Edema will surround an area of active chorioretinitis but disappears when the inflammation becomes inactive. Edema involves the retina diffusely in such conditions as hypertensive retinopathy, occlusion of the central retinal artery, or ocular contusion. When diffuse retinal edema is present, the gray discoloration is always more pronounced posteriorly, since the retina is thickest centrally. Edema is present in almost all acute retinal disorders, but is absent in chronic or inactive conditions.

Reflections. Retinal reflections are prominent in the healthy young eye and in areas of edema. Reflections are identified as such because they move as the position of the ophthalmoscope is changed, altering the incidence of light on the retina. In contrast, a definite pathologic condition, such as an exudate, will not move as do reflections. In a photograph, reflections and exudates may be indistinguishable.

Reflections are most prominent at changes of curvature (Fig. 10-50). Hence, reflections are normally seen along the course of retinal blood vessels, around the macula, and in the fovea centralis. Similarly, the edges of an area of inflammatory edema will cast characteristic reflections.

Delicate scar tissue may proliferate on the inner surface of the retina in chronic nutritional disorders, such as diabetic retinopathy or vascular occlusion. This scar tissue tends to shrink, producing a corrugated contour, somewhat like wrinkled cellophane. Although such scar tissue is invisible, its presence can be accurately inferred by recognition of the abnormal wrinkled pattern of retinal reflections.

Differential diagnosis of light-colored fundus changes

Ideally, light-colored fundus changes should be evaluated in a systematic sequence, such as has already been described for the accurate localization of hemorrhages. Unfortunately, such a large number of pale abnormalities exist that

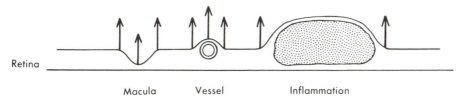

Fig. 10-50. Reflections are most prominent at changes of curvature, as seen along vessels, about the macula, and at the edges of edematous areas.

their classification in a foolproof diagnostic sequence is impossible. Hence, ophthalmoscopic diagnosis of pale lesions must proceed in a trial-and-error sequence that may be described as *hypothesis–evaluation–accept/reject*. In other words, the examiner selects a likely diagnosis, then looks more closely for the characteristic features that he knows will be present or that cannot be present in a given diagnosis. If the first diagnosis is rejected, a second is chosen and undergoes evaluation; this process continues until a diagnosis is found that is compatible with all the fundus findings.

Obviously, successful diagnosis of a pale fundus lesion requires knowledge of the various types of light-colored changes that may exist. Fortunately, the endless number of pale lesions can be reduced to perhaps nine relatively common entities. The remaining disorders (for example, tuberous sclerosis, retinoblastoma) are so rare that they are of little practical significance in a scheme of differential diagnosis. Diagrammatic representation of these nine common pale changes (Fig. 10-51) will help to indicate their diagnostic characteristics. A particularly noteworthy feature of this diagram is

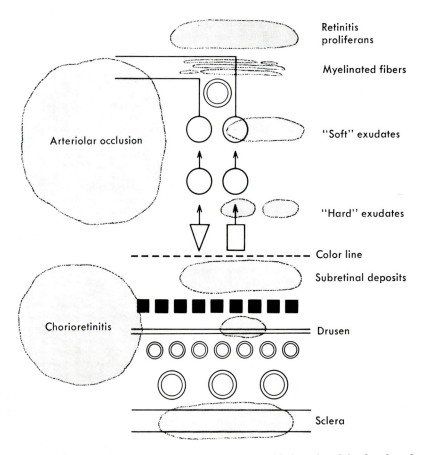

Fig. 10-51. Schematic drawing of representative types of light-colored fundus disorders.

the *color line*. Conditions anterior to this level do not cause melanin changes. Conditions posterior to this line characteristically result in recognizable proliferation or atrophy of pigment.

More accurate selection of a diagnosis for the original hypothesis can be made if some sort of rational process is followed. As an example, study the diagram above. A logical beginning is to note the *size* of the pale lesion. If it is very small (1 or 2 vessel diameters), it is probably either a hard exudate or a drusen. Note whether the lesion is faintly refractile or translucent (which indicates it is composed of hyaline material and is therefore a drusen) or whether it is light absorbing, somewhat like a piece of white blotting paper (which indicates it is a lipoidal deposit—a hard exudate).

Unfortunately, whether a pale lesion is of medium or large size is not very helpful because the size is so variable in individual cases.

Next consider *relationship to vessels*. If the lesion is entirely anterior to the retinal vessels, it is probably retinitis proliferans. This is a common finding in blinding diabetic retinopathy and consists of a fibrovascular new-formed membrane growing on the inner surface of the retina. If the white area is below the choroidal vessels, it represents sclera that has become exposed to ophthalmoscopic view by loss of the overlying pigment layers. If the white area is elongated and located in the area nourished by a retinal arteriole, it represents opaque, dead retina resulting from arteriolar occlusion.

Color (presence or absence of melanin change) should next be evaluated. If there is no melanin disturbance, a rounded pale lesion somewhat smaller than the disc is probably a soft exudate. If the lesion is striated, it is a patch of myelinated nerve fibers.

Obvious melanin disturbance suggests a chorioretinitis (which is almost always flat) or a subretinal deposit (usually a variant of macular degeneration), which is often slightly elevated.

Size

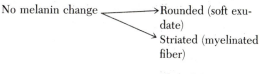

Relationship to vessels

Conceals retinal vessels→(retinitis proliferans)
Below choroidal vessels→(sclera)
Tributary to retinal arteriole→(occluded arteriole)

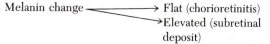

Macula

Most macular lesions (for example, hemorrhage, exudates, and edema) are comparable in appearance and course to the changes of similar cause that occur throughout the fundus. Because of the much higher visual acuity of the fovea, however, a tiny macular lesion may be disabling, in contrast to a considerably larger peripheral lesion that may pass almost unnoticed by the patient. Decreased visual acuity definitely indicates careful ophthalmoscopic examination of the macula. Dilation of the pupil with a mydriatic is often necessary for adequate macular visualization.

Many normal variants exist at the macula. Quite frequently the pigment is clumped into a peculiar granular distribution. A circular reflection, resembling edema, commonly surrounds the macula. The macula is usually slightly darker than the surrounding retina.

Senile macular degeneration is a relatively common disorder unique to the macula. This condition is slowly progressive and will ultimately destroy central vision. The peripheral retina remains unaffected. The ophthalmo-

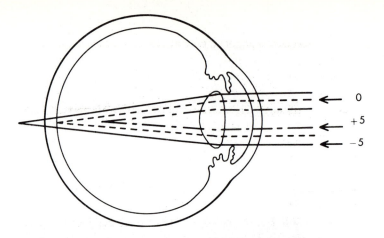

Fig. 10-52. Dioptric focusing of ophthalmoscope within the eye.

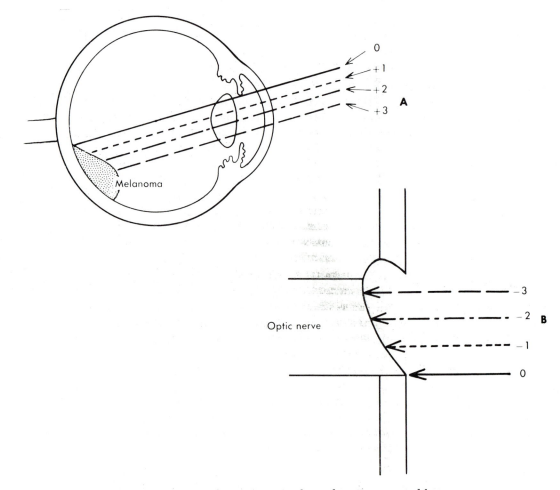

Fig. 10-53. Dioptric focusing on, **A**, elevated or, **B**, excavated lesions.

scopic appearance of senile macular degeneration is subject to great individual variation and may closely simulate chorioretinitis, hemorrhagic diseases, or even neoplasm. Hyperpigmentation, depigmentation, hemorrhages, exudates, scar tissue, elevated masses, cysts, or retinal holes may be seen in various forms of senile macular degeneration. Such gross discrepancies may exist between the changes observed with the ophthalmoscope and the degree of visual loss that prediction of visual acuity on the basis of fundus observation is never safe. Neither is it safe to assume that all such changes do indeed represent an untreatable macular degeneration.

Determination of depth

The simplest quantitative measurement of depth within the eye is the dioptric focusing of the ophthalmoscope. In the emmetropic eye, the zero lens focuses on the fundus (excluding accommodation by patient or examiner). Plus lenses focus forward within the eye, whereas minus lenses focus backward (Fig. 10-52). Three diopters of lens power represent 1 mm. of distance. The height of a raised lesion, such as a melanoma (Fig. 10-53, *A*), or the depth of an excavation, such as a glaucomatous cup (Fig. 10-53, *B*), can be measured dioptrically.

Parallax, a nonquantitative method of determining elevation, is extremely valuable in recognizing slight elevation of a structure within the eye. As illustrated in Fig. 10-54, deliberate movement of the ophthalmoscope in any direction (this movement is limited by pupil size) will cause recognizable shifting of the background behind any elevated detail. No such background shift will occur if the detail is not elevated. Parallax is a useful method of proving the elevation of a foreign body or hemorrhage within the vitreous or of demonstrating the elevation of a vessel within a detached retina above the underlying choroid.

An extremely precise method of determining depth within the fundus utilizes relationships to structures of known depth. The most con-

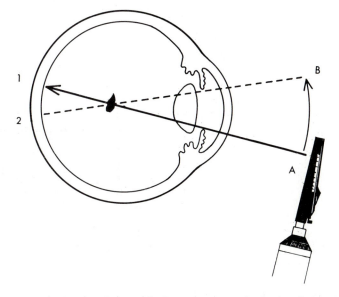

Fig. 10-54. Parallax movement of elevated object against its background. Movement of the ophthalmoscope from position *A* to position *B* will result in background shift from *1* to *2*.

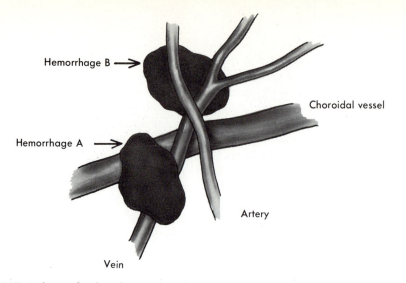

Hemorrhage B →

Choroidal vessel

Hemorrhage A →

Artery

Vein

Fig. 10-55. Relative depth judgment based on concealment of deeper details by overlying structures.

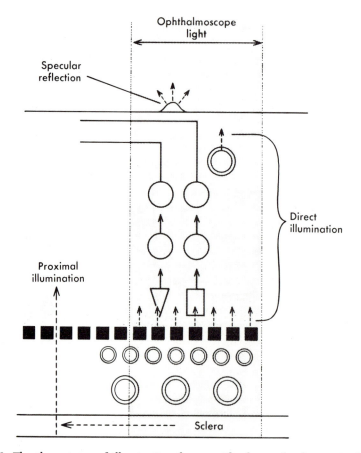

Ophthalmoscope light

Specular reflection

Direct illumination

Proximal illumination

Sclera

Fig. 10-56. The three types of illumination that provide the total information that can be gained from ophthalmoscopy.

venient such reference points are the retinal and choroidal vessels. For example, a hemorrhage that conceals the retinal vessels (Fig. 10-55, *A*) must be anterior to them. Conversely, a concealed hemorrhage (Fig. 10-55, *B*) must be posterior to the vessels.

Illumination techniques

Almost everyone just aims the ophthalmoscope light steadily at the detail under observation. This technique is wrong. Ophthalmoscopy consists of evaluation of the fundus by three separate methods: direct illumination, proximal illumination, and specular reflection. The light should be *moved* during examination of every noteworthy detail so that all three methods of illumination are employed. As shown in Fig. 10-56, direct illumination evaluates the surface of opaque structure, such as retinal pigment, retinal vessels, disc, or opaque pathology *anterior* to the pigment layer.

Proximal illumination scatters sidewise through the sclera and returns to the observer from *behind* the pigment. Abnormal density or rarefaction of pigmentation is recognizable at an early stage by proximal illumination. Of course, gross pigment changes are recognizable by direct illumination. Properly used proximal illumination reveals whether a lesion is anterior or posterior to the important diagnostic color line (Fig. 10-51). In proximal illumination the ophthalmoscope light is directed *adjacent* to the area under observation.

Specular reflection is a mirror reflection of light from the anterior retinal surface, within the directly illuminated area. It is the most delicate method of evaluating surface detail. Exaggerated specular reflections exist in edema and in gliosis of the retina, two of the most common pathologic responses of this tissue.

To illustrate the use of these techniques, direct illumination would be best for the examination of an arteriovenous crossing in search of the "nicking" of the vein characteristic of arteriosclerosis. Specular reflection would be the best way to examine the area adjacent to the disc in papilledema in an attempt to confirm the diagnosis by recognizing the presence of edema adjacent to the disc. Proximal illumination would be best for the examination of the macula in search of the faint pigment rarefaction characteristic of early senile macular degeneration in an older person complaining of failing vision.

Diagnosis of individual diseases

Further detailed description of the ophthalmoscopic appearances of various ocular and systemic diseases, together with their cause, symptoms, course, and treatment, is inappropriate in this text. However, the student should know that such ophthalmoscopic diagnoses are possible on the basis of the types of abnormality recognized within the fundus and their distribution. For example, the diagnosis of partial occlusion of a venous branch (Fig. 10-57) is made by recognizing that disease exists within the tributary area of a venous branch.

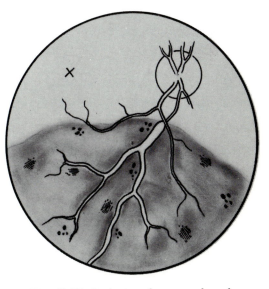

Fig. 10-57. Occlusion of a venous branch.

This occlusion is characteristically peripheral to an arteriovenous crossing that shows recognizable arterial compression of the vein. Venous caliber is typically enlarged peripheral to the site of partial occlusion. Within the tributary area are characteristic intraretinal hemorrhages (both linear and small rounded), as would be expected in a region of venous congestion. Hard and soft exudates may also be found in this tributary area. With time, microaneurysms and neovascularization develop. The implications of retinal venous branch occlusion extend, of course, beyond the eye. Such occlusions do not occur in healthy individuals and are a manifestation of rather severe vascular or thrombotic disease (for example, polycythemia, hypertension, or diabetes). Life expectancy is significantly reduced in a patient who is suffering from spontaneous retinal venous occlusions.

Proficiency in ophthalmoscopy is gained only through practice. Examine the eyes of every patient. This will soon lead to a considerable degree of skill in ophthalmoscopy. Remember, a greater variety of diseases can be diagnosed with the ophthalmoscope than by any other single examining instrument except one—the autopsy surgeon's scalpel!

SELECTED READINGS

Adler, F. H.: Gifford's textbook of ophthalmology, ed. 7, Philadelphia, 1962, W. B. Saunders Co.

Havener, W. H.: Synopsis of ophthalmology, ed. 5, St. Louis, 1979, The C. V. Mosby Co.

CHAPTER 11

EARS, NOSE, AND THROAT

Examination of the ears, nose, and throat is basically a study of epithelium. Using brilliant illumination the physician is able to inspect directly or indirectly most parts of the upper respiratory passages. A few parts, such as the nasal accessory sinuses and the middle ear, cannot be directly visualized. Nevertheless the examiner is usually able to infer the condition of these cavities by the appearance of adjacent mucous membranes.

A great many lighting systems are used. Some are entirely inadequate, such as the flashlight or otoscope (when used anywhere except in the ear). Others, such as electric headlights, are of variable worth, depending on their brightness.

The light par excellence is that reflected from the otolaryngologist's head mirror. The mirror should have a focal length of about 10 inches, certainly no more than 12 inches. A clear 150-watt light bulb provides the light source and is placed just behind and to the right of the patient.

To adjust the head mirror, first place it well down over the left eye so that the back of the mirror actually touches the skin or glasses (Fig. 11-1). Then close the right eye and focus the light on the patient's face to a small, brilliant

spot. Too often the beginner fails to keep the light bright by neglecting to move his head toward or away from the patient. Obviously, since the focal length of the mirror is fixed, the only way the examiner can maintain a sharp focus is by adjusting his head position. Once the left eye is focused, the right eye may be opened for binocular vision.

After a little experience, focusing becomes automatic and preliminary monocular focusing is not necessary.

The tongue depressor is held in the left hand so that the right hand is free to hold other instruments (Fig. 11-2). Tongue blades may be of either the wooden or metal type. Most examiners prefer the wooden ones.

The blade is best placed on the middle third of the tongue. If placed too far anteriorly, the blade causes the posterior part of the tongue to mound up so as to obscure rather than to expose the pharynx. On the other hand, most patients gag if the blade touches the posterior third of the tongue.

The correct maneuver depresses the tongue and scoops it forward at the same time. The blade is held in the corner of the mouth so that it will not be in the way of the instruments held in the right hand. The examiner should be

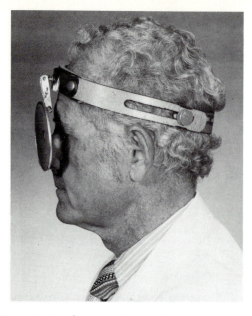

Fig. 11-1. Head mirror. Notice that it is very close to the eye. A common mistake is to wear mirror away from face, which markedly reduces the field of vision.

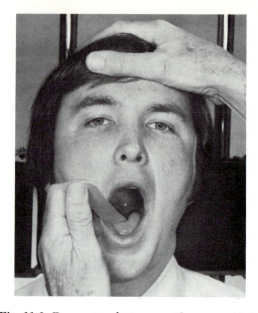

Fig. 11-2. Depressing the tongue. The tongue blade is held in the left hand, which leaves the right hand free for positioning of the head and the use of other instruments. The hand is braced on the patient's cheek as the tongue is depressed and scooped forward.

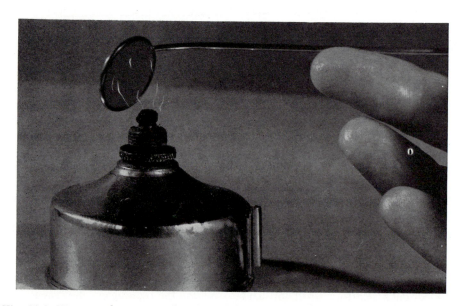

Fig. 11-3. Warming the mirror. The glass surface is placed directly over the flame. (From DeWeese, D. D., and Saunders, W. H.: Textbook of otolaryngology, ed. 5, St. Louis, 1977, The C. V. Mosby Co.)

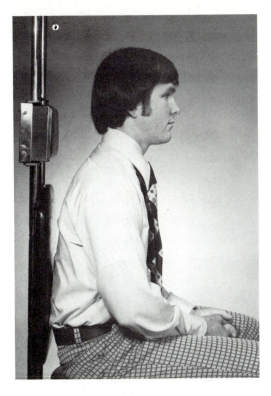

Fig. 11-4. Proper position of the patient; head drawn forward, back away from chair, and knees together. Notice that the headrest is not used.

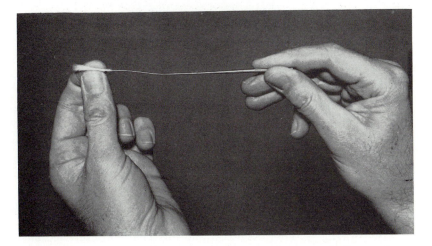

Fig. 11-5. Winding a cotton applicator. A wisp of cotton is wrapped around the end of a metal applicator. Notice that the tuft is small and the metal applicator tip is not at the very end.

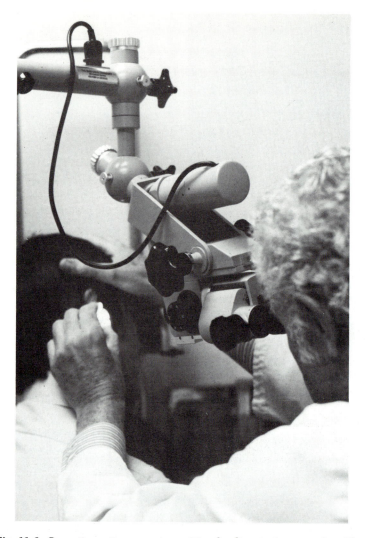

Fig. 11-6. Operating microscope in position for diagnostic use in the office.

careful not to press the patient's lower lip against the teeth.

The tongue is a strong, muscular organ. The examiner need not (and occasionally cannot) depress the entire tongue at one time. Sometimes, in order to press more firmly, two tongue blades may be used, one placed on top of the other.

Warming the mirror to be used in examining the nasopharynx or larynx in the flame of an alcohol lamp prevents fogging (Fig. 11-3). The glass surface of the mirror is placed directly into the flame for a few seconds. The back of the mirror is then tested for warmth on the examiner's hand. In examining children, rather than using the open flame from an alcohol lamp, which may be alarming, simply dipping the mirror in a container of warm water will help to prevent fogging.

The patient's position is very important in otolaryngic examinations. He should sit very erect with his head 10 to 12 inches forward from the back of the chair (Fig. 11-4). Many patients tend to slump and to slide their hips forward in the chair. The use of headrests is discouraged because they fix the head in one position and hinder the adjustments of the head position, which are constantly required. The correct position is not restful, but the examination is not so long as to be tiring.

The cotton applicator is one of the most useful instruments in otolaryngic examination. The examiner must learn to prepare his own, because commercial applicators are never satisfactory (Fig. 11-5). A stiff wire applicator is used, and a small piece of loose cotton is wound around it. The tip of the applicator is placed in the center of the cotton, and the cotton is twisted onto the applicator. This method leaves a small tuft at the end. The tuft may be firmed or left loose, as the situation demands. Beginners tend to make their applicators too thick, or fail to have a very small tuft at the tip.

The operating microscope (Fig. 11-6) has become an important instrument for careful examination of the ears. It provides brilliant lighting, useful magnification from about 4.5 to 16 times, and, very importantly, *binocular vision*. The expense of this instrument takes it out of reach of the occasional examiner, but its worth should be appreciated by all. Manipulations in the ear canal, myringotomy, and aspiration of pus or removal of polyps from the middle ear are greatly facilitated.

The operating microscope, which is used in modern aural surgery, is being used more and more in laryngeal endoscopic procedures. It is also used occasionally in physical examination of the nose and larynx in the physician's office.

EARS

Inspection of the external ear is so obvious that it is frequently neglected. It should require only a few seconds. Occasionally *tophi*, which are small white deposits of uric acid crystals caused by gout, are seen along the margins of the auricle. The gnarled, thickened *cauliflower ear* is the result of repeated trauma to the cartilage. Evidence of injury and congenital malformation are usually obvious.

Next the examiner inspects the external auditory canal and the tympanic membrane. In physical diagnosis the tympanic membrane, or eardrum, may be regarded as a translucent membrane through which the otologist views normal anatomy and also pathologic processes in the middle ear.

Cleaning the ear canal. The most important step in preparing for examination of the eardrum is making sure that the ear canal and surface of the drumhead are clean. Wax, particulate matter, pus and secretions must be meticulously removed. This precaution seems obvious, but neglect of this preliminary step is the rule. Actually, an experienced examiner may take several minutes to remove debris from the ear canal before he is ready to study the eardrum.

There are several methods of cleaning the ear canal. The most common method is to remove particulate matter with a cerumen spoon or cotton applicator by direct vision through the ear speculum (Figs. 11-5 and 11-7).

Irrigation (Fig. 11-8) is also important. Tap water at body temperature is used because water at any other temperature stimulates the inner ear and causes dizziness. If the cerumen to be removed is solidly impacted and especially if it is dry and hard, then irrigation may not be successful unless preceded by having the patient instill a few drops of mineral oil, or so-called "sweet oil," in the ear for three or four nights. This softens the cerumen and makes it easy to remove by irrigation.

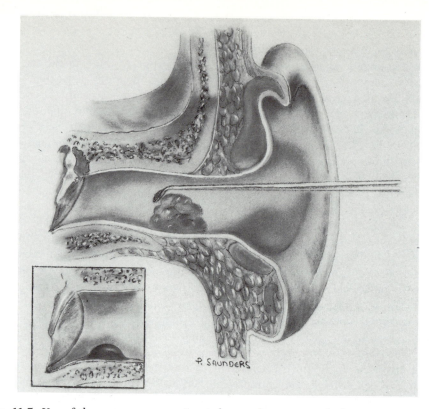

Fig. 11-7. Use of the cerumen spoon. Inset shows a hematoma, which is easy to produce unless care is taken. (From DeWeese, D. D., and Saunders, W. H.: Textbook of otolaryngology, ed. 5, St. Louis, 1977, The C. V. Mosby Co.)

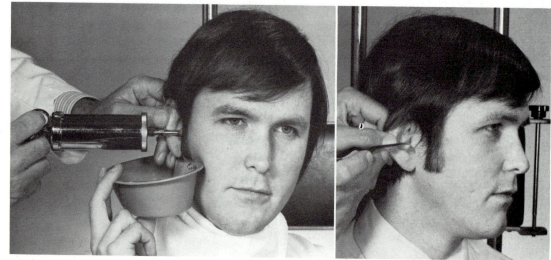

Fig. 11-8. A, Aural irrigation using tap water at body temperature. **B,** Drying the ear canal after irrigation.

A No. 5 or No. 7 angulated suction tip may be employed to aspirate semiliquid cerumen or pus. This method is gentle, since the end of the suction tip actually need not touch the epithelium of the ear canal or drumhead. Suction is of no use for removing dry cerumen or most other solid material.

A good way to begin the examination is to pull the auricle upward and backward and the tragus forward (Fig. 11-9). This maneuver opens the meatus and may even provide a good view of the drumhead. It also allows the examiner to select a proper-sized aural speculum.

Examination with the aural speculum. Most otologists employ a metal ear speculum and a head mirror to examine the eardrum. Most other practitioners use an electric otoscope (Fig. 11-10). Whichever method is used, the principles of examination are the same. The speculum selected should be the *largest* that will fit the canal. The student usually makes the mistake of choosing a small speculum when he could use a large one.

The speculum is inserted to straighten and slightly dilate the cartilaginous ear canal (Fig. 11-11). About halfway to the eardrum the cartilage ends and the supporting wall becomes osseous. Here speculum pressure is painful. The epithelium lining the bony portion of the canal is very thin and exquisitely sensitive. One must be very gentle when cleaning the inner half of the ear canal, even more so than when cleaning the outer surface of the drumhead. In adults the ear canal may be straightened by pulling upward and backward on the auricle; in young children and infants it is straightened by pulling the auricle downward.

The position of the patient's head is most important in aural examination (Fig. 11-12). It might be thought that with the patient's head perfectly upright the examiner could look directly into the ear canal and see the drumhead. This is a common error. Because of the oblique direction of the ear canal, the patient's head must be tipped sidewise (toward the opposite shoulder) for easy examination of the canal and drumhead. Students who neglect this step find that they are looking at the wall of the ear canal and not at the drumhead. It is usually necessary to *change the head position several times*

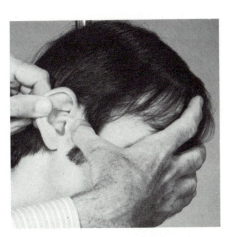

Fig. 11-9. Spreading the meatus—a preliminary step.

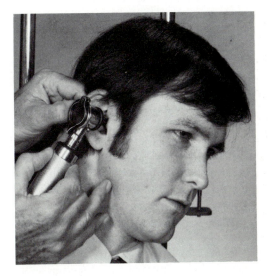

Fig. 11-10. Electric otoscope. Traction on the auricle straightens the canal.

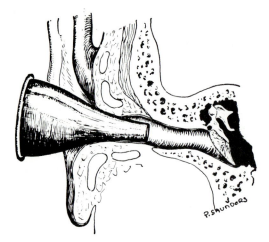

Fig. 11-11. The speculum dilates and straightens the cartilaginous ear canal. If it is pressed against the bony canal, it causes pain. (From DeWeese, D. D., and Saunders, W. H.: Textbook of otolaryngology, ed. 5, St. Louis, 1977, The C. V. Mosby Co.)

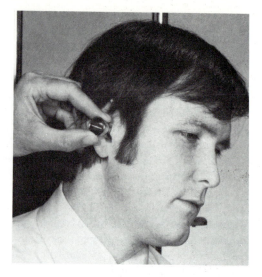

Fig. 11-12. Note the head is tipped to one side. Also note how one hand holds both the speculum and auricle.

in order to visualize all parts of the tympanic membrane.

Layers of drumhead. There are three layers in the drumhead: an outer squamous epithelium, an inner cuboidal epithelium, and a middle fibrous layer. This is the structure of the *pars tensa*, which comprises almost all of the drumhead. In a very small part superiorly, known as the *pars flaccida*, the middle fibrous layer is absent. When perforations heal in the drumhead, the area of perforation is often very translucent or even transparent. The reason is that the perforation repairs without a fibrous layer. The healing also leaves this portion of the drumhead flaccid and therefore more easily moved by pneumatic pressure (through an otoscope) than the rest of the drumhead.

Color of drumhead. The color of the drumhead is very important because it is relatively constant in health. The normal drumhead is usually described as pearly gray. In disease the color may be yellow or amber (serum in the middle ear), blue (*hemotympanum*), dead

white (pus in the middle ear), or red or pink (*myringitis*, or infection of the drumhead). Ordinarily the tympanic membrane is quite shiny.

Dense white plaques seen in some drumheads represent a process called *tympanosclerosis*, a result of healed inflammatory disease. Other patients have less distinctly marked deposits of tympanosclerosis, producing white flecks scattered throughout the pars tensa. Ordinarily these deposits cause no significant change in hearing unless they are associated with more extensive deposits in the epitympanum (attic), which fuse together the malleus and incus or fuse one of these bones to the wall of the epitympanum.

Position of drumhead. The position of the drumhead is oblique with respect to the ear canal (Fig. 11-13). The upper posterior part of the drumhead is closer to the examiner's eye than is the lower anterior part. This obliqueness is more pronounced in infants than in adults. Sometimes all of the drumhead cannot be seen because the floor of the ear canal is at

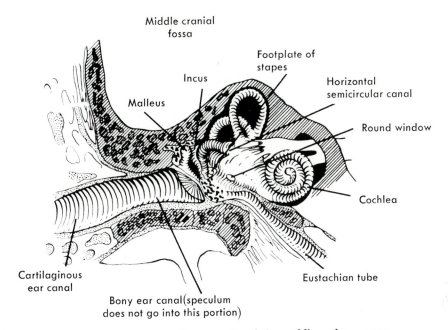

Middle cranial fossa

Footplate of stapes

Incus

Horizontal semicircular canal

Malleus

Round window

Cochlea

Cartilaginous ear canal

Eustachian tube

Bony ear canal(speculum does not go into this portion)

Fig. 11-13. External auditory canal and the middle and inner ear.

a higher level than the lowermost part of the drumhead. Also, the anterior part of the drumhead may be hidden by prominence of the bony wall of the ear canal.

The drumhead is also very slightly conical with the concavity external. When pus forms in the middle ear because of otitis media, intratympanic pressures are raised and the drumhead actually bulges outward. Sometimes this bulging is in one part of the drumhead only; at other times the entire drumhead bulges so that none of the landmarks are seen.

A "retracted" drumhead occurs when intratympanic pressures are reduced. Then the entire drumhead is pressed inward by outside atmospheric pressure, and the malleus is left in sharp outline. The malleolar folds are accentuated. This alteration of tympanic pressure is common. It occurs when the eustachian tube is obstructed (because of adenoiditis in the child, for example, or too rapid descent during air

travel in the adult). Whatever the cause, the tube no longer ventilates the middle ear properly, and oxygen is absorbed from the middle ear and mastoid air cells into the bloodstream. A partial vacuum results. A transudate of blood serum then partially fills the middle ear to relieve the vacuum, and the drumhead appears yellow. An air-fluid level may also be seen, or bubbles of air may appear in the amber fluid.

Landmarks. The landmarks visible in the normal drumhead vary with differences in translucency of the drumhead (Fig. 11-14). The *malleus* is the primary landmark. At the upper end of the malleus the lateral, or short, process stands out as a tiny knob. The manubrium, or the handle, of the malleus extends downward from the short process to the *umbo*. Both the short process and the manubrium are embedded in the eardrum.

When bulging of the drumhead occurs, the manubrium and short process become less and

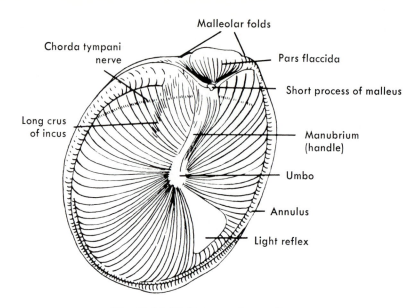

Fig. 11-14. Right tympanic membrane.

less well seen until they finally disappear. On the other hand, when the drumhead is retracted, the malleus stands out very prominently, and the short process shines chalky white through the drumhead.

The *anterior* and *posterior malleolar folds* are seen superiorly and enclose between them the *pars flaccida*. These folds of epithelium become more prominent when the drumhead is retracted.

The *annulus* is the peripheral fibrous ring of the tympanic membrane that fits in the tympanic sulcus. It looks whiter or denser than the rest of the drumhead. It is complete except superiorly, where it is deficient between the anterior and posterior malleolar folds. The importance of the annulus in aural diagnosis cannot be stressed too much. It is at the periphery of the drumhead that important perforations often occur, and they will not be found unless the annulus is systematically examined.

The *light reflex* or cone of light reflects from the anterior-inferior quadrant when the drumhead is in normal position and its outer epithelium is normal. The light reflex extends inferiorly and anteriorly from the umbo. Sometimes the reflex becomes broken or muddled, and sometimes it is missing altogether. Such changes usually indicate a disease state, but too much emphasis should not be placed on variations of the light reflex alone.

The *long process of the incus* is frequently visible posterior to the manubrium of the malleus. Whether or not it can be seen depends on the translucency of the tympanic membrane and the shape of the posterior wall of the bony ear canal.

Also seen in some ears is the *chorda tympani nerve*. It crosses transversely behind the drumhead at about the level of the short process of the malleus.

EXAMINATION OF HEARING

A hearing test should be part of every physical examination. Although precise measurement requires use of elaborate instruments, a

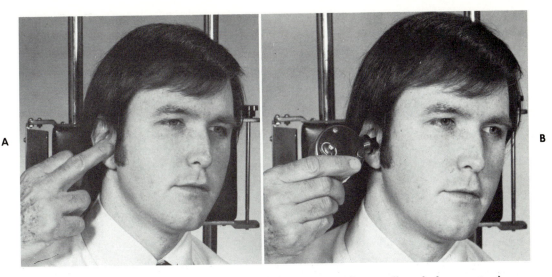

Fig. 11-15. Masking the ear not being tested. **A,** A moving finger will mask the examiner's whispered or low voice but not a loud voice. **B,** A Barany noisebox used to mask more intense sound. A loud noise in one ear usually has little effect on the hearing of the other ear.

reasonably accurate estimate of hearing can be made by any physician who understands a few basic principles. For testing hearing in the office or at the bedside the only instruments needed are one or two tuning forks, a masking device, and the examiner's own voice.

Types of hearing loss

Conductive. Conductive hearing loss occurs in patients with external or middle ear disorders. Their inner ears are expected to be normal. Examples of conditions that cause conductive hearing loss are cerumen impacted in the external auditory canal, perforation of the tympanic membrane, serum or pus in the middle ear, fixation of the stapes in the oval window (otosclerosis), and adhesions between the middle ear bones. Conductive hearing loss is always only a partial loss. Consequently these patients hear *perfectly* if the sound level is raised sufficiently to transmit sound pressure to their inner ears.

Sensorineural or perceptive. In patients with nerve or perceptive hearing loss the external and middle ears are normal, but there is disease in the inner ear, the auditory nerve, or the brain. Sensorineural loss contrasts sharply with conductive loss. For one thing, in sensorineural loss there is no effective medical or surgical treatment. Also, even though sound is increased in intensity so that the patient can hear, he may still fail to *understand* clearly the spoken word.

Mixed. Mixed loss means a combination of middle ear and sensorineural types of hearing loss and is common.

Importance of masking

In testing hearing it is extremely important to make certain that only one ear is tested at a time. In other words, the *opposite ear must be excluded from test* by masking it with noise. No one makes the error of failing to cover a patient's right eye when testing the left eye, but it is commonplace for an examiner to fail to mask the right ear when testing the left ear. If proper masking is not used, sound presented to the poorer ear is transmitted through the head or around the head and is heard in the better ear. The result is that the patient receives credit for better hearing than really exists in his poorer ear.

There are many ways to mask an ear. A moving finger in the external auditory meatus will mask a whisper or low voice or even a moderate voice. Rubbing the palm of the hand vigorously on the auricle is also effective. A sheet of paper placed against the ear and rubbed by the examiner's hand makes a loud noise in one ear. A stream of air from a hose directed into the external auditory meatus produces a good masking effect. Similarly a stream of water (body temperature) is effective. One of the most convenient devices is the *Barany noisebox*. This device is held in the examiner's hand, and the earpiece is fitted into the patient's external auditory meatus. A loud buzzing noise masks one ear against almost any sound presented to the opposite ear (which is under test) (Fig. 11-15).

For the most part, masking one ear has little effect on hearing acuity in the opposite ear. *But failure to mask the better ear often results in a grossly erroneous measurement of hearing acuity in the poorer ear.*

Testing

Voice tests. The examiner's own voice is of great use in obtaining a ready estimate of the patient's hearing. However, the physician must himself mask the ear not under test since he cannot rely on the patient to mask his own ear. Using his finger, or his hand, or the Barany noisebox to mask one ear, the physician whispers or speaks near the other ear to gain a reasonable estimate of the patient's hearing. Begin by testing with a very low whisper with the lips 1 or 2 feet from the patient's ear and directed

toward his ear (Fig. 11-16). Exhale and then whisper. In a quiet room, a patient with normal hearing can repeat what is said. If he cannot understand a low whisper, the examiner uses a medium whisper, and finally a loud whisper. A spoken voice is then used in the same manner as the whisper—at first low, then medium, then loud. The examiner should not ask questions that can be answered yes or no but should give the patient numbers to repeat or ask nonsense questions such as, "Do guns shoot bullets or flowers?"

Patients with perceptive or sensorineural types of hearing loss hear a spoken voice better than they do a whispered voice. The reason is that they usually have a high-tone hearing loss, and whispers are composed of high tones that these patients cannot hear. The intensity of a whisper may actually be just as great as that of the spoken voice.

Care must also be taken that the patient does not read the examiner's lips. On the other hand, after hearing is checked a test for lip-

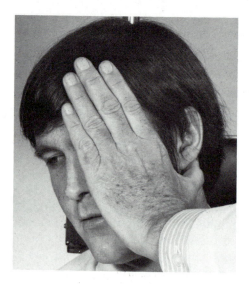

Fig. 11-16. Voice test. The examiner's hand shields the eyes of the person being tested to make certain he does not lip read.

reading ability may be given to obtain information regarding the patient's adjustment to his hearing loss. To do this the examiner speaks below a level at which the patient can hear, allowing the patient to closely observe his lips.

Another technique for testing hearing and one that is commonly used but that has the *serious disadvantage* of requiring the patient to provide his own masking is for the examiner to maintain a constant intensity for whispered or spoken voice and to vary his distance from the patient. Thus his report might read as follows: whispered voice—left ear, 3 feet; spoken voice—left ear, 6 feet.

Watch tick. The watch tick, which provides a high-frequency sound, is useful in testing patients for high-frequency hearing loss. Many patients first discover their hearing loss when they find themselves unable to hear a watch tick. Because it tests only part of the hearing range, the watch tick is a poor method to use exclusively. If a patient can hear the tick of a wristwatch at a normal distance, then he has a 98% chance of hearing all lower frequencies normally. In other words his perception of speech is normal since the frequency of a watch tick is well above most frequencies in the speech range (300-3,000 double vibrations per second).

Tuning fork tests. By using the tuning fork (500 or 1,000 cycles per second), an examiner can determine in most instances whether his patient has a conductive or a nerve-type hearing loss and can estimate the degree of hearing loss in the important speech frequencies (roughly 500 to 2,000 CPS). These forks are used because they represent the most important frequencies for speech and because their vibrations are not so likely to be felt as are the vibrations of a low-frequency fork.

Most beginners strike the fork too hard or strike it on a hard surface and produce overtones. Hearing tests should be done near threshold levels since the patient may become fatigued if he must wait too long or answer too often while a strongly activated fork dies down. Usually it is enough to stroke the fork between the thumb and index finger or to tap it gently on the knuckle (Fig. 11-17).

Normal patient. The patient with normal hearing hears a tuning fork placed in the midline of the head equally loud in both ears. He hears the fork better by air conduction (opposite the external auditory meatus) than he does when the fork is placed on the mastoid bone. Normally a tuning fork is heard twice as long by air conduction as by bone conduction. The reason is that when the patient listens by air conduction the route of hearing is through the middle ear, the more efficient route. Bone-conducted sound circumvents the middle ear and thus is not heard as loudly by the normal ear.

Weber test. In the Weber test, which makes use of bone conduction, the fork is placed on the midline of the skull or on the upper teeth (Fig. 11-18). If the patient has a middle ear disorder in one ear (conductive hearing loss) and normal hearing in the other ear, he will hear

Table 11-1. Summary of tuning fork tests

Hearing loss	Weber (bone only)	Rinne (air-bone)	Schwabach (bone only)
Normal	Not lateralized	"Positive" AC > BC	Equal
Conductive loss	Lateralized to poorer ear	"Negative" BC > or = AC	Patient hears longer than examiner
Sensorineural loss	Lateralized to better ear	"Positive" AC > BC	Examiner hears longer than patient

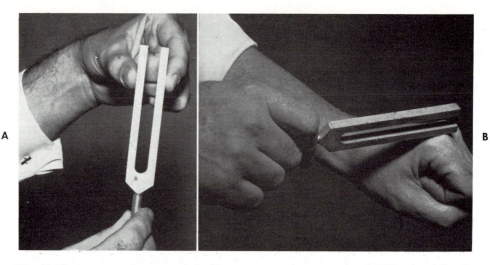

Fig. 11-17. Activating the tuning fork. Hearing is tested at *near threshold levels* so that the fork should be made to ring softly. **A,** "Stroking" the fork. **B,** Tapping the fork gently on the knuckle. (From DeWeese, D. D., and Saunders, W. H.: Textbook of otolaryngology, ed. 5, St. Louis, 1977, The C. V. Mosby Co.)

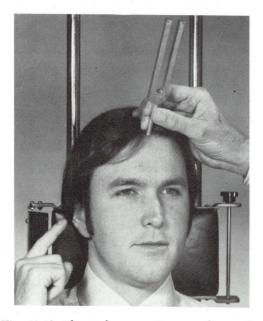

Fig. 11-18. The Weber test. Patient indicates the sound is heard louder in the right ear. This may mean either a conductive loss in the right ear or a sensorineural loss in the left ear. Another good place to hold the fork is on the maxillary teeth.

the fork in the poorer ear. One reason is that ordinary noise, always present in the usual testing situations, tends to "mask" the normal ear, but the poorer ear with conductive loss, not hearing such noise, has a better chance to hear bone-conducted sound. The Weber test may not "lateralize" in a completely quiet room. When a patient has sensorineural loss in one ear and the opposite ear is normal, the Weber test is heard in the better ear.

To better understand the Weber test, try it yourself. Occlude your left ear canal tightly with your finger to produce a conductive loss. Now touch a ringing tuning fork to the midline of your skull. The sound will be heard in the left ear (if you have normal hearing in the right ear). You have not increased your hearing acuity, but you have eliminated some of the ever-present environmental sound (ambient noise) from one ear.

Rinne test. In the Rinne test the tuning fork is presented to one ear alternately by air conduction and bone conduction (Fig. 11-19). The normal ear hears twice as long by air conduc-

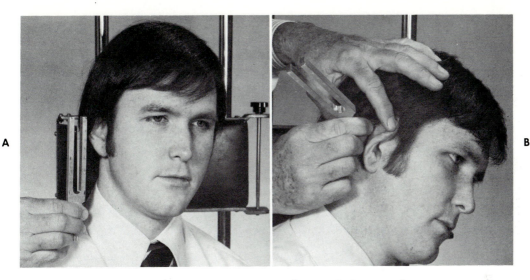

Fig. 11-19. The Rinne test. **A,** Air conduction. **B,** Bone conduction.

tion as by bone conduction. In middle ear disease the ratio between air and bone conduction changes in favor of bone conduction. In other words, in moderate conductive loss the patient hears about as long by bone conduction as by air conduction; in severe conductive loss he hears even longer by bone conduction than by air conduction. Arbitrarily this is called a "negative" Rinne test. The result is "positive" when the patient hears longer by air conduction than by bone conduction.

The patient with a sensorineural loss hears longer by air conduction than by bone conduction, but he hears poorly either way. In other words, the normal ratio is maintained, but hearing is reduced by both routes.

Schwabach test. In the Schwabach test the examiner compares his own normal bone conduction with that of the patient (Fig. 11-20). The tuning fork is pressed alternately to the examiner's mastoid and the patient's mastoid. If the patient has normal hearing, both the examiner and the patient will cease to hear the fork at about the same time. If the patient has middle ear disease (conductive hearing loss),

he will hear the fork longer than the examiner because room noise does not mask his ear as it does the examiner's. If the patient has sensorineural loss, he will hear the fork less long than will the examiner because his inner ear or auditory nerve is weak and cannot pick up signals readily.

No single hearing test is valid or completely informative. Speech tests and tuning fork tests must be used together for accurate estimation of hearing loss. More precise measurements are made with the calibrated electric audiometer.

Common errors in auditory testing. Common errors in testing are as follows:

1. Failure to mask the ear not under test is the most common and most serious error.

2. The correct tuning forks must be used. The examiner should not use the same low-frequency fork for testing hearing that he uses to test vibratory sensation. A low-frequency fork is heard well by many patients even though they may have a loss in speech frequencies. Also, low-frequency forks confuse some patients who report vibrations as "hearing."

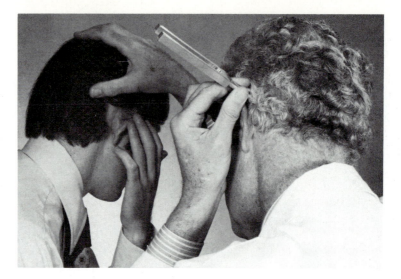

Fig. 11-20. The Schwabach test compares the examiner's and the patient's hearing by *bone conduction*.

3. Most beginners ring the fork too loudly. The fork should ring softly because the purpose is not to determine how intense a sound the patient can tolerate but rather the point at which he can just hear.

Special examinations

Function of the eustachian tube. Eustachian tube function may be demonstrated by looking at the drumhead under magnification while the patient holds his nose and swallows. This maneuver reinforces the opening of the eustachian tube which usually occurs during swallowing. At the moment of swallowing the eardrum can be seen to flick outward and then inward again, a movement indicating patency of the eustachian tube. Also the patient feels a sensation of pressure in his ears at the height of the swallow.

Demonstration of tubal patency is important in some patients who have certain symptoms (hearing loss, tinnitus, or dizziness) that may be caused by occlusion of the tube.

Use of the pneumatic otoscope. The pneumatic otoscope is a useful device that enables the examiner to compress air in the ear canal. This procedure exerts pressure against the drumhead, which moves in and out as a bulb in the examiner's hand is alternately squeezed and released (Fig. 11-21). Certain drumheads will be found more flaccid than normal (usually because of healed perforations), and others will not move at all because they are perforated. Adhesions in the middle ear may also prevent normal excursion of the drumhead. Another important cause of limited motion of the drumhead is the presence of fluid in the middle ear. The pneumatic otoscope is particularly useful in examining children suspected of having a middle ear effusion.

This device also can be used to suck down secretions from the epitympanum and mastoid antrum in patients having chronic mastoiditis or to evacuate the middle ear of fluid after myringotomy.

Temporomandibular joint. It is quite com-

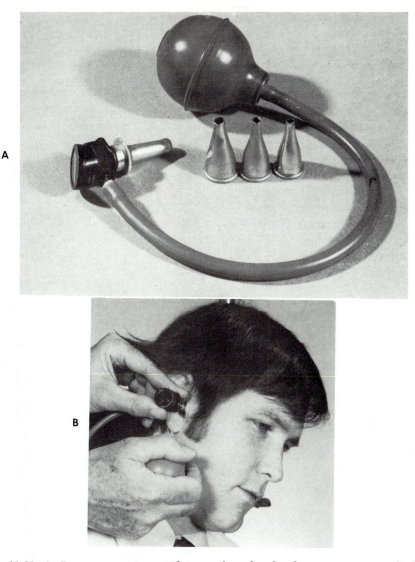

Fig. 11-21. A, Pneumatic otoscope. The speculum that fits this otoscope is attached. The usual type of speculum may also be used if only magnification is desired. **B,** The pneumatic otoscope in use.

mon to see a patient with ear pain that is the result of referred pain from the temporomandibular joint. By pressing the index fingers into the joint spaces as the patient opens his mouth widely, pain may be elicited (often only on one side) when he again closes his mouth. This pain commonly is referred to the ear and the patient complains not of a pain in the joint of his jaw but rather of otalgia. Common causes are of dental origin and have to do with malocclusion.

ORAL CAVITY

Tongue. The tongue is examined by both inspection and palpation. Palpation is necessary because some diseases of the tongue cause no surface manifestation and otherwise cannot be detected (Fig. 11-22).

Lingual papillae. The filiform papillae are the most numerous. Keratinization of these papillae produces the well-known "coated tongue." "Hairy tongue" is also common, and the appearance is caused by elongation and discoloration of the filiform papillae (Fig. 11-23). Fungiform papillae are scattered throughout the filiform papillae and are especially abundant on the sides and apex of the tongue. These papillae look like small red dots because the underlying vascular connective tissue shines through the thin epithelium. The circumvallate papillae are arranged in an inverted V at the posterior part of the tongue. The apex of the V is at foramen cecum. The circumvallate papillae are best examined with a laryngeal mirror.

Ventral surface. The ventral surface of the tongue toward the floor of the mouth is smooth and shows large veins. In older people these veins may become varicose.

Frenum. The frenum is found in the midline under the tongue. Rather rarely this structure is abnormally short and causes so-called "tongue tie." If the patient can protrude his tongue between his teeth, he should have no difficulty with speech.

Glossopalatine fold. The glossopalatine fold connects the tongue with the palate and is known as the anterior tonsillar pillar (Fig. 11-24).

Other structures associated with the tongue are the lingual tonsils, vallecula, and glossoe-

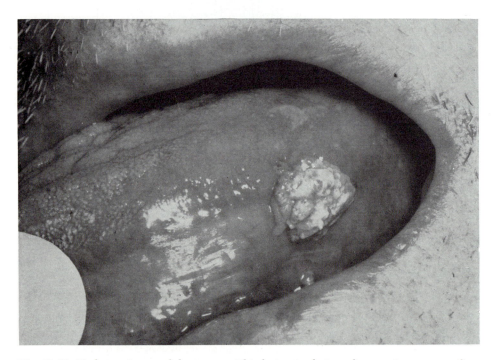

Fig. 11-22. Early carcinoma of the tongue. This lesion is obvious, but carcinomas are often not raised; therefore, palpation becomes important.

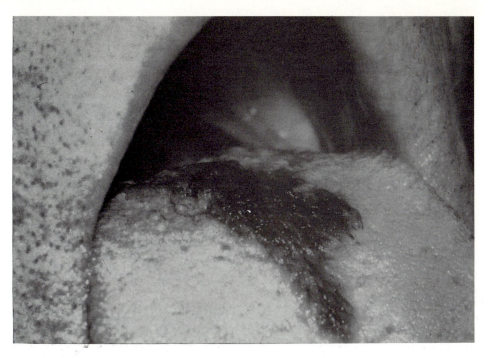

Fig. 11-23. Hairy tongue.

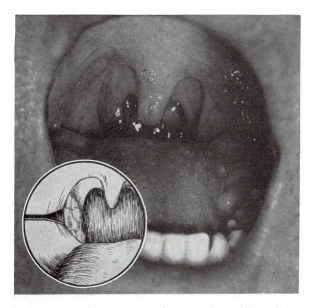

Fig. 11-24. Oropharynx. Note the anterior and posterior tonsillar pillars. Inset shows the pillar retractor withdrawing the anterior pillar. (From DeWeese, D. D., and Saunders, W. H.: Textbook of otolaryngology, ed. 5, St. Louis, 1977, The C. V. Mosby Co.)

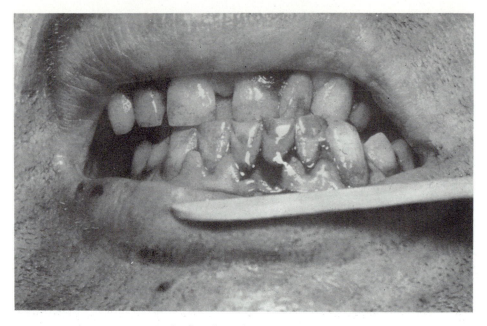

Fig. 11-25. Bleeding from the gums in aplastic anemia.

piglottic folds. These structures are best seen with the laryngeal mirror and therefore will be described in the discussion of laryngeal examination.

Floor of mouth. The floor of the mouth is another region where palpation is important. Tissues are loose, and neoplasms are sometimes detectable only by palpation. The submaxillary salivary ducts may contain calculi that are best felt by palpation. Bimanual examination, using one gloved finger inside the mouth and the other hand outside, is best.

Submaxillary salivary gland. The submaxillary salivary gland empties into the floor of the mouth on either side of the frenum of the tongue. The orifices of the ducts are quite small, but they may be seen as small dark spots from which clear fluid can be expressed by pressure over the submaxillary gland. Orifices of the sublingual glands are not seen.

Teeth and gingiva. There are 32 teeth in the full adult dentition. The teeth are inspected for evidence of caries and malocclusion. Sometimes it is worthwhile to percuss a tooth to elicit tenderness in patients suspected of having dental abscess.

The gums should be inspected and at times palpated. Bleeding from the gums is not unusual and many times is the sole cause of expectorated blood (Fig. 11-25). In adults the gums gradually recede from the teeth and expose a larger and larger amount of tooth root. In *pyorrhea,* an abnormal condition that starts as a simple gingivitis and is preventable in most instances, the teeth may actually fall out (Fig. 11-26).

Buccal mucosa. The parotid duct opens into the buccal mucosa opposite the upper second molar (Fig. 11-27). The orifice is larger than the submaxillary orifices and readily admits a probe. Pressure over the parotid gland produces a clear secretion.

In most adults yellowish glandlike structures may be seen shining through the buccal mu-

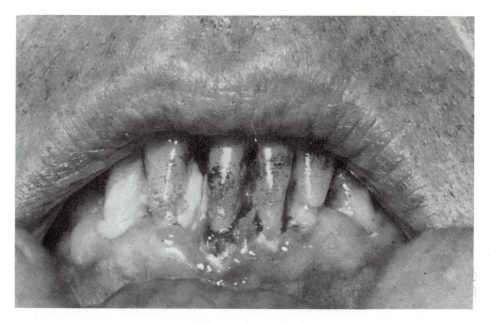

Fig. 11-26. Advanced pyorrhea.

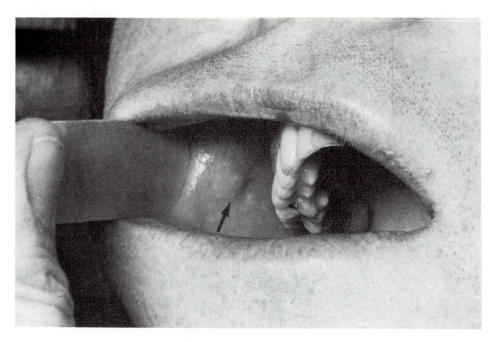

Fig. 11-27. Parotid duct.

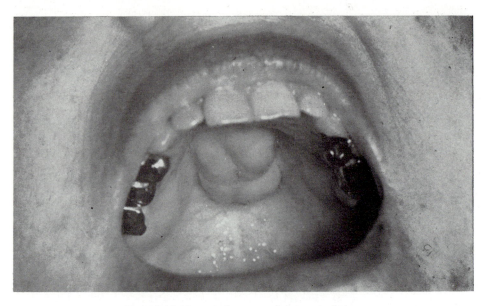

Fig. 11-28. Torus palatinus, a benign condition.

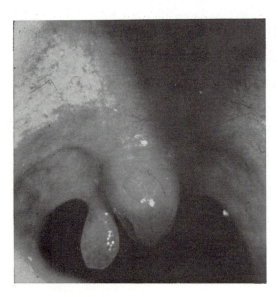

Fig. 11-29. Typical squamous papilloma. (**From** DeWeese, D. D., and Saunders, W. H.: **Textbook** of otolaryngology, ed. 5, St. Louis, 1977, The C. V. Mosby Co.)

cosa. These represent normal sebaceous glands lying directly under the squamous epithelium of the oral cavity.

A white line of parakeratin in the buccal mucosa just adjacent to the occlusal surfaces of the molar teeth results from invagination of the cheek between the teeth or from sucking on the cheek.

Palate. There is a distinct difference in color between the hard and soft palates. The soft palate is pink and shows fine vessels under the mucosa. The hard palate is whiter, more irregular, and has rugae running transversely. Scrutiny shows the orifices of ducts of mucous glands in the posterior part of the hard palate. In heavy smokers the duct orifices look like tiny red dots scattered throughout the hard palate. This is one form of nicotine stomatitis.

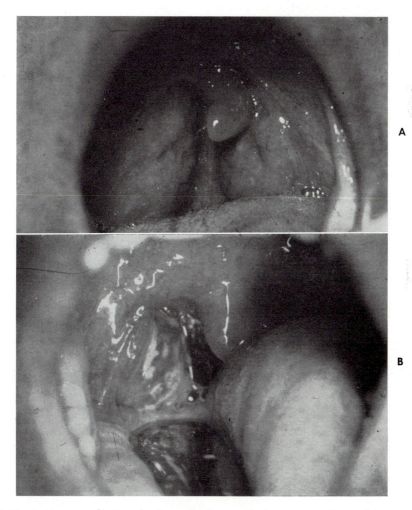

A

B

Fig. 11-30. **A,** Hypertrophic tonsils. Normally the tonsils do not protrude much beyond the margins of the tonsillar pillars. **B,** Acute follicular tonsillitis.

A common finding in the midline is *torus palatinus,* a bony protuberance or exostosis (Fig. 11-28).

Uvula. The uvula is a muscular organ that varies greatly in length and thickness. It is sometimes bifid. Frequently a small squamous papilloma is attached to the uvula, the free margin of the soft palate, or the anterior tonsillar pillar (Fig. 11-29).

Tonsils. Normally the palatine, or faucial, tonsils do not project much beyond the limits of the tonsillar pillars (Fig. 11-24). They are approximately the same color as the rest of the oral mucosa. There are crypts in the tonsils in which squamous epithelium exfoliates. Some patients have deep crypts, and plugs of epithelial debris push toward the surface, where they appear as white spots on the tonsils. When the tonsils become enlarged, they may extend considerably beyond the anterior tonsillar pillars, at times even to the midline (Fig. 11-30, *A*). At other times white spots on the tonsils may indicate follicular tonsillitis (Fig. 11-30, *B*).

It is sometimes helpful to retract the anterior tonsillar pillar for better visualization of the tonsil (Fig. 11-24). Palpation of the tonsil is important if neoplasm is suspected.

Tonsillectomy is common. Ideally the examiner should not be able to distinguish a tonsillectomized throat from one in which the faucial tonsils are extremely small. It is usually simple, however, to tell if a patient has had a tonsillectomy because of the changes in the anterior or posterior pillars that occur with healing. Also, lymphoid nodules may remain in the tonsillar fossa and form so-called tonsillar tags.

Posterior pharyngeal wall. The posterior pharyngeal wall is that part of the pharynx that is visible when the examiner uses only a tongue blade. Students are prone to speak of hyperemia or "injection" of the throat when they see vessels on the posterior pharyngeal wall. Usually these small vessels are normal and do not represent inflammatory changes. The same ap-

pearances may be seen on the tonsillar pillars and the soft palate.

Small, irregular spots of lymphoid tissue are common in the mucosa of the posterior pharyngeal wall. They are red or pink. The *lateral pharyngeal bands* are found behind the posterior pillars running downward from the nasopharynx toward the base of the tongue. These pink bands are also composed of lymphoid tissue. The lymphoid elements in the pharynx consisting of the adenoid, lateral band, faucial tonsil, and lingual tonsil are commonly known as *Waldeyer's ring.*

NASOPHARYNX
Technique of mirror examination

The best way to examine the nasopharynx is with the postnasal mirror. A No. 0 mirror is the correct size. Ordinarily children over the age of 5 years and most adults can be examined without difficulty. Because of the small size of

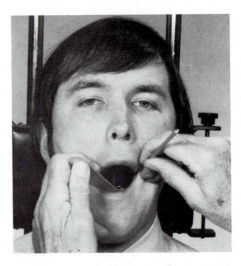

Fig. 11-31. Positioning the mirror for examination of the nasopharynx. Note maximum depression of the tongue. Both hands are braced on the cheeks. The mirror is held not by its handle but by its shaft. The patient should breathe through his nose or simply relax his throat.

the mirror, all of the nasopharynx cannot be seen at one time. Instead, the mirror is rotated slightly to bring successive areas into view.

First, after the mirror is warmed, the tongue is depressed to create a large space in which to place the mirror (Fig. 11-31). The light must be focused sharply in the space next to the uvula where the mirror will be placed. The mirror is placed to one side of the uvula and almost touches the posterior pharyngeal wall. The mirror is held in the right hand, and the fingers are braced against the patient's cheek to steady the hand. The tongue blade is held in the left hand in the corner of the mouth so that it will not obstruct the examiner's view of the oral cavity.

The patient is instructed to breathe quietly through the nose so as to allow the soft palate to drop away from the posterior pharyngeal wall. Often the patient will protest, "I can't breathe through my nose with my mouth open!" but quiet reassurance and encouragement help to accomplish the desired palatal relaxation.

The beginner is likely to make two mistakes:
1. He fails to depress the tongue adequately

so that there is insufficient space in which to place the mirror.
2. He fails to focus his light sharply on the mirror.

Choana. The choana is the posterior opening of the nose. Each choana is separated from the other by the posterior end of the vomer bone (Fig. 11-32). The posterior ends of the turbinates can be seen in each side. The turbinates (especially the inferior turbinates) vary greatly in appearance even in normal noses. Sometimes they appear engorged with blood and look swollen and bluish ("mulberry turbinate"). At other times the posterior tips are pale. Such changes may indicate an allergic or vasomotor disorder.

Posterior end of vomer. Unlike the anterior part of the nasal septum, the posterior end of the vomer is always in the midline. However, it is not unusual to see a thickening of the mucosa of the vomer caused by hyperplastic mucosa.

Middle meatus. The middle meatus is an important space clinically because it is here that pus may be seen running from the maxillary sinus. Pus runs from the ostium (not visible)

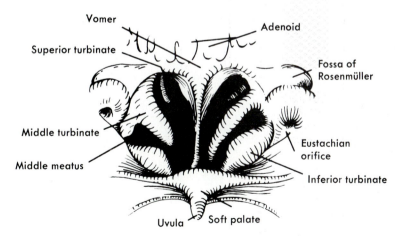

Fig. 11-32. Structures seen in the nasopharynx by posterior rhinoscopy.

into the middle meatus and then drips over the posterior end of the inferior turbinate—a pathognomonic sign of maxillary sinusitis. The frontal and anterior ethmoid sinuses also drain into the middle meatus, but more anteriorly, and their drainage is best seen using the nasal speculum.

Inferior meatus. The inferior meatus is not well seen and has no clinical significance as far as its visualization with the postnasal mirror is concerned.

Superior meatus. The superior meatus (above the middle turbinate) blends with the region known clinically as the sphenoethmoid recess and is the site of drainage of the sphenoid sinus and posterior ethmoid cells.

Eustachian tubes. The eustachian tubes open laterally into the nasopharynx just under the torus tubarius. Over the torus is the fossa of Rosenmüller. The orifice of the tube usually looks a little pale or yellowish and is about as large as the eraser end of a lead pencil. Normally the tube is closed, but it opens whenever the patient swallows or yawns.

Adenoid. The adenoid (pharyngeal tonsil) is a collection of lymphoid tissue present in every child and in some adults. The adenoid grows from the roof and posterior wall of the nasopharynx, extends into the fossa of Rosenmüller, and blends with that lymphoid tissue known as the lateral pharyngeal band. Sometimes the adenoid, particularly in adults, seems to be only a clump of lymphoid tissue centrally located.

In children the adenoid is prone to cause occlusion of the eustachian tube, which interferes with aeration of the middle ear. This causes partial hearing loss because of serous otitis media. Obstruction may also predispose toward middle ear infections. Large masses of adenoid also produce nasal obstruction and mouth breathing in infants and young children.

Posterior aspect of uvula and soft palate. The posterior aspect of the uvula and soft palate and the lateral wall of the pharynx are also visible in the postnasal mirror. Ordinarily no pathologic changes are found here except for nasopharyngitis, causing hyperemia and exudate formation. Many physicians fail to locate

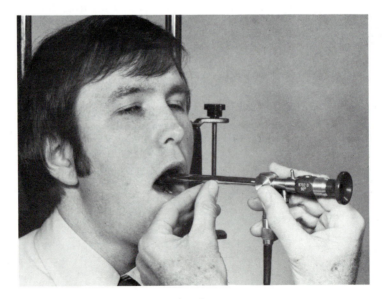

Fig. 11-33. The pharyngoscope.

the site of the patient's sore throat because they fail to examine the nasopharynx. They use only a tongue blade to inspect the oropharynx, but the oropharynx may be normal even when the patient has severe nasopharyngitis.

Other methods of examination

Nasal speculum. A nasal speculum may be used to see a small part of the nasopharynx by looking through the anterior nares. Such examination can be done in some patients without previous vasoconstriction, but in most patients a good view depends on careful shrinkage of the inferior turbinate. Anterior rhinoscopy is particularly useful in children who will not permit the use of a nasopharyngeal mirror. In adults it is a convenient route through which to take a biopsy of the nasopharynx.

Palpation of nasopharynx. The procedure of palpation of the nasopharynx is used in some instances. Usually, better and less distressing methods are available. If the examiner does use palpation, it is important to place several thicknesses of tongue blades between the patient's molar teeth or to invaginate the patient's cheek between his teeth with the index finger.

Pharyngoscope. The Ward-Hopkins (Fig. 11-33) pharyngoscope is an electrically lighted instrument that provides an excellent view of the entire nasopharynx. The instrument is introduced through the mouth, then the prism is directed either upward to view the nasopharynx or downward to view the hypopharynx and larynx. This instrument has largely replaced the older nasopharyngoscope that was introduced through the nose.

HYPOPHARYNX AND LARYNX

The approach to the patient is exceedingly important. The examiner must adopt a calm, reassuring attitude and yet conduct the examination with firmness. Admittedly it is difficult to cope with the "gaggy" patient, but annoyance on the examiner's part only worsens the situation.

Topical anesthesia, such as provided by 10% lidocaine (Xylocaine available in a spray bottle as Dental Xylocaine), 4% cocaine, or 1% tetracaine (Pontocaine), is permissible but is not often needed by the experienced examiner. The examiner should avoid spraying with compressed-air equipment because too much drug is likely to be administered in this way. The use of an atomizer and bulb is safer.

In an extremely "gaggy" patient, when all else fails, the intravenous administration of 5 to 10 mg. (1 to 2 ml.) of diazepam (Valium) over a 90-second period will secure cooperation almost without fail. The technique is safe and the "groggy" effect is over in about 15 to 20 minutes. The drug should be injected into a large vein because injection into a small vein may produce phlebitis.

The tongue is protruded as far as possible, and the examiner holds it firmly in a piece of gauze. He lays the gauze over the tongue and then wraps it under the tongue. This method keeps the gauze from wadding up on top of the tongue and obscuring vision. Then he holds the tongue between his left thumb and left middle finger and braces his index finger against the upper lip or upper teeth. If the patient cooperates and does not try to retract the protruded tongue, it is not necessary to actually pull on the tongue.

The No. 5 mirror is used in adults. The glass surface is warmed over an alcohol lamp, and the mirror back is tested on the examiner's hand for heat. The examiner holds the mirror midway along the shaft, not by the handle. He holds it like a pen and braces his fingers on the patient's cheek.

The mirror is inserted into the mouth so that the edge advances with the glass surface flush with the tongue. This means that the mirror is not introduced in its greatest diameter.

The mirror is placed with its backside against the tip of the uvula (Fig. 11-34). The uvula and soft palate are pressed upward in one smooth movement. Once contact is made, the mirror

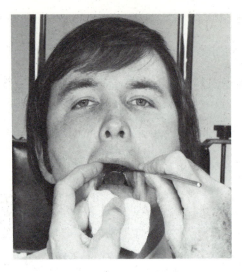

Fig. 11-34. Position of the laryngeal mirror. Note that the tongue and gauze do not obstruct the examiner's view. Both hands are braced against the cheeks, and the left index finger holds the patient's mouth open. The laryngeal mirror is held well up on the shaft.

is not shifted about to any extent, although slight changes in its position are necessary for seeing all of the larynx.

Touching the uvula and soft palate ordinarily does not cause gagging, but touching the back of the tongue does.

The patient is asked to breathe quietly through the mouth. He is told that as long as he breathes regularly he will not gag. Sometimes "gaggy" patients do best when asked to "pant in and out like a dog." After the examination has been completed during quiet respiration, the patient is asked to sound a high-pitched "e-e-e," "a-a-a," or best of all "he-e-e." Almost all patients phonate too low and too briefly and must be told to make the sound very high in pitch. A prolonged singing of "e-e-e" is desired and not a short utterance, which does not give adequate time for examination. The examiner always makes the same sound and, in effect, the two sing a duet.

Some patients when asked to phonate will remain aphonic, then shake their heads; others hold their breath. Careful explanation and quiet reassurance do much toward obtaining cooperation.

Examiner's common mistakes. The following are common mistakes made by the examiner:
1. Not explaining what he intends to do before he does it
2. Failing to position the patient properly
3. Failing to focus the light brilliantly on the mirror
4. Not elevating the uvula with the back of the mirror
5. Not insisting on a prolonged, high-pitched "e-e-e"

Hypopharynx

The hypopharynx is above the level of the larynx but below that part of the pharynx that can be conveniently examined using a tongue blade. The circumvallate papillae, lingual tonsils, valleculae, and epiglottis are the important structures seen in the hypopharynx when the examiner uses a laryngeal mirror.

Circumvallate papillae. These are arranged in an inverted V, with the apex at the foramen cecum. The papillae vary considerably in size and prominence, and patients sometimes mistake them for lingual tumors.

Lingual tonsils. The lingual tonsils, visible in most adults, lie on either side of the dorsum of the tongue. They vary greatly in size and sometimes are extremely large. Small white spots are frequently seen in the lingual tonsils. Such spots represent debris in crypts or, if the patient has active lingual tonsillitis, follicular exudate. When the lingual tonsils are enlarged, there is a deep cleft between them.

Valleculae. The valleculae are the cup-shaped spaces between the tongue and epiglottis. They are separated from each other by the median glossoepiglottic fold. Large veins are frequently seen in the valleculae. These are normal. Cysts may form here and are usually thin-walled and yellowish or white. To see the valleculae more distinctly, the examiner asks the patient to phonate.

Epiglottis. The epiglottis is cartilaginous, variously shaped, and of different sizes and thicknesses in different patients. Its color also varies. The free edge of the epiglottis is usually thin and slightly curved. Sometimes the entire epiglottis is furled, and laryngologists speak of an "omega-shaped" epiglottis. The lateral glossoepiglottic folds and median glossoepiglottic folds attach it to the base of the tongue; the aryepiglottic folds attach it to the arytenoid cartilages.

Because the epiglottis is usually in the way when the examiner wishes to see the anterior ends of the vocal cords, the patient is asked to phonate in a high-pitched "e-e-e" or "he-e-e." This maneuver draws the epiglottis anteriorly and out of the line of vision.

Up to this point the examiner has inspected the hypopharynx. Although it is not a routine part of the examination, *palpation* with one finger is done in certain patients. This is necessary not because visual examination is difficult but because tumors deep in the tongue may not cause visible mucosal alterations.

The lateral and posterior walls of the hypopharynx are inspected along with the rest of the hypopharynx. Ordinarily nothing in these areas confuses the examiner.

Larynx

In studying the larynx the beginner too often fixes his attention solely on the true vocal cords because these structures are so striking in their appearance and movement. But inspection of the true vocal cords is only part of the laryngeal examination.

False cords. The false cords lie directly above and a little lateral to the true cords. They are capable of contracting and closing the larynx, but generally they remain quiet during examination. Sometimes, however, the false cords are so active that they preclude a good view of the true cords. Ordinarily the false cords appear dull pink and look thicker than the true cords.

Laryngeal ventricle. Directly under the false cords is a space called the laryngeal ventricle. It is not well seen by mirror laryngoscopy, but more of it can be seen by having the patient tilt his head sideways (ear toward shoulder).

True vocal cords. The true vocal cords reflect light in such a way as to appear very white and sharp edged in the laryngeal mirror. However, their color is not really white, and the edges are actually rounded.

Anteriorly the cords meet in the midline, where they are attached to the thyroid cartilage. Posteriorly they are attached to the vocal processes of the arytenoid cartilages. The anterior attachment is fixed, but the posterior attachment is mobile and allows the cords to open and close during respiration and phonation.

Arytenoid cartilages. The arytenoid cartilages form the posterior attachments for the true vocal cords. They are mobile and swing in and out with phonation and respiration. Their color is a dull red, and they appear as small mounds at the posterior end of the glottis (the space between the cords). The arytenoids also attach to the epiglottis via the aryepiglottic folds. In the aryepiglottic folds are smaller cartilages, the cuneiform and corniculate cartilages. The aryepiglottic folds, the false cords, and the true cords are the sphincters of the larynx that protect the lower respiratory passages from foreign bodies and help to build up intrathoracic pressure for cough and other functions.

Pyriform recesses. The pyriform recesses are situated posterior and lateral to the arytenoids. They will dilate a little if the patient says "a-a-a" in a low voice. Secretions may gather here, but they should disappear on swallowing.

If they do not, the patient is said to have a "pooling" sign, which suggests obstruction or paralysis of the upper esophagus.

Laryngeal examination. The cords are first observed during quiet respiration (Figs. 11-35 and 11-36). They move only slightly or not at all, and the examiner notes their color, configuration, and position. He also looks between the cords at the anterior wall of the trachea. In most patients he can see all the way to the carina. He can see the carina best by kneeling on the floor in front of the patient and looking upward into the laryngeal mirror.

After the larynx has been inspected during quiet respiration, the patient phonates as previously described (Fig. 11-37). Phonation causes adduction of the cords, which can be seen to vibrate as sound is produced. They become more tense and appear elongated. Normally there seems to be perfect approximation of the cords, but in aged persons there is a small space that cannot be closed. This produces the quavering voice of the old man. If one vocal cord is paralyzed, it lies fixed while the opposite cord moves in and out.

Tumors of the true cords prevent accurate approximation during phonation and therefore cause hoarseness. For that reason malignant tumors arising on the true cords have a very favorable prognosis if the patient sees a physician as soon as he becomes hoarse and if the physician examines the larynx (Figs. 11-38 to 11-40).

The greatest difficulty in examining the larynx is seeing the anterior commissure, which is often hidden by the tubercle of the epiglottis. Rarely is it necessary to apply topical anesthesia and to use a retractor to displace the epiglottis. Usually proper phonation effects adequate retraction of the epiglottis.

The attachment of the true vocal cords to the arytenoid process causes a slight cup-shaped depression that is sometimes mistaken for abnormality. Pellets of mucus resting on the cords may look like small tumors. If the patient will cough, many of these "tumors" disappear.

Before examination is completed all parts of the larynx should be inspected during quiet respiration and phonation. Again the beginner is cautioned not to fix his attention on the true cords alone.

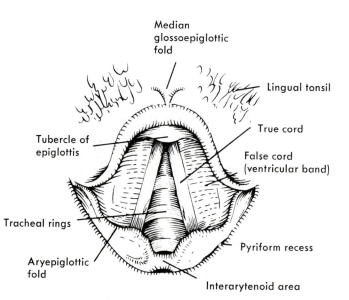

Fig. 11-35. Larynx in quiet respiration. Notice that the vocal cords are separated.

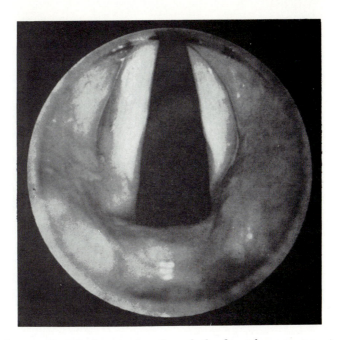

Fig. 11-36. Photograph of the larynx taken through the direct laryngoscope. Arytenoids are the mounds seen posteriorly. Anterior view is above. (Courtesy Dr. Paul Holinger, Chicago, Ill.; from DeWeese, D. D., and Saunders, W. H.: Textbook of otolaryngology, ed. 5, St. Louis, 1977, The C. V. Mosby Co.)

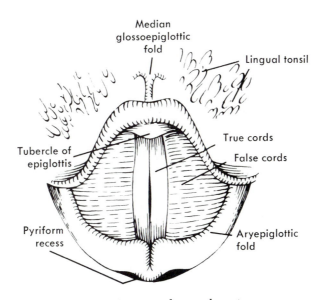

Fig. 11-37. Larynx during phonation.

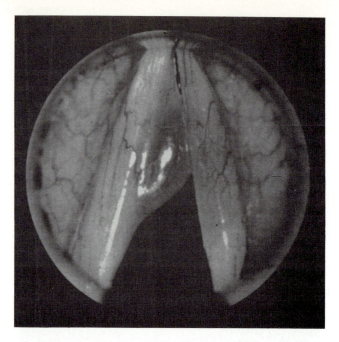

Fig. 11-38. Sessile laryngeal polyp. (Courtesy Dr. Paul Holinger, Chicago, Ill.; from De-Weese, D. D., and Saunders, W.H.: Textbook of otolaryngology, ed. 5, St. Louis, 1977, The C. V. Mosby Co.)

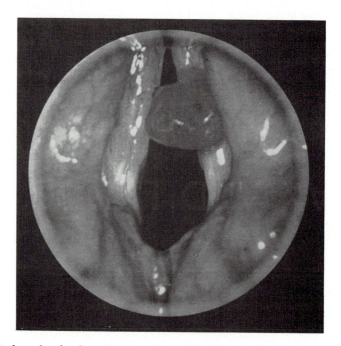

Fig. 11-39. Pedunculated polyp. (Courtesy Dr. Paul Holinger, Chicago, Ill.; from DeWeese, D. D., and Saunders, W. H.: Textbook of otolaryngology, ed. 5, St. Louis, 1977, The C. V. Mosby Co.)

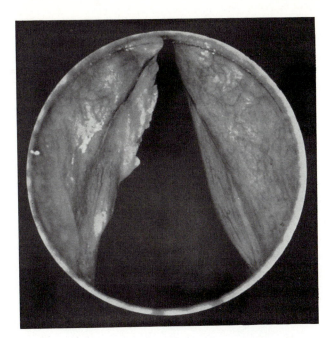

Fig. 11-40. Keratotic plaque. Such a lesion must be distinguished microscopically from leukoplakia and carcinoma. (Courtesy Dr. Paul Holinger, Chicago, Ill.; from DeWeese, D. D., and Saunders, W. H.: Textbook of otolaryngology, ed. 5, St. Louis, 1977, The C. V. Mosby Co.)

External laryngeal examination. Complete examination of the larynx calls for palpation of the neck. The shape of the thyroid cartilage is noted, and the space between the thyroid cartilage and the hyoid bone is palpated. This is a common site for a thyroglossal duct cyst. The space between the thyroid and cricoid cartilages is also palpated. Sometimes a lymph node is felt in patients with carcinoma of the larynx. The cricothyroid space is the site where an emergency tracheotomy may be done with the least bleeding.

Because the cricothyroid muscle is the only laryngeal muscle innervated by the superior laryngeal nerve, the function of that nerve may be tested by having the patient say "e-e-e" in a high-pitched voice. This action causes a contraction of the normal cricothyroid muscle, and the cricoid cartilage is drawn upward. This fails to happen if the superior laryngeal nerve is not intact.

Laryngeal crepitation is elicited by grasping the larynx (thyroid cartilage) between the thumb and index finger and rocking it vigorously from side to side. This maneuver should cause a crepitation felt on either side. If it does not, a postcricoid neoplasm may be present that cushions movements of the larynx across the vertebral column.

Palpation of the neck is an important part of the otolaryngic physical examination, but this subject is covered in Chapter 9 and will not be repeated here.

NOSE

The nasal chambers are examined by inspection. They are inspected anteriorly and posteriorly with the nasal speculum and the postnasal mirror, respectively. Either a metal applicator wound with cotton or a bayonet forceps provides a useful instrument for light intranasal palpation.

Lighting is the same as already described. It must be bright and focused to a small spot. Be-

cause the nasal chambers are several centimeters in length, the position of the examiner's head that allows him to focus sharply in the nasal vestibule will not provide a bright spot of light in the posterior nose. Therefore, the examiner must constantly alter the relationship

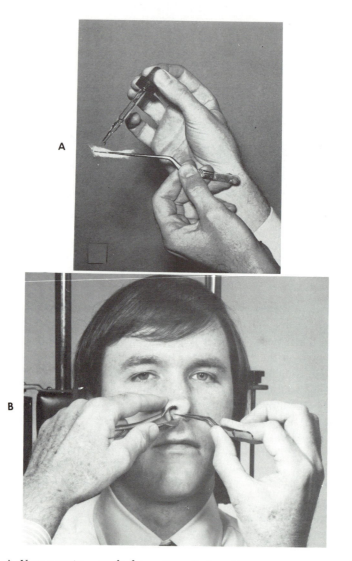

Fig. 11-41. A, Vasoconstrictor applied to cotton. **B,** Inserting cotton into nose. This maneuver should be done under direct vision. The cotton is placed alongside the inferior turbinate.

between the patient's head and his own to maintain adequate lighting.

Vasoconstriction is provided by topical application of 3% ephedrine in saline solution. Two percent cocaine has the added advantage of producing topical anesthesia. Shrinking the nasal mucosa (which means the inferior turbinates in most instances) is necessary in many patients before complete intranasal inspection can be done.

Ephedrine may be sprayed from an atomizer, or it may be applied on wisps of cotton that are wet with it, introduced along the inferior turbinate and left for several minutes (Fig. 11-41). Sometimes it is important to obtain vasoconstriction in other areas, such as about the middle meatus and middle turbinate.

The nasal speculum is held in the left hand

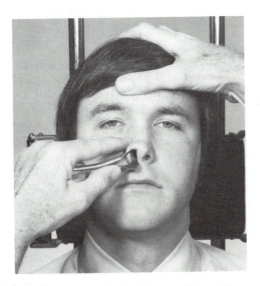

Fig. 11-42. Proper position for use of the nasal speculum. Note the right hand positioning the head. Position of the head must be changed several times as different parts of the nasal chamber are inspected. The speculum is opened as fully as possible. The blades should always be opened vertically. The index finger fixes the upper blade in the nares.

whether one is examining the left or right side of the nose (Fig. 11-42). The left index finger presses on the ala of the nose to anchor the upper blade of the speculum in place. The blades are inserted about 1 cm. into the vestibule. The speculum is opened vertically (and not transversely) to avoid painful pressure against the nasal septum.

The examiner's right hand is the real key to intranasal inspection because it positions the head. Except when used for instrumentation, the right hand is placed firmly on the top of the patient's head and is used to *change the head position from time to time*. Too much emphasis cannot be placed on this point. The examiner must look at small areas successively. For example, with the patient's head erect the examiner can see the floor of the nose and the inferior turbinate, but he cannot see the septum well unless he turns the patient's head sidewise. Similarly, he cannot inspect the middle meatus until the head is tilted back. The use of the headrest is discouraged because it fixes the patient's head and defeats proper use of the examiner's right hand.

Examiner's common mistakes. The mistakes every beginner makes are as follows:

1. He fails to adjust his head position to keep his light sharply focused.
2. He opens the nasal speculum too little. Actually, unless he opens the speculum as completely as the nose will permit (and often this means as fully as the speculum will open), it is better to use no speculum at all.
3. He fails to tilt and turn the patient's head with his right hand to see all parts of the nose.
4. He fails to use vasoconstrictors.

Vestibule. The vestibule of the nose is lined with skin and contains the nasal hairs or vibrissae. Except for folliculitis and fissures, no common diseases involve the nasal vestibule. The vestibule may be examined by tilting up the tip of the nose with the finger. A nasal speculum is also useful.

Mucosa. The nose is lined with respiratory mucosa except anteriorly where there is skin and far superiorly where there is olfactory epithelium. The nasal mucosa is redder than the oral mucosa; therefore, students are prone to call normal nasal mucosa "hyperemic" or "injected."

Nasal septum. The nasal septum is composed of both cartilage and bone. In virtually every adult the septum is not straight. Instead it gradually deviates from the midline to a greater or lesser degree, or it has developed a sharp projection (a "spur" or "ridge") or a more rounded projection (a "hump"). Sometimes the anterior end of the nasal septum is dislocated and projects prominently into one nostril (Fig. 11-43). In any case such irregularities of the nasal septum ordinarily cause no disturbance unless they are severe enough to obstruct the airway. Sometimes crusting occurs at the site of the nasal septal deviation or spur and bleeding results.

There is an anterior plexus of blood vessels in the mucosa of the nasal septum, and the examiner can often see small arteries and veins here. This is the most common site for *epistaxis* (nosebleed).

Lateral wall of the nose. The lateral wall of the nose consists of the inferior, middle, and superior turbinates and inferior, middle, and superior meati (Fig. 11-44).

The *inferior turbinate* is a separate bone; the middle and superior turbinates are parts of the ethmoid bone. The inferior, the largest turbinate, lies like a finger along the lower lateral wall of the nose. It is erectile and swells periodically. This swelling may cause alternating nasal obstruction that is especially troublesome at night to some patients who must turn from side to side to obtain decongestion of the dependent turbinate.

Both inferior turbinates are not the same size

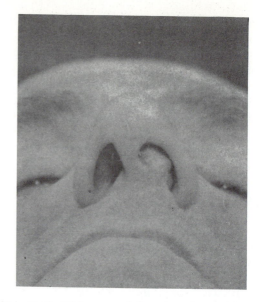

Fig. 11-43. Dislocation of the columellar end of the septal cartilage. (From DeWeese, D. D., and Saunders, W. H.: Textbook of otolaryngology, ed. 5, St. Louis, 1977, The C. V. Mosby Co.)

in most patients. When the septum is displaced to one side, the inferior turbinate on the opposite side is prone to swell and fill the concavity. Normally the turbinate is deep pink and similar to the color of the rest of the nasal mucosa, but in allergic states it becomes blue or pale and the tissue becomes boggy and swollen. Inflammation of the nasal mucosa causes a redness.

The *middle turbinate* is also seen by looking into the nose anteriorly. Sometimes a deflection of the nasal septum partially hides the structure. Occasionally the middle turbinate contains an air cell that enlarges its anterior end. Ordinarily the middle turbinate does not contribute seriously to nasal obstruction.

The inferior turbinate and the anterior end of the middle turbinate are sometimes mistaken for nasal polyps. Turbinates are tender, contain a bone, and are fixed in position; pol-

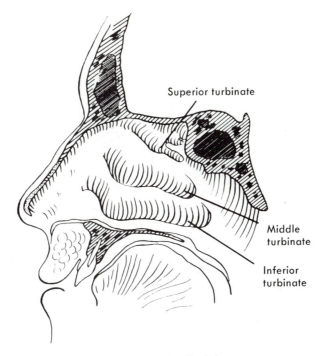

Fig. 11-44. Lateral wall of the nose.

yps are usually much paler, nontender, and movable.

The *middle meatus* is a very important area lying lateral to the middle turbinate. Appearing as a cleftlike space, often it is poorly seen because of encroachment by the adjacent middle turbinate. Vasoconstriction and careful positioning of the head will make the middle meatus visible. Secretions from the frontal, maxillary, and anterior ethmoid sinuses drain here. The ostia of the sinuses are not visible.

The *inferior meatus*, the anterior aspect only, can be seen. The nasolacrimal duct opening is not seen.

Nasopharynx. In most patients the examiner can look completely through the nose and inspect part of the nasopharynx. Sometimes this is possible on only one side because of a deflection of the septum or an unusually prominent inferior turbinate. The use of vasoconstrictors will greatly increase the number of patients who can be examined in this manner.

Having the patient say "kick" or "k" causes the soft palate to fly upward. This movement orients the examiner as to how far posteriorly he is seeing. It also provides information about the mobility of the palate.

PARANASAL SINUSES

Examination of the paranasal sinuses is done more indirectly than other otolaryngic procedures. The examiner cannot see into any of the sinuses and only rarely can he see a sinus ostium. Information about the condition of the sinuses is gained (1) by inspecting and palpating the overlying soft tissues (maxillary and frontal sinuses), (2) by noting secretions that may drain from the sinuses, and (3) by transillumination (maxillary and frontal sinuses only).

Palpation and percussion. Palpation and per-

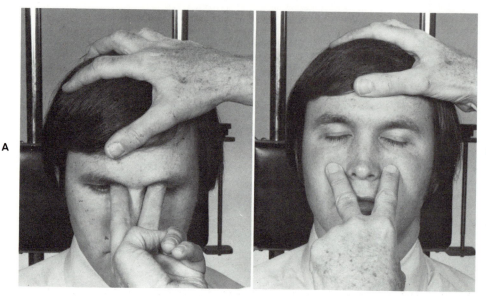

Fig. 11-45. A, Palpation for tenderness of the frontal sinuses. The examiner may percuss the anterior wall to elicit tenderness. **B,** Palpation of the maxillary sinuses.

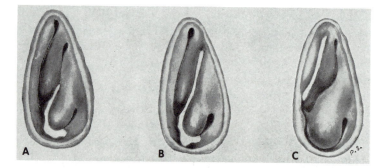

Fig. 11-46. Sites of purulent discharge. **A,** Maxillary sinusitis (low in middle meatus). **B,** Frontal sinusitis. **C,** Sphenoid or posterior ethmoid sinusitis (superior meatus). (From DeWeese, D. D., and Saunders, W. H.: Textbook of otolaryngology, ed. 5, St. Louis, 1977, The C. V. Mosby Co.)

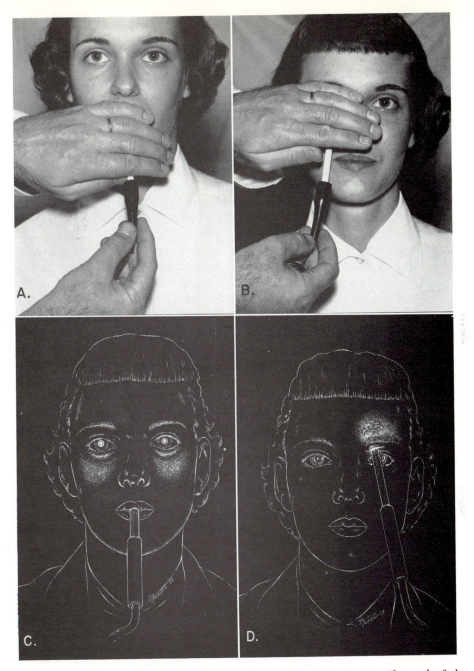

Fig. 11-47. Technique of transillumination of the maxillary sinuses. **A,** The end of the transilluminator aims toward the midline of the palate. Both maxillary sinuses are transilluminated at once. The hand shields light from the tube. **B,** Transillumination of frontal sinus. The hand should shield entire transilluminator. The procedure is repeated for the opposite frontal sinus. **C,** Drawing to show (1) the appearance of transillumination of the maxillary sinuses; note pink pupillary reflexes (patient should look from side to side); (2) diffuse pink reflex over the face of maxillary sinuses; (3) separate crescents of light under eyes. **D,** Transillumination of frontal sinuses varies greatly. Drawing represents a large frontal sinus with a relatively thin anterior wall.

cussion may be used over the maxillary and frontal sinuses. Simultaneous finger pressure over both maxillae will demonstrate differences in tenderness (Fig. 11-45, *B*). Palpation under the upper lip may demonstrate fullness not appreciated by inspection.

The frontal sinuses are palpated by finger pressure directed upward toward the floor of the sinus where the sinus wall is thin (Fig. 11-45, *A*). Tenderness may be elicited in this way. Swelling caused by tumors or retained secretions *(mucocele)* may cause a downward bulge in the floor of the frontal sinus. The ethmoid and sphenoid sinuses cannot be examined except by intranasal inspection.

Where sinuses drain. It is possible to tell which sinus is infected according to where a purulent discharge appears in the nose (Fig. 11-46). It is most important to use vasoconstrictors and a sharply focused light if the examiner is to see a small stream of pus in the nose.

1. Frontal and anterior ethmoid cells. Here the drainage is found well forward in the middle meatus and seems to come from high up.

2. Maxillary sinus. The ostium is somewhat farther back in the middle meatus, and drainage runs over the posterior end of the inferior turbinate. Therefore, pus from the maxillary sinus often is best seen by using the postnasal mirror.

3. Sphenoid and posterior ethmoid cells. The drainage is far posterior. The examiner sees secretions from these posterior sinuses by using either the nasal speculum or the postnasal mirror. The pus runs down between the middle turbinate and the septum.

Transillumination. The technique of transillumination of the paranasal sinuses is used less now than formerly because of greater use of roentgenologic diagnosis. Nevertheless, the technique is useful in certain situations and is described here. By shining a bright light in the mouth of a patient whose lips are closed about a special bulb, the examiner transilluminates the maxillary sinuses. The amount of light transilluminated varies greatly; therefore, differences in transillumination without other findings are not diagnostic. It is more important if one maxillary sinus transilluminates clearly and the other fails to do so than if both fail to transilluminate.

The frontal sinus is transilluminated by shining a shielded beam of light through the floor of the sinus. The ethmoid and sphenoid sinuses cannot be examined by transillumination.

The examiner should look for the following in sinus transillumination.

1. Frontal sinuses. As transillumination is done (one side at a time) the face of each sinus becomes light (Fig. 11-47, *B, D*). The frontal sinuses are rarely the same size, and so the examiner may see considerable difference in light reflex. Often neither side transilluminates well even in normal patients.

2. Maxillary sinuses. There are red pupillary reflexes and crescents of light under the eyes, and the faces of the sinuses glow pink (Fig. 11-47, *A, C*).

SELECTED READINGS

Becker, W., and others: Atlas of otorhinolaryngology and bronchoesophagology, Philadelphia, 1969, W. B. Saunders Co.

DeWeese, D. D., and Saunders, W. H.: Textbook of otolaryngology, St. Louis, ed. 5, 1977, The C. V. Mosby Co.

FILMS

The Ears—18 minutes, color, 16 mm., sound (Department of Health, Education and Welfare, National Medical Audiovisual Center, Atlanta, GA 30333).

The Nose—14 minutes, color, 16 mm., sound (Department of Health, Education, and Welfare, National Medical Audiovisual Center, Atlanta, GA 30333).

Physical diagnosis of the ears, nose and throat—28 minutes, color, 16 mm., sound (William H. Saunders, M.D., Department of Otolaryngology, The Ohio State University College of Medicine, Columbus, OH 43210).

CHAPTER 12

THORAX AND LUNGS

X-ray study of the lungs has become so widespread that it is now included routinely in every careful study of a patient, because the x-ray will reveal abnormalities in some instances that cannot be detected by physical examination. It is well recognized that some serious conditions can be detected by physical diagnosis only in their advanced stages, whereas the chest roentgenogram will reveal their presence much earlier, at a stage when the outlook for recovery is best. The superiority of chest roentgenography over physical examination in certain aspects has led all too often to the erroneous conclusion that x-ray films can detect everything that can be found as well as much that cannot be found by physical examination. The situation is analogous to watching television—the picture without sound leaves much to be desired and the sound without the picture may be meaningless. A friction rub, rales, and wheezing cannot be seen on x-ray films and can be detected only by our senses. In fact, the findings on the x-ray film in many instances can be interpreted intelligently only when coupled with the history and physical findings. *Careful examination should enhance our ability to interpret the x-ray films, and the chest film should serve as a check on the physical examination.*

Experience would indicate that the following order of procedure has much to recommend it: (1) inspection, (2) palpation, (3) percussion, and (4) auscultation. The adoption of a systematic approach, in which each stage is performed in sequence, helps to prevent oversight of any important aspect of the examination.

TOPOGRAPHIC ANATOMY AND THORACIC LANDMARKS

Before proceeding with discussion of examination of the thorax, it would be well to review the topographic anatomy of the thorax and some of the landmarks necessary to indicate (1) the location of the underlying structures and (2) the exact position of any abnormalities detected. For the sake of reference a number of lines and landmarks have been used to identify regions or locations on the thoracic wall. On the anterior surface the following vertical lines are commonly used: the *midsternal* and the right and left *midclavicular* (Fig. 12-1, A). The *midsternal* line is located in the middle of the sternum, and the *midclavicular* line runs directly downward from the midpoint of each clavicle. The nipple is not satisfactory as a landmark because of its inconstant location, even in the male.

On the lateral wall of the chest three vertical

189

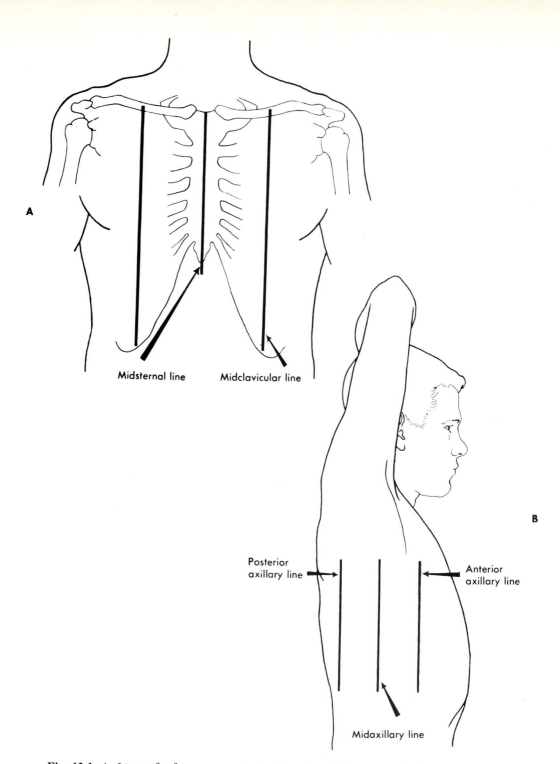

Fig. 12-1. A, Lines of reference on anterior thoracic wall. **B,** Lines of reference on lateral thoracic wall. In locating these lines the arm should be abducted directly away from the body and not more than 90 degrees.

lines (Fig. 12-1, *B*) are recognized: the *anterior axillary line*, drawn downward from the origin of the anterior axillary fold along the anterolateral aspect of the chest; the *posterior axillary line*, a continuation of the posterior axillary fold running downward along the posterolateral wall of the thorax; and midway between these two lines and running directly downward from the apex of the axilla is the *midaxillary line*. The arm must be abducted directly from the lateral thoracic wall in locating the above lines and should not be elevated more than 90 degrees. If the arm is moved either anteriorly or posteriorly as it is abducted or if it is abducted more than 90 degrees, the normal relationships of the axilla to the chest wall will be distorted.

On the posterior wall a valuable landmark is the *midspinal*, or *vertebral*, *line*, which runs down the posterior spinous processes of the vertebrae (Fig. 12-2). The *scapular line* runs parallel to the spine through the inferior angle of the scapula. Since there is considerable mobility of the scapula, this is a rather inconstant point of reference. When used, it should relate only to the position of the scapulae when the patient is erect with his arms at his sides.

For exact localization any abnormality should be described as being: (1) so many *centimeters medial* or *lateral* to the lines of reference, in (2) *a specific interspace* or *interspaces*. If described in this manner, there can be no question in anyone's mind as to the exact location of a lesion.

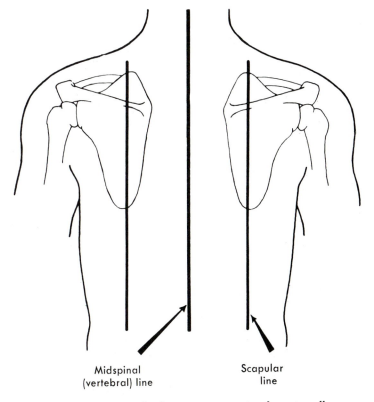

Midspinal
(vertebral) line

Scapular
line

Fig. 12-2. Lines of reference on posterior thoracic wall.

On the anterior thoracic wall the *manubrio-sternal junction* is a helpful landmark. This is a visible angulation of the sternum that corresponds to the second rib and serves as a convenient starting point for counting ribs. It is also significant in that it indicates the location of other important structures within the thorax that normally lie at the same level: (1) the fifth thoracic vertebra, (2) the bifurcation of the trachea, and (3) the upper level of the atria of the heart.

On the posterior thorax the *vertebra prominens* (seventh cervical vertebra) is usually found with ease at the base of the neck and serves as a convenient landmark to help identify the thoracic vertebrae and posterior ribs.

In addition, the student must have exact knowledge of the location of the underlying thoracic structures and those in the upper abdomen. The apices of the lungs extend for approximately 1½ inches above the clavicle on each side. On the right the fissure between the upper and middle lobes and the lower lobe (often called *right oblique* or *diagnonal fissure*) extends from approximately the fourth thoracic vertebra downward and laterally, where it crosses the fifth rib at the midaxillary line (Figs. 12-3, *A*, and 12-4). This fissure continues anteriorly and medially to approximately the sixth rib at its chondrocostal junction. In the anterior half of the chest this fissure separates the middle and lower lobes. The middle lobe lies between the upper and lower lobes but is present only in the anterior half of the thorax. The fissure between the upper and middle lobes (often called the *horizontal fissure*) arises

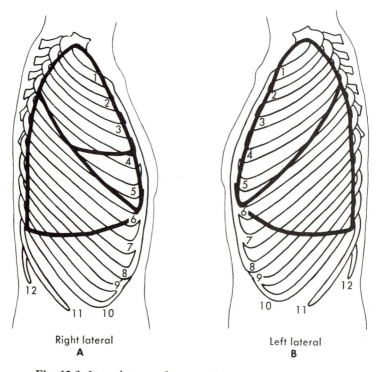

Right lateral
A

Left lateral
B

Fig. 12-3. Lateral views of topographic anatomy of the lungs.

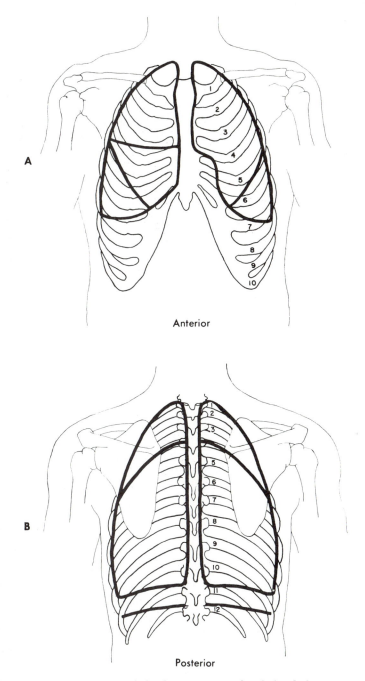

A

Anterior

B

Posterior

Fig. 12-4. Topographic anatomy of the lungs. Notice that behind the anterior thorax lie principally the upper lobes, whereas the lower lobes lie beneath most of the posterior thorax. The normal range of motion of the diaphragm is indicated in the posterior view.

slightly posterior to the midaxillary line at the fifth rib, from where it runs anteriorly in a horizontal plane to the third interspace.

On the left the fissure between the upper and lower lobes (the *left oblique* or *diagonal fissure*) is indicated by a line drawn from the fourth thoracic vertebra downward and laterally to the midaxillary line at the level of the fifth rib, continuing anteriorly and medially to the sixth chondrocostal junction (Figs. 12-3, *B*, and 12-4).

Thus, it will be seen that the anterior aspect of the right chest is composed principally of the upper and middle lobes, and the upper lobe lies beneath the major portion of the left anterior hemithorax (Fig. 12-4, *A*). On both hemithoraces the lower lobes present only a small portion anterolaterally and inferiorly. Posteriorly a very large proportion of the thorax is occupied by the lower lobes with only a small area of the upper lobes presenting superiorly (Fig. 12-4, *B*). While interpreting the chest roentgenogram, it is easy to assume that any lesion seen in the upper part of the lung fields is located in the upper lobes. This is a trap into which one can readily fall unless one keeps firmly in mind how high the superior segments of the lower lobes extend.

On the right the dome of the diaphragm is situated at a level approximating the fifth rib or fifth interspace at the midclavicular line. The dome of the left diaphragm is ordinarily about 1 inch lower than the right.

INSPECTION

Inspection of the chest, productive of the maximum amount of information, requires the following:

1. First and foremost, a definite desire to see and to appreciate every visible abnormality
2. The patient stripped to the waist
3. Good lighting
4. A thorough knowledge of topographic anatomy

5. The examiner and patient in a comfortable position throughout the examination. If either the physician or patient is uncomfortable, the examination may be hurried and consequently less thorough.

Since satisfactory inspection requires that the patient must be stripped to the waist, the room should be comfortably warm. If the patient is cold and shivering, inspection may be unsatisfactory, and the resulting sounds heard on auscultation may be confusing. For female patients, a disposable sleeveless paper gown serves admirably to prevent embarassing exposure and yet permit thorough examination.

Inspection is usually conducted while the patient is seated, except with those patients who are too sick to sit up. Slight differences in motility may be appreciated by looking from the side across the anterior aspect of the chest or down on the front of the chest in the patient who is seated. Examination of the supine patient is satisfactory. In fact, some examiners prefer the recumbent position for inspection. It is important that the patient be absolutely straight, whether seated or supine.

Good lighting is essential. It should be above and directly in front of the patient for inspection of the anterior thorax and above and behind for examining the posterior thoracic wall. Each of the lateral walls can be examined by the same light while the examiner is in the process of rotating the patient from front to back.

The student often finds inspection of the thorax difficult, partly because his powers of observation have not been developed. At times this may be true because his instructor attaches so much significance to auscultation and percussion that inspection and palpation are passed over lightly, as though unworthy of much attention. Once the art of critical inspection has been mastered, it requires little time and occasionally may prove to be very fruitful.

Normal thorax. The student should appreciate that in normal subjects there is a wide variation in the size and shape of the thorax. At times it is difficult to be certain where the normal variations end and definite pathologic changes begin. Although we expect that the shoulders normally will be at the same level, it will be noted frequently that one shoulder is slightly lower than the other. The clavicles should not be unduly prominent, but there is ordinarily a moderate depression of both the supraclavicular and infraclavicular areas. Although the two halves of the thorax anteriorly are seldom perfectly symmetric, they are nearly so. The right-handed person may show slightly greater muscular development on the right side of the anterior thoracic wall than on the left because of greater muscular development on the dominant side. The opposite would apply for those who are left-handed. Anteriorly each hemithorax, when viewed from above or below, projects farther forward than the sternum, which actually represents some depression between each side of the chest wall. The anteroposterior diameter of the thorax in the normal adult is definitely less than the transverse diameter. The thorax in the adult is roughly elliptic, whereas it is essentially cylindric in the infant. On inspiration there is both an upward and an anterior motion of the anterior thoracic wall, as well as outward expansion laterally.

On the posterior thoracic wall the scapular prominences are symmetrically located. The scapulae should be firmly applied to the underlying chest wall without "winging," and as a rule there is some depression between the medial scapular borders and the spine.

What to observe. First, the examiner should note the general nutrition and musculoskeletal development of the patient. Ordinarily he next observes the skin and breasts. A full consideration of the breast is found in Chapter 13. Normally the skin of the thorax is smooth, supple, and neither excessively dry nor oily. The adult male usually has a variable amount of hair. Lack of hair may be medically significant. As a rule the skin of the thorax reflects the general

character and coloration of the skin elsewhere in the body. It is heir to most of the disease conditions that may affect the skin in general (see Chapter 8). However, the *spider nevi* of cirrhosis of the liver (Fig. 15-3) are usually found only on the chest and shoulders, and *seborrheic dermatitis* commonly involves the hairy portion of the anterior thorax as well as the scalp.

The examiner should observe the anteroposterior diameter of the thorax. In those persons with pulmonary *emphysema* the anteroposterior diameter may be greatly increased so that it is as large as, and at times even greater than, the transverse diameter (Fig. 12-5). Next, the general slope of the ribs should be noted. Normally the ribs are situated at about a 45-degree angle in relation to the spine, but in patients with emphysema the ribs are more nearly horizontal. The width of the subcostal angle is noted; it is ordinarily less than 90 degrees and definitely widens during inspiration because of the lateral expansion of the thorax. In patients with emphysema this angle becomes abnormally wide, with little respiratory variation.

The presence of retraction or bulging of interspaces should be observed. *Retraction* of the interspaces, which may be noted on inspiration, is indicative of obstruction to the free inflow of air in the respiratory tract. *Bulging* of interspaces may occur in a massive pleural effusion, tension pneumothorax, and frequently is seen during forced expiration by the patient with emphysema or asthma. Occasionally, bulging may be noted in the thoracic wall as the result of tumor, aortic aneurysm, or marked cardiac enlargement in infancy and childhood.

Next, the examiner should observe the type, rate, and depth of quiet breathing. In the adult at rest the normal respiratory rate is approximately 16 to 18 breaths per minute and is quite regular in depth and rhythm. The normal ratio of respiratory rate to pulse rate is approximately 1:4. There is a definite increase in the

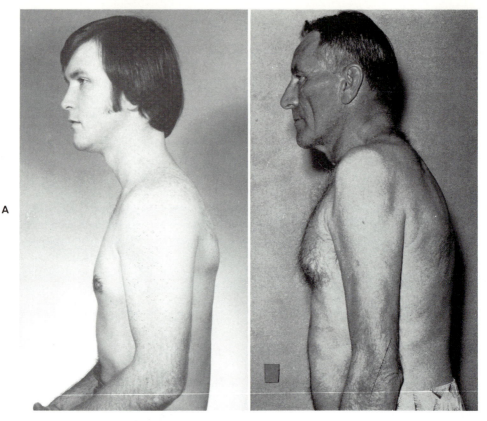

Fig. 12-5. Comparison of anteroposterior diameter of normal subject, **A,** with the obvious increase in diameter in patient with emphysema, **B.**

respiratory rate with fever, usually at the rate of approximately four additional respiratory cycles per minute for each degree above the normal temperature. Accessory respiratory muscles of the neck may be obviously participating in respiration in the person whose breathing is labored as the result of either strenuous exercise or disease. Under ordinary circumstances there is no evident use of the accessory respiratory muscles.

In the normal subject, the two sides of the chest move synchronously and expand equally, even though there may be great variation in rate and amplitude. Asymmetry may not be

seen during quiet respiration but may become quite obvious with forced inspiration. Consequently, expansion should be studied during both quiet and deep breathing.

Alterations in shape of the thorax include the following:

1. Unilateral retraction of the thorax in which, as the result of a thickened fibrotic pleura, one hemithorax is decreased in size and restricted in expansion as compared to the opposite side (occasionally seen in acute pleurisy or trauma to the chest wall, such as a fractured rib)
2. Pigeon or chicken breast (*pectus carina-*

tum), in which the sternum, instead of being lower than the adjacent hemithoraces, is protuberant, giving the thorax the configuration characteristic of fowl

3. Funnel chest *(pectus excavatum),* in which the sternum is abnormally depressed between each of the anterior hemithoraces. (At times the sternum is displaced so far posteriorly that it interferes with efficient function of the heart.)

The examiner must not forget that inspection of the chest includes examination of the posterior thorax. In general, the character of the skin of the posterior thorax is essentially the same as the anterior portion of the thorax except that growth of hair is usually less abundant. Acne is commonly observed in this area. The location of the scapulae and their range of motion should be noted. The spine should be straight, but when viewed from the side, there is normally a slight anterior concavity to the thoracic spine. A similar but opposite curvature is seen in the lumbar spine. An exaggerated thoracic curvature is called *kyphosis* and, when quite severe, is commonly termed *hunchback* or *humpback*.

Types of respiration. A number of terms have been used to describe the alterations that may be observed in breathing. Some of these terms are discussed here.

Dyspnea describes any status in which the patient becomes conscious of difficulty or effort in breathing. Ordinarily a person is not aware of any effort in breathing. Dyspnea is associated with definite uncomfortable sensations of not being able to get enough air and/or greater respiratory effort to satisfy the body's demands. Although dyspnea is an entirely subjective phenomenon, obvious respiratory effort may be observed, often including evident participation of the accessory respiratory muscles. Some patients become dyspneic only on exertion, whereas others, more severely dyspneic, may become quite short of breath with trivial effort

or may be so severely incapacitated that they are actually short of breath while at rest.

Dyspnea may be predominantly *inspiratory* or *expiratory*. *Inspiratory dyspnea* tends to occur primarily when there is obstruction, such as tumor, foreign body, severe laryngitis, or extrinsic compression of the trachea or major bronchi, resulting in an impediment to the inward free flow of air. Often this is accompanied by inspiratory retraction of the interspaces. Inspiratory obstruction, especially when located in the trachea or larynx, may be accompanied by low-pitched or crowing sounds, termed *stridor*. *Expiratory dyspnea* is associated primarily with obstruction in the bronchioles and smaller bronchi, as in asthma, bronchitis, and obstructive emphysema. Expiration is prolonged because of the obstruction to the outflow of air and may be accompanied by bulging of the interspaces.

Bradypnea is abnormal slowing of respiration (Fig. 12-6, *B*). *Apnea* is temporary cessation of breathing. *Tachypnea* indicates increased respiratory rate (Fig. 12-6, *C*). *Hyperpnea* is the condition in which there is actually an increase in the depth of respiration.

Hyperventilation is an abnormal increase in both rate and depth of respiration (Fig. 12-7, *A*). It is seen in diabetic acidosis, after vigorous exercise, and in highly emotional states. In emotional conditions it is termed the *hyperventilation syndrome*.

Pleuritic, or *restrained, breathing* is a type of respiration in which the inspiratory phase is suddenly interrupted as a result of pain associated with acute pleuritis. Consequently, people so afflicted have respirations that are quite shallow but more rapid than normal.

Periodic respiration (alternating hyperpnea and, apnea) is characterized by periods of rapidly increasing rate and depth of respiration, which within a matter of a few more respiratory cycles becomes shallower and shallower until respiration ceases (Fig. 12-7, *B*). This is fol-

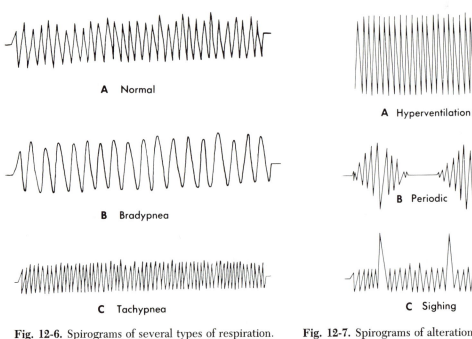

A Normal

B Bradypnea

C Tachypnea

Fig. 12-6. Spirograms of several types of respiration.

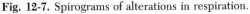

A Hyperventilation

B Periodic

C Sighing

Fig. 12-7. Spirograms of alterations in respiration.

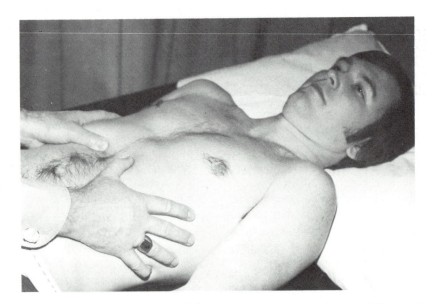

Fig. 12-8. Palpation in the evaluation of thoracic expansion. Note position of the examiner's hands, with the thumbs along each costal margin.

lowed by a period of apnea, which may last a few seconds to as long as 30 seconds. It is a common observation that the patient will sleep during the period of apnea but will become restless as respiration is resumed. Although observed occasionally in children and in the normal adult while asleep, periodic respiration may be present in many relatively severe disease states. In some instances the period of hyperventilation is followed by a period of quiet, shallow breathing rather than true apnea.

Stertorous respiration, a variety of noisy respiration, occurs frequently in the comatose patient and often is a terminal event. It is characterized by audible rattling and gurgling produced by the passage of air through secretions accumulating in the major bronchi and trachea of the patient who is so critically ill that the cough reflex is severely depressed or abolished. Because of its serious connotation it is commonly referred to as the *death rattle.*

Sighing respiration occurs when the normal respiratory rhythm is interrupted by a deep inspiration, which is followed by a prolonged expiration and ordinarily is accompanied by audible sighing (Fig. 12-7, *C*). Often called the "hallmark" of the neurotic, it is rarely associated with organic disease; instead it is almost always a manifestation of emotional tension.

Meningitic, or *ataxic, respiration* is an abnormality of breathing that is characterized by a gross irregularity of rate, rhythm, and depth. Seen only infrequently, it may be observed occasionally in meningitis and other forms of central nervous system disease and is of serious prognostic significance.

PALPATION

Often considerable information concerning the thorax and lungs can be obtained by palpation. Palpation may confirm or supplement the findings already noted during inspection.

Thoracic expansion

At times differences in expansion of one hemithorax in comparison with the other can be appreciated as well or better by palpation than by simple inspection. Variations in expansion are more readily detectable on the anterior surface where there is greater range of motion. The examiner's hands should be placed over the lower anterolateral aspect of the chest, with the thumbs along the costal margin, each pointing toward the xiphoid process, and the palms and fingers extended over the anterolateral wall (Fig. 12-8). Expansion should be tested during both quiet and deep inspiration. Expansion may be limited as the result of acute pleurisy, fibrous thickening of the pleura (fibrothorax), fractured ribs, or other trauma to the chest wall.

Fremitus

The term *fremitus* means vibration. In physical diagnosis the principal varieties that may be perceived by the hands as a vibratory sensation of the thoracic wall are vocal, pleural friction, tussive, and rhoncal fremitus.

Vocal fremitus. Vocal fremitus is a palpable vibration of the thoracic wall produced by phonation. The sounds that arise in the larynx are transmitted down along the air column of the tracheobronchoalveolar system into the bronchi of each lung, on through the smaller bronchi into the alveoli, setting in motion the thoracic wall that acts as a large resonator. Thus, vibrations are produced in the chest wall that can be felt by the hand of the examiner. Consequently, vocal fremitus is often called *tactile* fremitus.

In eliciting vocal fremitus the patient is directed to count "one, two, three"—"one, two, three," to repeat the words, "ninety-nine"—"ninety-nine," or to say "e-e-e, e-e-e, e-e-e." The patient should speak with a voice of uniform intensity throughout the examination so

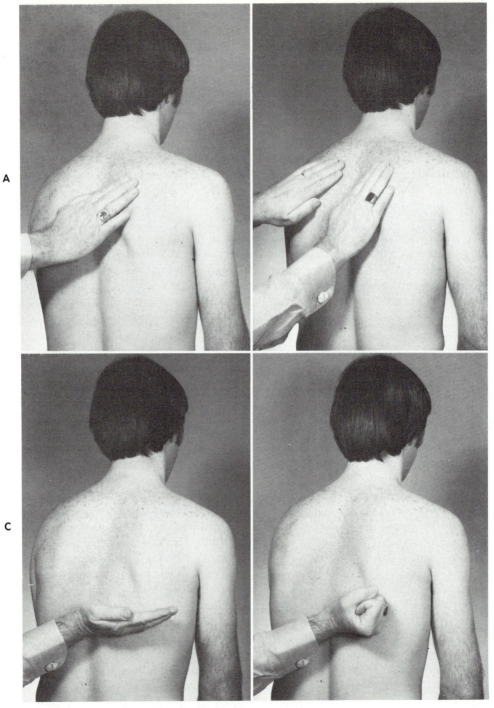

Fig. 12-9. Methods of detecting vocal fremitus. **A,** Palmar aspects of the fingertips. **B,** Simultaneous application of fingertips of both hands. **C,** Ulnar aspect of hand. **D,** Ulnar aspect of closed fist.

that the examiner can better compare the transmission of the femitus in different areas of the chest. If the fremitus is slight, it can be increased by having the patient speak in a louder, deeper voice.

The vocal fremitus is perceived by placing the palmar aspect of the fingers against the chest wall (Fig. 12-9). Usually both hands are used, placing them in corresponding areas so that simultaneous comparison of the two sides can be made. Some examiners prefer to use the ulnar aspect of the hand with the fingers extended or sometimes with the fingers closed in the palm. If only one hand is used, it should be moved from one place to the corresponding area of the other side to *compare* the transmission of sound.

Normal variations of vocal fremitus. The intensity of the vocal fremitus perceived in the normal subject is governed by the following:

1. Intensity of the voice
2. Pitch of the voice
3. Varying relations of the bronchi to the chest wall
4. Varying thickness of the thoracic wall

The tactile sensation of vocal fremitus is much more intense in subjects with deep voices and is less easily perceived in those with high-pitched voices. Low tones have a lower frequency and greater amplitude and consequently produce a vibration of the thoracic wall that is more readily palpable. Thus, it will be readily understood that vocal fremitus is ordinarily most intense in the slender adult male and that it is correspondingly less intense in women who possess voices with less volume and higher pitch.

In general, vocal fremitus is most prominent in the regions of the thorax where the large bronchi are the closest to the thoracic wall and tends to become less intense as one progresses farther from the major bronchi (Fig. 12-10). In the normal person the fremitus is found at maximum intensity over the upper thorax both anteriorly and posteriorly and along the course of the trachea and major bronchi anteriorly and posteriorly (between the scapulae and in the first and second interspaces just lateral to the sternum). It is least intense at the bases.

Also the intensity of the fremitus will vary with the thickness of the wall of the thorax. In a thin person the vibrations will be more intense than in the normally developed or obese patient in whom the normal or increased subcutaneous tissue has a damping effect on the fremitus. Likewise, it will be observed that, dependent on these same factors, there are changes in the vocal fremitus in different locations of the same subject, just as there is considerable variation from patient to patient.

It should be pointed out that only *gross changes* in the pleura and lungs give rise to perceptible changes in fremitus that are of diagnostic significance. It is not reasonable to expect that small patches of early tuberculosis or bronchopneumonia will be accompanied by significant changes of the vocal fremitus.

Alterations of vocal fremitus. Alterations of vocal fremitus include increased and decreased or absent fremitus. It will be recalled that a solid medium of uniform structure conducts vibration with greater intensity than does a porous structure composed of solid and air that is constantly undergoing variations in structure and density (as in normal lung tissue). Consequently, the transmission of sound will be greater than normal in any condition that tends to increase the density of the lung. Thus *increased vocal fremitus* occurs in conditions that are associated with a consolidation of the lungs, for example, lobar pneumonia. To produce exaggerated vocal fremitus the area of consolidation *must be in connection with a patent bronchus and must extend to the surface of the lung* where it may set the thoracic wall in motion.

Decreased or *absent fremitus* may occur when there is fibrous thickening of the pleura, when there is fluid in the pleural space, or

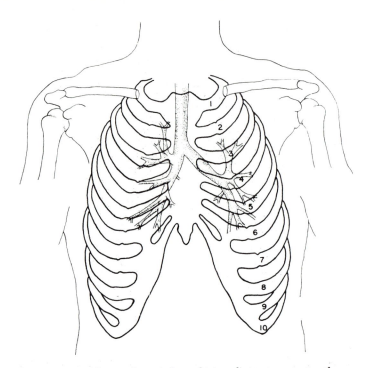

Fig. 12-10. Trachea and major bronchi in relation to anterior thorax.

when there is air in the pleural space (*pneumothorax*). When a major bronchus is obstructed, fremitus will be absent. This may result also from decreased intensity at the source of origin in the larynx, such as a decrease in voice. In large measure each of these conditions results from either a diminished production or transmission of the vocal sounds or from the interposition of an additional medium through which the sound must pass to reach the thoracic wall. Any condition that decreases fremitus may be sufficiently severe to cause the complete disappearance of fremitus.

Pleural friction fremitus. As the result of acute pleurisy, the inflamed pleural surfaces rub against one another, producing a *pleural friction rub* that may be detected by the examining hand. This palpable friction rub, known as *pleural friction fremitus*, gives a sen-

sation of "grating" that is synchronous with the respiratory excursion. When present, it is palpable usually in both phases of respiration, but occasionally it can be palpated only during one phase, most commonly inspiration. Friction rubs most commonly are felt as well as heard in the inferior anterolateral portion of the chest, the area of greatest thoracic excursion.

Other forms of fremitus. Other forms of fremitus include *tussive fremitus*, which is a vibration of the thoracic wall that is produced by coughing, and *rhonchal fremitus*, which is produced by the passage of air through thick exudate or an area of stenosis in the trachea or major bronchi. Pleural friction fremitus must be differentiated from rhonchal fremitus. As a rule, the latter can be eliminated by having the patient cough, since it is most commonly produced by the palpable rattling of exudate in the tracheobronchial tree. In contrast, the friction rub is not affected by coughing.

In addition, careful examination should include palpation of the thorax for areas of tenderness, pulsations, and masses. The texture of the skin also is noted.

Crepitation

Crepitation may be palpated when the subcutaneous tissues contain fine beads of air. This condition, known as *subcutaneous emphysema*, is caused by the escape of air from the lungs into the subcutaneous tissues as the result of injuries to or operation on the thorax. Crepitation is a coarse, crackling sensation that can be produced readily by pressing over the affected area. At times the crackling sound is actually audible. A somewhat similar sensation can be produced by rolling a lock of hair between the thumb and fingers.

PERCUSSION

Tapping various structures of the body in systematic fashion to produce a sound is known as *percussion*. There are two principal methods that may be used for percussion of the thorax, abdomen, or other structures.

1. *Mediate percussion* is that in which the examiner strikes a *pleximeter* (usually the middle finger of one hand) held against the thorax, thus producing a sound by setting the chest wall and underlying structures in motion. The *plexor* (the object striking the blow) is usually the middle finger of the other hand. This is the method in almost universal use today.

2. *Immediate percussion* may be useful in demonstrating changes in percussion note. This can be done by striking the chest with either the palmar aspect of the middle finger or the tips of all of the fingers held firmly together (Fig. 12-11).

Mediate percussion. The distal phalanx of the middle finger of one hand (usually the left if the examiner is right-handed) is pressed

firmly against the chest wall parallel to the ribs but with the palm and other fingers held *off* the skin (Fig. 12-12). A very short quick blow is struck at the base of the terminal phalanx of the pleximeter finger with the tip of the middle finger of the right hand. When properly performed, the forearm is virtually stationary, the entire movement being executed from the wrist. This maneuver may be practiced in either of two ways:

1. Placing the right hand and forearm flat on a table or the wall, cock the hand back at the wrist, strike the table or wall a quick blow with the tip of the middle finger, and then return immediately to the position of the "cocked wrist," ready to strike again.

2. Grasping the right distal forearm with the left hand to prevent any movement of the right forearm, cock the wrist, strike a sharp, quick blow with the tip of the middle finger, and return.

When the examiner strikes the chest, the entire chest wall and its contents will be set into motion. By percussing a localized site, he cannot limit the segment of lung that will be set in vibration. By striking a light blow, however, he can make deeper and more distant portions vibrate less and therefore produce less audible sound than the area receiving the immediate attention. Thus, the examiner is often able to make a sharper localization of changes in the lung underlying the area under study by *light* percussion than with a more forceful blow.

Practical experience has demonstrated that useful sounds produced by percussion probably do not penetrate more than about 4 to 5 cm. below the surface (Fig. 12-13). Hence any attempt to outline an organ or solid mass deeper in the chest is doomed to failure. Also a lesion must be at least 2 or 3 cm. in diameter to be detectable. Thus, it is obvious that percussion will only locate rather gross abnormalities.

In addition to the sound that is perceived by

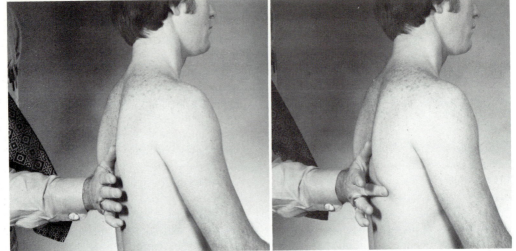

Fig. 12-11. Immediate percussion using the middle finger. **A,** The finger is poised to strike the thorax. **B,** The palmar aspect of the finger is striking the chest wall.

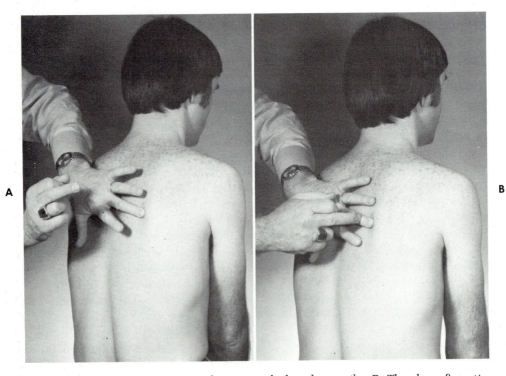

Fig. 12-12. Mediate percussion. **A,** The wrist cocked ready to strike. **B,** The plexor fingertip is striking the pleximeter finger. Notice that only the pleximeter finger touches the patient's thorax.

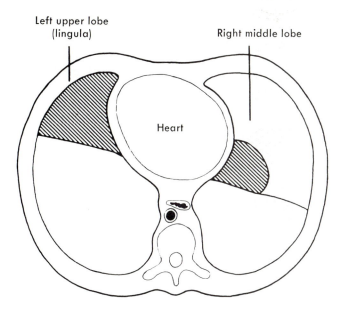

Left upper lobe
(lingula)

Right middle lobe

Heart

Fig. 12-13. A drawing illustrative of the limitations of percussion. Since the pneumonic consolidation seen in the lingula of the left upper lobe extends to the surface, changes in the percussion note might be present, but no changes could be expected over the central lesion in the right middle lobe because of its depth.

ear, the student should be aware that important vibratory sensations are perceived by the pleximeter finger. As the examiner becomes more expert in the art of percussion, the sensations palpated by the pleximeter finger will become virtually as important as the audible sound. In fact, if the room should happen to be sufficiently noisy to interfere with hearing the percussion note, a skilled examiner would still be able to perform a satisfactory percussion because he could rely on his cultivated sense of touch.

To obtain the maximum information from percussion:

1. The distal phalanx of the pleximeter finger must be pressed *firmly* on the chest wall; otherwise, a clear note is not obtained.

2. The plexor finger should *strike* the pleximeter finger only instantaneously and must be *immediately withdrawn*.

3. The examiner should also be *sensitive* to the *vibratory sensations* that are being received from the chest wall by the pleximeter finger.

4. The examiner must *compare one side* of the *thorax* with the *opposite* side as he proceeds with the percussion.

5. As the examiner listens to the sound elicited by percussion, a careful *analysis* should be made of all the characteristics of the tone so formed.

After the patient is properly positioned with the head and shoulders erect, the anterior thoracic wall is examined. Usually percussion is performed above the clavicles in the supraclavicular spaces, followed by percussion of the first interspaces, always comparing one side with the other. Examination is continued by percussing downward, interspace by interspace. Next, the patient should raise his arm and rest his hand on his head as each lateral wall is examined, beginning in the axilla and working down to the costal margin, with the pleximeter finger always parallel to the ribs— never across them.

In examining the back of the chest the patient should have his head inclined forward and the forearms crossed comfortably at the waist to move the scapulae as far laterally as possible, since percussion over a bony structure such as the scapula produces no useful information. Examination is started at the apices, where the percussion note as well as the width of the isthmus of normal resonance over the apex is determined (Fig. 12-14). Bounded medially by the neck muscles and laterally by the shoulder girdle, this band of resonance is normally about 5 cm. wide. The percussion is continued down-

ward, interspace by interspace, to the bases where the location and range of motion of each hemidiaphragm is ascertained.

Analysis of percussion tones. When we tap on the chest, the lung, the heart, and the thoracic wall are all set into motion and the waves pass from the vibrating chest through the air to the ear, producing a characteristic sound. The sound waves produced by percussion are influenced more by the character of the immediate underlying structures than by those more distant. Consequently the tone produced by percussion over the air-filled lung will be definitely different from the tone heard over a solid structure, such as the heart or liver. This is the basis for the scientific application of percussion to the study of the human body. Careful atten-

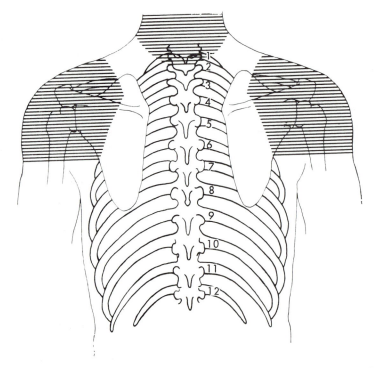

Fig. 12-14. A normal band of resonance over the apices is about 5 cm. in width and is bounded by dullness of the neck medially and the shoulder muscles laterally.

tion to the character of the percussion sounds will help to detect abnormalities as well as to locate normal structures.

Sound has four well-defined characteristics:

1. Intensity (amplitude). The intensity of a sound depends on the *amplitude* of the vibration, the loud sound having a greater amplitude of vibration than the soft tone. The tone produced by percussion over the porous lung is louder than that produced over the liver or heart because the lung is a more elastic tissue and, when struck, vibrates with greater amplitude.

2.Pitch (frequency). The pitch depends on the number of vibrations per second. The tone produced by percussion over the normal lung has fewer oscillations and therefore is lower in pitch than over a solid organ or consolidated lung.

3. Quality. The quality or timbre of a tone is very difficult to describe since it is purely subjective, but it is produced primarily by the associated overtones. However, it is the important characteristic that enables us to appreciate and distinguish sounds arising from different sources. For example, although the intensity and pitch of a given tone may be the same, it is the quality or timbre that permits us to readily differentiate tones produced by a violin from those produced by a piano.

4. Duration. An additional feature that helps in the analysis of the percussion sound is its duration. The normal or hyperresonant note is well sustained, whereas the dull note over pneumonic consolidation and the flat note over fluid or a solid organ are much briefer.

One of the most common mistakes of the beginning student in physical diagnosis is to pay attention to only one aspect of the sound—usually intensity—that is produced by percussion or heard on auscultation. As a consequence he neglects the other characteristics that may be of vital importance in the identification of variations in sounds. If the examiner overlooks the important changes in the pitch and quality as well as the duration of the tone, a normal percussion note of low intensity might be mistaken for the soft, high-pitched, brief note over a solid organ, pneumonic consolidation, or pleural fluid.

Percussion sounds. The sounds produced by percussion are generally classified as follows:

1. *Resonance,* the sound heard normally over lungs, although not loud, is usually heard with ease, is well sustained, and is moderately low in pitch. In addition, it has a characteristic quality. The composite normal resonant note can only be learned from personal experience, accomplished by percussion of many normal chests.

2. *Hyperresonance* is of lower pitch than normal resonance. It is a well-sustained sound that has a deep "booming" character. It is relatively intense and consequently is usually heard with ease. A relatively hyperresonant note is found normally in children. The hyperresonant note in the adult is commonly the result of emphysema and occasionally pneumothorax.

3. *Tympany* is a relatively musical sound in which the fundamental pitch can often be distinguished (somewhat similar to the sound of a drum). The sound, as a rule, tends to be higher than that of normal resonance, is only moderately well sustained in duration, and is moderate or loud in intensity. It results from air in an enclosed chamber (the stomach and bowel), and in general the greater the tension within the viscus, the higher the pitch. Tympany is the sound heard anteriorly and laterally over the abdomen except in the area of the liver. It never occurs in the normal chest, except below the dome of the left hemidiaphragm, where the underlying stomach and bowel will produce tympany.

4. *Dullness* is essentially the opposite of resonance and hyperresonance in that a dull note is short, high pitched, and is not loud (in other

words, it does not carry very far). The quality is difficult to describe but is most nearly compared to a dull "thud." Further, it should be noted that the pleximeter finger perceives relatively little vibratory sensation. Instead there often is a sense of increased resistance. This is in distinct contrast to the note of hyperresonance, such as encountered in the emphysematous chest, where there is considerable feeling of vibration. It should be emphasized that a dull percussion note is dull only as it compares with other percussion notes, not in terms of measurable scales of frequency and amplitude.

5. *Flatness* is the term used to describe the percussion note when resonance is absent. The sound and the feeling are very similar to striking a barrel or other container filled with wa-ter. Therefore, flatness is a more extreme manifestation of dullness.

Dullness tends to occur when there is considerable solid or liquid medium present in the underlying lung in proportion to the amount of air in the lung tissue. Thus, dullness will be found when there is consolidation of lung, such as occurs in pneumonia, or when there is a moderate amount of fluid in the pleural space with some underlying air-containing lung. Flatness will be present when there is a very large fluid mass, such as in an extensive pleural effusion with little underlying air-bearing lung to influence the sound, or heard over a solid organ such as the liver and heart.

A number of variations of the percussion note occur from patient to patient as well as in the same patient. Over the apices, where there

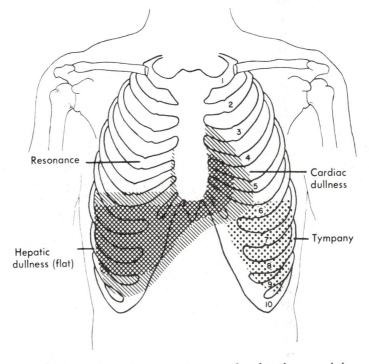

Fig. 12-15. Variations in the percussion notes found in the normal thorax.

are large amounts of muscle and bone with relatively little underlying resonant lung, the note is less resonant than over the bases, where there is a relatively greater amount of lung with less thoracic wall and muscle. The development of the pectoral muscles, the heavy muscles of the back, the breasts, and the scapulae, all tend to make the percussion note less resonant (duller). It should be noted that below the dome of the right diaphragm there is flatness because of the presence of the liver (Fig. 12-15). On the left there is ordinarily a relatively tympanic note that results from the presence of the partially air-filled stomach and bowel under the hemidiaphragm.

The change from resonance to flatness on the right and from resonance to tympany on the left is not immediate; instead, there is a zone of transition. Dullness from the liver is usually noted at approximately the fifth interspace in the midclavicular line, and this dullness soon gives way to flatness as that part of the liver not covered by the lung is reached. Also the change from pulmonary resonance to tympany over the left lower chest at about the sixth rib in the midclavicular line has the same general tendency to transition, not an abrupt change. There is also dullness to the left of the sternum, caused by the underlying heart, another solid organ. In the left fifth interspace this dullness normally extends to a point 1 or 2 cm. medial to the midclavicular line. Percussion of the heart is discussed in Chapter 14.

Effect of position on percussion sounds. Occasionally the patient is too ill to sit up to permit percussion of the posterolateral aspects of the chest. The anterior and anterolateral wall of the chest may be satisfactorily examined in the supine position. Under these circumstances the posterior and posterolateral thoracic wall must be examined with the patient rolled on his side. Although this is much less satisfactory than the upright position, reasonably accurate information can be obtained but only if the student is familiar with the changes that result from the patient lying on his side.

The lateral recumbent position causes the following changes:

1. Some curvature of the spine results, with a widening of the intercostal spaces in that portion of the thoracic wall that is against the bed and a narrowing of the interspaces on the upper side; this curvature can be counteracted to some degree if the pillow is removed and the head is allowed to rest on the bed.

2. Disproportionate elevation of the hemidiaphragm of the "down" side results from the pressure of the abdominal viscera.

3. The surface of the bed affects the percussion note by acting as a damper for the sounds.

As a result of these three factors, the following changes are observed (Fig. 12-16): (1) there is an area of relative dullness along the chest next to the bed; (2) above this area and at the base of the lung there is a roughly triangular area of dullness, with the base toward the bed and the apex approaching the spine; (3) on the upper side there may be some relative dullness at approximately the tip of the scapula, which is caused by changes in the lung as a result of the crowding of the ribs.

After rolling the patient on one side, inspection, palpation, percussion, and auscultation are performed on the "up" side, and then the opposite side is turned up and examined in the same manner.

Diaphragmatic excursion. The respiratory excursion of the diaphragm may be estimated by percussion. First, the patient is instructed to take a deep inspiration and hold it. Second, the lower margin of resonance (which represents the level of the diaphragm) is determined by percussion from the normal lung, moving downward until a definite change in tonal quality is heard. Third, the patient is instructed to

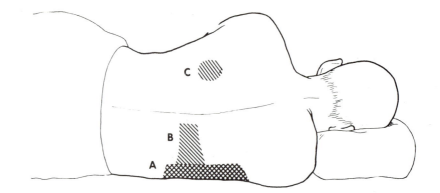

Fig. 12-16. Effect of lateral recumbent position on percussion note. **A,** Zone of relative dullness next to bed. **B,** Zone of dullness caused by pressure of viscera. **C,** Area of dullness at approximately the tip of the scapula.

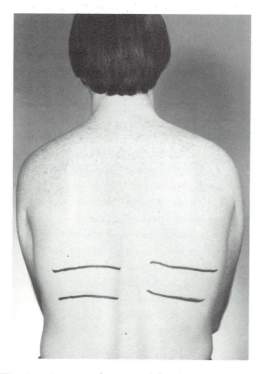

Fig. 12-17. Range of motion of the diaphragm as detected by percussion.

exhale as far as possible and to hold his breath, and the percussion is repeated. The distance between these levels indicates the range of motion of the diaphragm (Fig. 12-17). This procedure is repeated for the opposite hemidiaphragm. The normal diaphragmatic excursion is about 3 to 5 cm. It is decreased in patients with pleurisy and severe emphysema. The diaphragm is unusually high in any condition that causes an increase in intra-abdominal pressure, such as ascites or pregnancy, and lower than normal in pulmonary emphysema. In the recumbent patient the level of the diaphragm is approximately one interspace higher than in the upright position.

AUSCULTATION

Auscultation, which is the act of listening to sounds produced within the body, may be accomplished in two ways: (1) with the unaided ear *(immediate auscultation)* or (2) with the stethoscope *(mediate auscultation)*. The modern binaural stethoscope, consisting of a bell or diaphragm connected with rubber tubing to earpieces, is designed for the clear transmission of sound from the patient to the ear of the examiner and to exclude as far as possible all extraneous noise.

There are two principal types of stethoscopes: the bell and the diaphragm. From a clinical point of view it would appear that the diaphragm type of chestpiece is more receptive to the high-pitched tones than is the bell type, whereas low-pitched sounds are often heard better through the bell type. Perhaps the best examples are the murmur of mitral stenosis— a deep, low-pitched rumble, which is often heard better with the bell, and the relatively high-pitched, soft murmur of aortic regurgitation, which is heard better with the diaphragm. Stethoscopes that are combinations of the bell and diaphragm have been devised to take advantage of the acoustic qualities of each type.

It is essential that the earpieces fit properly and comfortably so that the examiner can use the stethoscope for hours at a time, if necessary, without discomfort. Although the earpieces must fit snugly to exclude extraneous sounds, they should not be so tight that they become uncomfortable. Often earpieces are too small and tend to slip into the auditory canal, virtually occluding all sound. The stethoscope should not exceed 20 inches in length (the shorter, the better); the tubing should have an internal diameter of $^3/_{16}$ inch or more with a thick plastic or rubber wall. Acoustically, double tubing is superior to a single tube.

The stethoscope should be placed *firmly* against the chest wall to exclude as much extraneous sound as possible, as well as to eliminate any sounds that may result from light contact with the skin during respiratory excursion. Sufficient pressure should be exerted so that when the examiner removes it after listening to two or three breaths, a definite blanched ring will be seen on the skin where the bell has been located. Care must be taken to avoid movement of the stethoscope on the skin, since such movement will produce confusing noises. Breathing on the tubing or moving or sliding the fingers on the chestpiece will also cause extrinsic sounds. The pressure of the stethoscope on hair on the chest can produce sounds that may resemble rales, since both are rather crackling in character.

The patient should be instructed to breathe a little deeper than usual with his mouth open. Breathing through the open mouth minimizes the sounds produced in the nose and throat. Although breath sounds will be more readily audible if the patient breathes a little deeper than usual, deep forced inspiration tends to introduce muscle sounds that may be confusing to the student.

Corresponding areas of each side are auscultated as the examiner goes from top to bottom, just as in percussion.

In general, auscultation consists of the following:

1. *Analysis of the breath sounds* themselves, comparing respiration and expiration for the following:
   a. Pitch (frequency). It must be clearly understood that when a breath sound is described as high or low in pitch it is: (1) high or low principally in relation to the pitch of other breath sounds, or (2) the pitch of expiration and inspiration may be high or low as contrasted to one another.
   b. Intensity (amplitude). Again it is to be emphasized (1) that breath sounds are loud or soft in relationship to other breath sounds or (2) that one phase of respiration is loud or soft in relation to the other.
   c. Quality. Quality of each phase should be ascertained.
   d. Duration. The relative duration of the expiratory and inspiratory phases should be noted.

2. *Transmission* and *alteration* of the spoken and whispered voice
3. Detection of any *adventitious sounds*

Careful attention to all the features just mentioned is essential if the examiner is to obtain the maximum information from all of the audible sounds.

Breath sounds—normal

As the result of the movement of air in the tracheobronchoalveolar system, relatively soft sounds are produced that are termed the *breath sounds*.

Vesicular. The vesicular breath sound is believed to be the result of movement of air in the bronchioles and alveoli. Variously described as sighing or a gentle rustling, vesicular breathing is a soft, relatively low-pitched sound (Fig. 12-18, *A*). The normal vesicular respiration is longer in the inspiratory than in the expiratory phase by a ratio of approximately 5:2, in contrast to the ratio of the respiratory thoracic motion, which is 5:6. It should be emphasized that expiration as heard in vesicular

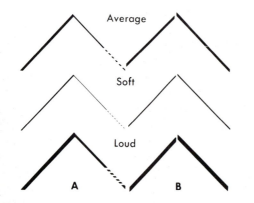

Fig. 12-18. A, Schematic representation of vesicular breath sounds. Inspiration (left arm of drawing) is definitely louder, longer, and higher pitched than expiration (right arm of drawing). **B,** Bronchovesicular breath sounds. Inspiration and expiration are very much the same.

breathing is not actually shorter than inspiration—only that much of expiration is not audible. Inspiration is higher in pitch and louder than expiration. In fact, expiration occasionally may be inaudible. *Vesicular breath sounds are heard normally over most of the lungs.*

Bronchovesicular. In certain areas where the trachea and major bronchi are in proximity to the chest wall, there is heard a mixture of both tracheobronchial and vesicular elements that is termed *bronchovesicular breath sound* (Fig. 12-18, *B*). This type of breath sound is heard *normally* on each side of the sternum in the first and second interspaces, between the scapulae, and over the apices anteriorly and posteriorly, but are more prominent on the right than on the left. *When heard in other locations, bronchovesicular breathing is abnormal and is indicative of some disease process.* In bronchovesicular breathing the inspiratory phase resembles that of normal vesicular breathing, except that it is slightly louder and higher pitched. The expiratory phase is longer, and increased in pitch and intensity, with a slightly tubular quality, as compared with the vesicular sound, but it is still somewhat shorter, softer, lower in pitch, and less tubular than in true bronchial breathing. A very brief pause may be noted between inspiration and expiration. In essence, the expiratory and inspiratory phases are very similar as to duration, pitch, intensity, and quality.

Vesicular and bronchovesicular are, therefore, the two types of breath sounds heard *normally* over the lungs. There is no better way to become familiar with the normal breath sounds than to listen to the chests of many different healthy persons.

Breath sounds—abnormal

Although in the different types of breath sounds—normal and abnormal—there are definite variations in the inspiratory phase, greater changes occur in the expiratory phase. Consequently, particular attention should be paid to the alterations that occur during expiration.

Bronchial breathing. This abnormal breath sound has a blowing, hollow character, more so during expiration than inspiration (Fig. 12-19). Bronchial breath sounds are in general higher in pitch than vesicular or bronchovesicular sounds. Expiration usually surpasses inspiration in length. Although it is usually louder than normal, at times it may be relatively quiet and can be recognized only by careful attention to its other qualities. Thus, as a rule, expiration is longer, louder, higher pitched, and more hollow or tubular than inspiration. Also, there is a short but definite pause between the two phases. Often it has another characteristic in that it seems to be very close, almost as though the sound were actually right in the very end of the stethoscope.

Bronchial breathing is not normally heard over the lungs, although a very similar sound is heard over the trachea. Therefore, *its presence over the lungs always indicates disease*. It occurs only with pulmonary consolidation, whether total or partial. Classically, it is heard in pneumonia and other conditions accompa-

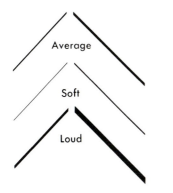

Fig. 12-19. Schematic representation of bronchial breath sounds in which the expiratory phase is longer, louder, higher, and more tubular, or hollow, than inspiration.

nied by consolidation of lung parenchyma—in other words, an increased conducting mechanism.

Bronchovesicular breathing. Bronchovesicular breathing is abnormal when heard in any area of the lungs that normally have vesicular breath sounds. An admixture of consolidated and aerated lung produces a mixture of bronchial and vesicular breathing—bronchovesicular breath sounds. To evaluate the pathologic significance of bronchovesicular breath sounds, the examiner must know accurately the areas where they are heard normally.

Asthmatic breath sounds. In asthmatic breathing expiration is markedly prolonged, is usually louder than normal, and is accompanied by wheezing sibilant rhonchi. Although expiration is definitely prolonged, in contrast to bronchial breathing there is no hollow or tubular component to the expiratory phase of the asthmatic breath sound. At times it is readily heard without the stethoscope. This type of breath sound is heard not only during asthmatic attacks but also may be present in emphysema and bronchiolitis.

Decreased or absent breath sounds. Breath sounds may be decreased in intensity without change in fundamental type as the result of several conditions. In some instances the breath sounds may be entirely absent.

1. One of the most common causes is fluid in the pleural space. The fluid may be blood (*hemothorax*), inflammatory (*pleural effusion*), pus (*pyothorax* or *empyema*), or transudate (*hydrothorax*). Here the diminution in breath sounds is the result of the interposed liquid medium as well as a definite decrease in ventilation of the underlying lung.

2. In the same manner air in the pleural space (*pneumothorax*) causes a diminution in the breath sounds.

3. If there is thickened pleura caused by fibrosis—which may follow effusion, hemothorax, and empyema—or by actual tumor in-

volvement of the pleura, decrease in breath sounds is noted.

Whether fluid, air, or solid in the pleural space, all interfere with the conduction of breath sounds so that they are decreased or even absent.

4. Breath sounds are commonly decreased in emphysema because of the decreased air velocity and sound conduction.

5. Breath sounds are markedly diminished or absent in complete bronchial obstruction.

6. If there is definite decrease in expansion, such as that commonly noted in painful pleurisy with its attendant shallow breathing, the breath sounds are diminished because of the decreased ventilation.

Voice sounds—normal

Vocal resonance. Vocal resonance is produced in the same fashion as vocal fremitus. The vibrations produced in the larynx by phonation are transmitted via the tracheobronchoalveolar tract to the thoracic wall, where the voice sounds can be heard with the stethoscope. The words spoken are not as loud and clear as when heard directly, and the syllables are not distinguishable; that is, one cannot understand what the patient is saying. The spoken voice as heard over the normal lung is termed *vocal resonance*.

Vocal resonance varies in exactly the same fashion as does vocal fremitus. It is heard loudest near the trachea and major bronchi and is less intense at the extreme bases.

Voice sounds—abnormal

Bronchophony. Bronchophony indicates vocal resonance that is increased both in intensity and clarity. It should be noted that the syllables are *not* distinguishable in bronchophony. It is usually associated with increased vocal fremitus, dullness to percussion, and bronchial breathing, and as a rule indicates the presence of pulmonary consolidation.

Whispered pectoriloquy. Although pectoriloquy can also apply to the spoken voice, its use in ordinary practice is limited to the study of the transmission of the whispered voice. To be of practical significance the sounds must be actually whispered; softly spoken words that require the use of the vocal cords are not suitable. In the normal subject the whispered voice is heard only faintly and indistinctly throughout the chest except anteriorly and posteriorly in the regions overlying the trachea and primary bronchi—in other words, those areas that correspond to the regions in which bronchovesicular breath sounds are normally heard. Even here the sounds are normally indistinct and the syllables cannot be clearly understood. At the bases the whispered voice may be entirely inaudible.

Pectoriloquy implies that there is definite recognition of words—the syllables are understood as they are whispered. It may be quite faint, but more often it sounds as though the words were being whispered directly into the end of the stethoscope. Although pectoriloquy is only a form of exaggerated bronchophony, at times it is more easily detected than bronchophony. Pectoriloquy is never normal, and its presence always indicates consolidation of the lung. Occasionally whispered pectoriloquy may be obvious before bronchial breath sounds develop over an area of pneumonia.

Egophony. Egophony is a modified form of bronchophony in which there is not only an increase in intensity of the spoken voice but its character is altered so that there is a definite nasal or "bleating" quality. It is occasionally heard over an area of consolidation, over the upper portion of a pleural effusion, or where there is a small amount of fluid in association with pneumonic consolidation. The exact reason for this modification of bronchophony is not known. It is most readily elicited by having the patient say "e-e-e." If egophony is present, the spoken "eeee" will sound as though the patient is saying "āāāā." "E" is a relatively pure tone. As one phonates "ā" it has a somewhat nasal character. It is the change from the "e" that the patient speaks to the "ā" heard with the stethoscope that indicates the presence of egophony.

Decreased vocal resonance. Vocal resonance is decreased under the same circumstances that the vocal fremitus and the breath sounds are decreased or absent—where there is interference in the conduction of vibrations produced in the thorax, such as is found with pleural thickening, pleural fluid, pneumothorax, adiposity, or complete bronchial obstruction. It should be noted that, although the vocal resonance and vocal fremitus are usually diminished over a pleural effusion, occasionally they may actually be increased at the upper level of the fluid as the result of compression of the lung or if there is pneumonic consolidation of the underlying lobe, provided the bronchus supplying the area is patent.

Adventitious sounds

Adventitious sounds are those that are not heard normally over the chest. They do *not* represent alterations in sounds normally present in the thorax but are sounds *that are superimposed on the breath sounds, and that may be normal or abnormal.* The most common adventitious sounds are the various types of rales and rhonchi and the pleural friction rub.

Rales and rhonchi. There have been many classifications of the abnormal sounds that may be heard in the alveoli or bronchi or both as the result of passage of air through narrowed passageways. The sounds so produced are most simply divided into two main varieties: *rales* and *rhonchi* (Fig. 12-20). Some systems of classification are very complicated and are quite confusing to the student. Although the following may represent an oversimplification of rales and rhonchi, practical experience indicates that it does have the advantage of simplicity and ease of comprehension, and gives some indication of the part of the pulmonary system that is primarily involved.

Rales. "Râle" (French) means "rattling" and is pronounced with a broad "a." Rales are a shower of discrete sounds of varying degrees of coarseness heard during respiration. They are also referred to as crackles or discontinuous sounds. They result from the passage of air through secretions in the respiratory tract and from reinflation of the alveoli and bronchioles, the walls of which have become adherent as the result of moisture. Rales, therefore, are produced by air flow plus abnormal moisture. According to the size of the air chamber involved (trachea, bronchi, bronchioles, and alveoli) and the character of the exudate, rales vary in their size, intensity, distribution, duration, and persistence. Rales are most often heard in the terminal phase of inspiration and are more pronounced when the patient is instructed to breathe deeply. Rales are very similar to the sound heard over a recently opened

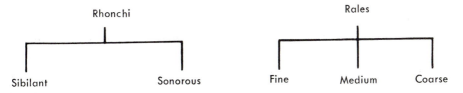

Fig. 12-20. Diagram of two forms of adventitious sounds: rhonchi, which are relatively continuous sounds, and rales, which are more or less discrete sounds.

carbonated drink; even though the sound seems to be continuous, it is actually composed of thousands of discrete sounds, each from the rupture of a small bubble—in other words, they are *monopolar* in origin. Rhonchi differ very fundamentally from rales in that the former are continuous sounds, similar to the sound produced by blowing a reed instrument or playing a violin. Rales may be divided roughly into three categories: fine, medium, and coarse.

Fine rales have a fine, crackling quality that may be simulated by (1) holding a lock of hair close to the ear and then rubbing it between the thumb and forefinger or (2) by separating slowly the thumb and forefinger after they have been moistened with saliva. Both maneuvers will produce a burst of sharp crackling sounds that resemble fine rales. The examiner will appreciate that rales are actually a series of relatively discrete sounds—not a continuous sound

(Fig. 12-21, *A*). They most commonly occur at the end of inspiration and are not cleared by coughing. Although fine rales do have a crackling, dry character, they are the result of moisture in the alveoli. Fine rales indicate inflammation or congestion involving the alveoli and bronchioles. Consequently they may be heard in pneumonia, pulmonary congestion, and many other diseases.

Medium rales represent a gradation between coarse and fine rales in that they are not as coarse and bubbling or gurgling as coarse rales and are not as finely crackling as the fine rales just discussed (Fig. 12-21, *B*). They may be simulated by rolling a dry cigar between the fingers or listening to the "fizz" of a freshly opened carbonated drink. They tend to be the result of the passage of air through mucus in the bronchioles and small bronchi or the separation of the walls of these structures that have become adherent because of exudate. Medium

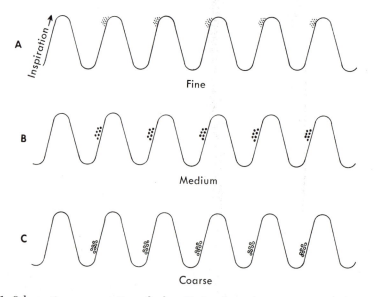

Fig. 12-21. Schematic representation of rales. Notice that rales are represented as a number of discrete sounds. Fine rales generally occur late in inspiration, whereas coarse rales tend to occur earlier in the inspiratory phase.

and coarse rales tend to occur earlier in respiration than do fine rales.

Coarse rales have their origin in the trachea, bronchi, and some of the smaller bronchi. They are relatively loud, coarse, bubbling, gurgling sounds that are produced by the passage of air through exudate (Fig. 12-21, *C*). Often they will clear, at least in part, as the result of a vigorous cough. They may be heard during the resolution of an acute pneumonia, at which time there is the production of relatively large amounts of thick exudate. In the moribund patient who has a definite depression of his cough reflex, there is often an accumulation of thick secretions, producing very coarse rales. At times these sounds may be audible without the stethoscope and are termed the *death rattle* because of their common presence in the seriously ill.

Not infrequently some rales that can be elicited only by coughing may be present in the presence of a tuberculous lesion. This is best done by having the patient give a little cough after exhaling all of his air. During or immediately after the cough, a shower of medium rales may be heard that cannot be elicited in any other way. These are termed *posttussive* or *latent rales;* and their presence, especially over the apices, may be very helpful in the early diagnosis of tuberculosis.

On the other hand, some fine rales heard during the first few respiratory cycles will disappear after several deep breaths have been taken. These represent the reexpansion of areas of lung that are underaerated (*atelectatic*). This phenomenon is most frequently noticed after a person has been asleep and in older patients.

Rhonchi. Rhonchi are continuous sounds produced by the passage of air through the trachea, bronchi, and bronchioles that have been narrowed, irrespective of the cause. Although there may be definite differences in the pitch, intensity, quality, and duration in the inspiratory phase as compared to the expiratory phase, it should be emphasized that rhonchi are continuous, or relatively so, through both phases of respiration. As long as air passes the obstruction, the sound will be produced. Rhonchi in general are more prominent during expiration than inspiration, although they are frequently audible during inspiration. Based primarily on the pitch, rhonchi are classified as *sibilant* or *sonorous*.

Sibilant rhonchi are high pitched, wheezing, squeaking, or musical in character. The wheezing quality often can be accentuated by forced expiration. They have their origin in bronchioles and smaller bronchi.

Sonorous rhonchi are low pitched and often moaning or snoring in character. They are produced by obstruction in the larger bronchi or trachea.

Rhonchi tend to vary greatly in intensity and character from time to time. In some instances they can be cleared, or partially so, by coughing.

Rhonchi are *bipolar* in origin, the sound being produced as air enters the area of obstruction and again as it leaves. They are produced as long as the air flows past. The two sources of sound are: (1) acceleration of air as it reaches an impediment and (2) deceleration as it leaves the narrowed area. The underlying obstruction or narrowing may be the result of a variety of causes: extrinsic compression as by enlarged lymph nodes or mediastinal tumor or by intrinsic narrowing as in bronchogenic carcinoma, exudate, mucosal inflammation or edema, and bronchiolar spasm (asthma). In each instance there are narrowing and irregularity in the tracheobronchial tree, with resultant turbulence of the air producing the sound (Fig. 12-22).

With turbulent flow the pressure gradient necessary to produce flow varies with the square of the flow rather than directly as it does with laminar flow. Therefore, the resis-

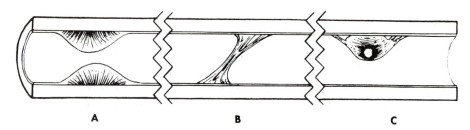

Fig. 12-22. Diagram illustrating methods of production of rhonchi. **A,** More or less annular narrowing, such as inflammatory thickening, stenosis, and tumor. **B,** Strings of thick secretions that vibrate with the passage of air. **C,** Unilateral encroachment on lumen, as in tumor, extrinsic compression by enlarged lymph nodes, or globule of thick, tenacious mucus.

tance to the movement of turbulent air is much greater than with nonturbulent flow. This is a significant factor in increasing the work of breathing in asthma, bronchitis, and emphysema, in which there is considerable bronchospasm, bronchiolar narrowing, and turbulent airflow.

Pleural friction rub. Normally the visceral and parietal surfaces of the pleura glide noiselessly over one another during respiration. However, when these surfaces become inflamed, as the result of pleurisy, pulmonary infarct, or underlying pneumonia, the rubbing of the roughened surfaces during respiration produces a very characteristic sound that is known as the *pleural friction rub*. It has a relatively characteristic creaking or grating quality, often described as the creaking of leather. The characteristics of a friction rub can be imitated by pressing the palm of one hand over the ear and then lightly and slowly rubbing the back of the hand with the fingers of the other hand. A pleural friction rub has a relatively superficial character, sounding as though it originated in the end of the stethoscope. It is usually heard during both phases of respiration. If audible in only one phase, it is most commonly heard during inspiration, particularly at the end. At times friction rubs are not heard during quiet breathing but are only audible when the patient takes a deeper breath.

The most common site for a friction rub to be heard is the lower anterolateral chest wall, the area of greatest thoracic mobility. A friction rub is seldom heard over the apex alone because its respiratory excursion is less than the lower portion of the thorax.

Sometimes it is difficult to differentiate a pleural friction rub from muscle sounds or very coarse rales. However, if the examiner considers that in general the friction rub is heard best over the lateral or anterolateral portion of the chest, that it is present during both phases of respiration, that it has an aspect of definite proximity to the surface, that it does not disappear with coughing as coarse rales will often do, and that cough is usually attended by discomfort, he usually can identify it with certainty. Furthermore, an increase in the intensity of the friction rub may be noted with firm pressure of the stethoscope over the thoracic wall.

ASSESSMENT OF PULMONARY ABILITY

Although precise pulmonary function studies are often not considered a part of the routine examination of the thorax and lungs, an assessment of the patient's ventilatory ability should be an essential part of every thorough physical examination. Respiratory flow rates and most of the lung volumes can be accurately determined with a recording spirometer (Fig. 12-23).

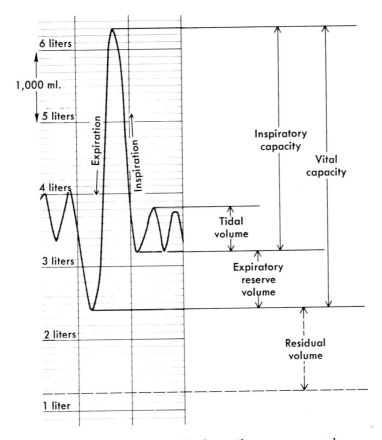

Fig. 12-23. The subdivisions of the lung. Flow rates are not shown.

The normal individual can exhale 76% or more of his vital capacity within a second and should be able to exhale 95% or more in 3 seconds (Fig. 12-24). Patients with obstructive pulmonary disease, such as asthma or emphysema, will require considerably longer to empty their lungs, as clearly illustrated in Fig. 12-24, which shows the contrasting spirographic patterns of the normal patient and those observed in patients suffering from obstructive pulmonary disease.

In contrast, individuals with restrictive pulmonary diseases such as diffuse fibrosis, sarcoidosis, or silicosis will be able to empty their lungs at the normal rate but will have a reduced vital capacity. If there is both a reduction in air flow rates and in the vital capacity, a combination of restrictive and obstructive disease may be suggested (Table 12-1).

An estimate of the ventilatory ability can be accomplished by having the patient take as deep a breath as he can and then expel it as rapidly and completely as possible. Observation of the volume of air expelled and the time necessary to exhale *completely* will give a rough estimate of both the vital capacity and the expiratory flow rate, although this is obviously quite crude as compared with use of the spirometer.

The Snider test is a useful bedside procedure to judge the adequacy of pulmonary ventilation. The patient is asked to blow out a match

Timed expiratory capacity

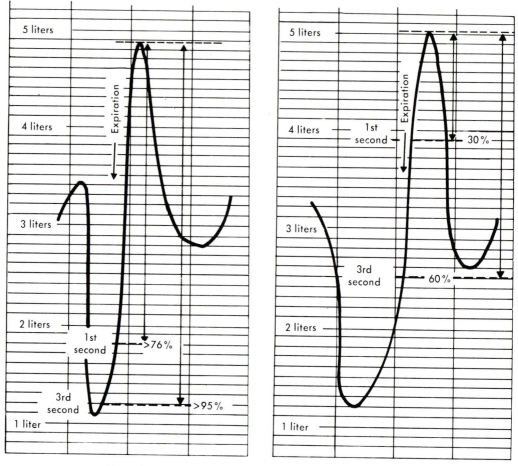

Normal   Obstructive lesion

Fig. 12-24. Spirograms illustrating the expiratory flow rates for 1 second, 3 seconds, and total time for expiration in the normal subject, as contrasted to the emphysematous patient with marked obstruction to expiratory flow.

Table 12-1. Expiratory flow rate and vital capacity in disease conditions

Type of abnormality	Expiratory flow rate	Vital capacity
Obstructive disease (asthma, emphysema, and others)	Reduced	Normal or slightly reduced
Restrictive disease (fibrosis, pleural effusion, and others)	Normal	Reduced
Combined obstructive and restrictive disease	Reduced	Reduced

held 6 inches from his *open* mouth. Pursing of the lips must be avoided; false teeth should be removed. A forced expiratory volume of approximately 1,000 ml. and a peak flow rate of 130 liters per minute or more are required to extinguish the flame. Inability to blow out the match under these conditions suggests ventilatory insufficiency.

MAJOR ALTERATIONS OF THE LUNGS

While pursuing the clinical examination of a patient, it is important to remember that our senses do not lie but that our interpretation of what we perceive with our senses may be erroneous. In the foregoing material, mention has been made of several abnormal conditions that may alter the physical findings. In each instance these may be the result of several disease processes causing the same general abnormality. A brief description of some of the major alterations and the more frequent causes follows.

Atelectasis. Atelectasis is a condition in which a portion of the lungs is unexpanded. It may involve a whole lung, lobe, or only small patches within a lobe. Atelectasis may be either congenital, functional, or acquired.

Congenital atelectasis is the failure of the lungs to expand fully in the immediate neonatal period.

Functional atelectasis results from the fact that the lungs may not completely inflate during ordinary quiet respiration. Occasionally fine rales will be noted in the axilla and over the extreme lower margin of the lungs when the patient breathes more deeply. These result from the inrush of air into small areas of unexpanded lung. After a few deep breaths the involved areas will become fully expanded, and the rales will disappear. As a consequence these fine rales are commonly called *atelectatic rales*. They are more frequently found in older patients or in those confined to bed.

Acquired atelectasis may be either obstructive or compressive:

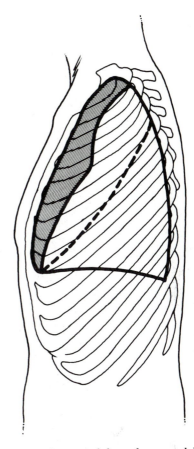

Fig. 12-25. Atelectasis of the right upper lobe. The dotted line indicates the normal location of the fissure between the upper and lower lobes, and the solid area indicates the marked decrease in the volume of the atelectatic upper lobe.

1. *Obstructive atelectasis* is the result of some obstruction of the trachea or bronchi (Figs. 12-25 and 12-26). It may be the result of aspiration of foreign body, tumor mass inside or outside the bronchus, or exudate. The fact that the bronchus or bronchi to the affected area are obstructed will produce abnormal physical findings—diminished expansion over the area involved, absence of vocal fremitus, dullness to percussion, absence of breath sounds, and absence of whispered and spoken

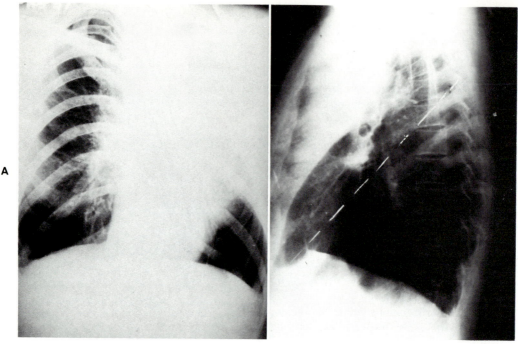

Fig. 12-26. A, Anteroposterior radiogram showing atelectasis of left upper lobe caused by cancer of the lung. Note the homogenous "ground-glass" appearance that characterized atelectasis. **B,** Lateral view. The normal diagonal fissure is drawn to show that it moves anteriorly and upward as the size of the left upper lobe decreases.

voice sounds. Rales will not be present since there is no significant flow of air to produce them. When there is a large area of atelectasis, it is often termed *massive collapse* in which the heart may be displaced toward the affected side.

2. *Compressive atelectasis* is the result of compression of the lung by fluid or air in the pleural or pericardial space, a large intrathoracic tumor, or elevation of the diaphragm. In this instance where the bronchus is patent, the physical findings will be limitation of expansion, decreased vocal fremitus, dullness, bronchial breath sounds, decreased spoken voice sounds, and occasionally egophony. Rales may or may not be heard. In some instances it will

be noted that the heart will be displaced to the opposite side. Often the signs of the condition producing the compression will predominate.

Emphysema. Although there are actually several varieties of emphysema, the type mentioned previously is the so-called *obstructive* (less properly *hypertrophic*) *emphysema* that usually results in enlargement of the thorax known as *barrel chest*. There is distention of the air sacs that produces considerable increase in the volume of the lungs. It is most commonly the result of long-standing, chronic bronchial irritation or infection and usually requires many years to develop into the more advanced stages that produce dyspnea and barrel chest (Figs. 12-5 and 12-27).

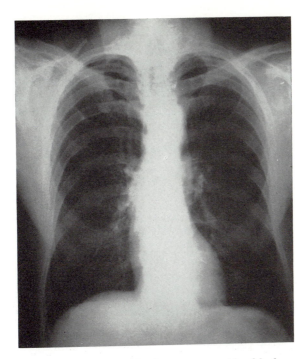

Fig. 12-27. Emphysema. Note that the diaphragm is considerably lower and flatter than usual as the result of the increased volume of the lungs. The heart is long and narrow. The lungs are hyperradiolucent (darker than usual) and appear quite voluminous.

The physical findings that accompany emphysema are increase in anteroposterior diameter of the chest (Fig. 12-5), fixation of the chest with the ribs in a more nearly horizontal plane, obvious participation of accessory respiratory muscles, normal or decreased vocal fremitus, hyperresonance, depressed diaphragms with decreased respiratory excursion, and decreased or absent breath sounds with diminished transmission of the whispered and spoken voice. Breath sounds are usually definitely prolonged during expiration and often accompanied by sibilant rhonchi.

Consolidation. Although the signs of consolidation may occasionally be found over a lung abscess or a large area of pulmonary embolization, the most common cause is lobar pneumonia, which may be the result of a variety of bacterial infections (Fig. 12-28 and 12-29). The most important causative organisms are the pneumococci, streptococci, and klebsiellae. Consolidation is infrequent in viral infections. Signs of consolidation may be found at times over areas of confluent bronchopneumonia, which is usually characterized by one or more patches of pneumonia.

The signs of consolidation are limitation and lag of expansion of the side involved, often palpable limitation of expansion, increase in vocal fremitus, dull percussion note, and bronchial breath sounds with fine or medium rales at the end of inspiration. Bronchophony and pectoril-

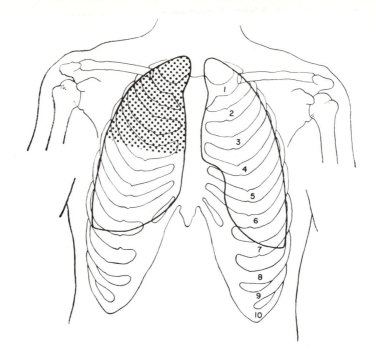

Fig. 12-28. Penumonic consolidation of the right upper lobe.

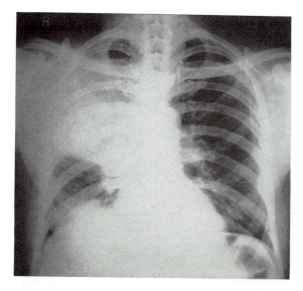

Fig. 12-29. Lobar pneumonia. There is obvious dense consolidation of the right upper lobe. This lobal pneumonia was caused by the pneumococcus, as demonstrated by sputum and blood cultures.

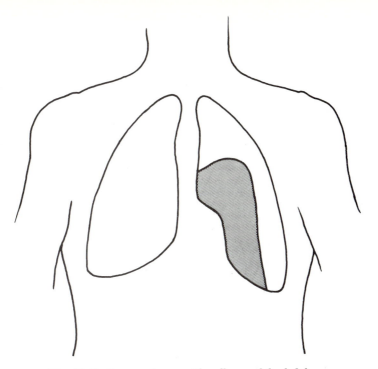

Fig. 12-30. Pneumothorax with collapse of the left lung.

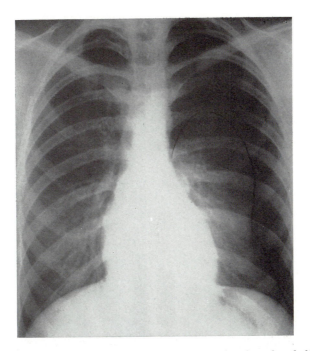

Fig. 12-31. Pneumothorax on the left. The lung is collapsed to less than half of normal size because of the spontaneous pneumothorax produced by the rupture of an emphysematous bleb on the surface of the lung.

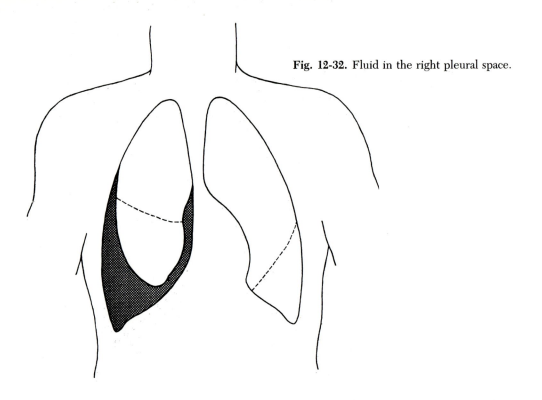

Fig. 12-32. Fluid in the right pleural space.

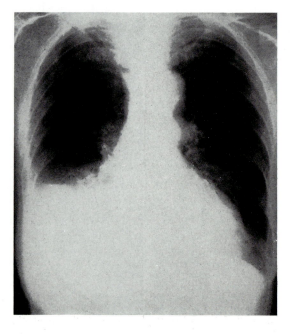

Fig. 12-33. Pleural effusion. As compared to the left, there is an obvious density of the lower right that is caused by considerable pleural fluid.

oquy may be heard, and occasionally egophony is present. A friction rub is occasionally audible.

Pneumothorax. Pneumothorax is present where air enters the pleural space, permitting partial or total collapse of the lung (Figs. 12-30 and 12-31). The most common cause is emphysema, in which air escapes into the pleural cavity because of rupture of a distended bleb on the surface of the lung. Occasionally pneumothorax will be the result of laceration of the lung from fracture of a rib, puncture wounds, or tuberculosis. The lung is an elastic structure, expansion of which is maintained by the negative intrapleural pressure. With the entrance of air into the pleural space (neutralizing the negative pressure), the lung will collapse.

Physical findings on the side involved will be decreased expansion, decreased or absent vocal fremitus, hyperresonant percussion note, diminished or absent breath sounds, and decrease in transmission of the spoken and whispered voice. If the pneumothorax is small, the alterations may be minor or even absent.

Pleural fluid. Fluid in the pleural space may be an inflammatory effusion, congestive hydrothorax, hemothorax, or empyema (Figs. 12-32 and 12-33). Although the fluid may be the result of a variety of causes, the physical findings will be the same—decreased respiratory excursion on the side involved, decreased or absent vocal fremitus, dullness to flatness, depending on the amount of fluid present, and decreased or absent breath sounds and vocal transmission. Adventitious sounds are ordinarily not present.

SELECTED READINGS

Baum, G. L.: Textbook of pulmonary diseases, ed. 2, Boston, 1974, Little, Brown and Co.

Comroe, J. H., and others: The lung, ed. 2, Chicago, 1962, Year Book Medical Publishers, Inc.

Felson, B.: Chest roentgenology, ed. 2, Philadelphia, 1973, W. B. Saunders Co.

Fraser, R. G., and Paré, J. A. P.: Diagnosis of diseases of the chest, ed. 2, Philadelphia, 1977, W. B. Saunders Co.

Snider, G. H., and others: Simple bedside test of respiratory function, J.A.M.A. **170:**1631, 1959.

CHAPTER 13

BREASTS

Evaluation of the breast is an important part of the physical examination because of the high incidence of disease in this organ. The breast is the most common site of cancer in the female. In addition it is often plagued with *chronic cystic mastitis*, inflammation of the breast, and other benign lesions that must be differentiated from cancer. Inflammatory processes, especially in the postpartum period, are much less frequent today than in the preantibiotic era, but they still occur and require careful consideration.

It is just as essential to examine the breasts in the male patient as in the female. Carcinoma of the male breast occurs comparatively infrequently, constituting about 1% of all breast cancers. However, it is important to know that it does occur and has the same general physical characteristics as in the female breast. Also, the male may be afflicted by *mastitis* and *gynecomastia* (enlargement of the male mammary gland).

An adequate investigation of the breast necessitates a definite, organized routine, which should include not only the breasts but the lymphatic drainage sites as well. Haphazard palpation of only the area designated by the patient may result in the failure to detect disease

of possibly even greater significance in another location. Whether the patient is seen in the hospital or in the office, it is important that adequate exposure be obtained (Fig. 13-1). The patient should disrobe to the waist. However, the breasts may be kept covered by a towel, except during the actual examination, to avoid unnecessary embarrassing exposure. The patient should be examined in the sitting as well as in the supine position. The examination should include thorough inspection and palpation.

INSPECTION

Breasts. In inspection of breasts special attention should be given to symmetry, superficial appearance, nipple, and skin retraction.

Symmetry. It is not uncommon to notice some difference in size of the two breasts (Fig. 13-2). At times this is sufficient to create a serious psychologic problem. With the patient sitting erect, obvious asymmetry will be evident. Although asymmetry is usually the result of difference in development of the breasts, an increase in size of one of the breasts may denote congenital anomaly, cyst formation, inflammation, or tumor.

Superficial appearance. A good light is essential for adequate inspection of the breasts. Erythema may be associated with inflammation or may indicate involvement of the superficial lymphatics by a neoplastic process, referred to as *inflammatory carcinoma* (Fig. 13-3). This latter type of redness represents a local reaction of the skin to the underlying invasive or necrotic cancer. An increased superficial vascular pattern may indicate accessory blood supply of a neoplasm.

Edema of the breasts, manifested by the fact that hair follicles and follicular openings are more pronounced or noticeable, may denote inflammation or neoplasm. Although the pathologic basis for these two types of edema is different, it may be impossible to distinguish them by physical examination. The edema associated with carcinoma is caused by mechanical blocking by cancer cells in the lymphatic channels in the skin. Edema that is caused by obstruction of lymphatics is termed *lymphedema*. The edematous appearance of the skin as-

sociated with inflammatory carcinoma of the breast has been frequently described as "orange peel" or "pig skin" (Fig. 13-4). Inflammatory edema is caused by extravasation of serum into the intercellular spaces. This occurs because of the increased capillary permeability caused by the action of the irritant. Notations should be made as to the exact location of edema found on the surface of the breast.

During pregnancy the breasts become enlarged; the areolae become larger in diameter and more pigmented. In addition, the axillae may appear full and at times give the impression that a mass is present. In some instances the breast tissue extends to the apex of the axilla. Usually this fullness is symmetrical, but occasionally one axilla is larger than the other. The increase in size of the breasts and axillary areas is caused by hypertrophy of the breast tissue in preparation for lactation.

Nipple. The size, shape, and general appearance of the nipple should be noted. It is not

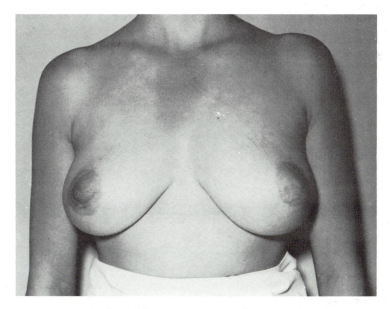

Fig. 13-1. Patient properly draped for examination. A short gown is worn or a towel is used to cover the breasts until the examination begins.

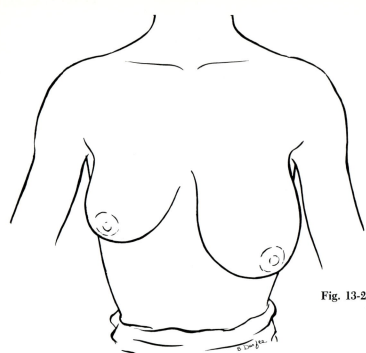

Fig. 13-2. Asymmetric development of breasts.

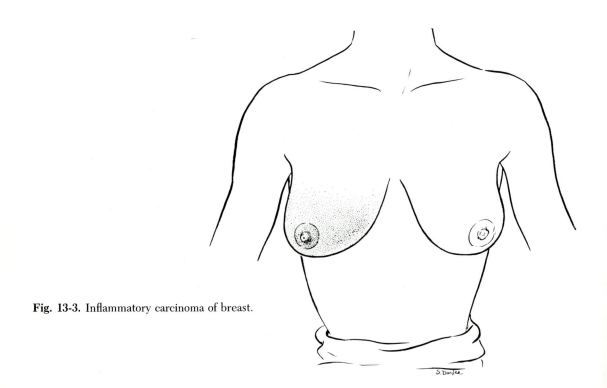

Fig. 13-3. Inflammatory carcinoma of breast.

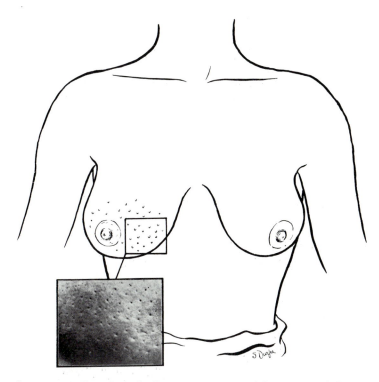

Fig. 13-4. "Orange-peel" or "pig-skin" appearance caused by tumor cell blockage of lymphatics.

uncommon that some asymmetry may be observed. Inversion may be present, but it is significant only if it is of recent origin. Ulceration of the nipple may indicate a malignant process of the breast *(Paget's disease)*. This is most important when only one nipple is ulcerated, since bilateral involvement usually denotes a benign dermatologic disease. The character of any discharge appearing at the nipple should be noted. This may be serous, bluish, yellowish, greenish, or sanguineous. A discharge of any kind denotes disease along the ductal system. Bleeding is most often caused by the presence of benign intraductal papilloma. Sanguineous discharge occurs in only about 1% of all patients with carcinoma of the breast. Nipple secretions, varying from clear to green, blue, or yellow, usually indicate chronic cystic

mastitis. During pregnancy the nipples become larger and more mobile. This should be taken into account during inspection.

Skin retraction. The phenomenon of *retraction* is one of the most important findings to note in examination of the breast. Retraction is manifested by a variable degree of *dimpling* of any part of the skin of the breast or nipple. Anatomically the breast lies between the superficial and deep layers of the superficial fascia. The suspensory ligaments, which are actually the fascial septa of the breast, traverse the breast between these two layers of fascia (Fig. 13-5, *A*). Because of the proximity of breast tissue to the skin, any process that is infiltrative or space consuming may exert an abnormal traction on some of these ligaments, causing dimpling of the skin overlying the lesion (Fig.

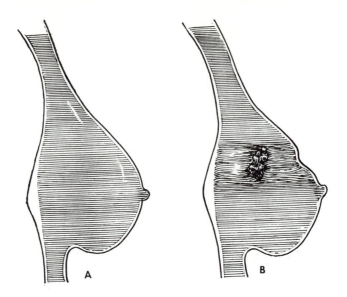

Fig. 13-5. A, Diagrammatic representation of suspensory ligaments in normal breast. **B,** Tumor producing shortening of suspensory ligaments, with resultant retraction of the overlying skin.

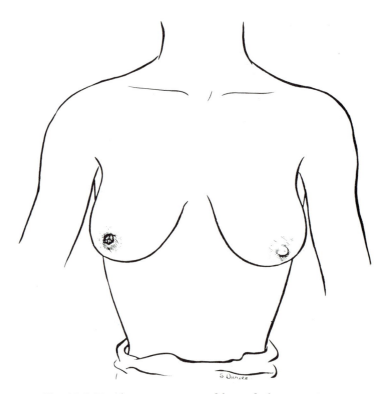

Fig. 13-6. Nipple retraction caused by underlying carcinoma.

13-5, *B*). If the involved ligaments supply a part of the nipple, there will be retraction of a portion of it, so that the nipple will point toward the site of the lesion (Fig. 13-6).

The pathologic process responsible for the retraction may be simple fat necrosis, which is usually traumatic in origin. As a result of the necrosis, fibroblastic proliferation produces shortening of the ligamentous fibers in the area involved. Any acute inflammatory process may cause the same type of retraction. However, it should be emphasized that *if the breast does not present definite evidence of acute inflammation, skin retraction indicates the presence of a malignant tumor*. In advanced carcinoma the other findings of tumor mass, skin fixation, and ulceration are so obvious that the diagnosis can be made without difficulty. In very early lesions and especially in the patient whose breasts are obese, a small degree of skin retraction may be one of the earliest physical findings suggesting the diagnosis.

In order to elicit an early retraction phenomenon, it is necessary to subject the patient to various gymnastics that will exert a pull on the suspensory ligaments of the breast. First, the patient should be examined while sitting erect. After a careful inspection of the breasts has been made, she is asked to raise her arms directly overhead (Fig. 13-7). This movement usually results in the equal elevation of both breasts. If there is a lesion that has caused shortening of some of the suspensory ligaments, a certain amount of retraction will occur, varying from a small dimple to flattening of a large segment of the breast as the arms are raised (Fig. 13-8). If the nipple is deviated by this maneuver, it will point toward the site of the lesion.

The phenomenon of retraction not seen when the arms are elevated may be produced by other methods. Any maneuver that causes a contraction of the pectoral muscles is an excellent way to elicit retraction. When the pectoral

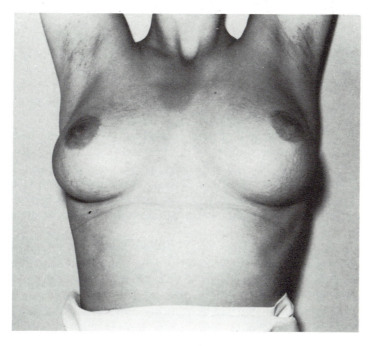

Fig. 13-7. Inspection with arms overhead.

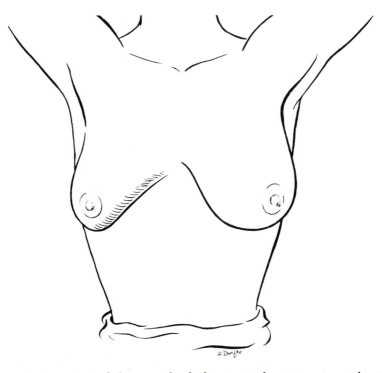

Fig. 13-8. Retraction on medial aspect of right breast noted on inspection with arms overhead.

muscles contract, there is ordinarily a general traction on the breast tissue. If there is shortening of the suspensory ligaments, contraction of the pectoral muscles exaggerates the retraction phenomenon. The patient places the palms of both hands together and then, at the command of the physician, pushes the hands together (Fig. 13-9, *A*). The same effect is produced if the patient places her hands on her hips and pushes forcibly against them (Fig. 13-9, *B*). She should be asked to do either of these procedures several times so that all parts of the breasts can be inspected. Next, the patient is instructed to lean forward at the waist with her hands placed on an object or the examiner's shoulders to determine if the pull of the breasts as they fall away from the thorax will cause unequal traction of certain ligaments. If the lesion is obvious, the patient need not be subjected to these procedures. However, if the small early malignant lesion is to be found, it is essential that all of these methods be executed.

Axillae and supraclavicular regions. Thorough inspection of the breasts includes observation of the axillary and supraclavicular regions, since these are the most important lymphatic drainage areas. Any bulging, retraction, discoloration, or edema should be described.

PALPATION

After a thorough inspection, the breasts, axillae, and supraclavicular regions are systematically palpated. It makes no difference in which order the examiner elects to palpate these structures, but it is difficult to overemphasize

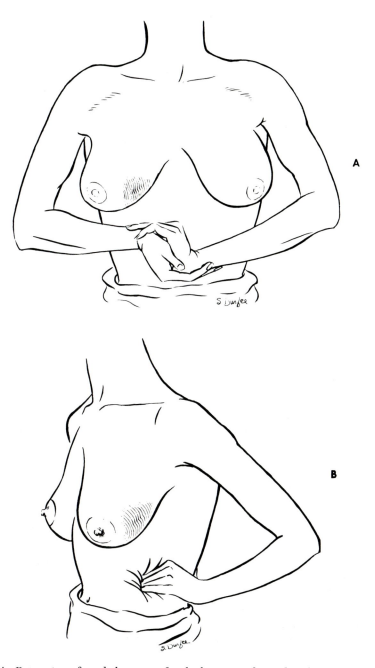

Fig. 13-9. A, Retraction of medial aspect of right breast made evident by patient pressing palms together. **B,** Retraction of lateral aspect of left breast made evident by the patient exerting pressure on both hips with her hands.

the importance of having a definite system of examination.

Breasts. The breast extends from the second or third rib to the sixth or seventh costal cartilage and from the edge of the sternum to the anterior axillary line. The axillary portion of the breast is quite variable in size; sometimes this portion will produce a visible bulge in the axilla.

It is important to realize that normal breasts vary greatly in their "feel." The breast tissue of older women is commonly stringy and nodular, whereas in younger patients it will be softer and more homogeneous. The breast is made up of lobules of glandular tissue. When felt as actual lobules, these should not be misconstrued as tumor masses. The amount of subcutaneous fatty tissue will alter the "feel" of the breast. The characteristic "feel" of the normal breast will be acquired with time and experience.

As palpation is being performed, the physician should keep in mind the monthly cyclic physiologic changes that occur in the breast. The breasts become engorged, lobular, and sensitive prior to the menses and decongest promptly thereafter. As a result of the cyclic changes that occur year after year, chronic cystic mastitis may develop. In this condition the breast has a granular consistency, feeling as though there were an accumulation of "shots" or nodules of varying size. These "shotlike" areas represent dilatations of the ductal system. At times they may become completely encysted and vary in size from a few millimeters to several centimeters in diameter.

During pregnancy the breasts become firmer and larger and the lobulations become more distinct. Sometimes the lobules become so well defined that they may be confused with tumor masses.

A recommended procedure of examination is to start at the upper lateral aspect of each breast. First, gently palpate the left breast, using the palmar aspect of the fingertips, with a rotary or to-and-fro motion. Remember that light palpation will yield more information than examination with a heavy hand. Then each portion is more deeply explored. The palpation proceeds in a clockwise direction until the breast has been completely examined, after which attention is focused on the nipple. Any masses, induration, or loss of elasticity in the nipple should be noted. A subcutaneous mass in the areolar area may represent a sebaceous cyst or, if deeper, an intraductal papilloma. Gentle pressure over a papilloma situated in the major mammary ducts beneath the nipple will produce a serous or sanguineous discharge. The right breast is examined in similar fashion, proceeding counterclockwise.

For thoroughness, the breast should be palpated with the patient in both the upright and supine positions. With the patient in the sitting position, the breasts are examined first with the patient's arms at the side, and then with her arms overhead (Fig. 13-10). When examining a patient in the supine position, it is well to elevate the shoulder on the side under study with a small pillow (Fig. 13-11). This allows the breast to rest more symmetrically over the chest wall, permitting more accurate examination. Then palpation of each breast, as described, is repeated.

If the patient complains of tenderness or a lump in one breast, the *opposite* breast should be palpated first. The examiner then turns his attention to the involved breast, and finally the suspected site should be most thoroughly evaluated. When the patient complains primarily of one portion of the breast, she will usually point out the area to the physician. If the examiner's attention is directed to that particular spot at first, especially if obvious disease is present, he may neglect other parts of the breast unless he has adopted a routine manner of examination. Instances are known in which patients have complained of a lump that proved to be insignificant, only to have a malignant lesion discovered elsewhere in the breast.

The examiner should not palpate the breast

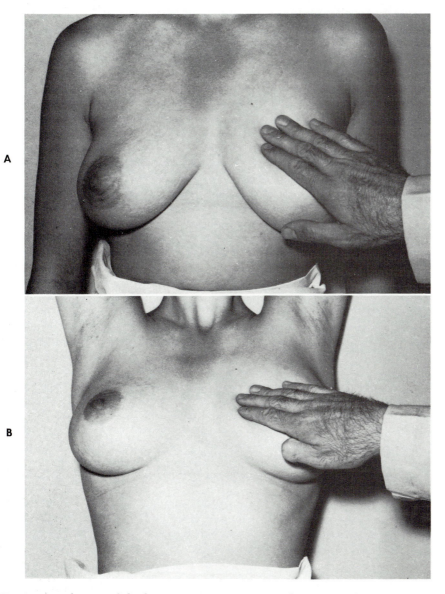

Fig. 13-10. Palpation of the breast. **A,** Patient sitting with arms at side. **B,** Patient sitting with arms overhead.

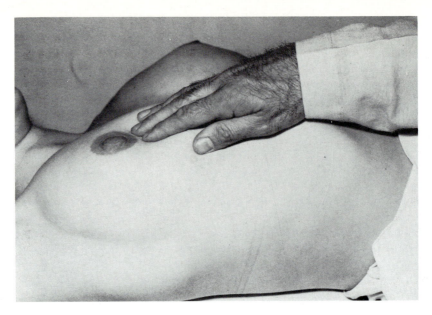

Fig. 13-11. Palpation of breast with patient in supine position.

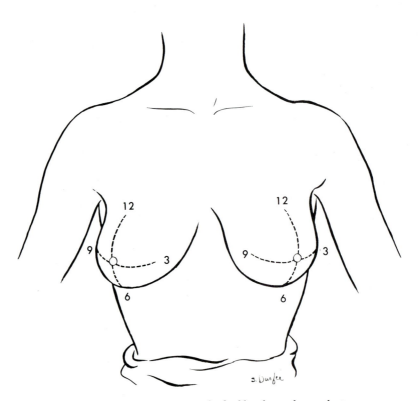

Fig. 13-12. Diagrammatic method of localizing breast lesions.

noninvasive lesions. If the margin or boundaries of the mass are difficult to determine, the process is more likely to have the properties of malignant invasion. In general, discreteness speaks for a benign process, whereas a lack of this quality suggests inflammation or cancer.

Axillae. After the breasts have been examined, it is essential to palpate the axillae. The axilla should be thoroughly explored with one hand while the examiner's opposite hand holds the ipsilateral arm of the patient (Fig. 13-13). The axilla may be considered to have an apex and four walls: (1) lateral; (2) anterior, which is formed by the pectoralis major muscle; (3) thoracic; and (4) posterior, which is composed of the teres major and latissimus dorsi muscles. Each of the above axillary areas should be palpated with the patient's arm at her side, and again while the arm is taken through a full range of motion to uncover any lesions that might have been hidden under a muscle or in subcutaneous fat. At times, by moving the patient's arm, it is possible to palpate enlarged lymph nodes that cannot be felt when the arm is at the side. The opposite axilla is examined in similar fashion.

Supraclavicular regions. Both supraclavicular areas should be palpated (Fig. 13-14). If an inflammatory process is present in the breast, it is possible to have adenitis extending into the supraclavicular lymph nodes. After this area has been carefully examined, particular care should be taken to thoroughly examine the deep jugular chain of nodes, since this is a frequent route of metastatic spread of breast cancer.

SELECTED READINGS

Haagensen, C. D.: Diseases of the breast, ed. 2, Philadelphia, 1974, W. B. Saunders Co.

Hytton, F., and Leitch, I.: The physiology of human pregnancy, ed. 2, Philadelphia, 1971, F. A. Davis Co.

CHAPTER 14

CARDIOVASCULAR SYSTEM

ARTERIAL BLOOD PRESSURE

Determining the systemic arterial blood pressure should be a routine procedure in every physical examination, and along with the recording of the temperature, pulse, and respirations, should be ascertained at the beginning of each examination. A combination of these data is generally referred to as *vital signs*.

Since the blood pressure as well as the pulse and respirations may be influenced by physical exertion and emotional tension, it is obvious that the patient should be physically relaxed and emotionally at ease prior to their determination. A patient's first visit to a physician may in itself be sufficiently frightening to result in both an increase in pulse rate and an elevation of blood pressure. This fact can be readily confirmed by taking the pulse and blood pressure at the onset of the physical examination and then repeating these determinations after the patient has relaxed and gained confidence in the examiner.

Two types of manometers, mercury and aneroid, are in common use for recording blood pressure. It actually makes little difference as to which instrument is used, provided it is ac-

curately calibrated and properly employed. The patient should be seated or reclining during this examination, and the arm should be at the heart level, relaxed, slightly flexed, and supported on a firm surface. When the patient is tense and apprehensive, it is often helpful if the physician engages him in conversation to distract his attention away from his medical problems. The patient is then more likely to be relaxed, enabling the examiner to obtain a more reliable measurement of pulse and blood pressure.

The blood pressure cuff should be deflated prior to its application on the arm. The cuff is evenly and firmly wrapped about the arm, with the center of the inflatable portion over the brachial artery and the rubber tubing along the medial aspect of the arm. Failure to apply the cuff properly results in bulging and slipping, especially in those patients who have obese extremities. The lower margin of the cuff should be placed 2 to 3 cm. above the antecubital fossa.

The radial pulse is palpated and the pressure in the cuff is rapidly increased to a level of about 30 mm. Hg above the point at which the radial pulse disappears. As the cuff is slowly deflated, a point is reached at which the pulse reappears. The pressure reading at this point is termed *palpatory systolic pressure*.

In determining the auscultatory blood pressure the bell or diaphragm of the stethoscope is placed in the medial aspect of the antecubital fossa over the brachial artery. To avoid producing adventitious sounds, it should not touch the cuff or rubber tubing. In using this method the examiner inflates the cuff so that the pressure is 30 to 40 mm. Hg above the level at which the radial pulse disappears. It is then gradually deflated, several millimeters at a time, until the first sound is heard through the stethoscope. This point is referred to as the *systolic blood pressure*.

As the blood pressure cuff is further deflated, the sounds undergo changes in intensity and quality. As the cuff pressure approaches diastolic, the sounds often quite suddenly become dull and muffled and then cease. The point of complete cessation of sounds is the best index of the diastolic pressure. Under those conditions in which no cessation of sounds occurs, the point of muffling, if distinctly heard, should be taken as the diastolic pressure and recorded as the point of muffled sounds. When no clear demarcation of the muffling is heard, the diastolic pressure should be left indefinite and so indicated, for example, 150/30.

In the process of determining the systolic pressure by the auscultatory method, the examiner may first detect the sounds at a high level only to have them suddenly disappear and then reappear at a lower level. This is referred to as the *auscultatory gap*. For example, the sounds may be heard first at 190 mm. Hg, disappear at 170 mm. Hg, and reappear at 130 mm. Hg. If the examiner inflates the cuff only to 150 mm. Hg before deflating, he then will assume that 130 rather than 190 mm. Hg is the systolic pressure. Failure to bear this possibil-

ity in mind may result in labeling a patient normotensive when actually he is definitely hypertensive.

A comparison of systolic pressure by the palpatory and auscultatory methods is always advisable in adults. As a rule, systolic pressure determined by the auscultatory method is higher than the pressure at which the radial pulsations are first palpable. Should the palpatory reading be higher than the auscultatory reading, several maneuvers may be undertaken to improve conditions for hearing the sounds. These include adjusting clothing to prevent constriction of the arm and avoiding inflation of the cuff when the arm is pendent. If, despite such efforts, the palpatory reading continues to be higher, it should be accepted as the reading for the systolic pressure.

In the initial examination of any patient it is advisable to determine the blood pressure in both arms. Under normal circumstances there is little or no significant difference in the blood pressure in the two upper extremities. In certain instances—for example, aortic aneurysm or obstruction of the innominate artery—there may be a significant discrepancy in the blood pressure in the upper extremities. If the patient has a history of syncope, it is essential that the blood pressure be measured with the patient standing as well as reclining. Normally there is a fall in cardiac output on standing, and this results in a fall in the systolic pressure of a few millimeters of mercury. In the presence of orthostatic hypotension and syncope there may be a precipitous fall in the blood pressure when the patient stands erect.

The blood pressure can be determined in the lower extremities by placing the cuff around the lower third of the thigh and the chestpiece of the stethoscope over the popliteal artery. Generally, a cuff larger than standard, ideally 20 cm. wide, should be used in measurement of blood pressure of the lower extremities in an adult. Ordinarily, the systolic pressure is slightly higher in the lower extremities than in the upper because of the larger muscle masses in the thighs that produce an increased resistance to compression of the artery. Because it is not customary to routinely obtain the blood pressure in the legs, it is important to remember that this procedure should always be done when the femoral and popliteal pulses are either weak or absent and in any child or young adult with hypertension in order to rule out *coarctation* (congenital narrowing) of the *aorta*. Coarctation is characterized by an elevated systolic pressure in the arms and a lower systolic pressure in the legs because the brachial arteries originate above and the femoral arteries originate below the stenosed segment of the aorta.

The so-called normal or average blood pressure is somewhat variable and depends on sex, race, and climatic conditions. As noted previously, the blood pressure in any given person will vary with physical activity and emotional tension. Obese extremities will often cause an erroneous high systolic reading because the pressure applied to the cuff must overcome the resistance of the tissues before compressing the brachial artery. Most life insurance companies accept 150 mm. Hg systolic and 90 mm. diastolic as the upper limits of normal blood pressure. In persons under 40 years of age the systolic pressure is usually 110 to 140 mm. Hg and the diastolic pressure is 60 to 90 mm. Hg. Many patients are unduly alarmed by their physicians concerning the presence of low blood pressure. Systolic pressures of 90 to 100 mm. Hg, unless accompanied by significant symptoms, are of no clinical importance and thus require no specific treatment. Some serious causes of low blood pressure *(hypotension)* include Addison's disease, acute myocardial infarction, hemorrhage, and shock. Among the causes of high blood pressure *(hypertension)* are essential hypertension, chronic glomerulo-

nephritis, pheochromocytoma, renal artery stenosis, and coarctation of the aorta. In some instances, as a result primarily of an increase in cardiac output, the systolic pressure is high, whereas the diastolic pressure is usually normal or even below normal. This is frequently the situation in anemia, hyperthyroidism, aortic regurgitation, and arteriovenous fistula. In elderly persons the most common cause for an elevated systolic and normal diastolic pressure is aortic atherosclerosis or arteriosclerosis of the peripheral arteries.

PULSE PRESSURE

The *pulse pressure* is the difference between the systolic and diastolic pressures and normally amounts to 30 or 40 mm. Hg. For example, if the systolic blood pressure is 120 mm. Hg and the diastolic pressure is 80 mm. Hg, the pulse pressure then is 40 mm. Hg. The pulse pressure may be increased in atherosclerosis of the aorta and large arteries, hyperthyroidism, aortic valve regurgitation, arteriovenous fistula, vigorous exercise, and fever. The pulse pressure may be decreased in aortic stenosis, mitral stenosis, heart failure, and massive pericardial effusion.

VENOUS BLOOD PRESSURE

The venous pressure can be measured directly using a manometer connected to a vein, by which technique the venous pressure with the arm at the level of the atrium is normally 40 to 80 mm. of water. The venous blood pressure may be estimated indirectly by the following methods:

1. With the patient sitting or reclining at 30-degree elevation or more with his arms in a dependent position, the veins on the dorsum of the hands are observed. The hands are then gradually elevated to the level of the shoulder and the examiner notes the point at which the hand veins collapse (Fig. 14-1). Normally these

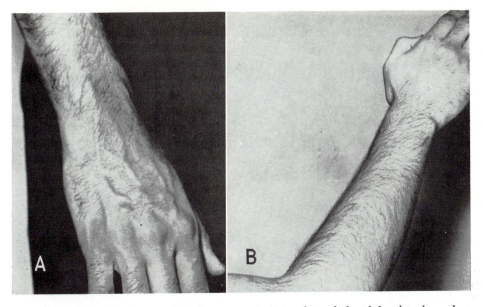

Fig. 14-1. Estimation of venous blood pressure. **A,** Veins distended with hand in dependent position. **B,** Veins collapsed with hand in elevated position.

veins will collapse when the hands are elevated to the level of the atrium (manubriosternal junction). This technique has less reliability than observation of the jugular veins.

2. The jugular veins reflect pressure and volume changes within the right atrium. Careful examination of these vessels enables the physician to infer physiologic events in the right side of the heart and thus permits more accurate estimation of the venous pressure. Significant distention of these veins is frequently seen in right heart failure or cardiac tamponade (Fig. 14-2). Further, observation of the venous pulse waves in the neck may assist in the diagnosis of pulmonary hypertension, complete atrioventricular heart block, tricuspid valve disease, and constrictive pericarditis.

The venous pulse can be readily evaluated by inspecting the external and internal jugular veins. Major abnormalities of the external jugular vein may occur, such as obstruction or kinking at the base of the neck. Consequently, it is quite important to delineate the internal jugular vein, which lies beneath the sternomastoid muscle.

When the venous pressure is markedly elevated, the cervical veins are best examined with the patient sitting erect. However, when the venous pressure is slightly or moderately elevated, the neck veins should be inspected with the patient reclining and with his trunk elevated 45 degrees from the horizontal. Constrictive clothing should be removed from the neck and thorax. The patient's head may rest on a pillow, but it is important that his head be in the same plane as the thorax and that his neck not be flexed (Fig. 14-3). In this position the jugular pulse should rise not more than 1 or 2 cm. above the level of the manubrium. If the level ascends over 4 cm., it should be considered as definitely abnormal. When the venous pressure is markedly elevated, the jugular

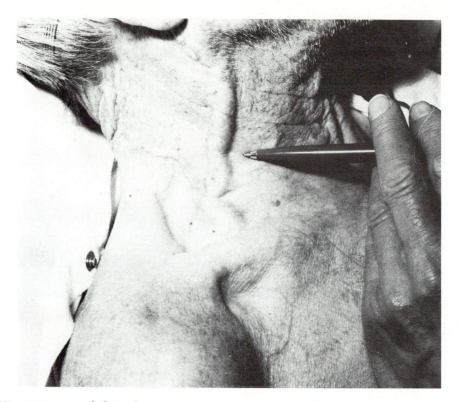

Fig. 14-2. Distended jugular vein in patient with severe right heart failure and marked elevation of venous pressure.

veins may be distended as high as the angle of the jaw when the patient is sitting completely upright (Fig. 14-4). The venous pressure is elevated in right heart failure, constrictive pericarditis, cardiac tamponade, tricuspid stenosis, and obstruction of the superior vena cava. In obstruction of the superior vena cava one usually sees dilated collateral veins over the upper thorax, the hepatojugular reflux is absent, and the distended neck veins do not pulsate. When examining the right jugular pulses, elevate the patient's chin slightly and tilt it to the left, thus exposing the right supraclavicular fossa. The internal jugular pulse waves then can be seen to rise and fall over the sternomastoid muscle or immediately behind its border. Occasionally it

is easier to detect the external jugular pulse waves as the vein crosses the sternomastoid muscle. During the period of ventricular ejection, the jugular pulses normally exhibit their negative phase. It is this phase that is readily recognized and can be appreciated by simultaneously observing the right side of the neck and listening to the heart or palpating the left carotid artery. The negative waves, x and y are more pronounced during inspiration. The veins are best examined with the use of tangential lighting. It is well to examine the veins on both sides of the neck. If the venous pressure is elevated, the jugular vein should be distended on both sides of the neck.

The pulsations of the internal jugular vein

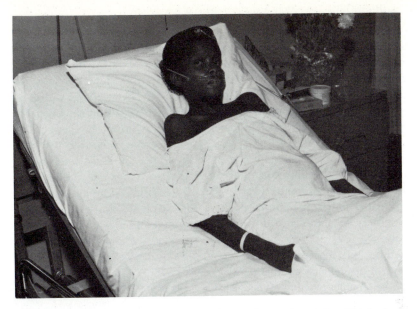

Fig. 14-3. Position of patient when examining the jugular venous pulse. The bed or examining table should break at the hips with the upper torso elevated 45 degrees from the horizontal. Patient's head may rest on pillow, but it is important not to flex the neck.

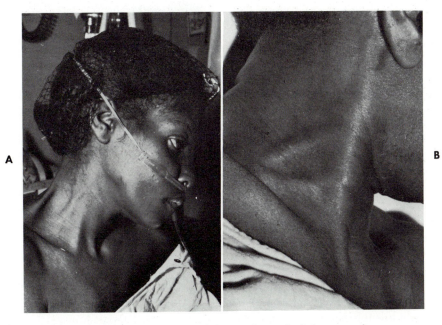

Fig. 14-4. Patient with chronic right heart failure and a marked elevation of venous pressure. Note distention of external jugular vein to angle of jaw with patient sitting erect. **B,** Patient with severe congestive heart failure. Note distention of both the internal and external jugular veins.

are frequently confused with those of the carotid artery, and these may be differentiated by several criteria:

1. The level of visible pulsation in the neck veins descends on normal inspiration and rises on expiration. Respiration does not alter the carotid pulse.

2. Slight pressure over the jugular vein, with the finger or a tongue blade, just above the sternoclavicular joint, will eliminate the jugular pulse. It requires much greater pressure to eliminate the carotid artery pulse.

3. The carotid artery pulse has only one phase. In the presence of normal cardiac rhythm, the jugular venous pulse has three positive waves.

4. In the presence of right heart failure, compression of the upper abdomen for 30 to 45 seconds will result in a rise in the venous pressure. The jugular pulses will become more prominent as the result of this procedure, and the level of filling of the neck veins will rise. This phenomenon is known as the *hepatojugular reflux*.

5. Usually the cervical veins become more prominent when the patient assumes a recumbent position and less prominent when he sits upright. Carotid artery pulsations are not significantly affected by change in the patient's position.

In the presence of right heart failure, the hepatojugular reflux can usually be demonstrated. When this test is performed, the patient is positioned in such a manner that the cervical veins are distended one third to one half way up the neck. The examiner then exerts firm pressure with the palm of his hand for 30 to 60 seconds over the right upper abdominal quadrant (Fig. 14-5). Actually, if the liver area is tender similar pressure may be exerted on adjacent areas of the abdomen. It is important that the patient breathe normally during the

procedure and that the examiner does not exert pressure to the point of causing pain. Either abnormal breathing per se or the production of pain, which interferes with breathing, will result in a Val-salva maneuver that will cause the veins to distend. When breathing is normal and pressure is applied to the abdomen as outlined, the examiner determines whether or not the neck veins distend and the level to which the venous engorgement ascends. If the level of the distention rises, the test is considered positive. In the normal individual the venous pressure either does not rise at all or not more

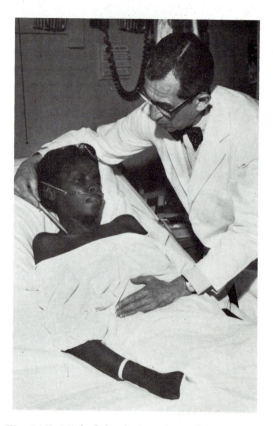

Fig. 14-5. Method for demonstrating hepatojugular reflux. Note hand of examiner exerting pressure in right upper abdominal quadrant.

than 1 cm. during the course of this procedure. The hepatojugular reflux occurs in the presence of right heart failure and constrictive pericarditis.

VENOUS PULSE WAVES

Careful inspection of the neck veins in subjects with normal sinus rhythm reveals three positive deflections—*a*, *c*, and *v* waves—and two negative components—*x* and *y* descents (Fig. 14-6).

The *a* wave is produced by atrial contraction and is usually the highest of the venous waves. The *a* wave begins just prior to the first heart sound. It can be identified by simultaneously observing the jugular pulse and auscultating at the apex; or it may be timed by palpating the carotid artery, in which case the *a* wave immediately precedes carotid pulsation. The *a* waves are absent in the presence of atrial fi-

brillation, in which case the atria do not contract in an organized manner. In the presence of atrial flutter, the *a* waves are replaced by smaller oscillating waves occurring at a rate of approximately 300 per minute. Atrial flutter can be best diagnosed at the bedside by close inspection of the jugular pulse.

The specific factors responsible for the production of the *c* wave are as yet unknown. Recent investigation has refuted the previously accepted concept; namely, that the *c* waves are produced by underlying carotid pulsation. This wave is related to bulging upward of the tricuspid valve at the onset of ventricular systole, and thus its time of occurrence approximates the start of ventricular systolic ejection. The *c* wave, which interrupts the downslope of the *x* descent, begins at the end of the first heart sound and reaches its peak very shortly thereafter. Being small in size and brief in duration

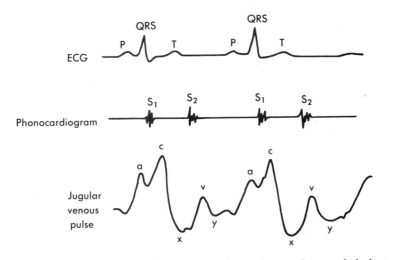

Fig. 14-6. Normal jugular venous pulse tracing with simultaneously recorded electrocardiogram and phonocardiogram. Note the three positive waves—a, c, and v—and the two descents—x and y. S₁ and S₂ represent the first and second heart sounds, respectively. The a wave occurs just prior to first heart sound and correlates with P wave on electrocardiogram (atrial contraction). The c wave begins at end of the first heart sound, and the v wave occurs in the latter part of systole. The x descent is related to atrial diastole, and the y descent to opening of the tricuspid valve.

the *c* wave is rarely seen under normal circumstances. Since the *a* wave corresponds to atrial contraction and the *c* wave corresponds to ventricular systolic ejection, the atrioventricular conduction time can be estimated from the *a-c* interval, providing the *c* wave is visible.

The *v* wave is produced as blood from the periphery enters the right atrium in the latter part of systole. It is actually a passive filling wave.

The *x* descent is a negative wave and is produced by atrial diastole.

The *y* descent follows the *v* wave and is also a negative wave. It occurs when the tricuspid valve opens, permitting the flow of blood from the right atrium into the right ventricle.

Abnormally large *a* waves occur when the right atrium has difficulty emptying into the right ventricle. Thus, they are seen in tricuspid stenosis (Fig. 14-7), severe pulmonary stenosis, and pulmonary hypertension. Also, large *a* waves occur in myocardiopathies, in nodal rhythm, or in prolonged *a-v* conduction time, wherein the atrium contracts at a time when the tricuspid valve is closed.

In addition to regular large *a* waves there may occur so-called irregular giant *a* waves, referred to as *cannon waves* (Fig. 14-8). These occur in the presence of complete atrioventricular heart block without atrial fibrillation. Such waves occur at irregular intervals, as mentioned, and specifically at those times when the atrium contracts against a closed tricuspid valve.

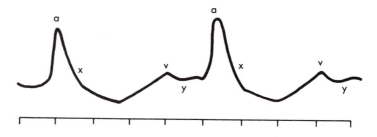

Fig. 14-7. Jugular venous pulse in tricuspid stenosis demonstrating regularly occurring large a waves.

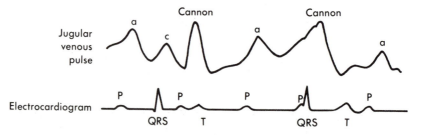

Fig. 14-8. Jugular venous pulse tracing and simultaneous electrocardiogram in complete heart block. Notice the giant a waves (cannon waves). These occur when the atrium contracts during ventricular systole, at which time the tricuspid valve is closed.

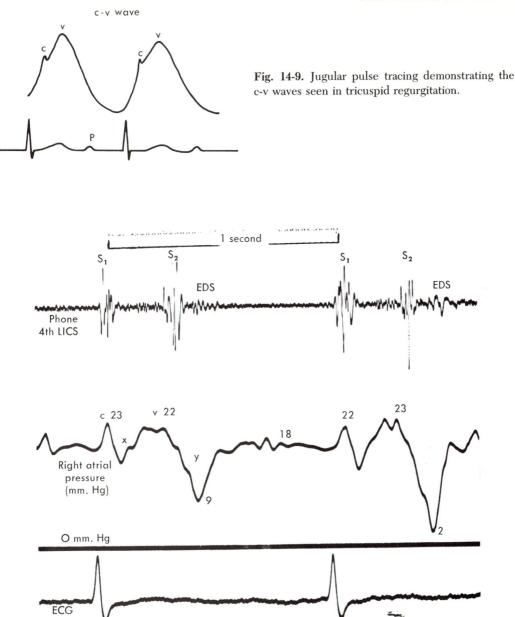

c-v wave

Fig. 14-9. Jugular pulse tracing demonstrating the c-v waves seen in tricuspid regurgitation.

Fig. 14-10. Electrocardiogram and phonocardiogram of a 58-year-old man with calcific constrictive pericarditis and atrial fibrillation. *Upper sound tracing,* external phonocardiogram, fourth left intercostal space: early diastolic sound (EDS) or precordial knock follows the second heart sound. *Right atrial pressure pulse* consists of c-v wave with a prominent y descent augmented with inspiration (second complex). The abrupt termination of early diastolic filling characteristic of constrictive pericarditis is reflected in the rise in atrial pressure after the nadir of the y descent. It is during this period that the early diastolic sound occurs. The jugular venous pulse would reflect the right atrial pressure pulse in this situation.

In the presence of generalized congestive heart failure, the right ventricle becomes dilated and the tricuspid valve becomes stretched, resulting in tricuspid insufficiency. Under such conditions or in the rarer form of organic tricuspid insufficiency, blood regurgitates into the right atrium during ventricular systole. This produces a large positive wave often called the *c-v* wave (Fig. 14-9).

In constrictive pericarditis the venous pressure is always elevated and the neck veins are markedly distended. In addition, the distention in these veins increases with inspiration, so the *x* and *y* descents are usually very prominent (Fig. 14-10).

PULSE

Palpation of the pulse should be a routine part of every physical examination. It is frequently executed as a mechanical maneuver without regard to the valuable information that this procedure may convey to the physician. The physicians of bygone years used their God-given senses in examining patients, and such things as the character of the pulse, the type of respiration, and peculiar aromas accompanying certain diseases often afforded these keen clinicians significant diagnostic clues concerning the patient's illness. In this mechanical age many of us neglect our senses of observation, palpation, and olfaction and instead rely unduly on various gadgets and instruments.

Normally the pulse is equal in the two upper extremities, but occcasionally the radial artery has an anomalous course on one side. Thus, one must check carefully before concluding that the pulse is absent. Thrombosis or embolism involving one subclavian, axillary, or brachial artery usually results in an absent radial pulse on the affected side. A cervical rib or scalenus anticus syndrome can be associated with impairment of the pulse in the ipsilateral extremity.

Information of great importance can be obtained from careful palpation of the pulse. The arterial pulse can be palpated at any point where the arteries lie near the surface of the body and where they can be compressed against a firmer surface, usually bone. Thus the examiner can detect the pulse over the radial, branchial, carotid, popliteal, femoral, dorsalis pedis, and other arteries; however, because of accesibility the radial artery over the radial and volar aspects of the wrist usually is selected. In taking the pulse at the wrist, the patient's hand is placed with the palm upward. The physician places his first three fingers on the patient's radial artery, with his index finger nearest the patient's heart. The radial artery is then gently compressed against the distal end of the radius. The pressure of the fingers flattens the artery during diastole, and the vessel regains its circular shape as it fills with blood during ventricular systole. When determining the rate, it is desirable to count the pulse for 1 full minute and not fractions thereof.

In examining the pulse it is important to bear in mind the following four points; rate, rhythm, character, and consistency of the arterial wall.

Rate

The pulse rate normally varies with age, sex, physical activity, and emotional status. In children it usually varies from 90 to 120 beats per minute and in adults from 60 to 90 per minute, being slightly higher in women than in men. In well-conditioned athletes a pulse rate of 50 beats per minute is not unusual. If the pulse is rapid during the initial examination, the patient should be permitted to rest, and the rate should be rechecked to ensure a more reliable reading. The rate is increased (*tachycardia*) in severe anemias, high fever, massive hemorrhage, various types of cardiac arrhythmias, hyperthyroidism, and at times in congestive heart failure. The pulse rate may be decreased *(bradycardia)* in increased intracranial pressure, obstructive jaundice, syncope, and complete heart block.

Rhythm

Rhythm, which applies to both the arterial pulse and heart, is discussed at this point for two reasons. First, the pulse should be investigated at the beginning of the cardiovascular examination prior to study of the heart itself. Second, the more common disturbances of rhythm can and should be detected by palpating the pulse. It is emphasized, however, that auscultation of the heart is the most accurate method for determining the rhythm. Whereas a number of alterations of rhythm can be diagnosed at the pulse and confirmed by cardiac auscultation, others can be identified only by listening to the heart. Some of the more complex arrhythmias can be diagnosed only by means of an electrocardiographic tracing.

Sinus arrhythmia. In the normal person the rhythm of the pulse is regular, and any deviation from this regularity is termed *arrhythmia*. In children, in young adults, and occasionally in older patients there may be detected a slight irregularity termed *sinus arrhythmia*. In this condition the pulse rate speeds up with inspiration and slows with expiration. It can be exaggerated by deep respiration. Although this is the most common alteration of rhythm, it is of no clinical significance and is important only in that it be differentiated from the abnormal arrhythmias.

Premature contractions. The second most common cause of the arrhythmias is premature contraction *(extrasystole)* (Fig. 14-11). This premature beat usually arises in the ventricle, atrium, or atrioventricular node and, as a rule,

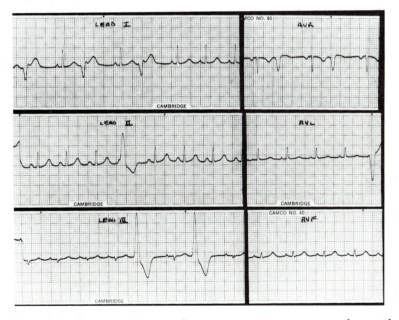

Fig. 14-11. Electrocardiogram of patient demonstrating premature ventricular systoles. The prolonged pause after each extrasystole is called the compensatory pause.

occurs in the absence of organic cardiac disease. However, the patient is often conscious of this arrhythmia and describes it as, "My heart turns a flipflop," "My heart stops beating occasionally," or "My heart skips beats." This arrhythmia may occur as the result of emotional tension, excessive smoking or alcoholic intake, excessive intake of digitalis, and also in some instances of organic heart disease.

Premature beats may stimulate ventricular contraction at a time when the ventricles have not had an opportunity to completely fill. Under such circumstances the ventricles contract on partially filled chambers and are unable to initiate a palpable peripheral pulse wave. In the diagnosis of premature contractions the examiner, by palpating the pulse, notes a general regularity except for scattered pauses that are followed by a resumption of the normal

rhythm. The palpating finger usually detects only the long pause and often misses the small beat, which is caused by the premature systole. Simultaneous auscultation at the apex of the heart will reveal the premature contraction that follows the normal beat, the subsequent pause, and then a resumption of the normal rhythm.

Atrial fibrillation. Atrial fibrillation constitutes a grossly irregular rhythm often described as an "irregular irregularity" (Fig. 14-12), and in the majority of persons it is so classic that it can be diagnosed by palpating the radial pulse. In this condition there seems to be neither rhyme nor reason to the rate, rhythm, or volume of the pulse. As the examiner palpates such a pulse he is immediately impressed with the fact that it is grossly irregular in rhythm, extremely variable in rate, and that there is great variation in volume. This condition differs

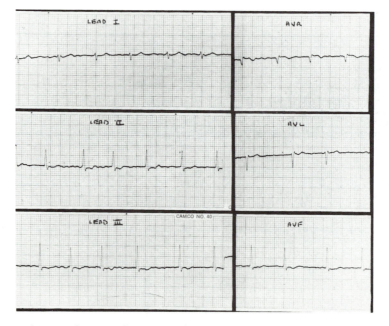

Fig. 14-12. Electrocardiogram of patient with chronic atrial fibrillation. Note the absence of P waves and variation of the R-R interval. The baseline is grossly irregular in contrast to that in normal sinus rhythm.

from premature contractions in that the latter have a regular rhythm altered at times by the extrasystoles, whereas atrial fibrillation has absolutely no regularity. On auscultation, a similar irregularity is heard over the heart itself. Often if the examiner simultaneously palpates the radial pulse and auscultates the heart, he will notice a disproportion of occasionally 5 to as many as 30 or 40 beats per minute. This disparity is referred to as a *pulse deficit* and is attributed to the fact that during some periods of diastole the ventricle has not completely filled. Thus, when systole occurs, the ventricle contracts on a partially filled chamber and is incapable of producing a palpable peripheral pulse wave. For example, the palpable pulse rate may be 90, whereas the apical rate may be 115. Pulse deficit may occur in other arrhythmias and is not pathognomonic of atrial fibrillation.

Atrial fibrillation usually indicates underlying disease, and it most commonly occurs in the presence of mitral stenosis, arteriosclerotic heart disease, and hyperthyroidism. Occasionally this arrhythmia will occur without any apparent cause and may be very transient in nature.

Bigeminal pulse. In a bigeminal pulse, beats are coupled or occur in pairs, with the second beat usually being weaker. This condition may be produced by two different mechanisms.

1. *Premature contractions.* If each normal beat is followed by a premature contraction, the premature contraction is in turn followed by a longer pause, and coupling of the beats will result. It is not infrequently caused by overdigitalization. Premature contractions are the usual cause of bigeminy.

2. *Partial, or second-degree, heart block.* When there is a defect in atrioventricular conduction, some of the atrial impulses fail to be conducted to the ventricles. Thus, only every second (2:1 block) or every third (3:1 block)

atrial impulse may reach the ventricle. If every third atrial contraction fails to reach the ventricle and cause it to contract, coupling will also occur.

Trigeminal pulse. In a trigeminal pulse there is a pause after every third beat. This, like the bigeminal pulse, may be produced by premature contractions occurring in place of each normal third beat, a pair of premature systoles and a pause occurring after a normal beat, or a heart block in which every fourth ventricular beat is missing.

Paroxysmal atrial tachycardia. When the pulse is regular and the rate is between 150 and 220, usually about 180 beats per minute (Fig. 14-13), paroxysmal atrial tachycardia should be suspected. Careful observation of the neck veins reveals a 1:1 ratio between their pulsations and the cardiac rate as determined at the apex. If pressure is exerted over the carotid sinus, the tachycardia will often terminate. In the presence of atrial flutter or sinus tachycardia, carotid sinus pressure only temporarily slows the ventricular rate.

Paroxysmal ventricular tachycardia. Usually paroxysmal ventricular tachycardia is a serious arrhythmia and often is difficult to diagnose accurately at the bedside by palpation of the pulse or auscultation of the heart. Frequently there are associated symptoms or signs suggesting the gravity of the situation. Usually dizziness, weakness, dyspnea, and precordial pain are present, the pulse rate is 150 to 160 beats per minute, and the rhythm is slightly irregular (Fig. 14-14). The ventricular rate does not change with carotid sinus massage. A suspected diagnosis should be confirmed by electrocardiography.

Atrial flutter. Atrial flutter is characterized by a rapid regular pulse with a ventricular rate of 140 to 160 beats per minute (Fig. 14-15). It may be confused with paroxysmal atrial tachycardia. However, in atrial flutter observation of

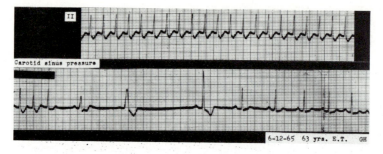

Fig. 14-13. Electrocardiogram of patient with paroxysmal supraventricular tachycardia (top strip). The cardiac rate is 176, and rhythm is regular. The lower strip demonstrates slowing with carotid sinus pressure and, finally, resumption of sinus rhythm.

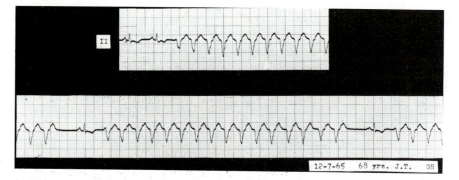

Fig. 14-14. Electrocardiogram of ventricular tachycardia. Note that the QRS complexes are widened and bizarre in shape. There is a slight variation in the interval between the ventricular complexes.

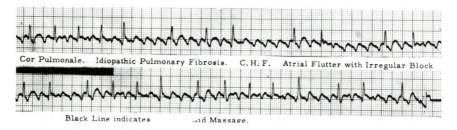

Fig. 14-15. Electrocardiogram of patient with atrial flutter and a variable ventricular response. Note the characteristic saw-tooth appearance of the baseline. Black line indicates application of carotid sinus massage, which fails to result in a conversion to sinus rhythm.

the neck veins will reveal flutter waves occurring at a rate twice that of the cardiac apex, whereas in paroxysmal atrial tachycardia the ratio is 1:1. Also, as mentioned, carotid sinus massage may be helpful in differentiating the two conditions.

Heart block. Atrioventricular (AV) heart block is divided into three types: first, second, and third degree.

1. *First degree AV block* is characterized by a prolongation of the P-R interval above the limits of normal (Fig. 14-16). In the adult the upper limit of the normal P-R interval is 0.2 second. Usually there are no significant physical findings associated with this condition except a decreased intensity of the first heart sound at the apex.

2. *Second degree AV block* is divided into two types:

    a. In the Wenckebach phenomenon there is a progressive lengthening of the P-R interval for a number of beats and finally one P wave fails to result in ventricular contraction. Following this, the P-R interval is shorter, and the entire sequence of events is repeated. On physical examination one may detect a dropped beat without an associated premature beat such as occurs in extrasystoles. In addition, there is a varying intensity of the first heart sound related to the varying P-R interval.

    b. In the other type of second degree block there is an alteration of AV conduction so that only every second, third, or fourth atrial impulse is conducted to the ventricles (Fig. 14-17). In a 2:1 block the atrial rate might be 80 and that of the ventricles would be 40. In a 3:1 block the atrial rate may be 120 and that of the ventricles will be 40. Also, the ventricular rhythm may be irregular when the block is variable rather than constant. This type of block may be suspected at the bedside by cor-

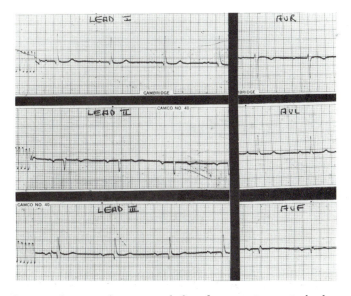

Fig. 14-16. Electrocardiogram of patient with first degree atrioventricular heart block. The P-R interval is 0.34 second.

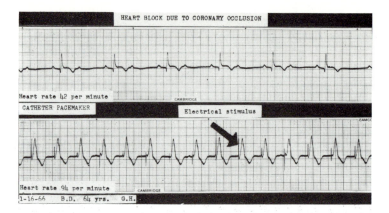

Fig. 14-17. Electrocardiogram of patient with second degree atrioventricular heart block. Top tracing demonstrates heart rate of 42; every second atrial complex is blocked at the AV node, resulting in a 2:1 block. Lower tracing reveals electrocardiogram of same patient following insertion of catheter pacemaker.

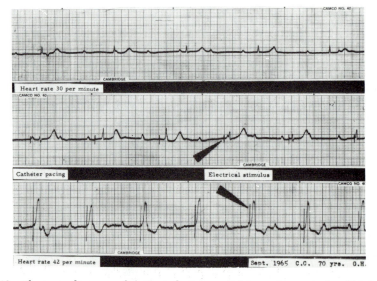

Fig. 14-18. Electrocardiogram of patient during complete atrioventricular (third degree) heart block. The atria and ventricles are beating at their own independent rhythms (top strip). The P waves and QRS complexes are completely disassociated. The middle and lower strips demonstrate electrocardiogram of same patient following insertion of transvenous jugular pacemaker.

relating the *a* waves in the jugular pulse, which represent atrial contraction, with auscultation at the apex to determine the ventricular rate.

3. Third degree heart block (complete heart block) is characterized by a lack of conduction of the atrial impulse through the AV node to the ventricle (Fig. 14-18). There is no specific relationship between the atrial and ventricular complexes. In other words, the atria and ventricles are beating, each at their own independent rhythm. On physical examination one may detect cannon waves in the jugular veins, as mentioned previously, and the *a* waves in the neck may be unrelated to the heart sounds as detected at the apex. The ventricular rate is usually less than 50 beats per minute, and there is a varying intensity of the first heart sound.

Quality and character of the pulse waves

The arterial pulse starts at the instant the aortic valve opens and left ventricular ejection begins. This results in an abrupt sharp rise in aortic pressure, since blood enters the aorta much faster than it flows to the more distal arteries. During the systolic phase of left ventricular ejection a large portion of the blood is temporarily stored in the proximal aorta. Once the aortic pressure reaches a peak it begins to fall as ventricular ejection slows, and blood continues its flow in the peripheral arteries. As the ventricle relaxes, there is a transient reversal of flow from the central arteries to the ventricle and the aortic valve closes. The aortic pressure continues to decrease during diastole as blood flow continues to the peripheral vessels.

The pressure wave is propagated by the action of molecules within the blood, which push each other forward as well as laterally. This results in a propulsive force as well as in disten-

tion of the arterial wall. Thus, as the blood flow progresses in the more peripheral and less distensible arteries, the velocity of the pulse wave increases.

The carotid pulse wave is detected approximately 0.03 second following ventricular ejection, when timed from the QRS complex of the electrocardiogram. Comparable delays in other arteries are as follows: brachial 0.06 second; radial, 0.08 second; femoral 0.075 second.

The character of the arterial pulse wave is dependent on the rate of change and the magnitude of the pulse pressure and can be studied readily in the carotid arteries. The examiner should palpate the carotid artery while simultaneously listening to the heart in order to identify the first and second heart sounds. The pulse wave is composed of an ascending limb, peak, and descending limb (Fig. 14-19). There is a small notch *(anacrotic)* near the peak of the ascending limb and a similar notch *(dicrotic)* on the descending limb.

The upstroke is prompt and smooth, but the anacrotic notch is not palpable in most normal persons. The peak of the pulse wave is rounded and smooth. The descending limb is more gradual and less steep than the upstroke. The dicrotic notch in most normal persons cannot be palpated as a definite notch but can be sensed as a change in the slope of the downstroke.

Pulsus magnus. A strong bounding pulse with a tall rapid ascending limb and an equally rapid descending limb characterizes *pulsus magnus* (Fig. 14-20). The peak of the pulse wave is sharp and very brief. Pulsus magnus is also called a *water-hammer,* or collapsing, pulse. A water-hammer consists of a glass tube about 12 inches in length, partially filled with water, in which the air has been expelled by boiling the water just prior to sealing the open end of the tube. When such a tube is rapidly inverted, the water falls suddenly through the

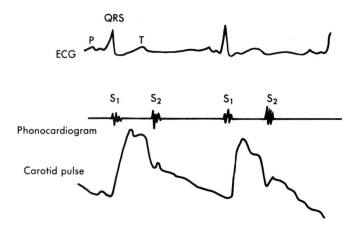

Fig. 14-19. Normal carotid pulse with simultaneous electrocardiogram and phonocardiogram. Note character of ascending limb, peak, and descending limb. S_1 represents the first heart sound, and S_2 the second heart sound.

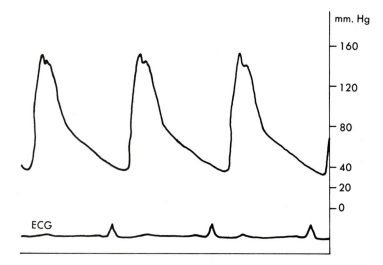

Fig. 14-20. Arterial blood pressure in aortic regurgitation. Note the elevated systolic and low diastolic levels, resulting in a wide pulse pressure and a pulsus magnus (water-hammer pulse).

vacuum, and the hand feels a sharp thud or shock. A similar sensation is transmitted to the fingers when palpating pulsus magnus. This type of pulse is usually associated with a wide pulse pressure, increased stroke volume of the left ventricle, and a decrease in peripheral vascular resistance. The more common causes are aortic regurgitation, hyperthyroidism, severe anemia, arteriovenous fistulae, and systolic hypertension. Occasionally, pulsus magnus may occur in normal persons during anxiety, exercise, or fever.

Pulsus parvus. A small weak pulse with a delayed systolic peak (Fig. 14-21) is characteristic of *pulsus parvus*. It occurs in the presence of a narrow pulse pressure, in situations where there is an increase in peripheral vascular resistance, and in those conditions where the stroke volume of the left ventricle is low. The more common causes for such a pulse are aortic stenosis, mitral stenosis, left ventricular failure

secondary to myocardial infarction, constrictive pericarditis, and cardiac tamponade.

Pulsus alternans. *Pulsus alternans* is characterized by a regularly alternating pulse, in which every other beat is weaker than the preceding beat (Fig. 14-22). Actually, there is an alternating series of high and low pulse waves caused by an alternating contractile force of the left ventricle. Since the weak beats are but slightly weaker than the strong beats, this arrhythmia may be overlooked unless the examiner is skilled or alerted to its possibility. It is more likely to be detected when the patient is sitting or standing. It must be distinguished from bigeminy. Pulsus alternans is entirely regular in rhythm, although variable in volume, in contrast to bigeminy, which is variable in both rhythm and volume. Pulsus alternans is best detected when taking the blood pressure. Only the stronger beats are heard at the top systolic level. As the pressure is lowered 10 to

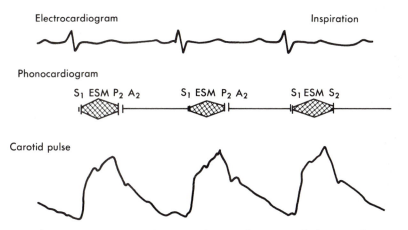

Fig. 14-21. Carotid pulse with simultaneous phonocardiogram and electrocardiogram in severe aortic stenosis. Note the anacrotic notch on upstroke of pulse wave; the systolic peak is delayed. S_1 and S_2 represent first and second heart sounds, respectively. P_2 and A_2 refer to pulmonary and aortic components of second sound. Note paradoxical split of second sound (closes on inspiration and splits on expiration). ESM represents the diamond-shaped systolic ejection murmur.

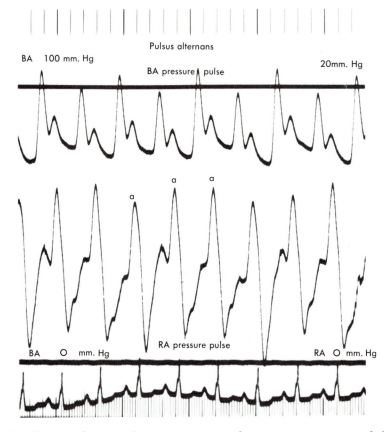

Fig. 14-22. Electrocardiogram of a young woman with severe primary myocardial disease, sinus tachycardia, functional classification. III. *Upper pressure pulse tracing:* brachial artery; scale 0—100 mm. Hg at left. *Lower pressure pulse tracing:* right atrial pressure; scale 0—20 mm. Hg at right. Brachial artery pressure pulse demonstrates pulsus alternans; right atrial pressure pulse shows prominent a waves and brisk x descent.

30 mm.Hg, the weaker beats will appear alternately between the stronger beats, and the rate is then doubled. Pulsus alternans occurs most frequently in severe arterial hypertension, coronary artery disease, and left ventricular failure. Consequently, it is a valuable indication of left ventricular failure and is accompanied frequently by a ventricular diastolic gallop sound (S-3) at the cardiac apex.

Bisferiens pulse. Bisferiens pulse is some-

times termed the *"double beating"* pulse and is characterized by two impulses occurring during systole (Fig. 14-23). The initial upstroke rises rapidly and is referred to as the *percussion wave*. This is followed by a small dip and then a second slower upstroke called the *tidal wave*. This type of pulse is found in combined aortic regurgitation and stenosis, functional hypertrophic aortic stenosis, and occasionally in pure aortic regurgitation.

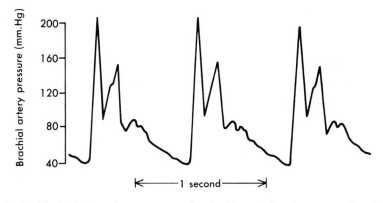

Fig. 14-23. Pulsus bisferiens demonstrating the double impulse during systole. This occurs in combined aortic stenosis and regurgitation and occasionally in pure aortic regurgitation.

Anacrotic pulse

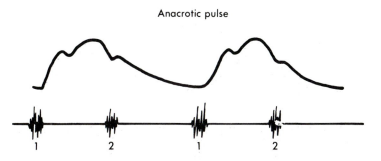

Fig. 14-24. Anacrotic pulse demonstrating an anacrotic notch on the upstroke or during systole. 1 and 2 refer to the first and second heart sounds.

Dicrotic pulse

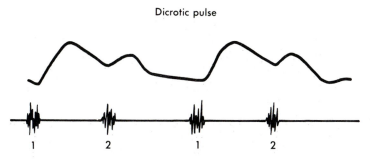

Fig. 14-25. Dicrotic pulse demonstrating a dicrotic notch on the downstroke or during diastole. 1 and 2 refer to first and second heart sounds.

Paradoxical pulse. *Paradoxical pulse* is characterized by a decrease in the amplitude or an actual imperceptibility of the pulse (*not* a decrease in its rate) that occurs during the inspiratory phase of respiration. In normal subjects this phenomenon can be produced by forced inspiration. When it occurs during quiet respiration, however, it is definitely abnormal. In normal individuals the systolic blood pressure may decrease 5 to 10 mm. Hg during inspiration. Generally this is either imperceptible or barely detectable by palpation of the peripheral arteries or while determining the blood pressure. This phenomenon is caused mainly by pooling of blood in the pulmonary circuit during inspiration, resulting from the expansion of the lungs and an increase in the negative intrathoracic pressure. In turn this results in a decrease in the return of blood to the left side of the heart, a decrease in left ventricular output, and thus a decrease in arterial blood pressure. When the systolic blood pressure falls more than 10 mm. Hg during inspiration, the pulse is referred to as paradoxical. The most accurate means of identifying a paradoxical pulse is with the use of a sphygmomanometer, since it can be easily overlooked while palpating the radial artery. The presence of a paradoxical pulse should suggest the possibility of massive pericardial effusion, constrictive pericarditis, and severe pulmonary emphysema.

Anacrotic pulse. *Anacrotic pulse* is characterized by the presence of two beats that are palpable during systole (on the ascending limb of the pulse wave). This type of pulse is rarely detected and even then only in severe aortic stenosis where it may be palpated in the carotid artery (Fig. 14-24).

Dicrotic pulse. In *dicrotic pulse* there are two impulses that are palpable during diastole (on the descending limb of the pulse wave). It usually occurs in the presence of high fever and may be palpated in both the carotid and peripheral arteries (Fig. 14-25).

Consistency of arterial wall

In addition to determining the rate, rhythm, and character of the pulse, it is important to identify the character of the wall of the artery itself. This is best accomplished by expressing the blood from a distal segment of the radial artery that has been occluded by digital pressure. The true consistency of this vessel can then be determined by means of palpation. Normally the wall of an artery under these circumstances is soft and pliable. In arteriosclerosis the wall offers more resistance to compression by the palpating finger, and the vessel may be rolled easily between the examining digits. This is often referred to as a "pipe stem" artery. The artery may be beaded in consistency and tortuous in its course. In elderly persons the examiner may actually visualize these snakelike pulsating arteries under the skin of the arms and forearms.

THE HEART

The heart lends itself readily to inspection, palpation, auscultation, and percussion. The first three of these procedures are of inestimable value in the clinical diagnosis of heart disease, but percussion has very limited application in the cardiac examination and is discussed briefly elsewhere in this chapter.

The twentieth century in all probability will be recorded in history as the mechanical and nuclear age. It has had its impact on all sciences, medicine included. We rely on vehicles instead of walking; use innumerable mechanical devices to perform our everyday duties; and insist on more and more contrivances to see, hear, and think for us. Physicians, like others, have become involved in this technologic and scientific revolution. We have become entirely too dependent on a host of instruments to make our diagnoses. We see but do not observe, hear but do not listen, and think but fail to concentrate. All too frequently careful physical examination is replaced by the electrocardiogram, roentgenogram, echogram, and phonocardiogram. To be sure, these are valuable diagnostic aids and have contributed enormously to our present knowledge of cardiac function. It should be emphasized that cardiac catheterization, phonocardiography, echocardiography, and angiocardiography have helped us to more accurately apply our clinical acumen at the bedside. As a result, clinical evaluation of the heart now becomes the most important single diagnostic tool available today. It is vital to perfect these diagnostic skills and to discipline ourselves to systematically and logically evaluate the patient.

The importance of physical diagnosis in its relationship to the heart is best illustrated by the five-fingered approach of W. Proctor Harvey, M.D. (Fig. 14-26). The thumb represents the history and in most situations constitutes the single most important element in establishing a cardiac diagnosis. Physical examination is represented by the index finger. The electrocardiogram, chest x-ray, and special laboratory procedures are represented by the remaining three fingers. Just as the thumb and index finger are the most essential digits of the hand, so are the history and physical examination the most important factors in arriving at a precise cardiac diagnosis. They in no way detract from the importance of the electrocardiogram and other laboratory procedures that, when added to the history and physical examination, serve to either establish or confirm the diagnosis.

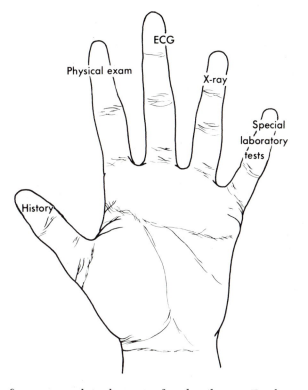

Fig. 14-26. Five-finger approach to diagnosis of cardiac disease. Emphasis is placed on the history and physical examination. (After W. Proctor Harvey, M.D.)

Prior to discussing physical examination of the heart, it is essential to have in mind the gross anatomy of the normal heart and its topographic relationship to the anterior chest wall.

Landmarks and topographic anatomy

Certain basic anatomic landmarks are helpful in localizing and describing the heart borders, valve areas, and great vessels. These are as follows:

1. Midsternal line
2. Midclavicular lines
3. Anterior, middle, and posterior axillary lines
4. Suprasternal notch (that area immediately superior to the manubrium)
5. Identification of the various ribs and intercostal spaces
6. Precordium (This refers to the area of the anterior thorax overlying the heart and pericardium.)

A brief review of the anatomy of the heart reveals that it has a base directed upward and toward the right and an apex directed downward and toward the left. It presents three borders: right, left, and inferior (Fig. 14-27). The largest portion of the anterior aspect of the heart is made up of the right ventricle, with the right atrium occupying a small area to the extreme right and the left ventricle occupying a relatively small area to the extreme left.

The base of the heart, formed by both atria,

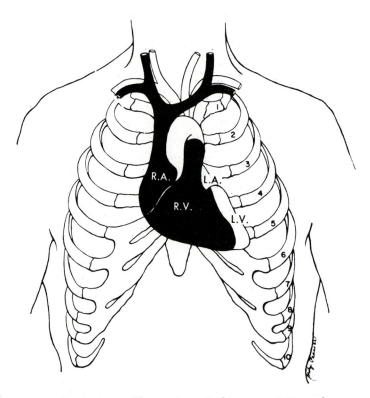

Fig. 14-27. Topographic anatomy of heart. R.A., Right atrium; R.V., right ventricle; L.A., left atrium; L.V., left ventricle.

corresponds to a line crossing the sternum obliquely from the lower border of the second left costal cartilage—at a point just to the left of its junction with the sternum—to the upper border of the third right costal cartilage—at a point 2 cm. lateral to its sternal junction.

The right border of the heart conforms to a curved line with its convexity toward the right, extending from the upper border of the third right costal cartilage 2 cm. lateral to its junction with the sternum, to the sixth right chondrosternal articulation.

The left border, formed largely by the left ventricle and superiorly by the left atrium, is represented by a curved line with its convexity directed upward and toward the left, extending from the fifth left intercostal space 1.5 cm. me-

dial to the midclavicular line, to the lower border of the second left costal cartilage 1 to 2 cm. to the left of its articulation with the sternum.

The inferior border, formed largely by the right ventricle and to a lesser extent by the left ventricle, is represented by a line drawn from the sixth right chondrosternal articulation to the site of the cardiac impulse in the left fifth intercostal space 1 to 2 cm. medial to the midclavicular line.

The cardiac valves all lie within a small elliptic area extending from the third left chondrosternal articulation to the junction of the sixth right costal cartilage with the sternum (Fig. 14-28). Within this area the pulmonary valve lies behind the third left chondrosternal articulation at the level of the upper border of the

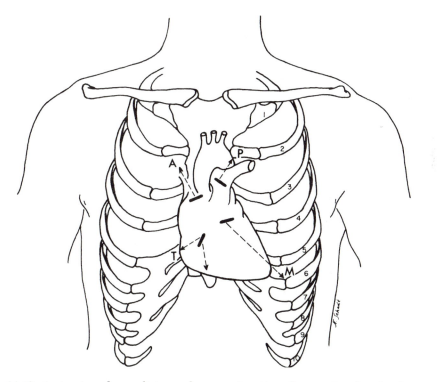

Fig. 14-28. Anatomic and auscultatory valve area. Location of anatomic valve sites is represented by solid bars. The arrows designate the transmission of the valve sounds to their respective auscultatory valve areas.

third costal cartilage. The aortic valve lies behind the sternum just to the right of the pulmonary valve at the level of the third intercostal space. The mitral valve lies behind the left sternal border at the level of the fourth costal cartilage. The tricuspid valve lies behind the body of the sternum midway on a line drawn obliquely across the mid-sternal line from the third left to the sixth right chondrosternal articulations. These areas are the *anatomic sites of the valves and do not correspond with the areas in which the valve sounds are best heard.*

Keeping these landmarks and anatomic relationships clearly in mind permits the examiner to describe his cardiac findings and to accurately localize them. For example, the left cardiac border in the third intercostal space might be 5 cm. from the midsternal line, or the cardiac border in the fifth left intercostal space may be located at the anterior axillary line. Such descriptions convey a mental picture of the cardiac configuration and are extremely important with regard to the patient's physical examination chart. For example, if the patient's left cardiac border 5 years previously was in the midclavicular line and is now located in the anterior axillary line, it would indicate obvious cardiac enlargement or a shift of the mediastinum.

The position of the heart, even when normal, varies considerably according to the configuration of the chest and height of the diaphragm. In the average person the heart occupies an oblique position in the mediastinum, with approximately one third of the organ lying to the right and two thirds lying to the left of the midline. In subjects who are short in stature and stocky in habitus the heart occupies a more transverse position in the thorax. In persons with an asthenic body configuration the heart is vertical in position and hangs like a pendulum in the midline.

INSPECTION AND PALPATION

Inspection and palpation are discussed together because there is an intimate relationship between these two processes in the course of the cardiovascular examination. In many instances those phenomena that are seen on the anterior chest also can be palpated. Generally, the outward movements over the precordium are best detected by inspection, whereas the inward movements are more readily palpable.

It is easy to overlook the various pulsatile and retractive phenomena associated with underlying cardiac pathology. In most instances inspection and palpation of the anterior chest are best executed with the patient lying flat on his back or with the upper third of the body elevated approximately 45 degrees.

The examiner should always observe the shape and contour of the patient's chest. Depressions of the sternum, kyphosis of the dorsal spine, scoliosis, and other thoracic deformities often alter the shape and position of the heart. In some instances, such as Marfan's syndrome, deformities of the thorax are accompanied by specific abnormalities of the heart.

Pulsations resulting from movement of the heart and great vessels are best seen with the use of tangential lighting; consequently, the examiner should observe the surface of the chest tangentially so that he may see the full range of the various pulsations. These pulsations are best visualized at the termination of normal expiration.

When pulsations are identified, their exact time of occurrence in the cardiac cycle must be determined. Thus, once the pulsatile movements are detected by inspection, palpation, or both, the examiner confirms their exact time in the cardiac cycle by simultaneous auscultation of the heart or by palpation of the carotid artery. In this manner one can determine whether the pulsations seen on the anterior chest wall occur in systole, diastole, or both.

Palpation serves either to confirm the observations of inspection or to detect those pulsatile movements that are not visible. Two procedures are advocated for palpating cardiac movements. The examiner may either place his fingertips in the appropriate intercostal space or place his fingers and the palm of his hand against the chest wall (Fig. 14-29).

In addition to pulsatile movements, palpation may reveal either thrills or friction rubs.

Thrills. *Thrills* are actually palpable vibrations, most commonly produced by the flow of blood from one chamber of the heart to another through a restricted or narrowed orifice. Thrills are palpable murmurs somewhat similar to the sensation one feels on the throat of a purring cat. Thrills occur principally with stenosis of a valve or a defect in the interventricular septum. When blood flows through the narrowed valve or septal defect, eddy currents develop distal to the narrowed area, and the walls of the chamber are set into vibration (Fig. 14-30). Thrills may occur in systole, diastole, or presystole and at times may be continuous.

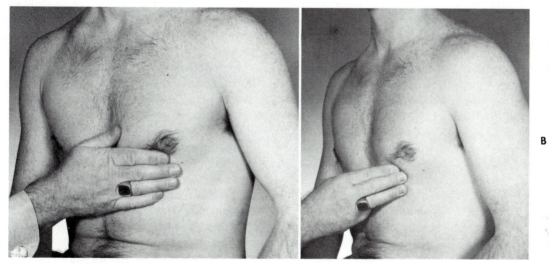

Fig. 14-29. Methods for palpating the point of maximum impulse. **A,** Palmar aspect of fingertips and hand. **B,** Fingertips.

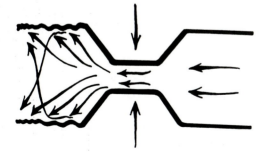

Fig. 14-30. Method of production of a thrill. Flow of blood from one chamber to another through a narrowed orifice.

Any thrill should be described as to its location, its time in the cardiac cycle, and its mode of extension or transmission. Timing a thrill may be very difficult and is best accomplished by relating it to either the apex beat or the carotid artery pulsations, both of which correspond to ventricular systole. The intensity of the thrill varies according to the velocity of the blood, the degree of narrowing of the orifice at which it is produced, and the difference in pressure between the two chambers of the heart. The greater each of these factors is, the greater the intensity of the thrill. The intensity of a thrill will decrease as the distance between the chest wall and the site of origin of the thrill is increased. The quality of a thrill depends on the frequency of vibrations producing it; rapid vibrations result in fine thrills, whereas slower vibrations produce coarser thrills.

Pericardial friction rubs. Although a *pericardial friction rub* may be palpated, it is best detected by auscultation. It is a to-and-fro grating sensation, which is usually present during both phases of the cardiac cycle. It is caused by a fibrinous pericarditis that may be the result of several disease processes. The rub may be intermittent, in which case it may be present at one moment and not perceptible several minutes later. The ability to palpate a pericardial rub depends to some extent on whether or not the visceral and parietal pericardial surfaces are in contact and rubbing against each other. Often rubs are more readily palpated with the patient sitting erect and leaning foward. In the presence of pericardial effusion the rub will usually disappear because of the separation of the visceral and parietal layers by the accumulated fluid. Although rubs may be detected over any portion of the precordium, as a rule they are best palpated in the left third and fourth intercostal spaces at the sternal border.

During the process of inspection and palpation it is advisable to concentrate on seven rel-atively specific areas: sternoclavicular, aortic, pulmonary, right ventricular, apical, epigastric, and ectopic (Fig. 14-31). This specific approach toward inspection and palpation of the heart was proposed by J. W. Hurst, M.D., and is the most informative method advocated to date.

1. *Sternoclavicular area.* The sternoclavicular area includes the sternoclavicular joints, manubrium, and the upper part of the sternum. Normally one detects little or no pulsation in this location. Abnormal pulsations in this area are produced usually by dissecting aneurysms of the aorta and aneurysms caused by atherosclerosis or syphilis. Slight pulsations in the region of the right sternoclavicular joint may be detected in the presence of a tortuous innominate artery or a right-sided aortic arch.

2. *Aortic area.* The aortic area is located in the right second intercostal space adjacent to the sternum. In the presence of valvular aortic stenosis one may palpate a systolic thrill in this area that may radiate toward the right side of the neck. A thrill in this area is best detected with the patient leaning forward and holding his breath in deep expiration. On occasions one may detect abnormal pulsations in this area attributed to aneurysmal dilatation of the ascending aorta or dilatation of the aorta caused by aortic regurgitation.

3. *Pulmonary area.* The left second intercostal space just lateral to the sternum is the pulmonary area. In pulmonary stenosis one may detect a systolic thrill in this area that at times radiates to the left side of the neck. Minimal pulsations may be detected in this location in normal children or in adults with thin chests; such pulsations are accentuated by the presence of anemia, fever, or pregnancy.

In those conditions where pulmonary artery pressure or pulmonary flow is increased, one detects abnormal pulsations in this area. In mitral stenosis or primary pulmonary hypertension, where the pulmonary artery pressure is increased, there is a slow, sustained, and forceful pulsation of the pulmonary artery. In conditions where the pulmonary artery flow is increased, such as atrial septal defect, the pulsations are vigorous, active, and less sustained.

4. *Anterior precordium (right ventricular).* The anterior precordium encompasses the lower half of the sternum and the adjacent intercostal spaces, both to the left and right. Slight pulsations in this area may occur in children or thin-chested adults and are accentuated by fever, hyperthyroidism, anxiety, and anemia.

Abnormal pulsations in this area are usually attributed to those conditions associated with right ventricular hypertrophy or dilatation. In right ventricular hypertension, the pulsations have a gradual lift or elevation and are well sustained. The more common conditions resulting in a pressure load on the right ventricle include pulmonary stenosis, mitral stenosis, repeated pulmonary emboli, cor pulmonale, primary pulmonary hypertension, severe pulmonary hypertension secondary to a left to right shunt, and pulmonry hypertension secondary to chronic left heart failure of any cause.

Atrial and ventricular septal defects are the most common congenital lesions associated with an increased volume load on the right ventricle. In such instances the pulsations over the anterior precordium are more rapid, vigorous, and less sustained than those associated

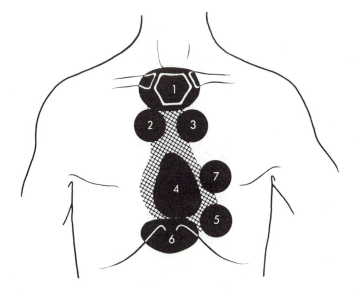

Fig. 14-31. Specific areas for cardiac examination. *1,* Sternoclavicular—includes the sternoclavicular joints, manubrium, and upper part of sternum. *2,* Aortic—right second intercostal space adjacent to sternum. *3,* Pulmonary—left second intercostal space adjacent to sternum. *4,* Anterior precordium (right ventricular)—lower half of sternum and intercostal spaces, both to left and right, adjacent to this portion of sternum. *5,* Apical—fifth left intercostal space in or slightly medial to midclavicular line. *6,* Epigastric—just inferior to xiphoid. *7,* Ectopic—left cardiac border midway between pulmonary and apical areas. (After J. W. Hurst, M.D., and R. C. Schlant, M.D., Department of Medicine, Emory University School of Medicine; courtesy American Heart Association.)

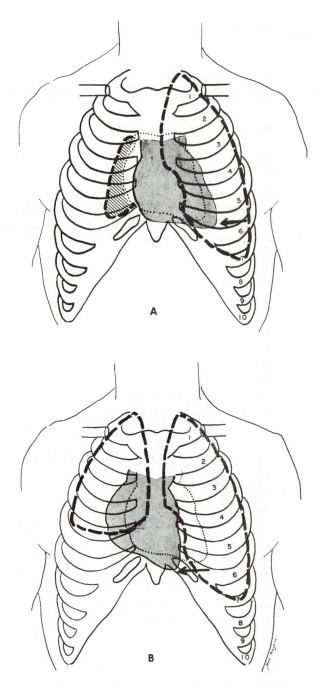

Fig. 14-32. Displacement of point of maximum impulse is designated by an arrow. Displacement of the heart is represented by a shaded area. Normal cardiac position is indicated by dotted lines. **A,** Effect of massive right pleural effusion or pneumothorax. **B,** Effect of massive right atelectasis.

with right ventricular hypertension. A systolic thrill in the left third, fourth, or fifth intercostal spaces adjacent to the sternum is strongly suggestive of ventricular septal defect. Occasionally tricuspid regurgitation will produce a thrill in this area.

5. *Apical area*. The detection and evaluation of the apical impulse is a most important facet of the cardiac examination. The examiner should pay particular attention to the location, size, and character of the impulse. In adults the apical impulse normally is located in the fifth left intercostal space, either at or slightly medial to the midclavicular line. In conditions such as pregnancy or a high diaphragm, which displace the heart to the left, the apical impulse may be located slightly lateral to the midclavicular line. Any disease resulting in a shift of the mediastinum may also result in displacement of the point of maximum impulse. For example, a massive right pleural effusion will displace the impulse to the left, whereas a massive atelectasis on the right will result in a displacement of this impulse toward the right (Fig. 14-32).

The apical impulse is normally 2 cm. or less in diameter. The early systolic outward movement of the apical area begins about the time of the first heart sound, lasts through the first third of systole, and is produced by the isovolumetric contraction of the left ventricle. At the end of the first third of systole there is an inward shift of the movement and it returns to a base line by the end of the first two thirds of systole. In the absence of heart disease, the apical impulse may have increased amplitude and duration in those persons with a thin chest wall, anemia, fever, hyperthyroidism, and anxiety.

The nature of the apical impulse is influenced by the presence of left ventricular hypertrophy, dilatation, or both. In left ventricular hypertrophy, such as occurs in pure aortic stenosis, the impulse may be normally located or slightly displaced to the left, but is very forceful and sustained throughout systole. In conditions such as aortic regurgitation, where the left ventricle is both hypertrophied and dilated, the apical impulse is usually displaced laterally, is very diffuse and forceful, and has great amplitude.

In early diastole one may at times feel or see the vibrations produced by a normal ventricular filling sound (third heart sound) or by a ventricular gallop. In late diastole, antecedent to the first heart sound, one may detect vibrations attributed to an atrial gallop. The presence of an atrial gallop is diagnostically significant in such conditions as ischemic heart disease, hypetension, and myocardial infarction.

A presystolic or diastolic thrill, attributed to mitral stenosis, is usually localized to a small area approximating the point of the apical impulse. The presystolic thrill occurs just prior to the systolic thrust of the ventricle and immediately precedes the first heart sound. In some cases of mitral regurgitation, a systolic thrill in this same location may be felt.

6. *Epigastric area*. Visible or palpable pulsations of the aorta may occur in the epigastrium in some normal individuals, as well as in the presence of fever, anemia, and hyperthyroidism. Unusually large pulsations of the aorta in this area may be produced by aortic aneurysms or aortic regurgitation. Hepatic pulsations may occur in this region, especially in the presence of tricuspid regurgitation or stenosis.

7. *Ectopic areas*. On occasion one may detect cardiac pulsations over the left cardiac border midway between the pulmonary area and the apical area. At times, either during an anginal attack or in the presence of acute myocardial infarction, one may see or palpate an abnormal outward pulsation of this area during systole. This pulsation results from a paradoxical outward bulging of the ischemic area of the

infarcted myocardium. In the presence of an anginal attack such pulsation is very temporary, whereas in acute myocardial infarction it may last several weeks. Should a ventricular aneurysm result, the paradoxical outward bulging is persistent.

PERCUSSION

Percussion is the least valuable of the four commonly practiced bedside techniques in the cardiovascular examination. Cardiac fluoroscopy or x-ray examination of the chest is far more precise in delineating the size and contour of the heart. If neither of these modalities is available, percussion may be helpful; however, the physician must appreciate its limitations.

At times the apical impulse is difficult to visualize or palpate. In such instances percussion may help to locate the left border of the heart. Under normal conditions it is impossible to detect the right border of the heart by this technique.

In the past it was considered appropriate to differentiate between absolute and relative cardiac dullness, the former being the percussion note detected over that area of the heart not covered by the lung. Experience has shown that this distinction cannot be made accurately and is of little importance. On the other hand, an actual decrease or absence of cardiac dullness per se is suggestive of pulmonary emphysema. Dullness over the base of the heart may also be increased in the presence of a substernal goiter or an anterior aneurysm of the arch of the aorta.

In the presence of pericardial effusion, percussion at times may be helpful in outlining the changing cardiac silhouette resulting from a change in the patient's position. When the patient reclines and the fluid gravitates toward the base of the heart, the area of dullness, particularly in the left second intercostal space and to a lesser extent in the right second intercostal space, may be increased (Fig. 14-33). When the patient sits erect or stands, the fluid gravitates inferiorly, resulting in a decrease in the area of dullness at the base of the heart and an increase in dullness over the lower aspect of the precordium.

AUSCULTATION

Satisfactory auscultation necessitates that the examiner concentrate on what he hears and that the patient be completely relaxed. A quiet room is essential, and the examiner should attempt to eliminate as much extraneous noise as possible. Conversation by both the patient and the physician should be avoided during the auscultatory procedure.

Heart sounds, in general, are low pitched (low frequency) and are in the range of sound to which the human ear is relatively insensitive. Thus, it is important to use every possible technique to improve audibility. The physician should be in a position that permits him to listen at ease and without strain. Right-handed examiners as a rule perform better at the right side of the patient. The patient should be disrobed from the waist up and should be properly gowned. It is important that the patient be made comfortable in the various positions required for auscultation of the heart.

Although the choice of stethoscope is an individual matter, it is advisable that both the bell and the diaphragm chestpieces be available in order to detect the low-pitched as well as the high-pitched sounds. The bell is more satisfactory for low-pitched sounds, whereas the diaphragm is preferable for those that are high pitched. It should be borne in mind that the most important segment of the auscultatory apparatus is that between the earpieces of the stethoscope. A keen sense of awareness, coupled with the knowledge gleaned from experience, constitutes the difference between hear-

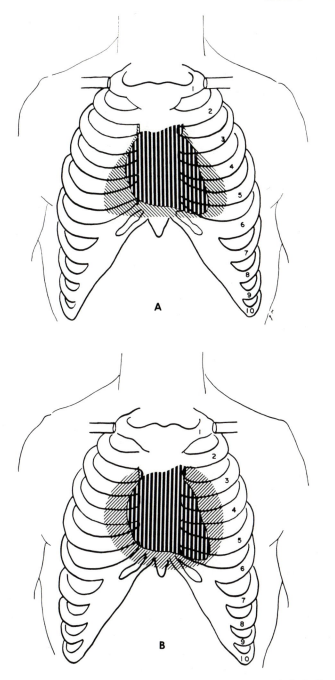

Fig. 14-33. Effect of position on cardiac outline in a patient with pericardial effusion. Vertical stripes represent normal cardiac silhouette, and diagnoal stripes represent pericardial effusion. **A,** Patient upright. **B,** Patient recumbent.

ing and actually listening; the latter implying analysis of sound by means of integration and correlation.

A systematic method of examination is essential. One may start at the apex and progress along the left sternal border to the pulmonary and aortic areas, or vice versa. In any case, the examiner should "inch" the stethoscope from one area to the other and eventually encompass the entire precordium and other areas of the thorax whenever indicated.

The student must learn to listen specifically to the various components of the heart cycle. He must concentrate on a specific aspect of the cycle and make a careful analysis of it. The first heart sound should be identified and then evaluated regarding its intensity, whether it is split, and for variations of its intensity. The second heart sound is then analyzed relative to its intensity and as to the type and degree of splitting caused by aortic and pulmonary valve closure. It is important to know whether the second sound is single or split, and if split, the degree of splitting and its relationship to inspiration and expiration. The examiner listens for sounds in systole, such as ejection sounds or systolic clicks. Following this he listens for sounds in diastole, such as opening snap, ventricular gallop, atrial gallop, or a normal third heart sound. Finally the examiner concentrates and listens for murmurs in systole and then for murmurs in diastole. In this manner each component of the cardiac cycle can be fully analyzed. Thus, for adequate auscultation one must listen specifically to the various components of the heart cycle and not attempt to listen to everything at once.

Initially, the patient is examined lying on his back. Then the patient is asked to turn in the left lateral position, and the apical area is auscultated—not only when the patient is supine and after he has turned to the left, but also while he is actually turning—using the bell of

the stethoscope lightly applied to the chest wall in order to detect low-frequency sounds or murmurs over the apex. After the patient has been examined in the reclining and left lateral positions, he is requested to sit upright and lean slightly forward. With the patient in this position the examiner listens particularly over the pulmonary and aortic valve areas and along either sternal border, in both phases of respiration. The patient is then requested to exhale and hold his breath in deep expiration, and the diaphragm of the stethoscope is pressed firmly against the chest wall to detect the possible presence of the high-pitched blowing diastolic murmurs of aortic or pulmonary origin. In the presence of pulmonary emphysema, one should listen with the patient in the upright position and also over the xiphoid or upper epigastric region in order to avoid interference by the emphysematous lung.

Recent investigation has demonstrated that in some instances a mitral systolic murmur can be detected only when the patient is standing erect and that it disappears when he reclines. Further experimentation has shown that some of these murmurs are of organic origin. Thus, in those situations in which the patient relates a history of cardiac symptoms or a previously diagnosed systolic murmur and such murmur is not heard when he is reclining, it is advisable to have him stand and to auscultate again.

Auscultatory valve areas. In auscultation of the heart it is customary to listen over each of the four valve areas and the precordial region in general. Depending on the underlying disease, it is necessary to listen over other areas of the thorax. Although it makes little difference whether the examiner starts at the aortic valve region and progresses to the mitral valve area or vice versa, it is important to adopt a routine procedure for auscultation. The aortic area is located in the second right intercostal space just lateral to the sternum (Fig. 14-28).

The pulmonary valve area is in the second left intercostal space just lateral to the sternum. The mitral valve area is in the fifth left intercostal space, 1 or 2 cm. medial to the midclavicular line. The tricuspid valve area is located at the junction of the xiphoid process and the sternum. As indicated in Fig. 14-28, the auscultatory valve areas do not correspond with the anatomic location of the valves themselves.

Rate and rhythm. Rate and rhythm have been discussed previously in the section on pulse. In addition to careful palpation of the pulse, however, the examiner should always determine the rate and rhythm of the heart by

means of auscultation. There may be a discrepancy between the palpable pulse rate and that heard over the heart itself, especially in certain arrhythmias accompanied by a pulse deficit. As mentioned earlier, some alterations of rhythm are recognized more readily by auscultation than by palpation of the pulse.

Heart Sounds

The proper identification of the various heart sounds and the characterization of their quality and intensity is of extreme importance in a well-executed cardiac examination. Unless the physician properly identifies the first and sec-

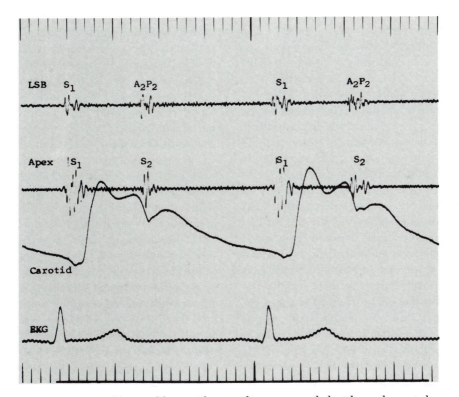

Fig. 14-34. Patient with normal heart. Phonocardiogram recorded with one horn at the cardiac apex and the other at the left sternal border (LSB). S_1 and S_2 represent the first and second sounds, respectively; A_2 and P_2 represent the aortic and pulmonic components of the second heart sound. Notice the absence of any murmurs.

ond heart sounds, he is unable to correctly locate a murmur in the cardiac cycle.

Identification and evaluation of the heart sounds can be accomplished best if the student learns to concentrate on each of the heart sounds at each valve area. Only after the identification and evaluation of each sound has been completed is the student ready to listen to the intervals between these sounds.

In most normal individuals there are four heart sounds. The first and second sounds can be heard with ease in normal subjects. However, the third and fourth sounds are frequently inaudible.

Characteristics of heart sounds. The first heart sound is synchronous with the apical impulse and corresponds with the onset of ventricular systole (Fig. 14-34). This sound has been likened acoustically to the syllable "lubb." The second sound occurs at the termination of systole and corresponds with the onset of ventricular diastole. The second sound has been compared acoustically to the syllable "dup." Both sounds are usually clearly audible over all valve areas and together acoustically resemble a "lubb dup." When the heart beats slowly and regularly, the two sounds can be readily differentiated from one another. This differentiation is facilitated by recognizing that there is a longer pause between the second sound and the subsequent first sound (diastole) than between the first and second sounds (systole). When the heart is beating rapidly, the diastolic interval becomes shorter, at times approximating systole in length, and consequently the differentiation of the systolic from the diastolic inerval may be very difficult. It may be necessary to identify the first sound by synchronous palpation at the apex or over the carotid artery. Because of the time lapse in the pulse wave, it is impossible to time these sounds by correlation with the radial pulse.

The third heart sound, being low in both fre-

quency and intensity, is best heard with the bell of the stethoscope. It occurs in early diastole approximately 0.12 to 0.14 second after the second heard sound (Fig. 14-35). Thus it occurs during the phase of early diastolic filling. This sound is heard in most children and some adults. When an adult with heart disease develops a third sound not previously present, it is considered to be definitely abnormal.

The fourth heart sound is also low in frequency and intensity. Like the third sound, it is best heard at the apex. This sound occurs late in diastole or just prior to the first heart sound and is temporally related to atrial contraction (Fig. 14-35). It is rarely heard under normal conditions.

Origin of heart sounds. The first heart sound is produced by several factors (ventricular contraction, alteration in pressure and flow) that are temporally related to closure of the atrioventricular valves. Thus, it is a composite sound resulting from the closure of both the mitral and tricuspid valves. Usually the ventricles contract asynchronously and thus the two valves close asynchronously. Mitral valve closure precedes slightly that of the tricuspid valve (Fig. 14-35). Normally the first heart sound is of lower frequency and longer duration than the second sound.

The second heart sound is produced by closure of the semilunar valves. It, too, is a composite sound resulting from closure of both the aortic and pulmonary valves. Normally aortic valve closure precedes pulmonary valve closure by 0.04 to 0.06 second during inspiration and by 0.02 to 0.04 second during expiration. The second sound is higher in frequency and shorter in duration than the first sound (Fig. 14-34).

In some patients with pulmonary emphysema or a very muscular chest wall, all heart sounds may be distant because of the actual physical separation of the heart and stethoscope. Conversely, in those persons with a poorly developed or a relatively thin thoracic wall, all heart sounds may be accentuated because of the proximity of the heart and the stethoscope.

Physiologic principles related to the cardiac cycle. It is essential to have a thorough knowl-edge of the pressure curves in order to under-stand the various events that comprise the car-diac cycle. By superimposing the left atrial pressure pulse curve and the aortic pressure pulse on the left ventricular pressure pulse curve, it is possible to correlate the acoustical events on the left side of the heart (Fig. 14-35).

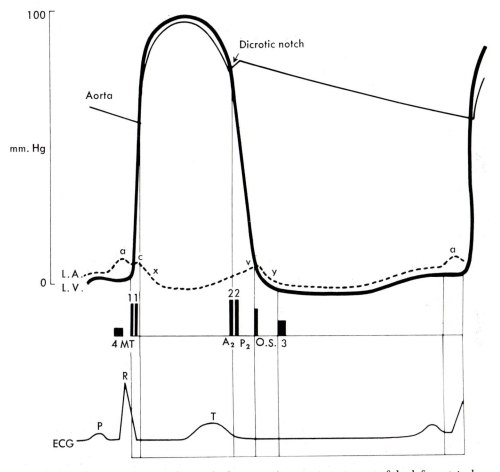

Fig. 14-35. Diagram of the cardiac cycle demonstrating pressure curves of the left ventricule (L.V.), left atrium (L.A.), jugular pulse waves, electrocardiogram (ECG), and relationship to heart sounds and valve closure. MT represents mitral and tricuspid components of the first heart sound. A_2 and P_2 represent the aortic and pulmonary components of the second heart sound, respectively. 3 and 4 represent the position, in the cycle, of the third and fourth heart sounds. The third sound occurs in early diastole, and the fourth sound in late diastole (presystole). O.S. represents the time of occurrence of the opening snap when it is present.

The left ventricular curve is initiated by a small presystolic wave that is produced by atrial contraction. This is followed by an even, sharply rising ascending limb, a rounded peak, and finally a descending limb that falls rather rapidly to the base line.

The left atrial curve is characterized by three positive deflections, a, c, and v waves, and two negative components, x and y descents (Fig. 14-35). The a wave is caused by contraction of the left atrium, and the c wave is caused by bulging upward of the mitral valve into the left atrial cavity at the onset of left ventricular systole. The x wave is caused by left atrial relaxation (diastole) and attains its lowest level at the time of maximal ejection of the ventricle. The v wave, a passive filling wave, is produced by a rising pressure in the left atrium at the time when the mitral valve is closed. The y descent results when the mitral valve opens and the atrial contents empty into the left ventricle.

The aortic pressure pulse very closely follows the outline of the left ventricular curve from the initial crossing to that point where the ventricular and aortic curves again cross (Fig. 14-35). Because of a slight pressure gradient the aortic curve lies below the ventricular curve. The aortic curve declines abruptly immediately prior to where it crosses the ventricular curve for the second time. Immediately following the second crossing is a notch (dicrotic notch) produced by closure of the aortic valve and in turn followed by a sudden brief rise in aortic pressure and then a gradual decline in pressure during diastole.

When the electrocardiogram and heart sounds are superimposed on the preceding pressure pulse curve, one can temporally correlate the acoustical events within the cardiac cycle (Fig. 14-35).

The a wave, representing left atrial contraction, begins at the crest of the P wave. The QRS complex, resulting from depolarization of the ventricular muscle, antecedes mechanical contraction. Contraction of the left ventricle begins at the peak of the R wave; and right ventricular contraction, which occurs later, synchronizes with the descending limb of the R wave. The T wave represents repolarization or recovery of the ventricles; it is concluded while the ventricles are still contracting.

The mitral component of the first heart sound (M-1) is produced by closure of the mitral valve as the result of a sudden elevation in left ventricular pressure and a resultant gradient between the left atrium and left ventricle (Fig. 14-35). The tricuspid component of the first heart sound (T-1) follows M-1 and is produced by closure of the tricuspid valve. M-1 coincides very closely with the peak of the R wave on the electrocardiogram.

When left ventricular pressure exceeds aortic pressure, as noticed on the ascending limb of the ventricular pressure curve, the aortic valve opens (Fig. 14-35). This does not result in any acoustical phenomenon except in certain instances, such as aortic stenosis where one may hear systolic ejection sounds.

The phase between closure of the mitral valve and opening of the aortic valve is referred to as isometric contraction, and both valves are closed at this time.

Following the opening of the aortic valve the aortic pressure increases and finally exceeds left ventricular pressure, as noted on the descending limb of the ventricular pressure curve (Fig. 14-35). At this point the aortic valve closes and is thus responsible for the aortic component of the second heart sound (A-2). The pulmonary component of the second sound (P-2) immediately follows A-2 and is produced by closure of the pulmonic valve. Both components of the second heart sound coincide with termination of the T wave on the electrocardiogram.

The interval between the opening and closing of the aortic valve is the phase of left ventricular ejection. The early period of ventricular ejection is rapid because of increasing ventricular pressure, whereas the late phase is slow as the result of a fall in ventricular pressure.

Following the closure of the aortic valve, left ventricular pressure falls and finally is exceeded by left atrial pressure as noted by the *v* wave on the pressure curve (Fig. 14-35). At this point the mitral valve opens, and under normal circumstances this is a silent acoustical event. In the presence of mitral stenosis one hears an opening snap (O.S.) at this time.

The phase between closing of the aortic valve and opening of the mitral valve is referred to as isometric relaxation, and once again both valves are closed.

Following the opening of the mitral valve blood flows rapidly from the left atrium into the left ventricle as a result of the pressure gradient between the two chambers. This is referred to as the period of rapid ventricular filling. It is in this period that one may hear a normal third heart sound or its pathologic counterpart, the ventricular (S-3) gallop sound (Fig. 14-35).

During the later phase of diastole, which corresponds with atrial contraction and is referred to as presystole, the pressure gradient between the left ventricle and left atrium is much less than in the earlier phase. It is in this period that under rare conditions one may detect a fourth sound and in various abnormal circumstances the atrial (S-4) gallop sound (Fig. 14-35).

Similar pressure pulses occur on the right side of the heart. However, acoustical and mechanical events in the left and right heart are not synchronous.

Physiologic principles regulating the timing of closure of the heart valves. The onset of left ventricular contraction precedes the onset of right ventricular contraction. However, the isometric contraction period of the right ventricle is very brief in relation to that of the left ventricle; therefore, right ventricular ejection actually commences prior to left ventricular ejection. Ejection terminates earlier in the left than in the right ventricle.

The sound of mitral valve closure normally precedes the sound of tricuspid valve closure, and the sound of aortic valve closure precedes the sound of pulmonary valve closure. The duration of ejection of each ventricle determines the timing of closure of the semilunar valves and, therefore, the timing of the two components of the second heart sound.

The terms A-2 and P-2 refer to closure of the aortic and pulmonary semilunar valves, respectively. In the past, these same terms have been erroneously applied to mean the second heart sound over the aortic and pulmonary valve areas.

A-2 may be heard anywhere over the precordium and is not necessarily best heard in the aortic valve area. A-2 is often best heard at the apex and on many occasions very distinctly over the pulmonary area, where it is readily distinguished from the later occurring P-2. The second heart sound in the pulmonary area is split into an earlier aortic and later pulmonary component. The split is most evident at the end of inspiration because inspiration increases right ventricular filling and prolongs right ventricular ejection. This mechanism delays pulmonary valve closure (the pulmonary component of the second heart sound, or P-2). Since left ventricular filling is not affected to this extent, aortic valve closure is almost constant in timing. Thus, auscultation over the pulmonary area reveals a second sound, which splits on inspiration and is single or closes on expiration, as P-2 moves back and forth from the more stationary A-2. Splitting of the second sound is best heard during normal, not forced, inspiration.

Abnormalities of the first and second heart sounds. It is extremely important to pay specific attention to each of the two main heart sounds, noting their intensity, splitting, and the effect of respiration.

First heart sound. The principal factor responsible for the intensity of the first heart sound is the position of the atrioventricular valve at the onset of ventricular contraction. When the valve leaflets are widely open, their closure results in large vibrations and produces a loud sound; when the leaflets are in close apposition at the moment of ventricular contraction, the vibrations are small and the first heart sound is less intense. The relationship of the P-R interval of the electrocardiogram to the in-

tensity of the first heart sound is well established. The P-R interval on the electrocardiogram represents the period between the beginning of detectable electric excitation of the atrial muscle and the onset of detectable excitation of the ventricular muscle. The variation of intensity of the first heart sound in relationship to the P-R interval is dependent on several factors, the most important of which are position of the atrioventricular valves at the time of ventricular systole and the magnitude of ventricular pressure. When the P-R interval is short, namely 0.10 to 0.14 second, the atrio-

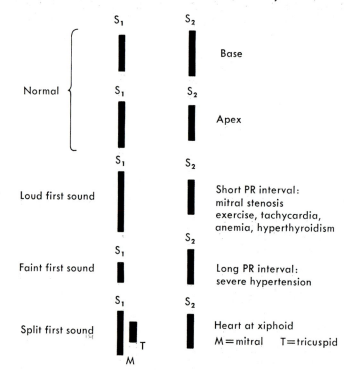

Fig. 14-36. The first heart sound under normal conditions and in the presence of various physiologic as well as disease states. S_1 and S_2 refer to the first and second sounds, respectively. At the apex S_1 is normally louder than S_2; over the base of the heart S_2 is louder than S_1. The figure lists the more common conditions responsible for either increasing or decreasing the intensity of S_1. M and T refer to the mitral and tricuspid components of the first heart sound. In some instances the first sound is normally split, in which case the mitral component (M) is louder than the tricuspid (T).

ventricular valve leaflets are widely open at the onset of ventricular contraction, and this results in a loud first heart sound. When the P-R interval is prolonged, such as 0.21 to 0.24 second, the valve leaflets are closely apposed at the onset of ventricular contraction, and this results in a faint or soft first heart sound (Fig. 14-36). In fact, a decrease in intensity of the first heart sound may be the first clinical indication of a first degree heart block.

Tachycardia, anemia, fever, exercise, and hyperthyroidism may be associated with an increase in the intensity of the first heart sound (Fig. 14-36). In the presence of a normal ventricular rate of 60 to 80 per minute, a loud first heart sound should make one suspicious of the possibility of either mitral stenosis or a shortening of the P-R interval. When a loud first heart sound is accompanied by an accentuated second sound over the pulmonary area and by an opening snap, the examiner should be further alerted to auscultate carefully for the diastolic rumble of mitral stenosis.

In the presence of complete heart block where there is a frequent changing of the P-R interval, there will be an accompanying variation in the intensity of the first heart sound. The first sound may also vary in intensity in the presence of atrial flutter, when treatment has been instituted to control or revert the flutter. The first sound is frequently diminished in intensity in acute myocardial infarction and in other conditions accompanied by a decrease in cardiac output.

Splitting of the first heart sound may occur normally with mitral valve closure preceding tricuspid valve closure (Figs. 14-35 and 14-36). The degree of splitting normally varies and usually is not wide; at times it may be single. A widely split first heart sound at the apex or over the lower left sternal border should suggest the possibility of a bundle branch block—either right or left, but more commonly the former. At times an atrial or fourth sound occurring just before the first heart sound or an early systolic ejection sound may be misinterpreted as a split. When the first heart sound is split, the mitral or first component is usually the louder of the two. If the tricuspid or second component is louder, one should suspect the possibility of an atrial-septal defect.

Second heart sound. Careful analysis of the second heart sound as part of the total clinical cardiovascular evaluation is of diagnostic importance. The second sound may be accentuated in some healthy individuals as well as in some ill patients. An accentuated second sound over the pulmonary area without any evidence of disease is of no significance. An increase in pressure in the peripheral arterial system or on the pulmonary arterial side may result in an accentuation of the corresponding aortic or pulmonary valve closure. The second sound becomes louder, with an increase in pressure in the aorta, such as occurs in arterial diastolic hypertension or coarctation of the aorta. Abrupt closure of the aortic valve, such as occurs in aortic regurgitation may accentuate the second heart sound.

There is an accentuation of pulmonary valve closure in pulmonary artery hypertension that may be caused by atrial-septal defect, ventricular-septal defect, patent ductus arteriosus, primary pulmonary hypertension, and recurrent pulmonary emboli.

In children and adolescents, pulmonary valve closure normally may be accentuated. The pulmonary component of the second sound may also be accentuated in congestive heart failure and in various types of heart disease where increased pressure develops in a pulmonary artery following prolonged congestion in the lungs.

A decrease in intensity of the second sound over the aortic and/or pulmonary valve area may be caused by stenosis of the related semilunar valve. In acquired aortic stenosis the second sound is often faint to absent; however, it may be normal in intensity or occasionally even accentuated. In congenital aortic stenosis the second sound is normal or accentuated. In severe pulmonary stenosis the pulmonary component of the second sound is delayed and faint, and the aortic component may be masked by the accompanying murmur associated with the valve defect.

Splitting of the second heart sound is of great practical importance. Since the second sound is the result of closure of the aortic and pulmonary valves with the aortic valve closing first and followed by pulmonary valve closure, slight to marked asynchrony of closure should then result in various degrees of splitting. Splitting of the second sound is best detected

over the pulmonary valve area or third left intercostal space adjacent to the sternum. Most normal individuals have a split-second sound over these areas, the split being either very close or single on expiration (Fig. 14-37). Because of the normal increase in venous return to the right side of the heart on inspiration, the right ventricle requires a slightly longer period to empty itself. The pulmonary valve closure does not occur until the ventricle has emptied itself. The widening of the splitting of the second sound coincides with inspiration and is a normal finding.

Conditions that cause a delay of contraction or emptying of the right side of the heart also cause a delay in pulmonary valve closure. Such conditions include complete right bundle branch block and atrial-septal defect. Right

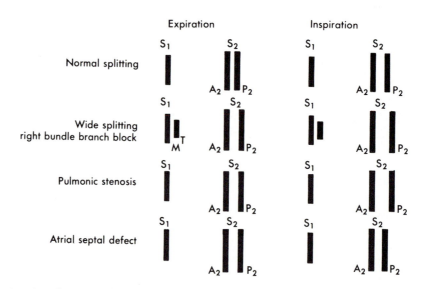

Fig. 14-37. Splitting of the second heart sound, as related to respiration, under normal conditions and in the presence of specific defects. S_1 and S_2 represent the first and second sounds, respectively. A_2 and P_2 refer to the aortic and pulmonary components of the second sound. In the normal heart S_2 is either single or slightly split on expiration, and the split increases during inspiration. M and T refer to the mitral and tricuspid components of the first heart sound, which are often split in right bundle branch block. In atrial septal defect there is a wide fixed split of S_2.

bundle branch block results in a wide splitting of the second sound even with expiration (Fig. 14-37). With inspiration there is a further widening of the split. In right bundle branch block this alteration is the result of electric delay of activation of the right side of the heart. If there is a wide split of the second sound with the patient in the reclining position, the examiner should ask him to sit erect and should recheck the sound. If the split of the second sound decreases, it has less significance; on the other hand, if the second sound remains widely split when the patient is erect, this is further evidence of the underlying cause.

In complete left bundle branch block, the order of valve closure may be reversed. There is a delay of activation of the left ventricle, and on expiration pulmonary closure occurs first and is followed by aortic valve closure. During inspiration the pulmonary valve closure is normally delayed, with increased filling on the right side of the heart, and aortic valve closure normally may occur earlier. The two components then move closer together on inspiration and may be single. This is referred to as paradoxical splitting of the second heart sound (Fig. 14-38).

In the usual case of atrial-septal defect, the second heart sound over the pulmonary area is widely split, with little or no change in the degree of splitting during either phase of respiration. This is referred to as fixed splitting (Fig. 14-37).

Gallop rhythm. The term "gallop rhythm" refers to that condition in which three and occasionally four heart sounds are spaced to audibly resemble the canter of a horse. The mere detection of the presence of an additional heart sound or sounds during diastole is inadequate for an accurate diagnosis. The examiner should determine the relative position of the additional sound within the diastolic phase of the cardiac cycle. When the extra sound occurs soon after the second heart sound, it is termed *protodiastolic*. When it occurs late in diastole or just prior to the first heart sound, it is termed *presystolic*. Although the term gallop rhythm suggests a rapid sequence of auscultatory events, tachycardia is not a necessary component. Gallops may occur in the presence of normal and even slow heart rates.

Ventricular gallop. The ventricular gallop (protodiastolic) is a brief low-pitched sound, usually heard near the end of the first third of diastole or approximately 0.15 second following the aortic component of the second heart sound (Figs. 14-39 and 14-46). If the heart rate is rapid, it may approach middle diastole in posi-

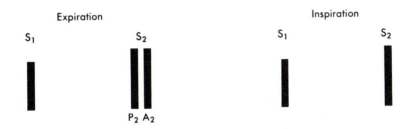

Fig. 14-38. Paradoxical (reversed) splitting of the second heart sound may occur in aortic stenosis, left bundle branch block, and patent ductus arteriosus. S_1 and S_2 refer to the first and second heart sounds, respectively. P_2 and A_2 refer to the pulmonary and aortic components of the second sound. Note that, contrary to normal, the second sound is single on inspiration and splits during expiration; the pulmonary precedes the aortic component.

tion. It is the pathologic counterpart of the third heart sound and occurs at the time of rapid diastolic ventricular filling. It is usually heard at the apex and is often accompanied by a palpable precordial heave. The ventricular gallop sound is produced by an overdistention of the ventricle in the rapid filling phase of diastole, caused either by an excessive volume of blood or by a load much too great for a diseased ventricle with impaired compliance. It is associated with an increase in ventricular diastolic volume and pressure. Consequently, ventricular gallop is usually heard in mitral or tricuspid regurgitation, left to right shunt, and left or right ventricular failure from any cause. A differentiation between the physiologic third

heart sound and its pathologic counterpart, the ventricular gallop sound, depends on the cardiac context in which the sound is heard. In most instances a physiologic third heart sound will disappear within 20 to 30 seconds after an individual has assumed an upright position, while ventricular gallop sounds will persist.

Gallops may originate from either side of the heart. As in the case of murmurs, variations in intensity of the gallop during the respiratory cycle will suggest which side of the heart is responsible for its individual production. A ventricular gallop that increases in intensity during normal inspiration is likely to originate from the right ventricle; and when unaffected by inspiration it usually originates from the left ven-

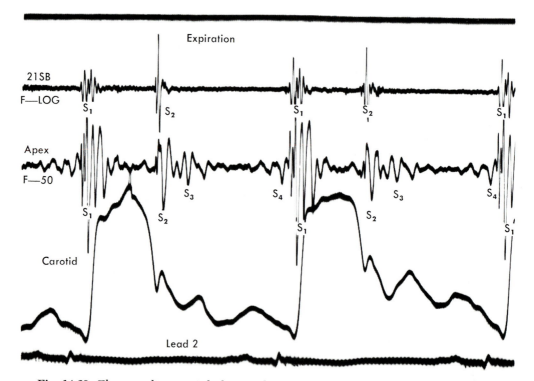

Fig. 14-39. Electrocardiogram and phonocardiogram of a 71-year-old man with arteriosclerotic heart disease; prominent S_3 (ventricular) gallop at apex; S_4 (atrial) gallop also present. S_1 and S_2 represent the first and second heart sounds, respectively.

tricle. The presence of right or left ventricular hypertrophy, as well as other underlying pathologic conditions, may be helpful in determining the specific origin of the gallop.

Atrial gallop. The atrial gallop sound (presystolic) occurs in late diastole and is temporally related to atrial contraction (Fig. 14-39). This is the pathologic equivalent of the sometimes normally occurring fourth heart sound. Atrial gallop occurs after the beginning of atrial contraction during the later phase of ventricular filling. Evidence indicates that the production of atrial gallop is favored by those factors that increase resistance to ventricular filling in late diastole. Such factors may be reversed by lowering the ventricular end diastolic tension

and pressure, by reducing venous return to the heart, or by lessening the force of atrial contraction.

Atrial gallop occurs principally in those conditions associated with systolic overloading of either ventricle where the ventricular diastolic pressure is elevated; namely, in systemic or pulmonary hypertension and in aortic or pulmonary stenosis. Atrial gallop may also occur wherever the distensibility of the ventricle is impaired, such as in acute myocardial infarction and cardiomyopathies. Also, it is frequently present in hyperthyroidism and severe anemia.

In all probability, the detection of an atrial gallop is the earliest auscultatory abnormality

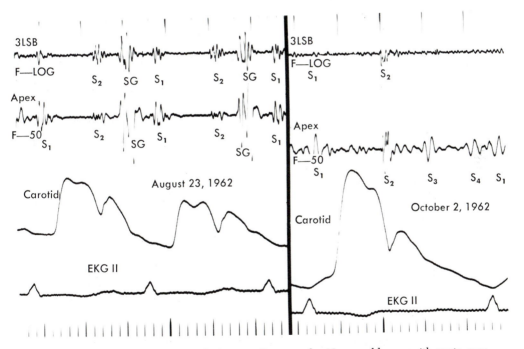

Fig. 14-40. Electrocardiogram and phonocardiogram of a 38-year-old man with acute myocarditis and congestive heart failure. *Left:* August, 1962—sinus tachycardia, diminished amplitude of the first heart sound, pronounced summation gallop (SG). *Right:* October, 1962—following therapy, heart rate was slower, S_3 (ventricular) and S_4 (atrial) gallops are apparent.

detectable in hypertensive heart disease, and it may even precede the signs of left ventricular hypertrophy. The presence of an atrial gallop does not necessarily indicate heart failure. An atrial gallop may be present for years in hypertensive heart disease without accompanying heart failure. When heart failure supervenes, a ventricular gallop may be added, resulting in either a quadruple rhythm or summation gallop.

Atrial gallop may be heard occasionally in patients with angina pectoris and thus is a useful sign in evaluating chest pain of an equivocal nature. Often it is heard in acute myocardial infarction, and if persistent following recovery, indicates a less favorable long-term prognosis. The atrial gallop sound is low pitched, is of short duration, and is best heard when the bell of the stethoscope is applied lightly to the chest wall.

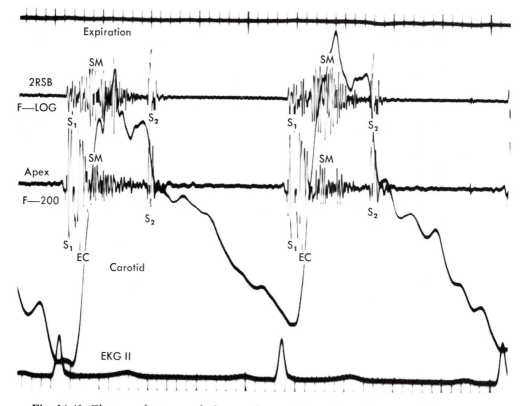

Fig. 14-41. Electrocardiogram and phonocardiogram of a 28-year-old man with isolated valvular aortic stenosis, congenital. Poststenotic dilatation present; aortic valve not calcified. *Upper sound tracing,* second right intercostal space: systolic ejection murmur (SM) with peak amplitude in midsystole. *Lower sound tracing,* apex: prominent vibration (after initial vibrations of first sound) represents an aortic ejection click (EC). Prominent ejection click and accentuated aortic closure sound are frequently present with noncalcific aortic valvular stenosis.

Summation gallop. When both the protodiastolic and presystolic gallop sounds are present, this results in a *quadruple* rhythm. For example, a presystolic gallop may be heard in a patient with uncomplicated arterial hypertension. When such a patient develops hypertensive heart disease and congestive heart failure, a protodiastolic gallop is frequently added to the preexisting presystolic gallop, resulting in the quadruple rhythm. If both gallop sounds are present and the heart rate increases, the diastolic interval shortens and the extra sounds come closer together. They may actually fuse, resulting in a *summation gallop* (Fig. 14-40).

Systolic ejection sounds and ejection clicks. The term "systolic gallop" has become obsolete, and the phrase "gallop sound" is now restricted to the diastolic filling sounds just described. Extra sounds heard in systole are referred to as *systolic clicks.* They may occur in early, middle, and late systole.

Early systolic clicks are termed "ejection sounds" or "ejection clicks" because they occur approximately at the time of onset of right or left ventricular systolic ejection (Fig. 14-41). Such clicks may be caused by the sudden tensing of the aorta or pulmonary artery as the result of ventricular ejection or by the actual

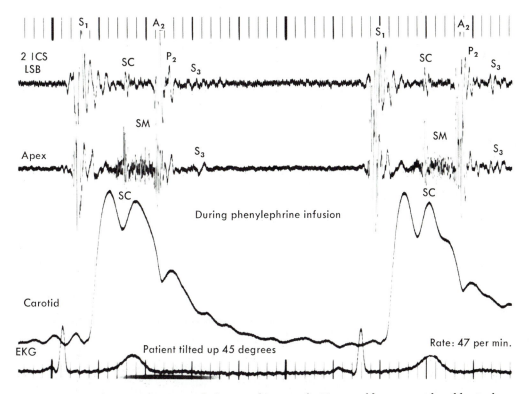

Fig. 14-42. Electrocardiogram and phonocardiogram of a 21-year-old woman with mild mitral regurgitation, familial occurrence, of midsystolic click, and late systolic murmur (SM). Both click and murmur were accentuated by vasopressor (phenylephrine). Systolic click (SC), which is seen in both recordings, was loudest at apex and was followed at the apex by a late systolic murmur.

opening of the semilunar valves in the presence of aortic or pulmonary stenosis. Pulmonary ejection clicks may occur in stenosis of the pulmonary valve, in pulmonary hypertension, and in those situations where the pulmonary artery is dilated. They are best heard over the pulmonary auscultatory valve area. Aortic ejection clicks occur in stenosis of the aortic valve, aortic regurgitation, coarctation of the aorta, aneurysms of the ascending aorta, and hyper-

tension with dilatation of the aorta. They are heard over the base of the heart as well as at the apex. Often they are louder over the apex.

In the past, ejection clicks heard in middle and late systole have been considered benign and extracardiac in origin. However, more recent investigation has shown that some middle and late systolic clicks occur just prior to or during a late systolic murmur (Fig. 14-42). The systolic click is probably related to termination

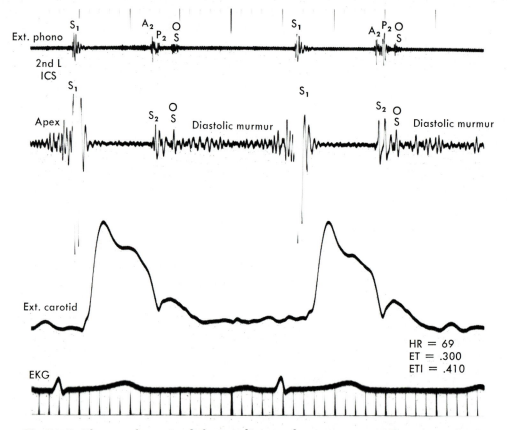

Fig. 14-43. Electrocardiogram and phonocardiogram of a young woman with severe, isolated, noncalcific mitral stenosis, sinus rhythm. *Upper tracing,* second left intercostal space: aortic and pulmonic components of the second heart sound are recorded with normal inspiratory splitting of the second heart sound components behind the opening snap (seen in the second complex). *Apex:* accentuated first heart sound, second heart sound, mitral opening snap (O.S.) followed by a diastolic murmur with presystolic accentuation.

of closure of the prolapsed mitral valve, and most likely arises from the chordae or exuberant leaflets. Following the termination of the prolapse, the late murmur is a reflection of late systolic mitral regurgitation.

Opening snap. The opening snap occurs soon after the second heart sound and is produced by opening of the atrioventricular valves (Figs. 14-35 and 14-43). Normally the opening of the atrioventricular valves is not audible. However, in mitral stenosis the valve forms a restrictive diaphragm, which bulges into the left atrium during systole and then springs into the left ventricle when atrial pressure suddenly exceeds ventricular diastolic pressure. Since the valvular diaphragm is actually tensed, it literally and loudly snaps into ventricular position shortly after the second heart sound. This sound is brief in duration and higher in pitch than other gallop sounds. It is heard best in the left third and fourth parasternal areas, with the patient in the left lateral position. The detection of the opening snap should alert the examiner to listen carefully for the other characteristic findings of mitral stenosis. Opening snaps are heard also in tricuspid stenosis and atrial tumors.

The proximity of the opening snap to the second heart sound is roughly related to the severity of mitral stenosis. The interval depends on the speed with which the valve is snapped into its diastolic position. When atrial pressure is high, the opening snap promptly follows the second heart sound. However, when there is less mitral valve obstruction and the atrial pressure is lower, the valve opens more leisurely, and the snap is slightly delayed in its relationship to the second heart sound.

Pericardial knock. In the presence of constrictive pericarditis, at times an extra sound in diastole is heard occurring shortly after the second heart sound (Fig. 14-10). This is referred to as the *pericardial knock*. It may be confused with a ventricular gallop or with the opening snap of mitral stenosis. Pericardial knock occurs earlier in diastole than does the ventricular gallop, is higher in frequency, and is transmitted widely. When the examiner hears an extra sound in early diastole and the other findings of constrictive pericarditis are present, the diagnosis is facilitated.

Adventitious sounds

Pericardial friction rub. This to-and-fro rubbing or grating sound may be heard over the entire precordial region or may be confined to a very small area. It is heard, as a rule, in both phases of the cardiac cycle. It is unaffected by respiration and is thus differentiated from a pleural friction rub. A rub may be readily heard at one moment and be absent several minutes later, depending on whether or not the involved layers of the pericardium are in contact at the time that the examiner is listening. The intensity of the rub varies with the position of the patient. It is usually increased when the subject is sitting upright and leaning forward. It is also increased when the examiner presses the stethoscope firmly against the patient's chest wall.

Mediastinal crunch. On rare occasions the examiner may hear a loud crunching sound over the precordium caused by the presence of mediastinal emphysema. This sound, which may also be synchronous with the heart sounds, is more irregular and inconstant than the pericardial friction rub. It is produced by air in the mediastinal tissues and is usually the result of a pneumothorax. The examiner must be careful not to misinterpret this sound as a pericardial friction rub.

Cardiac murmurs. Cardiac murmurs are abnormal sounds produced by vibrations within the heart itself or in the walls of the large arteries. They originate in the vicinity of the various valves and are usually heard most distinctly over the area of the individual valve responsible for their production. In order to be able to detect murmurs it is important to differentiate them from the heart sounds themselves. As a rule, murmurs are definitely longer in duration than are the accompanying heart sounds and are clearly of a different quality.

Mechanism of production. The production of murmurs is easily understood if you visualize fluid flowing through a flexible or pliable tube, such as a soft rubber hose. Murmurs can be produced in such a tube by increasing the rate or velocity of flow, by constricting the circumference at any point, by dilating a portion, and by inserting a taut membrane so that it will vibrate as the fluid flows past (Fig. 14-44). Various acquired and congenital diseases are accompanied by physical defects that are capable of producing any or all of these phenomena within the heart or vessels.

A decrease in the diameter of a heart valve or a constriction in one of the major arteries results in a sudden alteration of the blood flow and often produces a murmur. Conversely, a sudden increase in the diameter of a major vessel or a dilatation of a heart valve results in a derangement of blood flow and may produce a murmur. When any of these conditions is accompanied by a change in pressure gradient, the probability of the development of a murmur is considerably increased. Increased blood velocity, such as occurs in hyperthyroidism, exercise, anemia, and pregnancy, often results in the production of a murmur that would not exist in the same individual when these conditions have been either eliminated or corrected.

Method of detection. Students frequently experience difficulty in timing heart murmurs, that is, in placing them in their proper phase of the cardiac cycle. The examiner must develop the habit of listening for specific events individually. After he has determined the rate and rhythm and has identified the individual heart sounds, then he should listen carefully to systole (the interval between the first and second sounds), entirely disregarding diastole and the quality of the heart sounds. During this process the examiner should concentrate his entire attention on systole. After the systolic

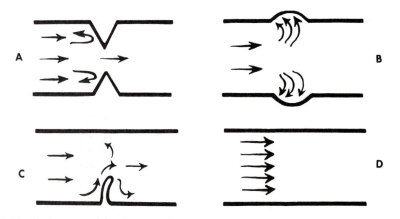

Fig. 14-44. Mechanisms of production of murmurs. **A,** Constriction of wall. **B,** Dilatation of wall. **C,** Partial impediment of flow, such as a taut membrane. **D,** Increased blood flow, represented by multiple arrows.

interval has been thoroughly studied, the examiner concentrates on diastole (the interval between the second and first sound), this time disregarding systole and the quality of the heart sounds. This procedure should be executed at all of the valve areas as well as along the left sternal border and over the great vessels. Only in this manner is it possible to analyze each of the events of the cardiac cycle.

Normally the interval between the heart sounds is entirely silent. If a systolic murmur is present, a noise should be heard during that phase of the heart cycle; namely between the first and second sounds. Systolic murmurs may be detected in any given segment of the systolic interval or may be audible throughout systole. Diastolic murmurs are identified in a similar manner.

Characterization of murmurs. When a murmur is found, it should be studied as to each of the following features.

1. *Location.* The examiner should describe the exact location of all murmurs. Some murmurs are localized to a small area, whereas others are heard over a large portion of the precordium. The location of a murmur is usually significant in determining its site of origin. Murmurs of valvular origin are usually best heard over their respective auscultatory valve areas. Murmurs caused by congenital septal defects and anomalies involving the great vessels may be best heard near the sternal borders and occasionally over the base of the heart and in the region of the neck.

2. *Timing.* Murmurs are timed according to the phase of the cardiac cycle during which they occur; thus, they are either systolic or diastolic, and at times they may be both. Systole and diastole may be divided into three parts: early, middle, and late. Systolic murmurs may begin with or after the first heart sound; they may be limited to early, middle, or late systole; and at times they may persist throughout systole *(holosystolic* or *pansystolic)*. The same is true of diastolic murmurs, although early diastole is often referred to as *protodiastole,* and late diastole is termed *presystole*.

The heart valves are considered to function normally and are referred to as being competent when they prevent the backflow of blood and at the same time permit the forward flow of blood. When the ventricles are in systole (contracting), the mitral and tricuspid valves are closed, preventing the regurgitation of blood from the ventricles into the atria. At the same time, during ventricular systole, the aortic and pulmonary valves are open, permitting the flow of blood from the ventricles into the aorta and pulmonary artery (Fig. 14-45). During ventricular diastole the situation is reversed—the aortic and pulmonary valves are closed, preventing regurgitation of blood from the aorta and pulmonary artery into their respective ventricles, while the mitral and tricuspid valves are open, allowing blood to flow from the atria into the ventricles (Fig. 14-45).

If a valve is incompetent, it fails to close completely in that phase of the heart cycle during which the cusps are supposed to be firmly apposed, so there is an aperture through which some blood flows from one chamber of the heart back into another. This regurgitation, or backflow, of blood results in a vibration of the valve and adjacent ventricular wall, producing a murmur of regurgitation. On the other hand, if the valve orifice is narrowed (stenosis), it is unable to open adequately in that phase of the heart cycle during which it should be widely patent. Thus, blood flowing through this narrowed orifice meets resistance and produces vibrations in the valves and ventricular wall, which results in a murmur of stenosis.

Certain systolic murmurs are produced by incompetence of the mitral and tricuspid valves or by stenosis of the aortic and pulmonary valves. Most diastolic murmurs are the result

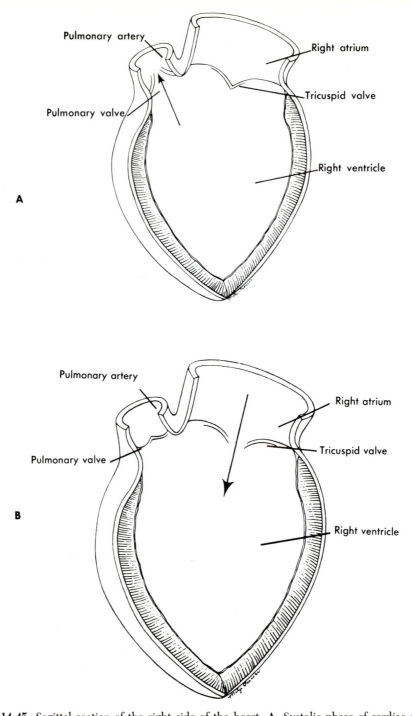

Fig. 14-45. Sagittal section of the right side of the heart. **A,** Systolic phase of cardiac cycle with pulmonary (semilunar) valve open and tricuspid (atrioventricular) valve closed. **B,** Diastolic phase of cardiac cycle with tricuspid (atrioventricular) valve open and pulmonary (semilunar) valve closed.

of stenosis of the mitral and tricuspid valves or incompetency of the aortic and pulmonary valves. The most common lesions encountered are mitral regurgitation, mitral stenosis, and aortic regurgitation. Other valve lesions occur but with less frequency. It should be pointed out that all murmurs are not necessarily the result of valvular defects, since some may be caused by congenital anomalies, some may be caused by alteration in velocity, some are on the basis of alterations within the large vessels themselves, and still others cannot be well explained.

3. *Quality.* On occasion the quality of heart murmurs may be of assistance in arriving at a more accurate diagnosis. It may be described as blowing harsh, rasping, rumbling, or musical. A blowing murmur resembles the sound produced by breathing forcibly through pursed lips. The louder murmurs are often harsh and rasping. The mid- and late diastolic murmurs increase in intensity just prior to the first heart sound and assume a rumbling quality. High-pitched blowing murmurs may resemble the sound of a whistle and at times are musical in character.

4. *Intensity.* Since there may be considerable difference of opinion as to the significance of some murmurs, it is important to grade them according to their intensity. Although several classifications are in use, a widely accepted scheme grades murmurs from I through VI, grade I being the least and VI the most intense. A grade I murmur is barely audible and is often missed on the first cardiac examination. A grade II murmur is usually readily heard and slightly louder than grade I. Grade III and IV murmurs are quite loud, and grade V is even more pronounced. A grade VI murmur may be heard with the stethoscope just removed from the chest wall. Adhering to this system of grading enables the physician to follow the progress of a given murmur over a pe-

riod of time, and in addition permits him to correlate the severity of the valvular defect with other clinical manifestations of cardiac disease. For example, if a grade I murmur increases over a period of years to a grade III or IV, it obviously indicates progressive valvular disease. If, on the other hand, a grade I murmur remains unchanged over many years, it is probably of little or no significance. Emphasis has been placed on gradation of intensity of murmurs rather than on their quality. Grade I murmurs are frequently encountered in persons without organic heart disease, whereas those of grade III intensity or louder seldom occur in a normal heart.

A murmur that increases in intensity after its onset is termed *crescendo*. If it decreases in intensity, it is referred to as *decrescendo*. If the first portion of a murmur is crescendo in character and the latter portion of the same murmur is decrescendo in intensity, it is then referred to as a *diamond-shaped murmur* (Fig. 14-41).

5. *Pitch.* Murmurs may vary in pitch just as they do in quality. The velocity of the blood flow is the main determining factor in the pitch. When the velocity is great, the pitch is high; when it is slow, the pitch is low. Murmurs are high, medium, or low pitched. For example, a low-pitched blowing murmur resembles the sound produced by air flowing through a large tube, whereas a high-pitched murmur of similar quality is likened to a shrill whistle.

6. *Transmission.* Some murmurs are transmitted with or in the direction of the bloodstream by which they are produced. This explains why the murmur of aortic regurgitation is heard so distinctly down along the left border of the sternum and over the apex. Other murmurs are propagated from their point of origin in many directions and on occasions even toward the bony structures in the upper ex-

tremities. For example, a loud murmur over the base of the heart may be audible over the carotid arteries or even transmitted to the apex. A murmur of maximum intensity, regardless of its origin, may be heard over the back of the chest, and on occasion is even detectable over the bony structures of the arms.

Classification of murmurs

Systolic murmurs. Systolic murmurs are those most frequently encountered in the daily practice. Since they are often misinterpreted, the patient with a systolic murmur is all too frequently labeled with the wrong diagnosis. Every heart murmur must be thoroughly evaluated as to its origin and cause. Systolic murmurs are divided into two categories: *ejection* and *pansystolic* (holosystolic).

Ejection murmurs. Ejection murmurs begin after the first heart sound, attain a climax or peak in early or middle systole, and terminate before the second heart sound. The systolic ejection murmur is short in duration and does not override or obscure either the first or second heart sound (Fig. 14-41). This murmur very definitely terminates prior to the second sound. Examples of systolic ejection murmurs are those heard in aortic stenosis, pulmonary stenosis, hyperthyroidism, and severe anemia. They also include the vast majority of so-called *functional* or *innocent* murmurs. Whenever a given murmur meets these criteria, it is always an ejection murmur, regardless of where it is heard—over the apex or in the neck or axilla, or elsewhere. Often loud ejection murmurs over the apex are misinterpreted as pansystolic murmurs of mitral regurgitation.

Ejection murmurs originate from the outflow tracts of the right and left ventricles and thus can be heard only when blood is being ejected from the ventricles; for example, an aortic systolic ejection murmur—the murmur cannot begin until the aortic valve opens. The aortic

valve opens only after left ventricular pressure exceeds aortic diastolic pressure, which can occur only after the mitral valve closes, since mitral valve closure occurs as soon as the ventricular pressure exceeds left atrial pressure. The aortic ejection murmur terminates prior to the second sound (closure of the aortic valve) because the aortic valve cannot close until ejection is complete.

Pansystolic murmurs. Pansystolic murmurs begin with the first heart sound and continue through the first part of the second heart sound. The pansystolic murmur of regurgitation is of longer duration than the ejection murmur and usually obscures the first and second heart sounds (Fig. 14-46). In contrast to the ejection murmur, in which there is a definite interval between the termination of the murmur and the second heart sound, there is no such interval related to the pansystolic murmur. Mitral pansystolic murmurs are high pitched, blowing in character, and frequently radiate toward the left axilla. In fact, when the left ventricle is markedly enlarged, the murmur may be best heard in the left axilla.

Pansystolic murmurs are usually associated with mitral regurgitation, tricuspid regurgitation and ventricular septal defects. They are produced by the flow of blood from a high-pressure chamber into one with lower pressure. The pansystolic murmur envelops the first heart sound because the same mechanism that is responsible for the production of the first heart sound (ventricular pressure exceeding atrial pressure at the onset of systole) is responsible for the regurgitation of blood when valvular insufficiency exists. Ventricular pressure remains above atrial pressure throughout systole. When the aortic and pulmonary valves close, the ventricular pressure is still well above the atrial pressure. Thus, the murmur of mitral and tricuspid regurgitation (from ventricle to atrium) or the murmur of ventricular

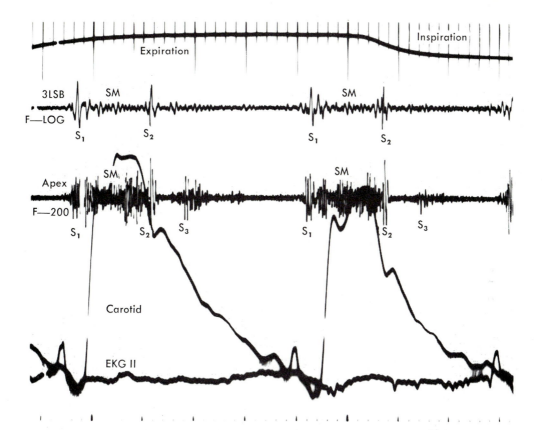

Fig. 14-46. Electrocardiogram and phonocardiogram of a 41-year-old woman with mitral regurgitation, probably rheumatic in origin. Holosystolic murmur at the apex (SM); S_3 (ventricular) gallop at the apex, surrounded by vibrations of a diastolic flow murmur.

septal defect (from left ventricle to right ventricle) is heard throughout systole and for a brief period following the second heart sound. This explains why the pansystolic murmur obscures the first and second heart sounds and why it is longer than the ejection murmur. In fact, one of the distinguishing factors between the pansystolic and ejection murmurs is the difference in their duration.

The intensity of systolic murmurs varies with respiration. Paying careful attention to the intensity as related to normal, not forced, respiration may be extremely helpful in determining the origin of the murmur. Murmurs that originate on the right side of the heart frequently increase in intensity during the course of inspiration. This fact may assist in differentiating tricuspid from mitral regurgitation and also in distinguishing between pulmonary and aortic ejection murmurs.

Diastolic murmurs. Diastolic murmurs are divided into two types—regurgitant murmurs resulting from semilunar valve insufficiency and ventricular filling murmurs. These diastolic murmurs can be distinguished readily on the basis of their location, quality, and time of occurrence in the cardiac cycle.

Regurgitant diastolic murmurs. The murmur of semilunar valve insufficiency is early in onset, beginning immediately after the second heart sound, is long in duration, and is pandiastolic in nature (Fig. 14-47). This murmur is classically high pitched, blowing in character, and transmitted along the direction of the regurgitant flow. For example, the murmur of aortic regurgitation is often heard best along the left lower sternal border. The intensity of the murmur varies with the pressure gradient across the valve and with the size of the valvular load. Because the intensity varies with the aortic-ventricular pressure differential, the murmur is decrescendo in character. The maximal intensity, like the maximal pressure differential, occurs immediately after the second heart sound and gradually diminishes as aortic diastolic pressure falls.

Regurgitant diastolic murmurs occur in either aortic or pulmonary regurgitation. At

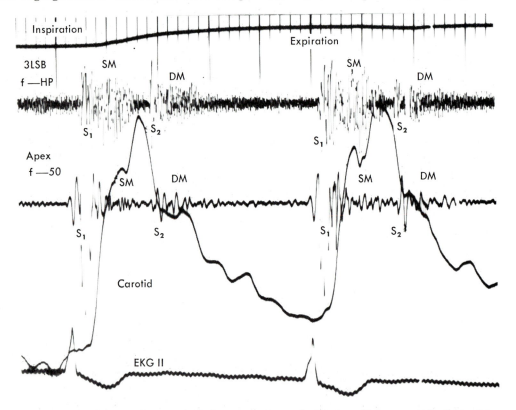

Fig. 14-47. Electrocardiogram and phonocardiogram of a 39-year-old woman with rheumatic heart disease and aortic valve disease with predominant regurgitation. At the third left intercostal space, left sternal border *(upper sound tracing),* a systolic ejection murmur (SM) ends before the second heart sound; a decrescendo diastolic murmur (DM) begins with aortic component of the second heart sound and persists throughout diastole. Example of a "to-and-fro" murmur associated with bidirectional flow at the aortic orifice.

times, differentiating these two valvular defects may be very difficult. The diagnosis of aortic regurgitation becomes simple when the murmur has all the classical features and when the peripheral pulse signs of aortic insufficiency are present. The diagnosis of pulmonary regurgitation also can be made with ease when pulmonary artery pressure is elevated and the peripheral signs of aortic regurgitation are absent. However, occasions arise when the differential diagnosis between these two valvular defects can be established only by angiography.

Diastolic murmurs of ventricular filling origin. The low-pitched diastolic murmurs of ventricular filling are produced by a column of blood as it rushes past the stenotic mitral or tricuspid valves, the leaflets of which are rigid and fixed as the result of the underlying rheumatic disease. On occasion one may encounter relative mitral or tricuspid stenosis.

In true mitral stenosis there is a definite delay in emptying of the left atrium. The pressure within the left atrium remains above left ventricular pressure throughout diastole. Thus, in mitral stenosis the flow of blood from the atrium into the ventricle is under constant pressure throughout diastole.

The mid-diastolic murmur of mitral stenosis is a decrescendo rumble. As the valvular obstruction becomes more severe and in the presence of a sinus rhythm, the murmur lengthens and terminates at the first heart sound in a presystolic crescendo accentuation (Fig. 14-43).

Relative stenosis of the mitral or tricuspid valve may occur in mitral regurgitation, aortic regurgitation, and in some cases of congenital heart disease with left-to-right shunt. This murmur, which is less intense and shorter in duration than its organic counterpart, is caused either by a very rapid and large ventricular diastolic inflow or by a normal flow entering a markedly dilated ventricle. A number of patients with mitral regurgitation have a diastolic rumble, which results when a large volume of blood that has regurgitated into the left atrium in systole rapidly empties back into the ventricle during the following diastole (Fig. 14-46). The nonobstructed mitral valve becomes relatively stenotic with respect to accommodating this large volume of blood.

SPECIFIC CARDIAC MURMURS

Mitral regurgitation. In mitral valve incompetence, blood is shunted back and forth between the atrium and ventricle. Mitral insufficiency may result from organic involvement of the valve (rheumatic valvulitis) or from dilatation of the valve ring. Rheumatic valvulitis may involve the cusps, chordae tendinae, papillary muscle or all three of these structures. Dilatation of the mitral valve ring may occur in the presence of a dilated left ventricle. On rare occasions bacterial endocarditis, congenital lesions, and myocardial infarction involving the papillary muscle or chordae tendinae will alter the structure of the mitral valve and produce organic mitral incompetence.

Classically the murmur of mitral regurgitation is pansystolic in time, is maximal over the apex, and is transmitted toward the left axilla, where at times it is loudest. The murmur begins with the first heart sound and extends through the aortic component of the second sound (Fig. 11-46). The persistently high ventricular pressure throughout systole and the resultant pressure gradient across the valve serves to maintain retrograde flow throughout systole and is responsible for the pansystolic murmur. Very often the first heart sound and the aortic component of the second sound are masked by the murmur.

The murmur is usually harsh or blowing (high frequency) because of the high velocity of the left ventricular systolic ejection jet. The murmur is often accompanied by a loud third heart sound probably produced by the rapid rush of blood into the ventricle under high pressure, which in turn expands the chamber and tenses the valve leaflets.

Variations of the typical murmur of mitral regurgitation occur; for example, the late systolic murmur of mitral regurgitation (Fig. 14-42). This latter murmur is usually associated with mild mitral regurgitation and is caused by disease involving the supportive structures of the valve. Investigations have shown that the actual cause of this murmur is a sudden prolapse of the mural cusp of the mitral valve into the left atrium late in systole.

Mitral stenosis. The three cardinal auscultatory findings in classical mitral stenosis are a loud first sound (S-1), an opening snap (O.S.), and a diastolic rumbling murmur, which in the presence of sinus rhythm has a presystolic accentuation. In some instances one or several of these findings may be absent. Mitral stenosis is usually a sequela of rheumatic fever and only in rare instances is it caused by a congenital abnormality.

Although a loud first sound may be the result of other causes, such as a short P-R interval or thyrotoxicosis, its presence should alert the examiner to listen carefully for the other auscultatory findings of mitral stenosis. When left ventricular pressure exceeds that in the left atrium, the rigid mitral valve snaps toward the atrium, resulting in an accentuated first heart sound. As the ventricle relaxes, its pressure falls below that in the left atrium, and the rigid mitral valve snaps in the direction of the left ventricle, producing the opening snap of the mitral valve. Thus, the opening snap, a high-pitched sound, occurs shortly after the second heart sound and often is best heard midway between the apex and the sternal border. Usually there is a relationship between the degree of left atrial pressure and the time of occurrence of the opening snap. The higher the atrial pressure (the more severe the stenosis), the closer the opening snap to the second sound. The sec-

ond heart sound over the pulmonary area is usually accentuated.

The mid-diastolic murmur of mitral stenosis is a very low-pitched rumbling sound occurring 0.02 to 0.04 second following the opening snap. Contraction of the atrium in the latter part of diastole intensifies the murmur, resulting in a presystolic (crescendo) accentuation (Fig. 14-43). Thus when both the mid-diastolic and presystolic components are present in the same patient, the murmur has a decrescendo-crescendo character.

The mid-diastolic murmur is the result of a passive pressure gradient between the left atrium and left ventricle and is independent of atrial contraction. The presystolic (late diastolic) murmur is produced by actual contraction of the left atrium just prior to ventricular systole, forcing blood from the left atrium through the stenosed mitral valve into the left ventricle. This murmur will disappear if atrial fibrillation supervenes because the atria no longer contract in organized fashion, whereas the mid-diastolic murmur will persist since it is not dependent on atrial contraction.

The diastolic murmur usually is well localized to the apex and may be inaudible just several centimeters away. Often it is best heard with the patient lying on his left side, which shifts the cardiac apex against the chest wall, or during the process of rotating the patient from the supine to the left lateral position. The murmur may be accentuated following exercise or acceleration of the heart rate. In many instances a diastolic thrill, at the apex, accompanies the murmur.

Aortic regurgitation. When the aortic valve cusps fail to close completely, the pressure gradient across the aortic valve causes blood in the aorta to regurgitate back into the left ventricle, and this results in the murmur of aortic regurgitation.

Aortic regurgitation is usually an acquired valvular deformity and may be the result of rheumatic fever, syphilis, bacterial endocarditis, or aortic dissection.

The murmur, which is high pitched and diastolic in time, begins immediately after the second heart sound and is decrescendo in character because of the progressive decreasing pressure gradient across the valve during diastole (Fig. 14-47). Although the murmur is heard well over the right second parasternal area, it is usually maximal over the third and fourth left intercostal spaces adjacent to the sternum. If the murmur is maximal to the right of the lower sternum, one should suspect that the cause of the regurgitation is other than rheumatic heart disease; for example, Marfan's syndrome, syphilis, or dissection of the aorta. Although the murmur is usually clearly audible when the patient is recumbent, there are occasions when it may best be heard with the patient sitting upright, leaning forward, and holding his breath following a deep expiraton.

One frequently hears an early systolic ejection sound in aortic regurgitation, and in the presence of severe valvular incompetence there may be an accompanying systolic ejection murmur.

Occasionally, when the patient has pure and usually severe aortic regurgitation (without organic mitral stenosis), there may be a presystolic murmur at the apex. This is referred to as an "Austin Flint murmur." It is probably caused by interference with normal mitral valve function as the result of blood regurgitating from the aorta.

Aortic stenosis. The valvular deformity in aortic stenosis may be the result of rheumatic fever but may also occur on the basis of a congenital defect or atherosclerosis. Calcific stenosis may occur when the underlying pathologic condition is either rheumatic or sclerotic.

In aortic stenosis, blood is forced under great pressure by the left ventricle through a narrowed aortic valve into the aorta. The combination of high velocity of blood flow and the narrowed valve orifice produces an eddy current, which results in a murmur that is systolic in time, loud, harsh, and usually has a crescendo-decrescendo character (Fig. 14-41). It is often referred to as being diamond shaped. The murmur is ejection in nature, beginning shortly after the first heart sound and ending just before the aortic component of the second sound. The more severe the stenosis, the later the onset of the murmur in systole. The murmur is heard over the right second interspace lateral to the sternum and radiates widely, frequently to the right side of the neck and especially to the apex. Regardless of where it is heard, it retains its diamond-shaped character.

In many instances an aortic systolic ejection click precedes the murmur and, when present, is usually accompanied by a good second sound. Since the ejection clicks are predicated on the basis of valvular mobility, they will not be detected when the valve is calcified. Thus, such clicks are rare in rheumatic stenosis but common in congenital aortic stenosis.

The aortic component of the second sound is delayed in most cases and is absent in a few. This delay is caused by prolonged left ventricular systole in an attempt to overcome the systolic pressure gradient across the narrowed valve. Consequently, there is either a single second heart sound, wherein the aortic and pulmonary elements are synchronous, or a reversed splitting of the second sound, the aortic component occurring after the pulmonary. In severe stenosis of the valve, usually a calcified valve, the aortic second sound is absent.

The murmur is often accompanied by a systolic thrill over the second right interspace lateral to the sternum. Both the murmur and thrill are frequently detected with greater ease when the patient sits upright, leans slightly forward, and holds his breath in deep expiration.

Pulmonary stenosis. Pulmonary stenosis is one of the more common congenital cardiac defects. The stenosis varies considerably in severity and is frequently associated with other cardiac lesions. In the uncomplicated case there is a systolic diamond-shaped murmur over the second left intercostal space lateral to the sternum. This is usually accompanied by a systolic thrill. Because of the delay in right ventricular ejection, the pulmonary component of the second heart sound is rather widely split. Also, a pulmonary systolic ejection click may be heard preceding the murmur.

Pulmonary regurgitation. Pulmonary regurgitation is a relatively uncommon valvular abnormality. Several recent studies have demonstrated that in organic pulmonary regurgitation this murmur occurs late in diastole and is crescendo-decrescendo in character.

In the presence of pulmonary hypertension, regardless of its cause, one may detect the murmur of relative pulmonary insufficiency (Graham-Steell) as the result of a stretching of the pulmonary valve ring. Because of the velocity of the regurgitant flow caused by the pulmonary hypertension, this murmur has a high frequency, similar to that of aortic regurgitation. Rarely, it may be of congenital origin or secondary to bacterial endocarditis.

Tricuspid regurgitation. Tricuspid regurgitation is a murmur closely resembling that of mitral regurgitation, and the two may be difficult to distinguish. The fact that the murmur of tricuspid insufficiency increases in intensity on inspiration is helpful in differentiating it from its mitral counterpart. The murmur is usually caused by dilatation of the right ventricle and tricuspid valve ring. On rare occasions it may be secondary to organic valvular disease.

Tricuspid stenosis. As a rule, tricuspid stenosis coexists with rheumatic mitral valve disease. The murmur, thrill, and opening snap are difficult to distinguish from those produced by mitral stenosis. The murmur is heard loudest closer to the sternum, whereas that of mitral stenosis is more distinct over the apex. In ad-

dition, the murmur of tricuspid stenosis usually increases in intensity during inspiration.

Ventricular septal defect. Ventricular septal defects are usually congenital in origin, but may be acquired as a result of trauma, bacterial endocarditis, or rupture of the septum following acute myocardial infarction. The classic murmur is pansystolic, beginning with the first heart sound and extending to or through the aortic component of the second sound. The murmur is heard best and is loudest in the left fourth and fifth intercostal spaces adjacent to the sternum. In the majority of instances the murmur is accompanied by a systolic thrill.

Atrial septal defect. Atrial septal defect may occur as an isolated anomaly or in association with other congenital defects. In the isolated defect one hears a systolic ejection murmur, which is loudest in the second left intercostal space beginning after the first heart sound and terminating before the pulmonic second sound. The second sound in the pulmonic area is split in both inspiration and expiration and is classically described as a fixed split because it does not increase with inspiration or decrease with expiration. As a rule, there is no thrill accompanying the murmur. In many instances there is a lift or heave just to the left of the sternum, indicating right ventricular enlargement. With large left-to-right shunts one may hear a mid-diastolic rumbling murmur over the left lower sternal border. The presence of the diastolic murmur, at times, may cause confusion with mitral stenosis. However, in mitral stenosis the mid-diastolic rumbling is heard over the apex and not the left lower sternal border, and there is no fixed splitting of the second sound over the pulmonic area.

SELECTED READINGS

Brest, A. N., and Moyer, J. H.: Cardiovascular disorders, Philadelphia, 1968, F. A. Davis Co.

Burch, G. E.: A primer of cardiology, ed. 4, Philadelphia, 1971, Lea & Febiger.

Butterworth, J. S.: Cardiac auscultation, including audiovisual principles, New York, 1960, Grune & Stratton, Inc.

Fowler, N. O.: Diagnostic methods in cardiology, Philadelphia, 1975, F. A. Davis Co.

Fowler, N. O.: Physical diagnosis of heart disease, New York, 1962, The Macmillan Co.

Friedberg, C. K.: Diseases of the heart, Philadelphia, 1966, W. B. Saunders Co.

Hurst, J. W., and Logue, R. B.: The heart, ed. 3, New York, 1974, McGraw-Hill Book Co.

Levine, S. A., and Harvey, W. P.: Clinical auscultation of the heart, Philadelphia, 1959, W. B. Saunders Co.

McKusick, V. A.: Cardiovascular sound in health and disease, Baltimore, 1958, The Williams & Wilkins Co.

Massey, F. C.: Clinical cardiology, Baltimore, 1953, The Williams & Wilkins Co.

Master, A. H.: Visual aids in cardiologic diagnosis and treatment, New York, 1960, Grune & Stratton, Inc.

Nadas, A. S.: Pediatric cardiology, ed. 3, Philadelphia, 1972, W. B. Saunders Co.

Ravin, A.: Auscultation of the heart, Chicago, 1967, Year Book Medical Publishers, Inc.

Rushmer, R. F.: Cardiovascular dynamics, Philadelphia, 1970, W. B. Saunders Co.

Schwedel, J. B.: Clinical roentgenology of the heart, New York, 1946, Paul B. Hoeber, Inc.

Segal, B. L., and Likoff, W.: Auscultation of the heart, New York, 1965, Grune & Stratton, Inc.

Segal, B. L., Likoff, W., and Moyer, J. H.: The theory and practice of auscultation, Philadelphia, 1964, F. A. Davis Co.

Wood, P. H.: Diseases of the heart and circulation, Philadelphia, 1968, J. B. Lippincott Co.

CHAPTER 15

ABDOMEN

Advances in scientific medicine have, on occasion, threatened to displace the history and physical examination in evaluating the patient. However, we usually discover that technologic advances serve to make the physical examination more rational and provide new understanding or objective documentation of long-appreciated physical findings. New techniques for evaluation of the intra-abdominal contents include many biochemical, isotopic, ultrasonar, and angiographic methods. These advances, although improving our ability to detect, document, and interpret physical findings, have not superseded the need for the skills involved in medical interview and physical examination. An orderly approach to the examination of the abdomen makes possible the analysis of the symptoms arising from the many organs of the digestive and genitourinary systems found in this region.

Certain features of the abdominal examination differ from those of other areas. Although most of the information acquired is obtained from palpation, there are many exceptions. Palpation may be very difficult in the obese, very muscular, or tense patient. For reasons to be described later, palpation is performed last.

The order of other techniques is also changed, but it must be recalled that the same basic steps of inspection, percussion, palpation, and auscultation are used in this area as in other areas.

Although a detailed analysis of abdominal pain is beyond the scope of this chapter, a few common examples that demonstrate the variable usefulness of different sources of information are worthy of note. The physical findings may be entirely negative in the presence of peptic ulcer disease, wherein a typical history of pain relieved by food will suggest the diagnosis. In the patient with jaundice, right upper quadrant pain, and tenderness the physical findings may not enable distinction between obstructive jaundice or hepatitis, but the history may be virtually diagnostic. Finally, when abdominal pain is referred from thoracic or vertebral sources, neither history nor physical examination confined to the abdomen will help unless integrated into the total clinical context.

Topographic anatomy

There have been several systems devised for dividing the abdomen into topographic segments, but only the one in most general use is described here. Other systems may be found in any standard textbook of anatomy.

The anterior surface of the abdomen is divided into four quadrants by two intersecting lines, one extending vertically from the xiphoid process to the symphysis pubis and the other extending horizontally across the abdomen at the level of the umbilicus (Fig. 15-1). This divides the abdomen into the right upper, right lower, left upper, and left lower quadrants. The term *epigastrium*, which is included here because of its frequent use in clinical medicine, is composed of the medial halves of the right and left upper quadrants. The student must know the structures located in each of these areas, the most important of which are the following:

Right upper quadrant
1. Liver
2. Gallbladder
3. Duodenum
4. Pancreas
5. Right kidney
6. Hepatic flexure of colon

Left upper quadrant
1. Stomach
2. Spleen
3. Left kidney
4. Pancreas
5. Splenic flexure of colon

Right lower quadrant
1. Cecum
2. Appendix
3. Right ovary and tube

Left lower quadrant
1. Sigmoid colon
2. Left ovary and tube

Midline
1. Bladder
2. Uterus

Position of patient

Before any attempt is made to examine the abdomen, care must be taken to see that the patient is relaxed and in a proper position. With the patient in a supine position, the head should be elevated on a pillow, and the arms should be placed across the chest. The patient should be assured that no sudden manipula-

tion or painful procedure will be carried out.

Since the structures under investigation are separated from the examiner's hand by a rather thick abdominal wall, adequate relaxation of the abdomen must be obtained before satisfactory examination can be performed. Details for obtaining relaxation of the muscular wall are discussed later in this chapter.

The examiner should resist the temptation to begin palpating the abdomen before adequate inspection is carried out. This is an excellent opportunity for the experienced clinician to make small talk to aid in the relaxation of the patient or even to restate briefly the digestive history to assure his own orientation to the examination. The patient should be suitably draped with the skin exposed from sternum to pubis. There should be adequate lighting, and occasionally oblique illumination will reveal features otherwise missed. The abdomen is observed first for general symmetry, visible masses, and the status of nutrition. The skin normally is the same as that noted elsewhere on the body. Silver striae (vertical, often wrinkled, streaks) are frequently seen in the lower quadrants of the abdomen following a large gain of weight or after pregnancy. Tight, glistening skin is often associated with ascites and edema of the abdominal wall. Exanthematous rashes and petechiae may be observed. The presence and location of any surgical scars should also be noted at this time, as well as any obvious pulsations. Frequently in slender patients, pulsations transmitted from the aorta may be seen in the epigastrium. Such pulsations may also represent masses in contact with major vessels or abnormalities of the vessels themselves.

Obvious asymmetry of contour may be an important finding. Lateral asymmetry will be noted only if one remembers to examine from above as well as from the side. The presence of masses or hernias may be suspected from this observation and confirmed later by palpation.

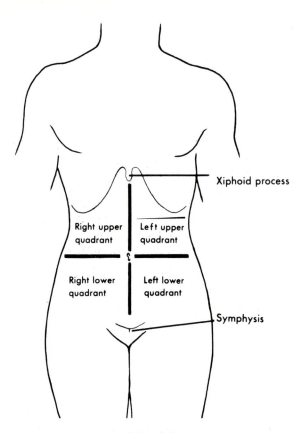

Fig. 15-1. Division of the abdomen into quadrants.

When observed from the side, the abdomen is usually flat from xiphoid to symphysis pubis, or symmetrically protuberant or scaphoid, depending on the nutritional status of the patient. The umbilicus is usually centrally located in the abdominal contour. Supraumbilical fullness may represent a mass originating in the upper abdominal structures, such as in the liver, pancreas, stomach, or transverse colon. Similarly, fullness in the lower abdomen may result from bladder distention, pregnancy, or masses arising from the ovaries, uterus, or colon.

Generalized symmetric abdominal fullness is a more frequent and often difficult diagnostic problem. This fullness is usually caused by *ascites* (free fluid within the abdomen, Fig. 15-2), obesity, or distention of the bowel with trapped gas. The distinction usually can be made from the history and related physical findings. Helpful information from inspection includes the overall nutritional status of the patient, bulging of the flanks caused by fluid accumulation, and the appearance of the umbilicus. The umbilicus is usually deeply inverted in obesity and flat or everted in long-standing ascites. When abdominal distention is accompanied by visible peristaltic contractions, it is almost diagnostic of intestinal obstruction. This finding is made more obvious when the abdomen is viewed by cross illumination.

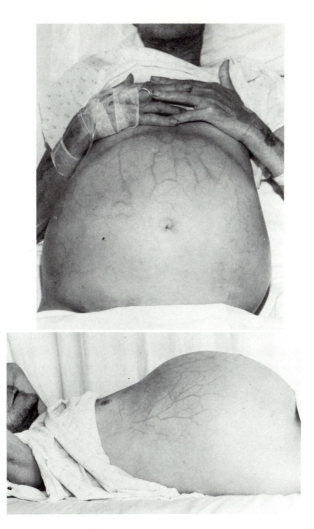

Fig. 15-2. Massive ascites. Note bulging flanks, dilated upper abdominal veins, and everted umbilicus.

Next the examiner may note the presence of distended abdominal veins. Prominence of these vessels indicates increased collateral circulation as a result of obstruction in the portal venous system or in the vena cava and may co-exist with ascites in the patient with cirrhosis. It is helpful to remember that the normal direction of flow in these vessels is away from the umbilicus, that is, the upper abdominal veins carry blood upward to the superior vena cava, and the lower abdominal veins drain downward to the inferior vena cava. The direction of blood flow in these collateral veins is easily assessed by a simple maneuver. A segment of vein in the epigastrium is emptied between two fingers to a distance of a few centimeters. One then allows blood to refill the vein from one direction by removing one compressing finger and observing the rate of refilling. The same segment is again emptied and filling from the opposite direction is estimated. Usually the rate of filling is obviously faster in one direction than in the other, indicating the direction of flow in that portion of the collateral venous system. The process is repeated in the hypogastrium, and the direction of flow in the lower abdominal veins is observed. In portal hypertension normal flow direction is maintained. In contrast, obstruction of the vena cava alters the flow direction in these veins. In obstruction of the superior vena cava, the flow direction in the upper abdominal venous collateral is reversed or downward. In inferior vena cava obstruction the direction is reversed in the lower abdominal veins, and they will drain upward.

When portal hypertension is present or when there is other reason to suspect liver disease, the examiner should make a careful inspection of the upper extremities, face, neck, and chest for the presence of *cutaneous angiomas (spider nevi),* which are found in asso-

ciation with liver disease. These may be distinguished from petechiae and other lesions by the fact that they blanch not only by pressure on the nevus but also by gentle pressure over the central arteriole that feeds this clump of dilated blood vessels, as illustrated in Fig. 15-3.

The abdomen is inspected for evidence of unusual pigmentation, such as jaundice. Disorders accompanied by hyperpigmentation also may be more notable on inspection of the skin of the abdomen, where changes caused by exposure of the skin to sunlight are readily separated from those caused by generalized increase in pigment. The tendency of these disorders to manifest increased pigmentation in areas of minor or persistent trauma to the skin may be especially evident at the belt line. Other pigment changes caused by intra-abdominal hemorrhage may be found. A bluish discoloration of the umbilicus occasionally is seen after major intraperitoneal hemorrhage. A similar discoloration of the flanks in the absence of trauma occasionally is seen following the ex-

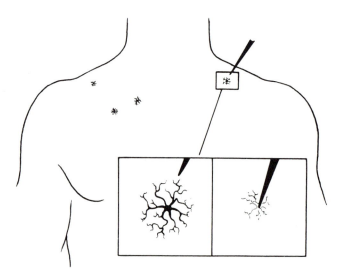

Fig. 15-3. Cutaneous angiomas, or spider nevi. Notice blanching produced by pressure on central arteriole.

travasation of blood from intra-abdominal organs into extraperitoneal sites, as in hemorrhagic pancreatitis.

Finally, hair distribution should be noted. In the normal female the pubic hair is roughly triangular with the base above the symphysis, whereas in the male it is in the shape of a diamond, often with hair continuing to the umbilicus. The distribution and quantity of hair may be altered by chronic liver disease and various endocrine abnormalities.

AUSCULTATION

Following inspection, the examiner should perform auscultation of the abdomen. Palpation and percussion usually follow inspection in the examination of the other body systems. This change in the order of examination is necessary because the auscultatory findings may be markedly altered by any manipulation of the abdominal wall. Consequently percussion and palpation which may increase or decrease peristaltic sounds, are deferred until auscultation has been completed.

The diaphragm of the stethoscope should be placed lightly against the abdominal wall in order to avoid artefacts resulting from friction and compression of vessels. First, one should listen to the sounds produced by intestinal peristalsis. These sounds are difficult to describe and are best appreciated from the experience of listening to the abdominal sounds in many normal individuals. Also, this exercise permits understanding of the normal wide variability of bowel sounds, which may be interpreted as evidence of disease by the inexperienced examiner. The recording of "slightly hypoactive" bowel sounds by the student usually represents an attempt to give significance to a normal finding.

Two abnormalities of the bowel sounds are significant. The absence of any sound or extremely weak and infrequent sounds heard af-

ter several minutes of continuous auscultation ordinarily represent the immobile bowel of peritonitis or paralytic ileus. In contrast, increased sounds with a characteristic loud, rushing, high-pitched tinkling quality often occur in mechanical intestinal obstruction and may be accompanied by waves of pain. The latter findings are caused by distention of the bowel and increased peristaltic activity proximal to the site of the obstruction.

Another sound that is unrelated to peristalsis may be heard in the appropriate setting and is known as a *succussion splash*. In cases of pyloric obstruction, with increased air and fluid in the stomach, this sound may be produced when the abdomen is rocked from side to side with one hand. A similar sound may be heard over the inferior sternum and epigastrium in the presence of a large hiatus hernia.

The early detection of vascular lesions in the abdomen has become increasingly important as vascular diseases of the abdomen have grown in recognition and treatment has improved. The most important physical finding indicating vascular disease is a bruit. A bruit in the abdomen is a systolic sound created by turbulence in the flow of blood through a partially occluded or diseased artery. One type of bruit is that which is heard over the abdominal aorta and is produced by atherosclerotic plaques or an aneurysm. Partial occlusion of other major abdominal arteries, either by congenital bands or by atherosclerotic plaques, may be detected by auscultation. Examples of these types of lesions are found in the celiac artery and superior mesenteric artery. Also, a bruit may be heard over diseased renal arteries. To be of significance a bruit must be heard consistently in the area if the patient is moved into various positions, and it must be heard with extremely light pressure on the diaphragm of the stethoscope.

Other sources of bruits in the abdomen include vascular malformations of congenital origin or those produced by distortion of vessels by tumor, cysts, or severe inflammation. Rarely, one may hear a bruit caused by an intra-abdominal arteriovenous shunt. Adequate auscultatory practice then must include listening in the epigastrium, above and lateral to the umbilicus on both sides, and over the liver. It is worth emphasizing that bruits often are soft and high pitched and require the same intensity of concentration as that required for the detection of grade I cardiac murmurs. Obviously, if the bowel sounds are very loud, significant bruits may be missed on casual examination.

Another vascular sound that may be heard is that of a *venous hum*. This is usually heard over the upper portion of the abdomen or liver and is associated with enlargement of the anastomotic veins most frequently associated with liver disease or with portal or splenic vein thrombosis. Congenital abnormalities of the umbilical vein will also produce this finding. This sound is softer than the arterial bruit and tends to be a continuous humming sound rather than systolic in time.

Occasionally, friction rubs may be heard over parts of the abdomen. A definite friction rub may be heard over the spleen in cases of inflammation of the spleen or with splenic infarction. Friction rubs may also be heard over the liver and almost always indicate either a primary or metastatic tumor of the liver. Since these sounds are quite soft and are associated with respiration, they must be separated from normal breath sounds. Care must be taken to avoid sounds from the skin.

PERCUSSION

Percussion of the abdomen is primarily used to establish the presence of distention, tumors, fluid, and enlargement of solid viscera. Light percussion is preferable, since it produces a clearer tone. It is well to establish an orderly

procedure for percussion. With the patient recumbent, the examiner should stand at the patient's right side. First, percuss down the lower left thoracic wall in the midaxillary line. This should produce a resonant note over the underlying lung in this area. Below the level of the left hemidiaphragm there is normally a tympanitic note caused by the splenic flexure of the colon. Any dullness extending above the ninth interspace in the left midaxillary line should make the examiner suspicious that there is enlargement of a solid organ in this area. This is most likely caused by the spleen, but occasionally may be mimicked by enlargement of the kidney or by marked enlargement of the left lobe of the liver. Consolidation of the left lower lobe of the lung or pleural effusion will invalidate this observation.

In the presence of lesser degrees of splenomegaly, another technique for percussing the spleen has been of value. Following percussion in the left midaxillary line, the procedure is repeated in the lowest intercostal space in the left anterior axillary line. Normally the percussion note here also is resonant. Percussion is continued while the patient takes a deep breath. In the absence of splenic enlargement, the percussion note should not change. With modest degrees of splenomegaly, the lower pole of the spleen moves inferomedially and is brought forward during inspiration. As it moves under the lowest intercostal space with inspiration it will produce a change in the percussion note from resonance to dullness.

Next, percussion of the liver should be performed in the right midaxillary and midclavicular lines. The normal upper limit of liver dullness in the midaxillary line varies from the fifth to the seventh interspace. Because of this variation, determination of the actual extent of liver dullness is more reliable. This is done by percussion in the right midclavicular line until the upper border is determined. One then percusses downward over the liver until the lower border of liver dullness is found. The normal lower limit of liver dullness is at the costal margin. Dullness extending into the normally tympanitic right upper quadrant indicates hepatic enlargement, a mass adjacent to the liver, or downward displacement of the liver. Measurement of the actual extent of liver dullness will help define these findings. The diameter may be checked by repeating percussion during full inspiration and again during full expiration, which should yield a range of about 2 to 4 cm. movement of both borders. The mean diameter of liver dullness is about 10 cm. with the normal upper limit being about 12 cm. Since these values vary somewhat with the sex, height, and body build of the patient, the overall size of the patient must be taken into account when using this method. Since estimates of liver size vary somewhat with the force of percussion, the student must learn that light percussion is most accurate.

There may be an absence of liver dullness following perforation of a hollow viscus, which allows free air to enter the abdominal cavity (Fig. 15-4). This indication of an intra-abdominal catastrophe must be correlated with the clinical situation, since on occasion interposition of the hepatic flexure of the colon between the diaphragm and the liver will produce the same finding with no clinical consequences.

The remainder of the normal abdomen is more or less tympanitic to percussion, depending on the amount of gas in the intestine. After percussion of the liver and spleen, one may percuss over any visible masses to determine whether they are dull (as with tumor or fluid-filled spaces) or tympanitic (as with distended bowel). Distention of the urinary bladder may yield an area of suprapubic dullness. If other masses are detected by palpation later in the examination, percussion may help to characterize them further.

The last thing to be noted on percussion is the presence or absence of free fluid in the ab-

dominal cavity (ascites). This may be detected by several maneuvers: (1) fluid wave, (2) shifting dullness, and (3) elbow-knee position.

Fluid wave. With the patient lying on his back, the examiner's left hand is placed against the patient's right flank. An assistant or the patient places the ulnar edge of one hand lightly against the middle of the abdomen to prevent the transmission of any wave through the tissues of the abdominal wall (Fig. 15-5). The examiner's right hand then lightly taps the left flank of the patient. In the presence of a significant amount of ascites, a wave will be transmitted *through the fluid* that will be felt against the examiner's left hand as a sharp impulse. This finding is present only when there is a reasonably large amount of fluid.

Shifting dullness. When the patient with ascites lies on his back, the fluid will migrate into the flanks, producing dullness laterally. At the same time the midabdomen is tympanitic because of the underlying bowel. When dullness is found in the flanks, a mark is made on the skin at the appropriate level (Fig. 15-6). The patient is then rolled onto his right side, and the percussion is again carried out toward each flank. In the presence of ascites the fluid will gravitate toward the dependent right flank (Fig. 15-7). Consequently it will be noted that the level of dullness on the right has moved toward the midline and that the bowel, which has been displaced upward by the fluid, results in a tympanitic note in the upper flank. This is repeated after rolling the patient to his left side. By this means an estimate of the amount of free fluid can be made.

Elbow-knee position. The presence of small amounts of fluid may be readily detected by placing the patient in an elbow-knee position and percussing from the flanks toward the most dependent portion of the abdomen. Free fluid, if present, will run from the pelvis and gutters of the abdomen into the most dependent area, which, if the patient is in the proper position,

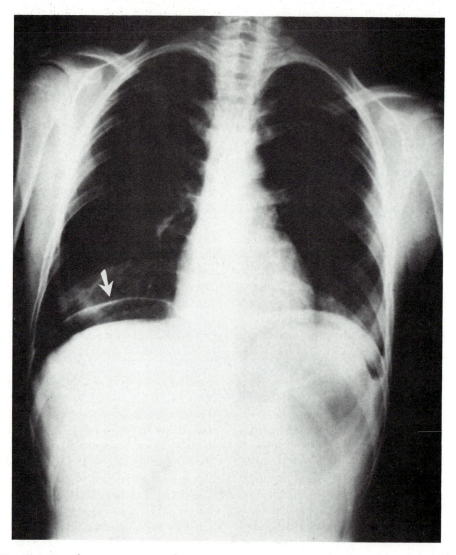

Fig. 15-4. Upright posteroanterior chest roentgenogram in a patient with no hepatic dullness to percussion. The roentgenogram confirms free air under the diaphragm (best seen under the right hemidiaphragm—arrow) caused by a perforated hollow viscus.

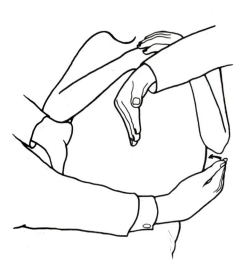

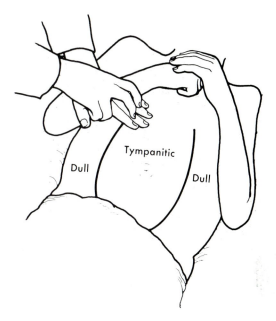

Fig. 15-5. Production of fluid wave. Examiner's right hand strikes the patient's left flank (arrow). Notice position of the assistant's hand, preventing transmission of the wave through the tissues of the abdominal wall.

Fig. 15-6. Shifting dullness. Draw the line at the level of dullness in each flank. Note central tympany caused by air-filled bowel.

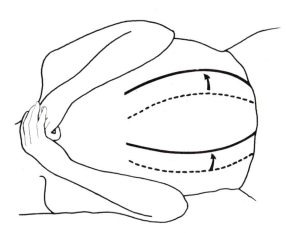

Fig. 15-7. Shifting dullness. Rotate patient onto his side. Notice that dullness has shifted toward the umbilicus on the dependent side. Tympanitic area has shifted toward the superior flank.

is located in the periumbilical region. The finding of dullness in this area indicates the presence of ascitic fluid. This technique is more sensitive for detecting small amounts of fluid than are the previously described methods.

PALPATION

The final step in the abdominal examination is palpation. This procedure is usually the most important and often the most difficult to perform accurately. Proper preparation of the patient and systematic application of the principles outlined will result in a satisfactory examination. Several different kinds of information may be obtained by palpation. One may elicit pain or discomfort on abdominal pressure, the nature of which may be of considerable value in arriving at a diagnosis. A related finding is a change in the tone of the abdominal wall, often caused by intra-abdominal irritative processes. One also may detect masses or organ enlargement, findings that ordinarily are of great importance in the evaluation of the patient.

Relaxation and positioning of the patient. During palpation the patient should continue to lie supine with arms relaxed on the chest or at the sides. The examiner should make certain that his hands are warm. He should assure the patient that he will make an effort not to cause discomfort and follow up this assurance by avoiding at the outset an area already described as painful. If the patient exhibits ticklishness, the examiner should disregard it and try to continue. If this proves unsuccessful, it is useful to have the patient place his own hand on his abdomen, since this never tickles. The examiner may tentatively exert pressure on the abdomen through the patient's own hand, and gradually increase the pressure, while assuring the patient that the examination will cause no discomfort. When the patient has relaxed, the examiner again places his own hand on the abdomen and allows the patient to maintain contact with his hand. This usually completes the relaxation of the ticklish patient, and the examination proceeds as usual.

The examination is begun with gentle exploration of the abdominal wall with no effort made to palpate deeply. The patient may be further relaxed by instructing him to breathe slowly and deeply. As with inspection, the initial step in palpation may be facilitated by distracting conversation or questions regarding the history. If the patient remains tense or if the abdominal wall is very muscular, better results may be obtained by having the patient flex the thighs and knees.

It should be emphasized again that during the preliminary stages muscle relaxation is the goal. At this time no attempt should be made either to elicit discomfort or to palpate for a mass or enlarged viscus. By light palpation some estimate may be made of the degree of muscle rigidity or resistance. If these are present, the examiner should determine whether the abdominal wall exhibits voluntary muscle tightening or actual rigidity. *Rigidity* of the abdominal muscles is manifested by increased tonus, which is reflex in nature and produced by irritative lesions involving the peritoneum. This muscle spasm cannot be relaxed by voluntary effort. *Voluntary tensing of the muscles,* on the other hand, is brought about through fear or nervousness and is not necessarily associated with an intra-abdominal lesion. This type of muscle tension can be overcome by proper technique, reassurance, and an effort to relax on the part of the patient.

A maneuver occasionally useful for confirming that increased muscle tone is caused by voluntary tension is to use the stethoscope for palpation. Having carried out auscultation without exerting pressure, the examiner may reapply it to several areas of the abdominal wall without comment. The patient does not associate the instrument with pain or pressure and will not react to it with muscle guarding. The examiner applies the head of the stethoscope lightly at first, then with increasing pressure. In voluntary tension one may apply considerable pressure in this way, often to find a much more relaxed abdominal wall. On the other hand, true increased tone caused by peritoneal irritation will be manifest by a response equal to that produced by manual palpation.

During deep palpation in the midepigastrium almost all patients will complain of tenderness, which accompanies pressure on the abdominal aorta. It is well to reassure the patient that this sensation is normal during deep palpation of this area. In fact, if the examiner is able to palpate the aorta and the patient does not experience some discomfort, this would probably be abnormal.

Locating painful area. After relaxation is obtained, the examining hand is first moved gently over the entire abdomen, and an estimate of the muscle tone in the various quadrants is made. Following general palpation an attempt should be made to detect and localize any painful area within the abdomen. Two types of pain may be elicited by palpation.

1. *Visceral.* This is pain that arises from an organic lesion or functional disturbance within an abdominal viscus. For example, it is the type seen in an obstructive lesion of the intestine in which there is a buildup of pressure and distention of the gut. This type of pain has several characteristics: it is dull, poorly localized, and difficult for the patient to characterize.

2. *Somatic.* This is similar to the distress noted in painful lesions of the skin. It is sharp, bright, and well localized. It is not caused primarily by involvement of the viscera; rather it indicates involvement of one of the somatic structures, such as the parietal peritoneum or the abdominal wall itself. It should be pointed out that an inflammatory process originating in a viscus will produce visceral pain that may ex-

tend to involve the peritoneum. Inflammation of the peritoneum would then result in somatic pain. This is best illustrated by appendicitis in which the pain is at first poorly localized, dull, ill defined, and primarily midline (when it is entirely visceral in origin). Later, as the inflammation spreads to the peritoneum, the pain becomes sharp, bright, and well localized in the right lower quadrant over the involved region.

After a painful area is located, the examiner should determine whether the pain is constant under the pressure of the examining hand or if it is transient, tending to disappear even though pressure is continued over the area. Pain caused by inflammation usually remains unchanged or increases as pressure is applied. Visceral pain as the result of distention or contraction of a viscus tends to become less severe while pressure is maintained.

Occasionally the examiner may have difficulty in distinguishing visceral pain from that arising in somatic structures, such as the spine and abdominal wall. An example of abdominal wall discomfort is seen in patients with fibrositis. These types of pain may be differentiated by having the patient tense his abdominal muscles, which may be accomplished by forcefully elevating his head while keeping his shoulders flat on the table. Under these conditions increased tension of the abdominal wall will accentuate the pain if it originates in somatic structures. On the other hand, discomfort from intra-abdominal sources will be less severe with the abdomen tense than when relaxed.

Rebound tenderness. When pain has been elicited, the examiner should test for the phenomenon of rebound tenderness. This is found only when the peritoneum overlying a diseased viscus becomes inflamed. Although it may be elicited in different ways, the most common is to press firmly over a region distant from the tender area and then suddenly release the pressure. The patient will feel a sharp stab of

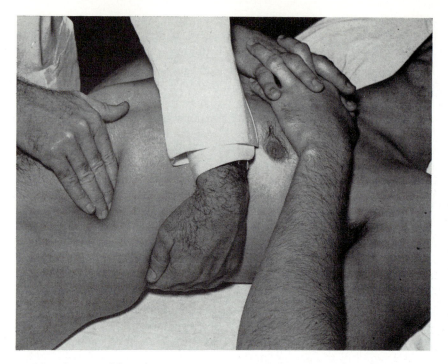

Fig. 15-8. Palpation of the spleen. Notice examiner's left hand pressing spleen anteriorly.

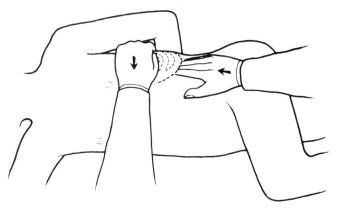

Fig. 15-9. Palpation of the spleen with the patient in right lateral decubitus position.

pain in the area of disease if true rebound tenderness is present. For example, pressure applied in the right lower quadrant and then suddenly released will cause a marked increase in pain over an area of diverticulitis in the left quadrant. Rebound tenderness may also be elicited by having the patient cough or by applying gentle pressure over the tender area and having the patient cough or strain. Marked tenderness to percussion in the area is usually seen in this situation. This type of tenderness indicates widespread inflammation of the peritoneum (*peritonitis*). At times, if the area involved is small, rebound tenderness may be elicited only over the most tender area of the abdomen.

Palpation of organs and masses. The examiner should palpate for enlargement of intra-abdominal organs, principally the spleen, liver, and kidneys. In examining for splenic enlargement, the examiner should stand at the patient's right side (Fig. 15-8). His left hand is placed over the patient's left costovertebral angle exerting pressure to move the spleen anteriorly. At the same time his right hand is worked gently under the left anterior costal margin. With the examiner's hands stationary in this position, the patient is instructed to take a deep breath. If there is significant enlargement of the spleen, it will be palpated as a firm mass that slides out from under the ribs, bumping against the fingers of the examiner's right hand. The spleen normally moves down with inspiration. If splenic enlargement is suspected from previous percussion but cannot be felt by the technique just described, the patient should then be rolled slightly toward the right so that the spleen may fall anteriorly (Fig. 15-9). The examining hands are again placed as described, and the procedure is repeated. Occasionally a spleen that cannot be felt with the patient in the supine positon may be palpated by this maneuver. When the spleen can be felt, it must be considered abnormal, since the normal spleen is not palpable.

One must be careful to avoid missing a spleen so large that the edge is well below the costal margin. Previous percussion of the left upper quadrant should prevent this error. If the edge is not felt under the left costal margin

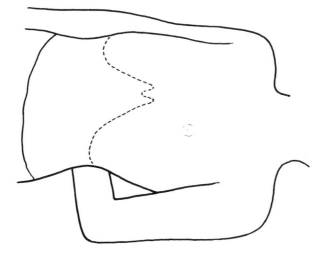

Fig. 15-10. Another position for assisting in palpation of the spleen.

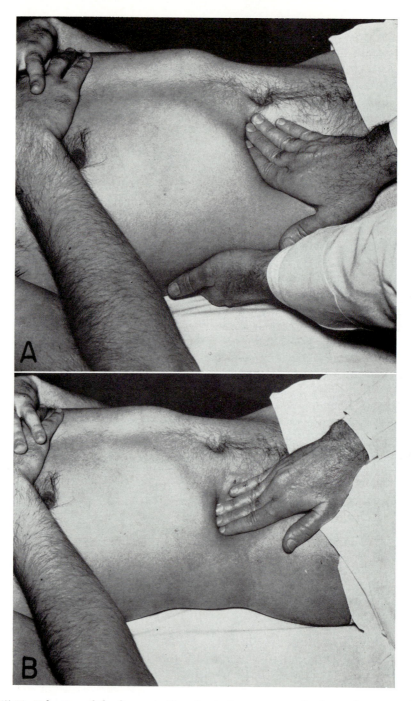

Fig. 15-11. Palpation of the liver. **A,** Examiner's fingers perpendicular to long axis of the patient. **B,** Examiner's fingers parallel to long axis of the patient.

but splenomegaly is suspected, the examiner should palpate more medially, then in the midaxillary line, and finally in the inferior portion of the left abdomen. A technique used in the obese or heavily muscled patient is for the physician to move to the patient's left side and face the lower abdomen, while the patient rests the small of the back on his left forearm. The examiner then may palpate with both hands over a large portion of the left abdomen while the patient takes deep breaths (Fig. 15-10).

Next, palpation for enlargement of the liver is performed. The right hand may be held either parallel or perpendicular to the long axis of the patient (Fig. 15-11). The fingers are gently worked deep into the right upper quadrant. With the examiner's fingers in place, the patient is again requested to take a deep breath. Ordinarily the liver is not palpable, although not infrequently the examiner may feel the edge of the normal liver at or slightly below the right costal margin. When the liver is palpated, a firm edge will strike the fingers on inspiration. When felt more than 1 cm. below the costal margin, however, the organ should be considered abnormally large. An exception is a congenitally large right lobe of the liver, which occasionally extends quite far into the right flank. Another exception is seen in severe, chronic emphysema, in which the diaphragms are depressed by the overexpanded lung, displacing the liver below the costal margin. In both instances the total mass of the liver is within normal limits. The findings on palpation should be predictable from the estimates made during percussion. The character of the surface of the liver should be described. Not infrequently large metastatic masses may be present and palpable in the liver (Fig. 15-12). In some persons with cirrhosis, the anterior surface of the liver will have a granular feel. This is easily felt in the thin individual.

The same precautions mentioned in the examination of the spleen also apply to the palpation of the liver. In some conditions the left lobe is predominantly enlarged, and palpation must include the epigastrium to appreciate that portion of the liver. If percussion suggests massive enlargement, one may need to explore a large area of the right abdomen to find the lower border of the liver, which occasionally may extend below the level of the umbilicus or even to the iliac crest. As in palpation of the spleen, it may be helpful to palpate from above using the palmar aspects of both hands in an attempt to feel the liver through the obese or very muscular wall.

A very common error in palpation of the upper abdomen is moving the palpating hand during inspiration.

Occasionally other normal structures may be felt in the abdomen. In thin persons the lower poles of the kidneys may be felt high in either flank by deep palpation. The kidneys will descend with inspiration. A distended bladder may be palpated in the suprapubic region. Often this is more readily detected by percussion. Confirmation that a mass felt in the suprapubic region is actually a full bladder may be obtained by again palpating the area after urination. In many persons the cecum may be felt as a soft, gas-filled mass in the right lower quadrant. It is easily manipulated by the examining fingers, and the gas may be expressed into the colon. By deep palpation in the left lower quadrant the examiner may feel the sigmoid colon as it rolls over the pelvic brim, where it is felt as a sausage-shaped mass that is freely movable and frequently tender.

It should be emphasized that careful palpation of the vascular structures of the abdomen has become an important part of the physical examination. In patients who are thin or have some anterior curvature of the spine, the abdominal aorta is normally felt as a soft pulsatile structure in the midepigastrium and extending down to the brim of the pelvis. Tenderness is elicited from pressure on this structure. In older individuals, aneurysms frequently occur in this vessel. These aneurysms are saclike enlargements of a segment of the abdominal aorta, are felt as pulsatile masses in the midportion of the abdomen, and are frequently associated with pain in the abdomen. If a pulsating mass is noted, the examiner must first decide if this is a pulsation transmitted through an overlying structure from the aorta. If the aorta appears to be the site of the enlargement, then its width should be estimated. Aneurysms may be multiple and involve not only the abdominal aorta but also the internal iliac vessels. Consequently, if the examiner discovers a pulsatile mass in the aorta, he also should palpate carefully in the region of the pelvic brim for other similar lesions.

Under normal circumstances the gallbladder cannot be palpated. However, in a jaundiced

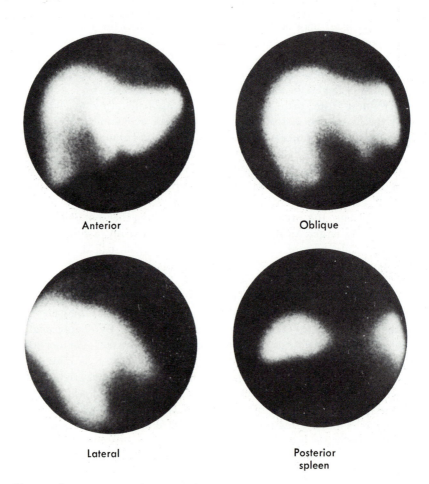

Anterior

Oblique

Lateral

Posterior
spleen

Fig. 15-12. Radioactive scintophotogram (liver scan) of a patient with a bruit and a palpable hard mass at the lower border of an enlarged liver. The scan shows a filling defect in the same area, proved by biopsy to be neoplastic.

patient the right upper quadrant should always be carefully palpated for a soft, cystic mass, approximately 6 to 8 cm. in diameter, that appears to be attached to the liver and moves with respiration. This is an exceedingly valuable sign in differentiating jaundice caused by cancer of the head of the pancreas or the common bile duct from that caused by gallstones. In the presence of tumor of the common bile duct or head of the pancreas, the wall of the gallbladder is normal, and consequently, the organ is capable of distending to the point that it is palpable. On the other hand, if the obstruction is caused by gallstones, the gallblad-

der wall is inflamed, and this diseased organ is not capable of distention; therefore, the gallbladder will not become palpable (Fig. 15-13).

Exceptions to this rule occur in nonjaundiced patients with inflammatory gallbladder disease. Patients with gallstone obstruction of the cystic duct and cholecystitis may develop hydropic distention of the infected gallbladder, which is palpable as a tender right upper quadrant mass (Fig. 15-13, *B*). The gallbladder may also become transiently palpable early in the course of an attack of biliary colic, only to recede with subsidence of the attack.

When one can palpate an abdominal mass

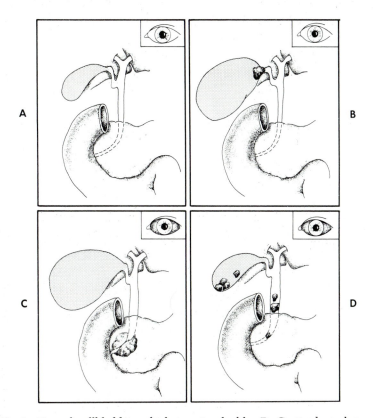

Fig. 15-13. A, Normal gallbladder, which is not palpable. **B,** Cystic duct obstruction (hydrops)—gallbladder enlarged, but jaundice is not present. **C,** Obstruction of common bile duct by tumor—gallbladder palpable and jaundice present. **D,** Common bile duct obstructed by stone—gallbladder fibrotic, not enlarged, but accompanied by jaundice.

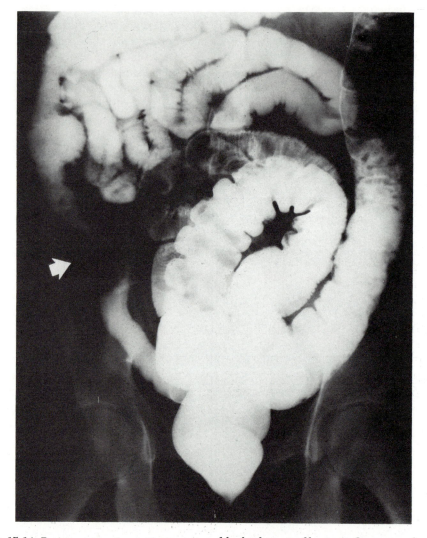

Fig. 15-14. Barium enema in a patient suspected by his history of having inflammatory bowel disease. Examination disclosed a 4 × 8 cm. firm, slightly irregular, mobile, tender mass in the right lower quadrant (arrow). This roentgenogram confirms the presence of abnormality in the ascending colon, with narrowing of the lumen of the cecum and displacement of adjacent bowel caused by the pathologic process responsible for the mass (Crohn's disease).

that is not clearly an enlarged organ, it should be characterized as to size, location, consistency, contour, mobility, and tenderness (Fig. 15-14). Masses in the abdominal wall may be distinguished from those of visceral origin by palpation during voluntary tensing of the muscles. When the patient lifts his head from the examining table, abdominal wall masses will remain palpable and even may become more evident as they are elevated by the tensed muscle. In contrast, intra-abdominal masses will be more difficult to discern after the wall is tensed. Finally, one should palpate the umbilicus for evidence of nodularity or a mass, the presence of which implies peritoneal seeding from an intra-abdominal neoplasm.

Abdominal hernias

Examination of the abdomen should include a careful search for the presence of hernias, which may be ventral, inguinal, or femoral. *Ventral* hernias are seen as soft masses that protrude into the anterior abdominal wall. Usually they occur in weak spots, such as in surgical scars, but they also may be seen in the umbilicus or other regions. Umbilical hernias are congenital in origin and are best seen when the patient coughs or strains. After the hernia has been reduced by gentle manipulation, a defect in the abdominal wall, usually large enough to admit the tip of an examining finger, will be found at the base.

An *epiplocele* is a defect in the abdominal wall in the midline above the umbilicus in which there is a small herniation of fat or omentum through or into the rectus sheath. When the abdominal wall is tensed, it will be felt as a small, tender nodule. It may or may not be associated with a separation of the rectus sheath, which is termed *diastasis recti*. This latter condition is often seen in obese persons or multiparous women and is of no particular clinical significance.

Most commonly seen is the *inguinal hernia*, which is a protrusion of peritoneum through the abdominal wall in the region of the inguinal canal. It may contain either bowel or mesentery. These hernias may be direct or indirect. An *indirect* hernia passes through both the internal and external inguinal rings and traverses the inguinal canal. The *direct* hernia passes through a weak spot in the abdominal wall in this region and thence into the external inguinal ring. Indirect hernias often become quite large and descend into the scrotum, at times producing a mass as large as a grapefruit. Direct hernias are usually smaller and do not enter the scrotum.

When palpating for inguinal hernias, the examiner should have the patient standing erect with the ipsilateral leg slightly flexed (Fig. 15-15). The examiner should be seated in front of the patient. Both inguinal areas are observed for evidence of bulging that might indicate the presence of a hernia. Following this the little finger of the right hand is inserted into the right external inguinal ring. This is done by picking up the loose skin on the side of the scrotum and pushing it ahead of the examining finger until the external inguinal ring itself is palpated. An estimate is made as to whether the ring is normally tight and small or abnormally large and relaxed. The patient is instructed to "bear down" and to cough while the abdominal muscles are tensed. An indirect inguinal hernia will be felt as a small, soft, sausage-shaped mass that pushes against the *tip* of the examining finger. The cough impulse is also readily transmitted to the finger. In a direct hernia the impulse and bulge will strike the *side* of the finger, since the sack comes directly through the abdominal wall instead of down the inguinal canal. The left little finger is used for examination of the left side. The examiner should not confuse an enlarged spermatic cord with an inguinal hernia.

Inspection is carried out just below the inguinal ligament and over the femoral triangle

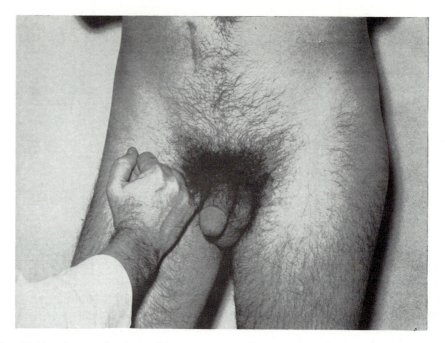

Fig. 15-15. Palpation for inguinal hernia. Notice that the ipsilateral leg is partially flexed. The right little finger is used to explore the right inguinal region, and the left little finger is used for the opposite side.

to detect the presence of a *femoral* hernia. This hernia presents on the anterior surface of the thigh, just below the inguinal ligament. On palpation a small soft mass will be felt, which becomes larger as the patient strains or coughs.

RECTAL EXAMINATION

The information obtained by the rectal examination is often of such great diagnostic importance that it is responsible for the saying, "If you don't put your finger in it, you'll put your foot in it." The rectal examination must be considered an essential part of a thorough physical examination and must be performed on every patient. If carefully done, this procedure causes little or no discomfort and often yields vital information.

Only a few pieces of equipment are needed for this examination. These include an adequate light source for inspection of the anus and perianal area, lubricating jelly, and either gloves or finger cots. Ordinarily no particular preparation is necessary. However, if the rectum is packed with feces, it is well to examine following a cleansing enema.

Positions of patient

1. *Left lateral.* The examination may be carried out with the patient in the left lateral position, lying on the left side with the thighs and knees flexed (Fig. 15-16). This is the most useful technique for the detection of masses within the rectum, since the rectal ampulla is pushed down and posteriorly in this position, making the mass more readily accessible.

2. *Knee-chest position.* The patient is on his

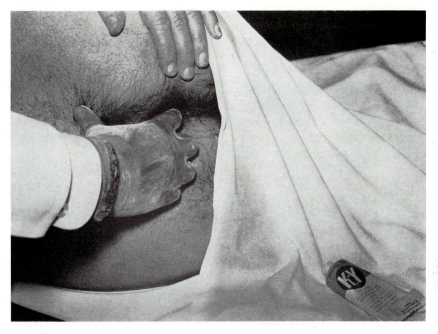

Fig. 15-16. Rectal examination with the patient in the left lateral position.

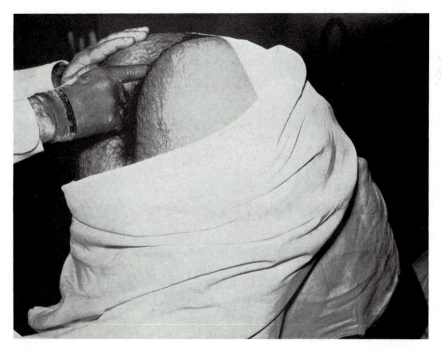

Fig. 15-17. Rectal examination with the patient in the knee-chest position.

knees with his shoulders and head on the examining table (Fig. 15-17). This position is particularly valuable in evaluating the size of the prostate gland.

3. *Bending over a table*. The rectal examination may be performed while the patient bends over a table, which should be about waist high. This position is widely used by urologists in prostatic evaluation and massage.

4. *Dorsolithotomy position*. In the female the rectal examination is done while the patient is in the dorsolithotomy position for examination of the pelvis. This position can also be used for rectal examination of the male, especially in the very ill patient.

Technique of examination

Following proper positioning of the patient, the area around the anus is first inspected for evidence of skin lesions, external hemorrhoids, fissure, or fistula. If a fissure or fistula is present, spreading of the buttocks and the immediate perianal region may result in considerable pain. Next, a small amount of lubricant is placed on the gloved index finger, which is then applied to the anal sphincter with gentle but steady pressure. After a few seconds there will be relaxation of the sphincter, at which time the finger will painlessly enter the anal canal and rectum. The examiner should note the tone of the anal sphincter and determine the presence or absence of stricture. Internal hemorrhoids cannot be felt unless thrombosis is present. The mucosa of the lateral and posterior walls of the rectum is palpated for tumor or polyps. The examining finger is then turned anteriorly, and an estimate is made of the size, shape, and consistency of the prostate. The examination of the prostate is discussed in Chapter 16.

After the examination of the palpable part of the rectum is completed, the patient is instructed to bear down. A mass that may not be felt under normal circumstances may be pushed down as much as 3 or 4 inches by this maneuver, making an otherwise inaccessible tumor palpable.

In the rectal examination of the female, the cervix presents as a small round mass in the anterior wall. The student should not confuse this normal finding with tumors or other lesions.

Cancer of intra-abdominal organs frequently spreads to the peritoneum anterior to the rectum. These malignant implants may be felt as hard nodules just above the prostate in the male and in the cul-de-sac in the female. These are known as "shelf" lesions.

Following the withdrawal of the finger, the character of any stool clinging to the glove should be noted. If it is very light tan or gray, it would suggest obstructive jaundice. If it is tarry black, the examiner should suspect upper gastrointestinal tract bleeding. In any event, the feces on the glove is an adequate specimen for a chemical test for the presence of blood, which should be performed after each rectal examination. If any abnormality is noted by digital examination, sigmoidoscopic examination is mandatory.

It has been variously estimated that routine sigmoidoscopy will disclose significant lesions in 5% to 10% of the individuals examined. The examining finger on a rectal examination will adequately cover the lower 6 to 8 cm. of the rectum. X-ray examination is satisfactory only above the level of 15 to 20 cm. This leaves a segment of 8 to 10 cm. in the upper portion of the rectum in which an adequate examination can be carried out only through the use of the sigmoidoscope. Since this is readily accessible to examination and is the site of many polyps and tumors, a physical examination should not be considered complete until this area of the bowel has been inspected by sigmoidoscopy, especially in patients over the age of 50. Sigmoidoscopy is a safe procedure and enables the examiner to detect many diseases in their early stage. In fact, the early detection of polyps and malignant lesions may be life saving.

EXAMINATION OF PATIENT WITH ACUTE ABDOMINAL PAIN

The physician is confronted with a particularly grave responsibility when examining a patient with acute abdominal pain. Speed is often essential, yet there are few events in clinical medicine where hasty and incomplete assessment have more adverse consequences. This situation, often referred to in medial jargon as an "acute abdomen" or "surgical abdomen," epitomizes the need for skill in physical diagnosis. Exceedingly important decisions often depend largely on clinical assessment supported only by a handful of relatively simple radiologic and laboratory aids. It is in this situation that the physician who has allowed sophisticated batteries of diagnostic tests to replace, rather than reinforce, his clinical assessment finds himself at a loss, since there is usually no time or place for these in the emergency case. Because of the special circumstances of these cases, it seems appropriate to include in this text introductory comments regarding the approach to such patients. As in the rest of this text, no attempt is made to cover disease entities in depth; therefore, the student should take care to study the unique historical and physical characteristics of these conditions as they are met later in his studies. It may be mentioned here that nearly all serious abdominal illness arises from inflammation, obstruction, infarction, perforation, or hemorrhage into or from one of the organs contained in the abdomen. Only a few pathophysiologic principles are involved in the evolution of most intra-abdominal illnesses, although the variety of clinical presentations, and overlap among them at first seems considerable. A systematic approach to the clinical assessment of patients with these illnesses helps in the application of these principles to individual diagnosis and management and clarifies the decision for early surgical treatment when appropriate.

History

The student should review the chapter on history and appreciate that the principles of collecting information are the same, even under emergency conditions. One should gather all relevant information in as concise a manner as appropriate, using friends or family, if available, to supplement information given by the patient. The patient's age, occupation, habits, previous medical history, and medication use may be pertinent, even in apparently new illness.

The pain should be characterized as completely as possible, beginning with nature and location at onset, and duration. It is almost axiomatic that most severe abdominal pains lasting six hours or more in patients previously well are caused by conditions requiring surgical therapy, hence the term "surgical abdomen." The exceptions can be defined only by prompt and continuing analysis of all signs and symptoms. The character of the pain and associated features—such as collapse or vomiting, change in location with time, radiation, recent bowel habits, diet, and medication—should be noted. In women the relationship to the menstrual cycle and abnormalities of the menses should be recorded. The relationship of the pain to vomiting, urination, defecation or passing flatus, inspiration, and changes in body position may be important.

Anatomic principles provide the basis for other axioms in the analysis of acute abdominal pain. Visceral pain originating in midline structures, or those that are embryologically derived from the midline, will usually be poorly localized at first, as seen early in cholecystitis, small bowel obstruction, and appendicitis, where early epigastric or periumbilical (midline) pain is the rule. When somatic pain follows as the condition evolves, its generalized or local nature will provide a clue to the location of the process as well as to the rate of progression. Because the examiner may first see the patient at variable times after the onset, a careful history of the sequential behavior of the pain is critical. Referral of pain often reflects the segment from which innervation is derived as well as the location of the organ. For example, diaphragmatic irritation of various etiologies (such as pleurisy, subphrenic abscess, or peritonitis caused by ruptured viscus) is often associated with shoulder pain because of afferent fibers in the phrenic nerve. Likewise, retroperitoneal inflammation in the pancreas or kidney may be felt in the back as well as the anterior abdomen.

Examination

Physical examination of the abdomen in acute conditions may be quite precise and is often the single most diagnostic maneuver. However, the same constraints regarding completeness and orderly examination mentioned before should not be abandoned here. In the urge to push on to abdominal palpation one should not omit first recording the vital signs and making serial observations of temperature and the state of the vascular system. Abnormal respiration may be a clue to underlying cardiopulmonary disease or impending collapse. Inspection of the patient can be completed by the experienced observer while taking the history, with pallor, sweating, abnormalities of mental status, state of hydration, and general health being noted. The immobile patient with peritonitis who resists moving in bed may be distinguishable from the patient suffering colic who is typically restless and agitated. The contour of the abdomen should be observed, and

if indicated, girth should be measured and recorded.

Auscultation again precedes palpation, but here the presence or absence of bowel sounds is the major concern, for peritonitis and bowel obstruction are major differential diagnoses. Percussion should then be carried out lightly, as an adjunct and preliminary to palpation, for the purpose of outlining organ enlargement and bladder distention, for evaluating fluid and air distribution in the abdominal contents, and for detecting local areas of tenderness.

Next, palpation of the abdomen is performed, with two major goals: to evaluate the tone of the abdominal wall muscles, that is, to detect rigidity, and to define areas of tenderness. Often rigidity and tenderness are maximal in the same area if generalized peritonitis has not developed. It often is not necessary to demonstrate rebound tenderness or to palpate deeply to elicit definite findings. It bears repeating that gentle examination of an apprehensive patient, who is assured that you will do nothing to cause him undue discomfort, is most fruitful. On occasion, the examiner should assess the effect of respiration on the abdominal findings, as when the descent of an inflamed gallbladder during inspiration and palpation sharply increases the local tenderness in the right upper quadrant.

A few additional comments are especially relevant to this situation. The pelvis should not be overlooked as a source of acute abdominal pain. However, innervation of the pelvis is not represented in the abdominal wall muscle, so pelvic inflammation may not be associated with abdominal wall rigidity or tenderness. Prostatitis and pelvic inflammatory disease may be associated with considerable hypogastric pain but present few findings on abdominal palpation. In contrast, rectal or pelvic examination may reveal tenderness, enlarged organ, or a mass. Also, the iliopsoas and obturator internus muscles may be affected by local intra-abdominal inflammation and their examination by two additional maneuvers is sometimes of value. Testing for iliopsoas rigidity by extending the thigh on the affected side while the patient lies on the opposite side is useful in some patients with posterior abdominal inflammation, such as retrocecal appendicitis. Similarly, stretching the obturator internus by rotation of the flexed thigh on the affected side will produce pain if this muscle is in contact with a local inflammatory lesion. Finally, the patient with an acute abdominal condition should be examined for hernia since it is a common cause of intestinal obstruction.

Culmination of these efforts usually leads to a working differential diagnosis and a decision regarding the imminent need for surgical intervention. It is, therefore, pertinent to end with a partial but representative list of nonsurgical conditions that may, on occasion, simulate abdominal catastrophes. Among the more commonly encountered conditions are acute food poisoning and gastroenteritis, diabetic ketoacidosis, pleurisy and pneumonia, myocardial infarction, pericarditis, congestive heart failure, and genitourinary tract infection. Less common considerations include acute intermittent porphyria, periodic peritonitis (familial Mediterranean fever), lead colic, tabes dorsalis, typhoid fever, and intestinal tuberculosis. Extravisceral conditions, such as acute vertebral osteomyelitis and herpes, may be included. These nonsurgical problems are mentioned to remind the student that not all "acute abdomens" are "surgical abdomens." Application of the preceding diagnostic principles guides the physician to the proper diagnosis.

SELECTED READINGS

Castell, D. O.: The spleen percussion sign, Ann. Intern. Med. 67:1265-1267, 1967.

Castell, D. O., and others: Estimation of liver size by percussion in normal individuals, Ann. Intern. Med. 70:1183-1189, 1969.

Cope, Z.: The early diagnosis of the acute abdomen, ed. 13, London, 1968, Oxford University Press, Inc.

Cope, Z.: A sign in gallbladder disease, Br. Med. J. 3:147-148, 1970.

Corman, M. L., and others: Proctosigmoidoscopy—Age criteria for examination in the asymptomatic patient, CA 25:286-290, 1975.

Sleisenger, M. H., and Fordtran, J. S.: Gastrointestinal disease, ed. 2, Philadelphia, 1978, W. B. Saunders Co.

Spiro, H. M.: Clinical gastroenterology, ed. 2, New York, 1977, MacMillan, Inc.

CHAPTER 16

GENITALIA

MALE GENITALIA

Inspection and palpation of the external genitalia in the male can result in a high degree of accuracy in the diagnosis of abnormalities. However, because of wide variation in the appearance of normal male genitalia, the examiner must rely on a careful history, inspection, and palpation to distinguish healthy, normal structures from those that are malformed or diseased. Diseases and disorders of the male genitalia vary widely and frequently are related to other systems of the body. In order to carry out a successful examination the patient should be put as much at ease as possible, especially if the patient is a child.

Penis

The foreskin, if uncircumcised, should be gently retracted and the penis examined for cleanliness and lesions of the prepuce and glans penis, including glandular adhesions, smegma collections, or any irregularities of the skin or glans, such as new growths or ulcerations that may be associated with systemic diseases, such as diabetes mellitus.

The normal foreskin should be soft and pliable without breaks in continuity. At times retraction of the foreskin is difficult, and this con-

dition, called *phimosis*, may require an incision to enable exposure of the glans penis. Phimosis, which is relatively uncommon in infants, is characterized by adhesions of the prepuce to the underlying glans penis, which prevent retraction. Normally these adhesions will separate spontaneously or can be broken by insertion of a probe beneath the foreskin. Care must be taken to avoid forced stretching of the prepuce, which may cause radial splitting of the foreskin resulting in inflammation, with subsequent scarring and contracture, and leading to an acquired phimosis (Fig. 16-1). This is frequently encountered in an adult who has developed irritation resulting from retained bacteria, urine, and cellular debris *(smegma)* beneath the prepucal sac.

The foreskin may be found retracted over the glans, swollen and inflamed, so that reduction of the skin forward to cover the glans becomes impossible. This is termed *paraphimosis* and may require an incision of the constricting ring, with local anesthesia, to allow replacement of the foreskin over the glans. The foreskin should always be replaced over the glans after examination, particularly in elderly men, in order to avoid this difficulty.

Ammoniacal dermatitis is seen frequently in

children but may also be encountered in the elderly or incontinent patient. This results from the breakdown of urea by bacteria, releasing ammonia, which causes a bright erythema of the penile skin and glans and, at times, the scrotum.

The penis should be inspected for size and position of the urethral meatus. In the young male the meatus, at times, is quite tight (*meatal stenosis*) as a result of the presence of a thin membrane at the meatal opening. Also, there may be an inflammatory reaction (*meatitis*) or slight ulceration about the meatus, especially in newly circumcised infants, because of ammoniacal wet diapers.

Hypospadias is one of the most common anomalies of the penis. In this condition the urinary meatus lies on the ventral aspect of the penis—and may be on the glans, penile shaft, scrotum, or perineum—because of failure of fusion of the genital folds (Fig. 16-2). Also, the prepuce is incomplete on the ventral surface and forms an excessive amount of foreskin of the dorsal side of the penis. This is the *hood*

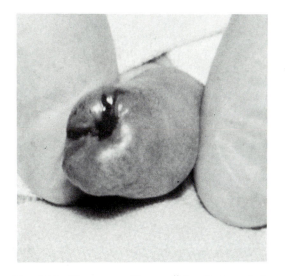

Fig. 16-1. Phimosis with a radial splitting of the foreskin caused by forceful retraction.

and should not be removed routinely by circumcision, since it will be needed for future repair of these defects. In the most extreme of these imperfectly formed phalluses the scrotum also must be thoroughly examined for the presence of gonads in order to rule out an intersex problem. In·the absence of testes chromosomal studies must be conducted for identification of the proper gender. There is frequently, but not always, an associated ventral curvature of the penis called *chordee* caused by a restricting band of tissue between the glans and the meatus (Fig. 16-2, *A*). These bands usually result from adherence of extracorporeal strands of inelastic tissue to the glans or to the corpora cavernosa. Rarely, a chordee may be present in the absence of a hypospadias (Fig. 16-3). There also may be an associated torsion or rotation of the penis, probably from the same developmental failure, wherein the median raphe of ventral penile skin is off to one side or the other (Fig. 16-2, *A*).

A similar defect of an entirely different embryologic origin may involve the position of the meatus on the dorsum of the penis. This is referred to as *epispadias*, a condition in which the opening is located on the glans or the dorsal shaft and may involve the puboprostatic urethra and the bladder neck (Fig. 16-4). In extreme or third degree epispadias there is absence of urinary sphincter control, with an associated failure of closure of the symphysis pubis similar to that seen in exstrophy of the bladder.

Exstrophy is a more extreme developmental failure in which the anterior wall of the bladder and the ventral wall of the lower abdomen have failed to close, and the bladder mucosa is exposed (Fig. 16-5). The umbilical cord is attached to the margin of the exstrophied bladder, and the umbilicus as such is absent. In the presence of these developmental anomalies the anal orifice is in a more ventral than normal position, the scrotum is flatter than usual, and

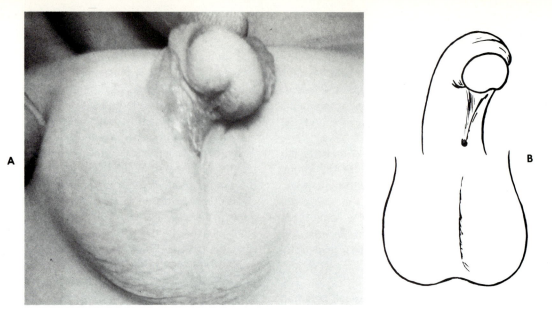

Fig. 16-2. A, Penoscrotal hypospadias with chordee and mild torsion of the penis. There is a dorsal hood present. **B,** A drawing of the penoscrotal hypospadias, showing the contracting bands of the chordee more clearly.

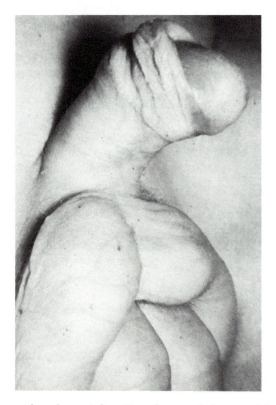

Fig. 16-3. Chordee without hypospadias. Note the partial absence of the ventral foreskin.

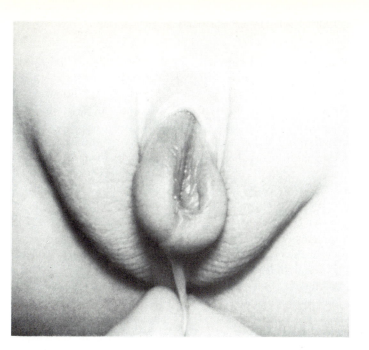

Fig. 16-4. Epispadias showing the failure of fusion of the dorsal surface of the penis and urethra. There is a ventral hood present.

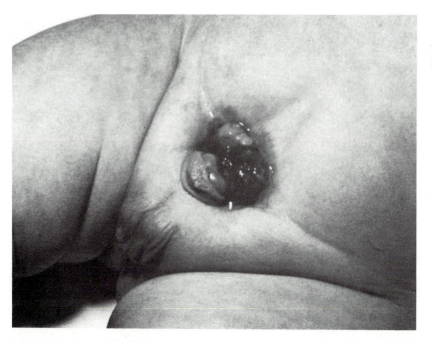

Fig. 16-5. Exstrophy of the bladder with a complete epispadias defect of the penis. The mucosal surface of the bladder is exposed.

the shaft of the penis is short with an epispadic urethra open to the glans. In the female the clitoris is usually bifid.

When the urethra does not appear at the tip of the glans, as in hypospadias or epispadias, the foreskin is not fully developed and appears as a hood attached either in a dorsal or ventral position on the penis.

In the United States most males are circumcised in the newborn period because of religious and family tradition as well as for hygienic reasons. It is of interest that the Committee on Circumcision of the American Academy of Pediatrics states that there is no good reason for routine circumcision and that it is contraindicated in prematurity, jaundice, and in the presence of developmental abnormalities of the penis, such as hypospadias. However, a good argument for routine circumcision can be made, for in countries where hygiene is inadequate, incidence of carcinoma of the penis is extremely high where circumcision is not practiced, while it is extremely low in areas where circumcision is routine.

Acquired lesions are usually seen in the adult as growths, tumors, and infections and should be carefully noted.

In the uncircumcised adult the foreskin may be normal, pliable, and easily retracted. On the other hand, there may be constriction of the foreskin, with or without inflammation, which prevents retraction. Occasionally there is a scarred area around the opening and splitting of the skin accompanied by varying degrees of inflammation. This cracking often occurs in diabetic patients. The glans in these patients may be raw, frequently as a result of yeast infections. Cultures for aerobic and anaerobic bacteria and for fungal infections should be made. If there is any urethral discharge, which may be gonorrheal or nonspecific in origin, cultures should be obtained. Any discharge should be placed on a clean glass slide for staining and microscopic examination to identify the infecting organism. Of the inflammatory conditions, *herpes progenitalis* is frequently present in the uncircumcised patient.

Primary syphilis produces a watery, at times ulcerated, firm, pale, nodular lesion either of the prepuce or along the coronal sulcus and at times involves the glans penis. The *chancre* can be scarified and a bit of fluid examined by darkfield microscopy for the presence of spirochetes (*T. pallidum*).

Epidermoid or *squamous cell carcinoma* of the penis may be seen in the coronal area and should be suspected in the presence of a raised, firm, at times ulcerated, lesion that also may involve the foreskin and glans (Fig. 16-6). Advanced lesions may be cauliflowerlike, fungating, and foulsmelling, with purulent discharge. Microscopic examination of a biopsy specimen is necessary to establish the correct diagnosis.

Precancerous lesions, which vary in their appearance, include *Bowen's disease, erythroplasia of Queyrat, leukoplakia*, and *Paget's disease*. These growths require biopsy to establish an accurate diagnosis. They must be differentiated from inflammatory lesions such as *condyloma acuminata* (venereal warts) of viral etiology. Other viral infections, such as *herpes simplex* and *herpes zoster,* also can occur on the penis.

Condyloma latum is the highly infectious manifestation of secondary syphilis characterized by flat mucoid lesions that may be seen on the glans penis as well as the foreskin and scrotum.

Other rare, and often difficult to diagnose, lesions that may involve the penis are *chancroid* (soft chancre), *lymphogranuloma venereum,* and *granuloma inguinale*.

Balanitis xerotica obliterans is a chronic inflammatory process resulting in sclerotic epithelial changes of the urethral meatus. It is characterized by a whitish perimeatal discoloration, with stenosis of the meatus, and also may involve the foreskin in uncircumcised males. This must be differentiated by a biopsy from leukoplakia, which is a precancerous condition.

Erection is the engorgement of the corpora, producing elongation and rigidity of the penis. Various conditions that may alter this normal state of erection can be detected by careful inspection and palpation of even a flaccid organ. In fact, the penile shaft is best examined in the flaccid state. The history may reveal that erections are only partial or incomplete and this, in fact, may be the patient's chief complaint. Un-

satisfactory erection may be caused by physiologic, psychologic, or anatomic causes. *Priapism,* a prolonged or sustained painful erection, may result from coexisting disease, such as sickle cell anemia (Fig. 16-7) and high spinal cord lesions, but may occasionally be from excessive sexual excitement and stimulation. Rarely, diabetes and drug ingestion may be associated with priapism.

Peyronie's disease results from a localized fibrotic thickening of the tissue about the corpora cavernosa. Plaques may be palpated along

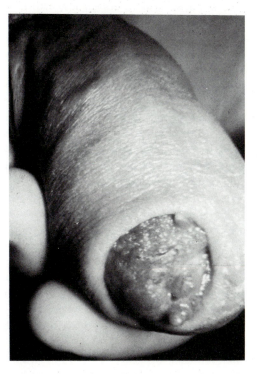

Fig. 16-6. Squamous cell carcinoma of the glans penis with an intact foreskin.

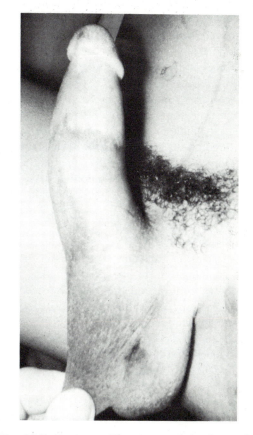

Fig. 16-7. Priapism. This is a prolonged, painful erection of the penis of a 15-year-old boy with sickle cell disease.

the penile shaft, usually on the dorsum but sometimes involving any part of the corpora cavernosa. Inelasticity produces angulation or curvature of the penile shaft on erection, which may be very painful. There is a high correlation between Peyronie's disease and Dupuytren's contracture of the palmar fascia. Differential diagnosis requires the consideration of fibrosis secondary to trauma, severe urethritis, late syphilitic lesions, penile infiltration with lymphogranuloma venereum, benign and malignant tumors, and congenital curvature.

Rarely, the corpora cavernosa exhibit nodular lesions metastatic from carcinoma of the prostate, rectum, or bladder. At times there may be a direct extension to the corpora from carcinoma of the urethra, characterized by a firm nodular area along the ventral penile shaft.

Urethral stricture produces an indurated area that may be identified by careful palpation along the penile urethra but can be more easily identified by the passage of a urethral sound or catheter. Occasionally strictures may be recognized by the presence of an indolent, firm, tender mass that may involve even the skin over the penile shaft.

Scrotum and its contents

The scrotum is a musculocutaneous pouch that contains the testes, epididymides, and spermatic cords. It functions as a thermal regulator, keeping the testes one to two degrees cooler than normal body temperature. Its external appearance varies under different circumstances. In the old and debilitated individual or when the scrotum is warm, it is elongated and flaccid; in the young and robust or when cold, it is wrinkled and short and firmly hugs the testes. The left scrotal sac usually hangs lower than the right due to the greater length of the left spermatic cord.

Normally both testes are in the scrotum at or shortly after birth. About 14% of testes are undescended at birth, but by 1 year of age only 4% remain so. The scrotum and its contents can be palpated with the patient in a standing or recumbent position; however, examination for position of the testes must be very gentle, for any stimulation of the scrotum or inner thigh may elicit the cremasteric reflex and cause the testes to be retracted into the inguinal canal *(migratory testis)*. In the presence of a very active cremasteric reflex in a child, he should be asked to take a knee-chest stance, and the testis will return to the scrotum. A hot tub bath may also relax the cremasteric muscle and allow the testis to descend into its normal intrascrotal position.

Congenital defects of the scrotum are not uncommon, particularly in association with intersex problems where there is ambiguity of the external genitalia. A *bifid scrotum* is usually associated with an extensive degree of hypospadias as well as other developmental anomalies of the penis. The scrotum is flat and anterior in the child with exstrophy of the bladder. In the child with undescended testes there may be no scrotal pouch development, or there may be unilateral failure of development. Both scrotal development and descent of the testes result from stimulation by androgenic hormones. Normal skin coloration may vary widely, as does pigmentation, which is usually more prominent in the virile male.

Dermatologic lesions that may be encountered on the scrotum are *hemangiomata, varicosities, sebaceous cysts, lipoma,* and varieties of *venereal warts (papular lesions* or *flat condylomata)*. Papillary tumors, even squamous cell or epidermoid, may involve the scrotal wall.

The scrotum and the inner aspects of the thighs are frequently affected by fungal infections, especially in hot, humid climates. The scrotum is prey to infections, and the skin may rapidly ulcerate or become gangrenous. Such infections are frequently streptococcal in origin and represent a serious problem because progression from cellulitis to gangrene may occur in 48 to 72 hours. On examination of a rather indurated, reddened area, careful inspection for a break in the skin is indicated. Exudate should be cultured and examined by gram stain for the offending organism. *Pseudomonas,* *Candida albicans,* and *Streptococcus* are frequent causes of soft-tissue infections. *Streptococcus,* the most frequent organism causing scrotal cellulitis, seldom has a discernible port of entry. In any case, fluid accumulates rapidly in the space between Colles and Buck's fascia, producing intense swelling of the scrotum. If this swelling is not immediately reduced, devascularization of the scrotum and penile skin occurs rapidly.

Edema of the scrotum may be the result of systemic or localized disease (Fig. 16-8). It can accompany chronic congestive heart failure, cirrhosis of the liver, and chronic nephritis. Carcinoma of the prostate, various localized conditions (such as torsion of the testes in young males), and debilitation associated with hypoproteinemia or malignancies may produce severe scrotal swelling. Scrotal edema in an older male that cannot be explained by some of the foregoing causes should arouse suspicion of carcinoma of the prostate, especially if the swelling is unilateral or associated with edema of the thigh. Massive scrotal swelling *(elephantiasis)* caused by lymphatic blockage with microfilaria *(F. bancrofti)* occurs in tropical climates. A nonfilarial lymphatic fibrosis also can produce scrotal edema.

Pathologic intrascrotal masses are frequently encountered. The most frequent mass is a *hydrocele,* which is an accumulation of fluid in the tunica vaginalis. This is a common finding, occurring in about 7.5% of all males. It is present most often in children, but it does oc-

cur in adults frequently enough to justify concern when a scrotal mass is encountered. Diagnosis is usually simple because the scrotum is thin, smooth, and elastic and the cystic character of the hydrocele is easily appreciated on palpation. Light is readily transilluminated through a hydrocele, except when thickening of the tunica vaginalis occurs on the basis of an inflammatory reaction.

Hydrocele may extend along the cord into the inguinal canal. Occasionally one encounters a hydrocele of the cord that is different from a

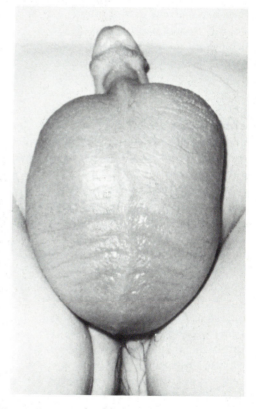

Fig. 16-8. Scrotal edema as seen with acute epididymitis. This amount of edema may be seen in torsion of the spermatic cord and other intrascrotal inflammatory lesions.

true scrotal hydrocele. In children the hydrocele may communicate with the peritoneal cavity through a patent processus vaginalis that accompanies the descent of the testis into the scrotum. A hydrocele may mask epididymal and testicular tumors and obscure normal scrotal masses, such as the testis. Aspiration of a hydrocele makes possible precise differentiation of the scrotal contents.

The testis is situated in the posterior, inferior portion of the scrotum below and behind the hydrocele. Differentiation of a hydrocele from a hernia may be difficult, especially if the hernia cannot be reduced. However, in the presence of a hernia, bowel sounds may be audible, and usually there is a much thicker cord that transmits an impulse on coughing.

Other fluid-filled scrotal masses include *spermatocele* and *cyst of the epididymis*. These too can be transilluminated. Aspirate from these cysts placed on a microscopic slide usually contains sperm.

Varicocele is characterized by abnormal dilatation and tortuosity of the spermatic veins so that the scrotum feels like a bag of worms when the patient is standing. The outline of these veins can be seen through the scrotal wall, to which they add a bluish tint when transilluminated. When the patient is placed in the supine position, the engorged veins disappear in a few minutes; however, they transmit an impulse on coughing or straining. A varicocele is rarely seen before puberty and is nearly always encountered on the left side because of the incompetence of the valves of the left spermatic veins. If the right scrotum is involved, spermatic vein obstruction is probably the result of extrinsic pressure from a retroperitoneal tumor, such as lymphoma or invasion by a neoplasm. In such cases intravenous pyelography should be carried out. Varicoceles are usually asymptomatic, but when the swelling is prominent, they may cause a dragging sensation or

dull pain in the scrotum and lower abdomen, especially on strenuous activity.

Testis

The normal testis may vary in size, shape, and consistency. It usually lies in the scrotum with its long axis in a vertical position, but may lie in a transverse position, in which case intrascrotal torsion is more likely to occur.

The consistency of a normal testis may vary from very firm and smooth to very soft, almost mushy. The softer testis is more apt to be present in the elderly male. Along the posterior border of the testis is a ridge of tissue, called the epididymis, which is usually adherent and has about the same consistency as the testis itself. Nodularity of either the upper or lower pole indicates the presence of chronic infection or fibrosis.

Epididymitis (specific or nonspecific) is the most common of all intrascrotal, inflammatory lesions in the adult male. In conjunction with orchitis or urinary infection it may also affect the prepubertal child. Acute infection of the epididymis produces a firm, exquisitely tender enlargement of the entire epididymal body, occasionally with extension along the spermatic cord. The scrotal wall usually is extensively swollen and reddened (Fig. 16-8). Acute epididymitis may be encountered at all ages but is seen most often in the vigorous young male. It rarely involves the testis. It appears in the upper pole (globus minor) and produces marked tenderness and swelling of the vas deferens.

In chronic epididymitis abscesses may result in suppuration of the testis and scrotal wall. There is central softening from which pus can be aspirated for culture. Staphylococcus and colon bacilli can usually be cultured from the urine. Gonorrheal infections should be considered when there is an associated urethritis. In a "cold abscess" that has been present for a long time, tubercle bacilli may be found. In tuberculous epididymitis the prostate, seminal vesicles, and vasa deferens are usually beaded or nodular.

Inflammation of the testis *(orchitis)* is rarely encountered in the absence of epididymal infection. Acute orchitis is usually seen 4 to 6 days after mumps parotitis and may occur in association with other systemic diseases, such as infectious mononucleosis. Pyogenic orchitis is encountered rarely, again usually in association with epididymitis. Central abscess formation may involve the scrotal wall and result in a palpable fluctuation.

Enlargement of the cord, epididymis, and testis also may result from trauma. Following vasal ligation as a means of birth control, a firm, nodular, somewhat tender mass may be palpable in the lower cord or epididymis because of a sperm granuloma. This can be diagnosed when there is a history of vasal ligation, but one must consider the possibility of testicular tumor.

A tumor of the testis may appear as a painless, asymmetrically enlarged, firm, heavy, and sometimes nodular scrotal mass (Fig. 16-9). The overlying skin is rarely attached to the underlying, primary tumor, although attachment may exist in lymphomatous involvement of the testis. Edema and redness seldom appear except as corollaries to inflammation and trauma.

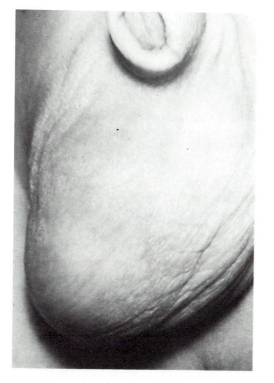

Fig. 16-9. Unilateral scrotal enlargement as seen with a right testis tumor. Notice absence of edema of the scrotal wall.

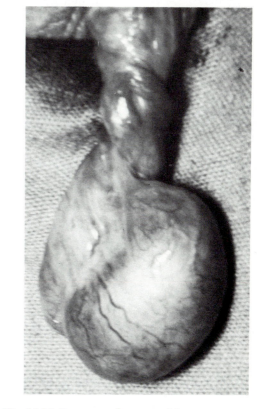

Fig. 16-10. Intravaginal torsion of the spermatic cord with testicular infarction.

The mass seldom, if ever, transilluminates light unless there is accompanying hydrocele that may mask the tumor's presence.

Torsion of the spermatic cord with infarction of the testis is a frequently misdiagnosed intrascrotal lesion and may be confused with an acute epididymitis (Fig. 16-10). If recognized early, the twisted testis may be rotated by a surgical procedure in time to prevent the loss of vital tissue of the testis. This condition is most frequently seen in children, but may be present at birth as well as in the elderly.

Torsion is caused by an anomalous investment of the tissues derived from the peritoneum and abdominal wall. Twisting can and usually does occur intravaginally, but can occur proximal to the investing tunica vaginalis (Fig. 16-11). The scrotum is swollen and reddened, and the testis is exquisitely tender, elevated, and cannot be transilluminated, making precise examination almost impossible. The patient is reluctant to stand and will grab the examiner's hand to prevent manipulation of the cord and testis. The newborn and very young seldom exhibit tenderness because of a lack of development of pyramidal tracts in the spinal cord.

The spermatic cord above the twist is quite tender but usually not swollen as is the case in epididymitis. Body temperature may be slightly elevated, and leukocytosis usually is present. Normally, the urine is clear. Torsion and infarction of other mullerian remnants, such as the appendix testis (hydatid of Morgagni), appendix epididymis, vasa aberrantia, or paradidymis, present similar findings but to a lesser degree.

Infection—acute, subacute, or chronic—may involve the spermatic cord (*funiculitis*), and while usually a complication of disease elsewhere in the urinary tract it also can be metastatic from foci elsewhere in the body.

Spermatocele and epididymal cysts are nontender, round masses palpable along the epididymis or cord. They are distinctly separate from the testis and can be transilluminated.

Spontaneous thrombosis of the pampiniform plexus of veins may resemble acute inflammation of the cord structures and is characterized by a history of sudden pain in the scrotum followed by an enlargement of the spermatic cord.

A frequently encountered scrotal mass is the indirect inguinal hernia, which is discussed in Chapter 15.

Prostate

A careful evaluation of the prostate is an essential part of any physical examination in the male. Digital examination can be made with the patient standing beside the bed or examining table, leaning forward with hands on knees or lying on the bed in a knee-chest position. A less satisfactory examination can be made with the patient in bed on his back with his knees drawn up or with his heels in stirrups on an examining table; however, this does permit a bimanual examination of the bladder region. In a debilitated patient a satisfactory prostate examination can be conducted with the patient lying on his side with his knees drawn toward his abdomen.

The gloved examining finger should be well

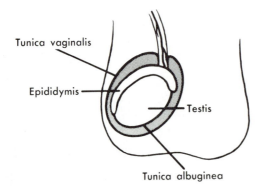

Tunica vaginalis

Epididymis

Testis

Tunica albuginea

Fig. 16-11. A complete intravaginal testis (bell clapper) that allows the rotation of the testis in the tunica vaginalis.

lubricated and introduced gently into the anal orifice. If this is carried out too rapidly or vigorously the procedure may be painful and result in sphincter spasm, in which case the examiner will have to allow the patient to relax before continuing the examination. Much more information can be obtained by performing this examination gently and tactfully. The examiner should first examine the lower rectum (Chapter

15), then the prostate, which can be palpated on the anterior rectal wall (Fig. 16-12).

Examination. The normal prostate is described by Dr. Reed Nesbit in a letter to his father as follows:

One gland in the adult is about the size and shape of a chestnut and weighs less than an ounce. The first part of the urinary passage where it leaves the bladder channels directly through this gland in

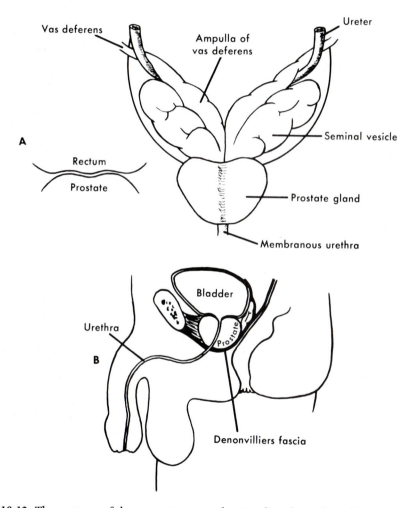

Fig. 16-12. The anatomy of the prostatic region showing the relationship of the normal prostate to the rectum, seminal vesicles, and base of the bladder.

such a way that the lining of the urethra at this point is comprised of the exposed inner surface of the gland. This arrangement explains why enlargements of the gland tend to encroach upon the urethral channel and cause obstruction to the normal flow of urine. . . . The location of the prostate gland is such that its posterior surface comes into close proximity with the rectum, so that it can be examined by touch when a finger is introduced into the rectum. Thus palpation of the prostate gland by rectum is an integral part of every complete physical examination carried out on the male, just as a vaginal examination is in the female.

Enlargement of the prostate gland, and resulting interference with urination (Fig. 16-13), occurs in about one third of elderly men. The enlargement may not be directly proportional to the degree of obstruction, since a very small gland may sometimes produce complete obstruction and a very large gland very little. The degree of obstruction cannot always be detected by digital examination alone, but must be demonstrated by x-ray or cystoscopic examination and by determination of the amount of residual urine in the bladder.

The prostate gland is rather smooth, elastic, discretely outline, and slightly movable (Fig. 16-12). A median groove or furrow that normally extends along the posterior surface up toward the base of the bladder is obliterated when the lobes of the prostate are hypertrophied or involved with carcinoma. Seventy-five percent of all carcinoma of the prostate arises in the posterior lobe, which is palpable on rectal examination. A notch is palpable at the base of the gland at the junction of the bladder neck. The seminal vesicles extend up laterally from the prostatic base beneath the bladder and usually are not palpable unless they are diseased. If any secretions are produced by prostatic palpation or massage, a specimen should be placed on a glass slide for microscopic examination to determine the presence of bacteria as well as cellular elements.

The consistency of the prostatic tissue is usually firm and rubbery, but may vary from a very soft, fluctuant texture that suggests prostatic abscess (Fig. 16-14), soft carcinoma, or congestive prostatitis to a stony hard nodularity that may involve small areas or the entire gland. These hard areas may not involve the entire gland, but usually are limited by the capsular margins and suggest granulomatous prostatitis, prostatic calculi, prostatic infarction, tuberculosis, or localized carcinoma (Fig. 16-15 and 16-16). Extensive carcinoma may involve the capsule and periprostatic tissues. Carcinoma of the prostate tends to extend up beneath the base of the bladder and the region of seminal vesicles to form a shelf or plateau (Fig. 16-17). Usually this periprostatic invasion is limited by Denonvillier's fascia, but once this barrier has been broken circumferential extension about the rectum occurs.

Various terms have been used to describe the size of the prostate gland. On rectal palpation the normal gland is roughly 2 to 3 cm. across its midportion, which is about twice the width of the examining finger. A slightly enlarged gland, classified 1+, is about three fingerbreadths across and a 2+ gland is about two times the normal breadth. A 3+ classification defines a considerably larger gland, while a gland termed 4+ occupies most of the anterior pelvic outlet, with marked encroachment of the posterior lobe on the rectal wall reducing the caliber of the rectal passage.

The consistency is described as first degree in the slightly softer than normal gland, second degree in the gland with benign hypertrophy (rubbery), and third degree in the stony hard gland (from carcinoma, prostatic calculi, and chronic fibrosis). These degrees of induration are designated by lines on the diagram of the prostate (Fig. 16-18): first degree, a single set of lines; second degree, crossed or two sets of lines; and third degree, three sets of lines.

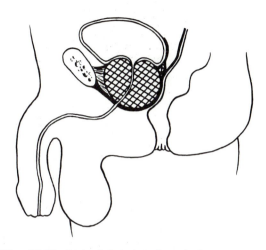

Fig. 16-13. Sagittal drawing showing benign prostatic hypertrophy projecting through the bladder neck into the bladder. This may produce varying degrees of obstruction of the bladder outlet.

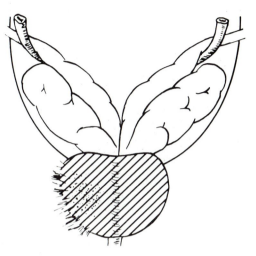

Fig. 16-14. Prostatic abscess showing some softness of the left prostatic lobe with periprostatic capsular adhesions.

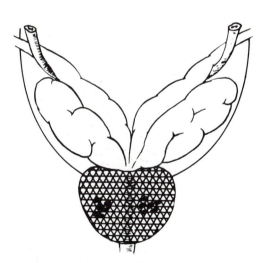

Fig. 16-15. Firm (third degree), nodular prostate with pockets of prostatic calculi. Crepitation may be felt on digital examination over these areas.

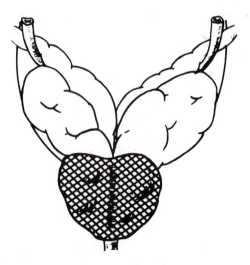

Fig. 16-16. Localized areas (nodules) of prostatic induration that may represent either areas of prostatic infarction, tuberculosis, or localized carcinoma.

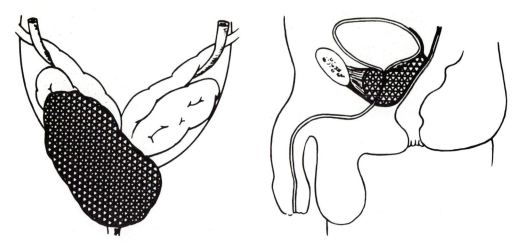

Fig. 16-17. Extension or shelving of the carcinoma of the prostate up beneath the bladder and seminal vesicles.

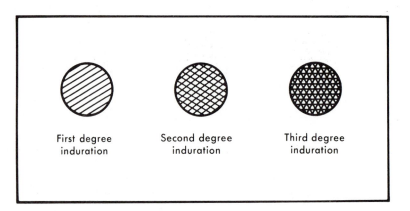

Fig. 16-18. Diagrammatic designation of degrees of prostatic induration.

Neurologic examination of genitalia

A neurologic examination of the external genitalia and anal sphincter may help to determine neural defects in these areas.

A careful history, revealing deficiencies in the patient's erectile capabilities, ability to ejaculate, urinary continence, and voluntary bowel control is of great value in focusing sus-

picion on the existence of a neurologic lesion of the sacral cord segments.

The patient's inability to perceive touch, pain, and temperature in the perineal and scrotal areas, as well as a lack of sensation of bladder distention are fundamental signs that suggest the presence of cord lesions.

Evaluation of the rectal sphincter tone and

the anal and bulbocavernosus reflex directs attention to a possible lesion at the level of the conus. A patulous anal sphincter reflects a defect at S3, S4, and S5, which also supply the urinary sphincters. The ability to voluntarily contract the anal sphincter on the examiner's finger indicates a normal neurologic status. A pinprick at the anal mucocutaneous junction will elicit a strong sphincter contraction, termed the anal reflex, that is mediated by S2, S3, S4, or S5. The bulbocavernosus reflex (S3-S4) is an anal sphincter contraction that can be elicited and evaluated by gently squeezing the glans penis or tugging on an indwelling Foley catheter while the examiner's finger is in the rectum.

Presence of reflex voiding or incontinence (neurogenic bladder) with a positive bulbocavernosus reflex indicates the possibility of a cauda equina lesion. Overflow incontinence can be indicative of either upper or lower motor neuron lesions.

Reflex incontinence usually indicates the presence of an upper motor neuron lesion. Continuous dribbling in the absence of obstruction, but with a distended bladder, usually indicates a lower motor neuron lesion. Diurnal or nocturnal enuresis that persists beyond the age of 8 to 10 years may reflect a neurogenic disorder or injury of the central nervous system, although it must also be ascertained that these symptoms are not of psychogenic origin.

Status of possible cord lesions may be further assessed by evaluation of the cremasteric reflexes (L1, L2) and the lower superficial abdominal reflexes, T11 and T12.

As a result of crowding of segments in the lower cord, a lesion of the conus medullaris usually involves multiple levels. Thus, the ankle jerks, (L5, S1) will be depressed or absent while the knee jerks (L2, L3) are normal or slightly increased. If the lesion is chronic, the legs are atrophic and often asymmetric.

Sensations of pressure and stretch in the fibers of the cauda equina arise from cord levels of L2 and below and at bone levels as high as T-10. Lesions in this area cause back pain, spasm in the paravertebral muscles, splinting of the back, and night pain resulting from relaxation of these muscles in sleep.

Upper motor neuron lesions responsible for incontinence and decreased bladder capacity in children may be reflected by shortened Achilles tendons, a tendency to tiptoe in early walking, and later a clumsy, spastic gait. Electromyographic studies contribute to more precise evaluation of the neural deficits in these areas.

FEMALE GENITALIA

In no other small space in the body are there so many interrelated physiologic functons—micturition, defecation, menstruation, ovulation, copulation, impregnation, and parturition. An abnormality in any one pelvic organ may easily produce signs, symptoms, or abnormal findings in another. During the pelvic examination the physician should take advantage of the opportunity to incorporate any additional important details of the history. This is particularly true in localizing areas or points of pain and tenderness and in the differentiation of adnexal, ureteral, and intestinal pain, as well as vaginal, uterine, rectal, and bladder discomfort. It must be remembered that abnormalities of pelvic organs, some of which are very serious, may be absolutely asymptomatic. The examiner must be cognizant of the fact that abnormal symptoms and findings within the pelvis may be produced by pathologic conditions of other systems outside the pelvis, such as the upper urinary and gastrointestinal tracts, the endocrine glands, the neuromusculoskeletal system, and perhaps as important, the psyche. Thus, it is essential in taking a history to correlate the complaint of pain with the functions of all of the organs within and including the bony pelvis.

In the pelvic area there are two general organ types. Part of the viscera are hollow and often are the source of colicky pain. Disease involving the solid organs usually results in continuous pain. The nerve supply of the pelvic organs is visceral, but pain symptoms caused by pelvic disease have fairly constant points of somatic reference.

In women of menstruating age, pain symptoms often are closely associated with various stages of the menstrual cycle. These associations should be recorded, since the pain of common disease processes of the female genitalia tend to follow characteristic cyclic patterns. For instance, the discomfort of pelvic inflammatory disease tends to become increasingly severe prior to menstruation and is relieved by the onset of the flow. The pain of endometriosis does not begin until the onset of menstruation and increases during the menstrual flow. Pelvic discomfort may be related to the patient's activity and indirectly to the time of day. In the case of uterine displacement, and especially prolapse of the uterus, pelvic discomfort and backache are more pronounced when the patient is on her feet; she feels best on arising in the morning. The longer she is on her feet, the greater the discomfort; thus, her symptoms are most pronounced in the evening. In the absence of prolapse, these symptoms suggest pelvic congestion caused by varicosities of the pelvic veins or congestion from other causes. Pelvic symptoms, whether pain, vaginal discharge, or bleeding, may have a direct relationship to defecation or urination. These relationships may also be influenced by the various stages of the menstrual cycle, by sexual intercourse, nervous tension, or physical exercise.

An accurate and complete history combined with a carefully performed pelvic examination usually result in a correct diagnosis of the gynecologic or obstetric condition. Treating the patient with kindness, sympathy, and respect and at the same time maintaining dignity will go far in establishing rapport with the patient. The examiner at all times must attempt to allay fear and apprehension on the part of the patient. During the examination, always inform the patient regarding the procedure to be performed. Always be gentle!

Preparation of the patient

The patient should not douche for at least 24 hours prior to the pelvic examination. Douching will interfere with proper evaluation of vaginal discharge, cytologic studies, and cultures or stained smears for microorganism identification. It is essential that the patient's bladder be emptied immediately prior to the pelvic examination. Since collection of a urine specimen is often indicated, it should be routine. It is desirable that the rectum be empty but it is not always mandatory. However, in certain instances it may be necessary to have the patient return for examination after emptying the lower bowel by enema or laxative.

The patient is placed on the examining table by a nurse and draped to permit adequate examination of the breasts, abdomen, and pelvis but also to avoid undue exposure and embarrassment. With a male physician a female nurse in attendance may furnish much comfort and assurance to the patient, and her presence may be important for the legal protection of the male physician. In addition, the nurse may be needed to assist the physician. It is absolutely essential to have a nurse in attendance during the pelvic examination of a psychotic patient or as a witness in the examination of a patient involved in an alleged criminal act. It should be borne in mind, however, that most female patients would rather not have a third person in attendance during the examination. In fact, they frequently take this opportunity to discuss with the physician problems of a more intimate and confidential nature, if they are not inhibited by the presence of the nurse.

The examination of the breasts is an integral part of the gynecologic examination and should never be omitted. (See Chapter 13.)

Pelvic examination

Positions. Pelvic examination may be performed in one of the four following positions:

1. The dorsolithotomy position is the most practical. With the patient lying on her back, the thighs are flexed and abducted, the legs are flexed, and the feet are supported in stirrups.

2. The knee-chest position may be used when the urethra or the anterior vaginal wall must be carefully inspected. It is also a useful position if the cervix or upper vagina is obstructed from view by uterine displacement or by marked redundancy of the vaginal walls.

3. The advantages of the knee-chest position can be obtained with the lateral prone (Sims) position, in which the patient lies on her left side with her chest inclining toward the table. Her left arm is behind her, her right thigh is flexed about 90 degrees, and the left thigh is slightly flexed. A single blade retractor is placed in the vagina, retracting the posterior vaginal wall.

4. The standing position is used to evaluate hernias, uterine prolapse, relaxation of the vaginal walls or pelvic supports, and stress incontinence of urine.

Abdomen. Examination of the female pelvic organs begins with the examination of the abdomen. This is done by utilizing the usual four methods: inspection, palpation, percussion, and auscultation. Variations from the normal amount and distribution of pubic hair should be noted. Inspection may reveal enlargement or obvious tumors that have characteristic appearances (Fig. 16-19). Splinting of certain

muscle groups in peritoneal irritation is often visible. Rigidity and tenderness are readily apparent on palpation. An attempt should be made to differentiate superficial and deep tenderness, generalized and localized tenderness, and rebound tenderness, both direct and referred. If a mass is palpated, one should determine whether it is solid or fluctuant, whether

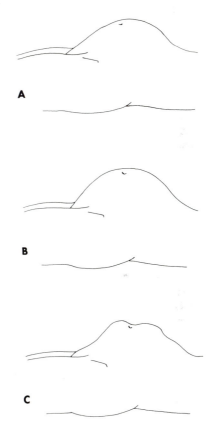

Fig. 16-19. Variations of abdominal contour. Notice in the lateral view of the contour of the abdomen distended by a large pelvic cystic mass (ovarian cyst or uterine pregnancy) that the drop in the upper portion of the curve is sharper, **A,** whereas in ascites the curve is more uniform, **B,** and the curve tends to be irregular in the presence of a solid intra-abdominal (pelvic) tumor, **C.**

its surface is rough or smooth, whether its outline is regular or irregular, its location, and its apparent point of origin. Examination of the abdomen should always include palpation of the femoral and inguinal lymph nodes.

Percussion is valuable in the differential diagnosis of free and encysted fluid within the abdomen. Usually the tympanitic bowel floats on free fluid and is found to be present in the midline or the most distensible part of the abdomen (Fig. 16-20). In contrast, encysted fluid, whether it be that within a pregnant uterus, a distended bladder, or a large ovarian cyst, presents dullness in the midline and tympany in the lateral portion of the abdomen (flanks). Shifting dullness is characteristic of free fluid. Demonstration of a fluid wave within a tense cyst will differentiate it from a solid tumor. Auscultation of the abdomen is important for detection and evaluation of bowel sounds, bruits, souffles, and fetal heart sounds.

Vulva and perineum. The examiner stands before the patient, who is in the dorsolithotomy position. If the physician is right-handed, a glove is worn on the left hand. The gloved hand is used to separate the labia during the inspection of the vulva (Fig. 16-21), and

the fingers of this hand perform the digital portion of the bimanual examination. Wearing a glove on the left hand and using this hand for the digital examination leaves the right hand free to handle instruments and to perform the abdominal portion of the bimanual examination.

The pelvic examination is begun by palpating the lower abdomen with the right hand. This should be gentle and superficial; deep pressure is avoided at this time. The patient must be encouraged to relax her abdominal muscles and, just as important, to relax the abductor muscles of the thighs. Her knees should be as far apart as possible, which is accomplished by relaxation of the patient, never by force of the examiner or an attendant. The patient should have her hands at her sides or her arms folded across her chest and should breathe slowly through her mouth.

Before the examining fingers touch the vulva or are inserted into the vagina, the patient should be informed regarding the procedure. The labia are separated with the thumb and forefinger of the gloved left hand (Fig. 16-21), and the vulva and vaginal vestibule are inspected.

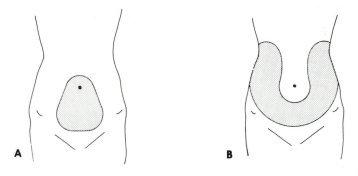

Fig. 16-20. A, Dullness on percussion (shaded area) is present in the middle portion of the abdomen in the instance of encysted fluid rising out of the pelvis. The lateral regions of the abdomen or the flanks may be tympanitic. **B,** Dullness is present in the flanks and lateral portions of the abdomen in ascites. The central part may be tympanitic.

The general development of the external genitalia is important to record. The labia majora are usually plump and well formed, whereas a scaphoid appearance of the perineum, as seen in a child, indicates a general hypoplasia of the genital tract. Distortion of the normal configuration of the vulva may be caused by ulcerative lesions, edema, varicosities, hernias, hydroceles, tumor masses, or lacerations. Most tumor masses of the vulva are nontender, except those caused by acute suppurative processes or more subtle, local cellulitis surrounding granulomatous, ulcerative, and malignant lesions. The skin of the vulva and perineum is subject to lesions just as is the skin found elsewhere on the body; in addition, there are some lesions characteristically localized to the vulvar area. In elderly patients the skin of the vulva is atrophic, and in some instances, if this condition is exaggerated, it results in shrinking and fibrosis, known as *kraurosis vulvae*. White, slightly raised plaques (leukoplakia) are seen commonly in this age group.

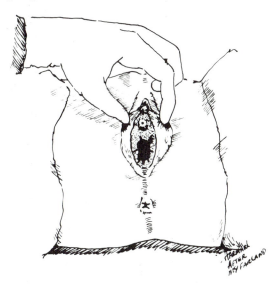

Fig. 16-21. Inspection of the vulva.

The size and development of the clitoris normally may be quite variable. True enlargement of the organ is obvious and represents some type of masculinization. If there is an associated anterior displacement of the urethral meatus, the clitoris may be interpreted as an hermaphroditic phallus with hypospadias. Inflammatory conditions of the clitoris or its prepuce are uncommon but may appear as cellulitis or abscesses. The tissue of the vestibule between the inner surfaces of the labia minora, of which the clitoris forms the anterior boundary, is the most common site of the granulomatous and ulcerative venereal lesions in younger women and of malignant changes in the elderly. Within the vestibulae, the skin is soft and much more delicate than that of the labia majora and the perineum. It is devoid of hair follicles but does contain sweat and sebaceous glands that may become inflamed or cystic. The lesser vestibular glands and the periurethral (Skene's) glands secrete mucus. These are often involved in acute and chronic gonorrhea; at times they are infected by nonvenereal organisms.

The external urethral meatus is inspected for evidence of inflammation, tumor, and prolapse of the mucosa. The prolapsed, outpouching mucous membrane of the urethra (caruncle) at times becomes infected, inflamed, and tender. The latter is a common finding in older women. Acute urethritis and acute suppurative suburethral adenitis may be demonstrated by "milking" the urethra from the bladder neck downward with the index finger. This requires only gentle anterior pressure as the finger is slowly withdrawn (Fig. 16-22). Any demonstrable discharge from the urethra or periurethral glands should be cultured, and a smear should be made for gram staining.

Following the inspection and palpation of any lesions of the vulva and skin of the perineum, the examiner notes the general appear-

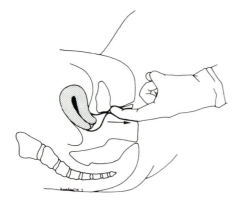

Fig. 16-22. Discharge is expressed from the urethra, the suburethral glands, and periurethral glands by gently pressing on the undersurface of the urethra and slowly withdrawing the finger.

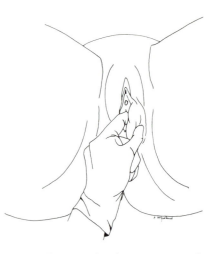

Fig. 16-23. Palpation of enlargements on the surfaces of the labia and within the labia is best accomplished by inserting the index finger into the vagina while making counterpressure with the thumb on the tissue in question. The swelling of the left labia is caused by an abscess of Bartholin's gland.

ance of the entrance of the vagina (introitus). In the nonparous individual, the labia minora lie together in the midline. If there is relaxation or laceration of the perineal muscles, they gape and fall to either side. The posterior vaginal wall may bulge into the introitus if the patient has a *rectocele,* or the anterior vaginal wall may present if she has a *cystocele* or *urethrocele.* In case of prolapse, the cervix may present at or even protrude outside the vaginal opening. The hymen or hymeneal remnants appear just inside the introitus. In the virgin this structure is quite variable, both in its thickness and in its restriction of the opening of the vagina. It normally will admit one finger, occasionally two fingers, and in some cases is impenetrable. The carunculae, or remnants of the ruptured or lacerated hymen, also normally vary in thickness and size in the nonvirgin. These structures may become quite red, tender, and obviously inflamed when associated with any form of acute vulvovaginitis.

The duct of the greater vestibular (Bartholin's) gland opens into the margin of the vaginal orifice just outside the hymen on either lateral side, slightly posterior to the horizontal midplane. Acute gonorrheal infection of this gland, its duct, and the duct opening is common when this disease is present in the vulva or vagina. With this or any other acute infection, the opening of the duct becomes easily obstructed, acute inflammation is common, and the resultant Bartholin abscess is easily visible on inspection of the vulva, even though the gland and its duct are rather deeply seated. The swelling appears to be beneath the labium majora and may involve the base of the labium minora; thus, obviously displacing the vaginal introitus toward the opposite side. Palpation of the inflamed gland, cyst, or abscess is accomplished best by introducing the index finger into the vagina. Light pressure on the labium with the thumb will determine the size, consistency, and tenderness of the mass (Fig. 16-23).

Papanicolaou smear. Because of its extreme value in the early detection of uterine cancer,

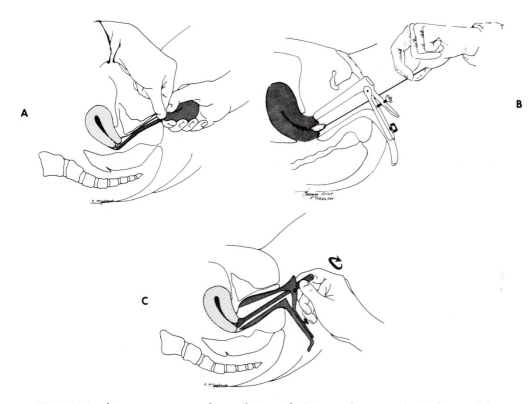

Fig. 16-24. Obtaining specimens for cytologic study (Papanicolaou smear). **A,** The tip of the aspirator is placed in the posterior vaginal fornix, and the pressure on the bulb is released as the aspirator is withdrawn. **B,** The saline-moistened, cotton-tipped applicator is inserted into the cervical canal and rotated. **C,** The cervical scraping is made under direct visualization of the cervix. The spatula is held with light pressure against the tissue surrounding the cervical os and is then rotated (in the direction of arrow) 360 degrees.

a simple screening test (Papanicolaou or exfoliative cytologic smear) must be considered a routine part of the pelvic examination. An aspiration of the exfoliated cells from the upper posterior portion (fornix) of the vagina is accomplished with a glass tube and bulb. The labia are separated with the thumb and index finger of the gloved left hand. The aspirator is held in the palm of the right hand. The bulb is deflated partially, and the tube is inserted (without lubricant) to the top of the vagina (Fig. 16-24). The pressure is released on the bulb and the aspirator is slowly withdrawn. The material obtained is placed on a ground-glass label slide. Another glass slide is placed on top of the material, and the two slides are separated by sliding them apart. The specimen slide is placed in an alcohol-ether fixative. Another preparation is made by means of a cotton-tipped applicator moistened with saline and rotated in the endocervical canal. A third preparation is made by scraping the squamo-columnar junction of the external os of the cervix with a spatula, which is described later.

Perineal and vaginal supports. The first and second fingers of the left hand should now be lubricated with a minimal amount of surgical lubricant. This should be spread lightly over the examining fingers and then on the inner aspect of each labium minora. The musculature of the perineum and the thickness and length of the perineal body are tested by inserting the first and second fingers of the left hand into the vagina. The integrity of the pelvic floor may be ascertained by having the patient attempt to tighten her perineal muscles about the fingers. If these muscles are intact, the examiner is able to feel pressure as the fingers are pressed against the pubic arch by the levators. Then the fingers in the vagina are separated, the perineal muscles are depressed posteriorly and the thickness of the perineal body is palpated. If the patient has had an extensive second-degree laceration of the perineum during childbirth, the perineal body will be shortened and thin. If there has been a neglected third-degree laceration (through the rectal sphincter or into the rectum), there may be a complete absence of the perineal body; the vaginal epithelium joins the rectal mucosa. To further evaluate the pelvic supports the perineum is depressed, and the patient is asked to strain or bear down as if attempting to empty the rectum. If there is a rectocele or weakness of the posterior vaginal wall, it will be felt as a bulge between the examiner's separated fingers. During this part of the examination any weakness of the anterior vaginal wall or the uterine supports will become evident. When the patient strains, the urethra may bulge downward as may the bladder floor, thus revealing an *urethrocystocele*. If there is marked weakness of the uterine supports or endopelvic fascia, the cervix will prolapse into view or an *enterocele* (herniation of the cul-de-sac) may be evident as a bulge of the top of the vagina behind the cervix. If, from the history, there is a question of differentiat-ing stress from urgency incontinence, a special test (Marshall-Marchetti) may be performed at this time and reevaluated later with the patient in the standing position.

As the fingers of the left (gloved) hand are introduced into the vagina, slight pressure should be made against the posterior portion of the introitus and the posterior vaginal wall. This avoids pressure on the urethra, which is normally sensitive. The extended examining fingers, the hand, and the forearm are held in a straight line, with no lateral or medial flexion of the wrist joint. The third and fourth fingers are completely flexed and the thumb is hyperextended. The hand should remain perpendicular to the floor (Fig. 16-25). It is important to maintain this position of the hand throughout the examination. The palm is *not* turned up. Keeping the wrist stiff and depressing the perineum posteriorly enhances the examiner's ability to palpate deeply into the pelvis. The dorsa of the flexed third and fourth fingers are pressed against the perineal body on deep palpation and will further depress the perineal floor. The most common error committed in doing the pelvic examination is turning the palm of the examining hand upward. If the palm is turned upward, the depth of penetration is halted when the back of the third and fourth fingers contact the pubic ramus. The only time the palmar surface of the hand should be turned up is when deep penetration is not necessary or when the anterior vaginal wall, the urethra, or bladder floor are being palpated.

Vagina. As the fingers are introduced into the vagina, any firmness, induration, or tumefaction of the vaginal walls is noted. Scars from previous perineal or vaginal lacerations may be tender. Tumors or cystic masses in the vaginal wall are easily palpated. The amount of relaxation or redundancy of the vaginal walls is noted. Congenital abnormalities are quickly ev-

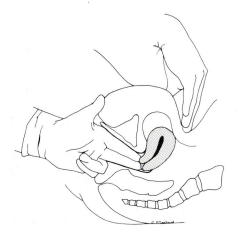

Fig. 16-25. Bimanual examination. Notice the position of the left hand and the fact that the wrist is not flexed laterally or medially and the hand is not supinated. The examining fingers here are palpating the cervix of a normally anteflexed uterus.

ident. A completely imperforate hymen is an uncommon anomaly. A partial or complete septum attached to the anterior and posterior walls of the vagina is often associated with a double or single cervix, a double uterus, or other anomalies of the genital or urinary tract. Partial or complete absence of the vagina is rare. With the finding of an imperforate hymen, a tight fibrous hymeneal ring restricting the entrance, or absence of the vagina, the internal genitalia must be evaluated by a rectoabdominal bimanual examination.

Bladder. The region of the bladder may be palpated for sensitivity, tumor induration, or stone. Inflammation of the bladder or bladder neck causes marked sensitivity on palpation. If the bladder is tender, there is frequently an associated reference of pain to the region of the umbilicus. The condition of the anterior rectal wall and the rectovaginal septum may be examined at this time, but a better evaluation can be made later by the rectovaginal examination.

Cervix. The size, shape, position, mobility, regularity, and consistency of the cervix are noted. The position of and direction in which the cervix points are quite variable. Normally, the cervix is found pointing posteriorly from the top of the anterior vaginal wall (Fig. 16-25). Usually it lies in the midplane of the pelvis with no displacement from the normal axis of the vagina, which is downward and backward (toward the hollow of the patient's sacrum) with the patient in the dorsolithotomy position. A change in the direction of the cervix that causes it to point upward usually signifies a retrodisplacement of the uterus. The cervix may show a marked change in its position as well as in its axis. This is usually the result of a tumor of the uterus changing the normal relationship or is caused by a tumor of some other intrapelvic organ displacing the body (corpus) of the uterus as well as the cervix. Inflammatory changes or tumor (usually cancer) in the parametrium may deflect the cervix to one side. Malignant infiltration or pelvic inflammatory disease may cause immobility of the cervix (fixation). Normally it is freely movable for 2 to 3 cm. in any direction. Motion of the cervix, especially from side to side, stretches the peritoneum in the lower pelvis. Thus, any irritation of the pelvic peritoneum that may be caused by bacterial invasion, blood, or a ruptured viscus is accompanied by exquisite tenderness on movement of the cervix. In uterine prolapse the cervix drops toward the perineum in the axis of the vagina.

By palpation, the examiner should note the length of the cervix and later compare it with the size of the uterine body. The normal adult ratio is 1:2. This is reversed in the child or in the adult with marked hypoplasia of the uterus. The external opening (os) of the cervix is normally small (3 to 5 mm. in diameter). Sometimes the cervical os may be patulous so as to admit the tip of the index finger if something has recently passed through it (abortion) or is about to (threatened or inevitable abortion, large polyp, or submucous fibroid). A cervical polyp is a soft, spongy mass, varying in size, usually from a few millimeters to 1 or 2 cm. in diameter and protruding from the cervical os. The cervix may be deformed by lacerations suffered during childbirth, by congenital defects, or, rarely, by instrumentation. The most common laceration sustained during childbirth is horizontal—from 9 to 3 o'clock.

The normal cervix is firm and smooth. It is hard if it has been invaded by cancer or is inflamed, but it becomes much softer during pregnancy. Smooth, firm nodules are felt frequently on the cervix; on inspection these prove to to be small cysts of the cervical (nabothian) glands. In addition to rendering the cervix much harder than normal, malignancy produces a rough, granular surface and is likened to both the feel and appearance of a cauliflower. Malignancy, extensive pelvic inflammatory disease, and endometriosis generally cause fixation and relative immobility of the cervix. With endometriosis and inflammation there is marked tenderness when the cervix is moved.

Parametrium. The parametrium (tissues adjacent to the cervix and lower segment of the corpus of the uterus) is normally pliable, soft, and nontender. This tissue extends laterally and posteriorly and is palpable in the lateral and posterior fornices of the vagina. It contains the vascular supply and the lymphatics draining the cervix. Therefore, the parametrium is indurated and tender if the cervix is inflamed. It is both indurated and immobile if involved by malignant tumor. The posterior parametrium, which includes primarily the uterosacral ligaments, may be nodular and cyclically tender in pelvic endometriosis. This posterior tissue is often involved when there is inflammatory or malignant infiltration from the cervix,

uterus, tubes, or ovaries. All of the parametrium is more easily palpated and its true condition is more accurately assessed by rectal than by vaginal examination.

Uterine corpus. The position, mobility, size, shape, and consistency of the uterus is palpated bimanually, the "abdominal hand" cooperating, as it were, with the "vaginal." The fingers of the right hand are placed on the abdomen about half way from the symphysis to the umbilicus. If the fingers make pressure too close to the symphysis, the abdominal wall is pressed downward in front of (or inferior to) the normally positioned uterus, making it impossible for the examiner to feel the intrapelvic structures. This is a common error of the beginner. It is better to begin with the abdominal hand fairly high (just below the umbilicus) and to bring the abdominal hand slowly downward toward the symphysis. As soon as pressure is made on the uterus, or any tumor within the pelvis, it is quickly perceived by the vaginal hand. The vaginal fingers should first survey the anterior vaginal fornix. The uterus in its usual position of anteflexion is palpable here. As it is steadied by the abdominal hand, its width, size, and regularity are noted by both the abdominal and vaginal fingers (Fig. 16-26). By depressing the anterior abdominal wall, pressure can be brought against the posterior portion of the lower uterine segment in most patients. It is normally firm and of the same consistency as the uterine fundus. In early pregnancy, it softens and is easily compressible. This is a dependable indication (Hegar's sign) of pregnancy and can frequently be elicited before there is significant enlargement and softening of the whole uterus (Fig. 16-27). Irregular enlargement of the uterine body is suggestive of fibroid tumors (leiomyomata). These tumors are firm, smooth, and rounded and more often appear as multiple nodularities within the substance of the uterus (Fig. 16-28).

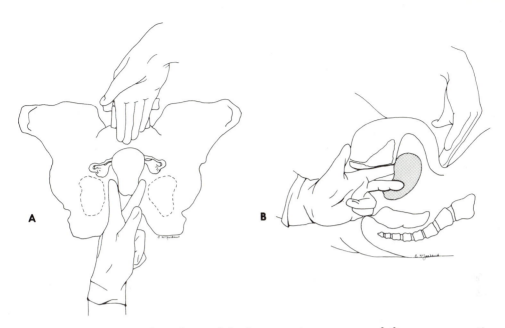

Fig. 16-26. The size and regularity of the lower uterine segment and the corpus are estimated by spreading the vaginal fingers—the index finger on the patient's right and the
second finger on the left. The vaginal fingers are pressing into the lateral vaginal fornices
and are moved up and down along the lateral walls of the uterus. While the vaginal fingers
steady the uterus, the abdominal hand recognizes enlargement and irregularities of the fundus. **A,** Anteroposterior view. **B,** Lateral view.

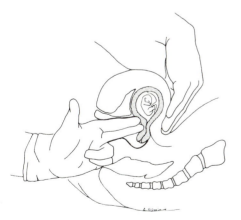

Fig. 16-27. Softening of lower uterine segment as an
early sign of pregnancy (Hegar's sign).

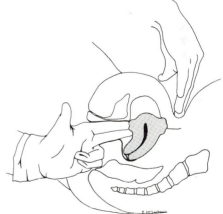

Fig. 16-28. In anteflexion of the uterus, tumors of
the anterior uterine wall are palpable by the vaginal
fingers and by the abdominal fingers if the tumors
are on the posterior surface.

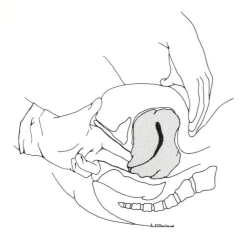

Fig. 16-29. The uterine mass is irregular in outline, smooth, and firm in the presence of leiomyomata. The cervix here is in the usual position; it may be displaced in any direction by fibroids or other intra-pelvic tumors.

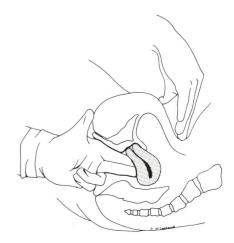

Fig. 16-30. Palpation of the retrodisplaced uterus on vaginoabdominal examination is performed primarily with the vaginal fingers.

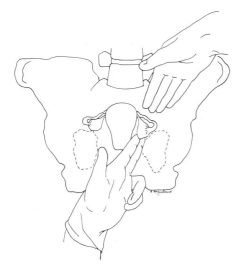

Fig. 16-31. Bimanual evaluation of the left adnexa. Notice that the ovary is between the palmar surfaces of the examining fingers.

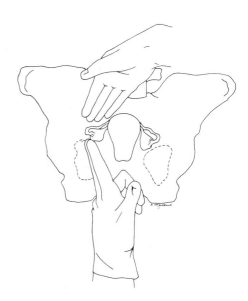

Fig. 16-32. Bimanual evaluation of the right adnexa. The position of and the direction of pressures of the examining fingers are changed from those used on the opposite side of the pelvis, but the ovary is palpated by the more sensitive palmar surfaces of the fingers.

They vary in size from 1 or 2 cm. in diameter to a size that enlarges the uterine mass to such an extent that it seems to fill the whole pelvic or abdominal cavity (Fig. 16-29). Such immense tumors are quite uncommon, but it is not rare to see fibroids 15 or 20 cm. in diameter that fill the pelvis and extend to or above the umbilicus. Soft compressibility of an irregular uterine mass is found in cystic degeneration of uterine fibroids. Uncomplicated fibroids are not tender. Areas of tenderness will be found in tumor masses when there is infarction, hemorrhage, or acute infection.

In approximately 20% of women the uterus is normally retrodisplaced. The fundus of the organ lies in the cul-de-sac and is palpable behind the cervix (Fig. 16-30). In the normal pelvis the body of the uterus is freely movable in any position. If gentle, steady pressure is made by the vaginal fingers, the uterus can usually be lifted out of the cul-de-sac. At times, it may be necessary to do this on rectal bimanual examination. True fixation of the uterus in this position suggests peritoneal adhesions caused by inflammatory disease, scarring and infiltration of endometriosis or malignancy. These pathologic processes will often cause fixation and immobility of the uterus in any position. In retrodisplacement, however, it may seem to be immovable because of tenderness.

Tube and ovary. Palpation of the tube and ovary, generally referred to as the uterine *adnexa,* is the most difficult part of the pelvic examination, especially for the beginner and occasionally for the expert. It should be stated at the outset that *the normal tube is not palpable.* The ovary is about 3 × 4 cm. in size and normally is sensitive to pressure. It is best palpated by the vaginal fingers. It lies deep in the pelvis above the lateral fornix of the vagina. On the patient's left, the external fingers should make deep pressure on the abdomen superior to the junction of the medial and middle thirds

of the inguinal ligament; the direction of the pressure should be slightly toward the midline. At the same time, the "vaginal" fingers in the lateral fornix should be directed slightly laterally and anteriorly to feel the ovary being pressed toward the palmar surface of the vaginal fingers by the abdominal hand (Fig. 16-31). On the patient's right, the vaginal fingers are directed deep and laterally, and pressure is made anteriorly and toward the midline. The abdominal fingers should make deep pressure toward the lateral pelvic wall. This again brings the ovary between the palmar surfaces of the palpating fingers (Fig. 16-32). Occasionally, if the examiner is not satisfied with his evaluation of the right adnexa, it is advisable to glove the right hand as the vaginal palpator and use the left hand on the abdomen. Enlarged ovaries may vary greatly in size and tend to lie in the posterior half of the pelvis. Because of the normal anatomic relationships, ovarian and tubo-ovarian masses usually lie posterior to the uterine body and tend to displace it forward within the pelvic cavity. At times they may fill the pelvis or, because of stretching of the ovarian pedicle, they may seem to float more or less freely in the lower abdomen. Ovarian tumors may be cystic, solid, or mixtures of both elements. The truly cystic tumors are compressible between the examining fingers, as would be a water-filled balloon (Figs. 16-33 and 16-34). They are usually smooth, may be quite tense or very soft, and are easily compressible. Solid enlargements are usually firm; they may be smooth or irregular and nodular. Nodular irregularities palpable on the surface of either a cystic or solid mass suggest malignancy. Cystic masses that lie in the anterior pelvis and tend to displace the uterus backward are usually found to originate in the embryonic remnants in the mesovarium, the epoophoron, and paroophoron, and are called *parovarian cysts.*

Marked tenderness of an adnexal mass is a

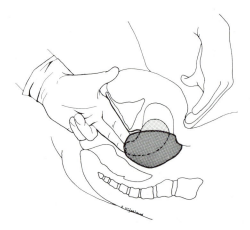

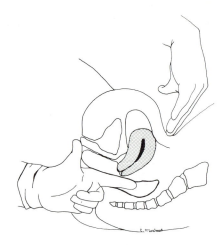

Fig. 16-33. Palpation of a cystic adnexal mass by vaginoabdominal examination. Size, shape, mobility, regularity, and consistency are noted.

Fig. 16-34. Rectoabdominal examination is useful in further determination of size and position of pelvic masses, especially when they seem to arise in the adnexa, broad ligament, or cul-de-sac.

characteristic finding in acute inflammatory change caused by tubo-ovarian infection, bleeding or degeneration within a tumor, ectopic pregnancy, or infarction caused by torsion of the pedicle of the mass that contains its blood supply. Acute tubal infection invariably involves the ovary. In such an instance, the two structures usually cannot be differentiated by palpation but appear to be a single, tender, indurated mass. Chronic inflammatory disease of the pelvis generally causes fixation of the adnexa and at times cystic enlargement of the tubes. Pain is caused by any attempt to mobilize the tubal or ovarian enlargement. Often confused with adnexal enlargements that are situated deep in the pelvis or cul-de-sac are masses originating in the sigmoid colon. These, of course, tend to be in the left side of the pelvis. Carcinoma and diverticulitis of the colon are the more common pathologic conditions to be differentiated. Tumors of the cecum and appendiceal abscess may present in the right side of the pelvic cavity but are higher and not so

easily palpable on bimanual vaginal examination. Occasionally a redundant cecum that extends down into the pelvis and becomes distended with gas is mistakenly interpreted as an adnexal enlargement.

A rectal examination should be made at this point. While the well-lubricated index finger of the left hand is inserted into the rectum, it is used to note any abnormality (see Chapter 15). Any weakness in the rectovaginal septum can be easily appreciated by exerting pressure toward the vaginal canal. A perineal hernia of the lower rectum allows bulging through the perineal body, and a rectocele is evident as a bulge above the perineal body. Induration of the rectovaginal septum may be palpated in posterior and inferior vaginal extension of carcinoma of the cervix.

Rectoabdominal examination

When it is impossible to insert a finger into the vagina because of a tight hymenal ring, atresia, or other malformation, the bimanual

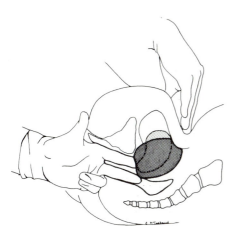

Fig. 16-35. Vaginorectoabdominal examination may provide much additional information if the vaginal introitus will admit but one finger. The examiner is able to palpate structures and pathologic changes much deeper in the pelvis than by a one finger vaginoabdominal examination.

examination is accomplished by the rectoabdominal approach (Fig. 16-34). The same general principles are followed as in the vaginal examination. The rectoabdominal examination performed in conjunction with the vaginoabdominal appraisal of the pelvis is very informative and, unless contraindicated, should be a part of the routine evaluation of the female pelvis. The areas of the cul-de-sac and uterosacral and transverse cervical ligaments are felt much more easily by rectal than by vaginal examination. If the vagina is shortened, as it may be following irradiation therapy of cancer of the cervix or surgical removal of the upper vagina, rectal examination is the only satisfactory method of appraisal.

The vaginorectoabdominal examination is also a useful source of information. This is carried out by inserting the index finger into the vagina and the second finger into the rectum (Fig. 16-35). The bimanual survey of the pelvic

structures is then accomplished as in the vaginoabdominal procedure. This examination is often used if the vaginal introitus will admit only one finger or if there is question of fixation of the upper vagina to the rectum. The method is particularly useful in palpating abnormalities in the cul-de-sac. Palpation of the rectovaginal septum may be performed most effectively by inserting the index finger into the rectum and the thumb into the vagina. The septum can then be palpated easily for tumor, inflammatory, or granulomatous masses.

Speculum examination

Whether the digital vaginal examination or the speculum examination is done first is a matter of personal preference by the examining physician. Since it is important not to contaminate cervical or vaginal scrapings for cytologic study with the surgical lubricant, many physicians believe the speculum visualization and cervical smear should be done before the bimanual examination. If only a very minimal amount of lubricant is used and is spread very thinly on the gloved fingers and in the vestibular area of the vulva, the problem of the lubricant interfering with cytologic studies will be avoided. There are distinct advantages to first performing the digital examination. The size of the introitus and vaginal canal can be judged, and the presence of obstructing anomalies can be discovered before an attempt is made to insert the speculum.

When the position of the cervix is ascertained first by digital examination, speculum visualization is facilitated and usually is accomplished with less discomfort to the patient. Areas of marked tenderness can be evaluated much better with the examining finger than with the blunt end of the steel speculum, thus minimizing discomfort to the patient.

The bivalve (Graves) speculum, which is almost universally used for vaginal inspection, is made in three standard sizes. There are several modifications of the original Graves speculum for special problems. The air endoscope (Kelly) is an ideal instrument for visualization of the vagina and cervix of children. When the proper speculum is chosen, it is important to be sure that the set screw that holds the two blades of the instrument together is tight. The set screw on the thumb rest should be loosened so the tips of the blades come together. Again, it is important to inform the patient what is to be done. The speculum is held in the right hand, and the labia are separated with the thumb and index finger of the left hand, or by pulling the skin of the left labium majora laterally with the left thumb (Fig. 16-36). With the first joint of the thumb against the underside of the thumb rest to hold the blades of the speculum tightly together, the handle of the speculum is turned approximately 45 to 60 degrees to the examiner's right (counterclockwise). The tip of the speculum is inserted into the posterior part of

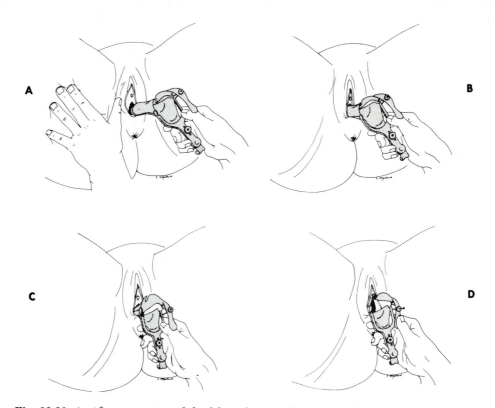

Fig. 16-36. A, After separation of the labia, the speculum is introduced into the posterior portion of the vaginal canal. The speculum has been rotated so that the wide part of the blades fits the configuration of the introitus. **B,** Introduction of the speculum continues downward and backward with slight pressure on the perineal body, thus avoiding the urethra. **C,** As the speculum reaches the top of the vagina the handle is restored to the anteroposterior position, and it is slightly elevated. **D,** As the thumb rest is depressed, so is the handle of the speculum.

the vaginal introitus that has been exposed, avoiding pressure on the external urethral meatus. The speculum is inserted gently to the top of the vagina, and at the same time the handle is elevated and rotated back to the axis of the midline. Again during this maneuver, slight posterior pressure should be made to avoid the more sensitive area of the urethra. Then the blades of the speculum are opened by pressing down on the thumb rest and at the same time depressing the handle of the speculum. When this is done, the cervix comes into view at the top of the vagina.

Another method of speculum insertion is done by introducing one or two fingers of the gloved hand through the introitus and depressing the perineal body backward. The posterior blade of the speculum is introduced into the vagina over the top of the fingers. This method also avoids pressure on the urethra.

Cervix. After insertion of the speculum specimens for culture, if indicated, should be taken from the cervical os. The cytologic smear should be taken from the endocervix with a saline-moistened, cotton-tipped applicator (Fig. 16-24, *B*). A scraping for cytologic study is taken from the squamocolumnar junction of the cervix. A tongue depressor or a slender wooden spatula made expressly for this purpose is used. It is placed against the cervix and with gentle pressure is rotated 360 degrees (Fig. 16-24, *C*). The material obtained is then transferred to a slide. If a smear for hormonal activity is desired, it is best obtained from the upper lateral vaginal wall with a separate spatula, and the material is placed on another slide.

The normal cervix is 2.5 to 3 cm. in diameter and extends into the upper vagina about the same distance. In children, in patients with uterine hypoplasia, and in the aged patient, the cervix is much smaller. It is cylindrical in shape and points posteriorly; but if the uterus is retrodisplaced, as it is in about 20% of women,

the cervix points anteriorly. It is normally covered by the same type of epithelium as the vaginal wall and its color is that of the vagina.

A somewhat cyanotic, bluish appearance of the cervix is an early indication (Chadwick's sign) of pregnancy. A beefy redness extending from the external os may be the result of so-called erosion. This is actually an extension of the columnar epithelium, which normally lines the cervical canal, on to the vaginal portion of the cervix. The margins of an erosion are ordinarily uniform and regular, whereas those of a carcinoma are usually irregular. Early carcinoma, however, has an appearance that cannot be well differentiated visually from erosion. In fact, the earliest malignancies may not change the appearance of the cervix from the normal. Extensive malignancy has a rough granular surface (cauliflower), which bleeds easily; but some cancers, particularly those arising within the cervical canal, may cause no abnormal appearance of the cervix.

If there is a fish-mouth deformity of the cervix from previous laceration, the endocervical epithelium is visible (eversion). When this condition exists, it may be complicated by chronic infection of the endocervical tissue, which is accompanied by a thick mucous or mucopurulent discharge. In this situation the cervix is enlarged, edematous in appearance, and often has multiple small cysts (nabothian) visible on the vaginal portion. Acute inflammation of the cervix causes a purulent discharge. If gonorrheal infection is suspected, a specimen for gram stain and culture should be obtained.

A dark cherry-red mass extending out of the cervix is usually a cervical polyp. These vary in size from several millimeters to 1, 2, or 3 cm. in diameter. They are smooth and uniform in contour and bleed easily. Endometrial polyps may present at the external cervical os, as may prolapsed submucous fibroids; the latter are usually larger and are often grossly infected or necrotic. If a large polyp or fibroid protrudes through the cervix, there is obvious dilatation of the canal and its external opening. Occasionally, the tumor may be so large as to obstruct the cervix from view.

Vagina. The lateral vaginal walls visible between the blades of the open speculum and in the fornices are inspected as to texture, color, support, and discharge. A more detailed inspection of the vagina is made as the speculum is slowly withdrawn. The vaginal walls of a child are smooth and delicate in appearance. In the normal adult the epithelium appears thicker and heavier, and it is obviously distensible because of its elasticity and the fact that it has many folds or rugae. In the postmenopausal patient, these rugae tend to disappear, and the epithelium takes on a thin, velvety appearance. The color of the vagina is normally pink and uniform. When the vagina is inflamed, the walls are markedly reddened and often coated with a discharge. In bacterial invasion of the vagina, a thin, yellow, purulent material is present. In the postmenopausal patient with nonspecific infection, the epithelium is frequently spotted with small petechiae. In trichomonas vaginitis the discharge is thin, yellow, often frothy, and has a rather characteristic peculiar musty odor. Further, the vaginal wall often has a "strawberry" appearance, with very small red spots seeming to show through the vaginal epithelium, which condition usually extends onto the portio vaginalis of the cervix. Monilial or yeast infection causes the formation of a thick, white, patchy, curdlike discharge that clings to the vaginal wall. The diagnosis depends on the identification of the causative organisms by smear and culture of the vaginal secretions.

The anterior and posterior vaginal walls are inspected by rotating the speculum in the long axis of the vagina. As the speculum is slowly withdrawn, the remainder of the vagina can be seen. After the blades of the speculum clear the cervix, the thumb screw of the instrument should be released, and the remainder of the vagina should be visualized by holding the speculum partially open with the thumb. Cystic or solid tumors come into view, as do ulcerations, injury, or fistulae.

As the speculum is withdrawn further to about the midpoint of the vagina, the patient is asked to bear down. If there is relaxation of the uterine supports, the cervix will protrude into the open speculum and may even follow it to the introitus. When there is relaxation of the anterior or posterior vaginal walls, the cystocele or rectocele bulges into the vaginal cavity. A rectocele may be confused with a concomitant herniation of the cul-de-sac (enterocele), which presents behind the cervix and may extend down the full length of the vagina. Even though she strains, the patient, while lying on her back, may not be able to demonstrate uterine prolapse or extensive vaginal relaxation to the examining physician. A useful method to determine the integrity of the uterine supports is by traction on the cervix. A long sponge forceps is used to grasp the anterior lip of the cer-

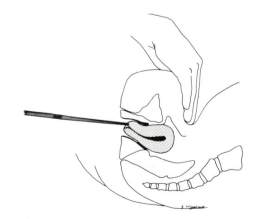

Fig. 16-37. Gentle traction on the cervical lip demonstrates degree of prolapse.

vix. A cervical tenaculum is used if the cervix cannot be grasped with a sponge forceps. As the patient bears down, gentle, steady traction is made on the instrument at the same time the speculum is slowly withdrawn. If the supports are weakened, the cervix will come into view at the vaginal opening or beyond (Fig. 16-37).

It may be desirable to study further the relaxation of the vaginal and uterine supports by examining the patient in the standing position. The patient stands with one foot on the floor—the leg is extended and straight—and the other leg slightly abducted with the foot on the step of the examining table. A clean glove is used, and the examining fingers are inserted into the vagina until the cervix can be palpated. The patient is asked to strain. The presence and degree of the prolapse of the uterus or the vaginal walls can be ascertained readily by this technique.

Special diagnostic tests

Wet smear. The wet smear is a simple test used to examine the vaginal secretions for specific organisms of trichomonas, monilia, or he-

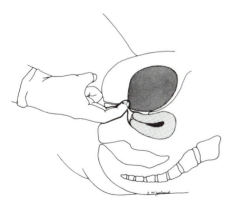

Fig. 16-38. The Marshall-Marchetti test is used to establish a diagnosis of bladder sphincter stress incontinence. The fingers make pressure on each side of the urethrovesical junction and not directly on this area.

mophilus vaginitis. Also, it may be used in cases of infertility as a method of evaluating sperm samples in the postcoital test and in suspected or alleged rape. With the speculum in place, a small amount of vaginal secretion is removed with an aspirator syringe or cotton-tipped applicator, and a drop or two is placed on a glass slide. To this is added a drop of normal saline solution, and the specimen is covered with a coverglass for microscopic examination. If monilia is suspected, 10% sodium or potassium hydroxide is often used instead of saline. The yeast organisms are seen more readily as the strong base destroys the desquamated vaginal cells. Some physicians prefer to take the specimen with a cotton-tipped applicator that is then placed in a test tube that contains 1 or 2 ml. of normal saline solution. The slide preparation can be delayed until a more convenient time. Occasionally the hanging drop preparation is more desirable.

Vaginal cytology for estrogen-progesterone effect. In the study of estrogen effect, as may be indicated in ovarian (follicle) failure from whatever cause or for progesterone effect as evidence of ovulation or pregnancy, a stained smear of vaginal cells is made for cytologic study. With the speculum in place and the blades open, the cells are scraped from the upper lateral vaginal wall with a spatula or tongue depressor. The specimen is placed on a slide by lightly stroking the slide with the spatula in the same manner as the cervical scrape for the Papanicolaou smear.

Marshall-Marchetti test. The Marshall-Marchetti test is used to establish the diagnosis of stress incontinence. The bladder is filled by catheter with 200 to 300 ml. of water, after which the patient is asked to cough or strain suddenly. If the water escapes from the bladder, the bladder sphincter is incontinent under stress. Then the first and second fingers of the gloved hand are introduced into the vagina with palmar surfaces to the anterior vaginal wall, and pressure is made anteriorly on each side of the urethrovesical junction, lifting the bladder neck to a position against the retropubic area (Fig. 16-38). The patient is again asked to cough, and it will be noted in cases of true stress incontinence that no water escapes from the urethra. If stress incontinence is suspected but no water is lost when the patient is lying down during the first part of the test, the examination should be repeated with the patient in a standing position.

SELECTED READINGS
Male genitalia

Aquino, J. A.: Peyronie's disease, J. Urol. 97:492, 1967.

Beggs, J. H.: Epidemoid carcinoma of penis, J. Urol. 91:166, 1964.

Grace, D. A., and Winter, C. C.: Priapism: an appraisal of management of twenty-three patients, J. Urol. 90:301, 1968.

Jewett, H. J., Bridge, R., Gray, G. F., and Shelley, W. M.: The palpable nodule of prostatic cancer, J.A.M.A. 203:403, 1968.

Mittemeyer, B. T.: Epididymitis, J. Urol. 95:390, 1966.

Moustofa, M. F. H.: Gangrene of the scrotum, Br. J. Plast. Surg. 20:90, 1967.

Nesbit, Reed M.: Your prostate gland (Letters from a surgeon to his father), Springfield, Ill., 1961, Charles C Thomas, Publisher.

Perry, H. O., and Greene, L. F.: Common diseases of the skin of the penis, GP 34:87, 1966.

Robson, C. J.: Testicular tumors, J. Urol. 94:440, 1965.

Schoenberg, H. W., and Murphy, J. J.: The differential diagnosis of intrascrotal masses, GP 25:82, 1962.

Smith, D. R.: Repair of hypospadias in the preschool child: report of 150 cases, J. Urol. 97:723, 1967.

Taylor, J. N.: Torsion of testicle, J. Urol. 94:680, 1965.

Winter, C. C.: Practical urology, St. Louis, 1969, The C. V. Mosby Co.

Female genitalia

Behrman, S. J., and Gosling, J. R. G.: Fundamentals of gynecology, ed. 2, New York, 1966, Oxford University Press.

Brewer, J. I., and DeCosta, E. J.: Textbook of gynecology, ed. 4, Baltimore, 1967, The Williams & Wilkins Co.

Taylor, E. S.: Essentials of gynecology, ed. 4. Philadelphia, 1969, Lea & Febiger.

Ullery, J. C., and Hollenbeck, Z. J. R.: Textbook of obstetrics, St. Louis, 1965, The C. V. Mosby Co.

CHAPTER 17

EXTREMITIES

A comprehensive and meticulous examination of the extremities not only can detect localized abnormalities but also is capable of identifying abnormalities associated with several systemic diseases. Thus, such illnesses as scleroderma, systemic vasculitis, diabetes, atherosclerosis, and acromegaly may display prominent physical signs evident during examination of the extremities. Similar to the peripheral joints, examination of the extremities is primarily accomplished by inspection and palpation. If possible, one should attempt to examine the extremities in conjunction with the peripheral joints since shared abnormalities are a frequent occurrence.

Proper examination of the extremities requires complete exposure and adequate lighting. Subtle unilateral abnormalities can be detected only by careful comparison with the contralateral extremity. Importantly, the recognition of subtle bilateral abnormalities requires that the examiner has a thorough knowledge of the variations existing among normal individuals. Thus, it is essential for the examiner to evaluate the extremities routinely as a part of every physical examination. The experience gained through the course of normal examina-

tions will definitely enhance one's ability to diagnose less apparent abnormalities.

Generally, inspection and palpation of the extremities are best performed as a systematic routine in conjunction with the peripheral joint examination. During inspection the following features should be observed: (1) size and symmetry; (2) muscle mass; (3) vasculature; (4) skin, hair, and nails; and (5) lymph glands.

In palpating the extremities, important characteristics to be noted include: (1) arterial pulses, (2) skin temperature and turgor, and (3) local tenderness.

A systematic approach is presented here for evaluating the extremities. Although specific disease states are not intended to be described in detail, certain abnormalities are presented to emphasize commonly existing defects.

UPPER EXTREMITIES

Size and symmetry. The size and symmetry of the upper extremities should be compared. Generally, right-handed individuals demonstrate slightly better muscular development of the right than left upper extremity. The opposite is true of left-handed persons. Obvious asymmetry is present in association with neurologic disorders, traumatic deformities, and congenital defects. A detailed history is quite helpful in defining the specific etiology.

Several diseases are associated with obvious abnormalities in the size and shape of the hands. In acromegaly, the hands are large, the fingers broad, and the palms wide (Fig. 17-1). Similarly, soft tissue enlargement secondary to myxedema can involve the hands in addition to other areas of the body (Fig. 17-2). Sarcoidosis can sometimes result in soft tissue swelling of the metacarpophalangeal, proximal interphalangeal, and distal interphalangeal joints (Fig. 17-3). Symmetric decrease in the size of the

upper extremities can be observed as a result of certain illnesses occurring during childhood. Juvenile rheumatoid arthritis and inflammatory bowel disease, especially when treated with corticosteroids, are associated with growth retardation. However, the decrease in the upper extremity growth usually is proportional to the diminished stature, and the cause is obvious from the taking of the history.

Unilateral or bilateral edema may be present in the upper extremities. Because excess fluids tend to accumulate in the more dependent lower extremities, upper extremity involvement is less common. Bilateral upper extremity

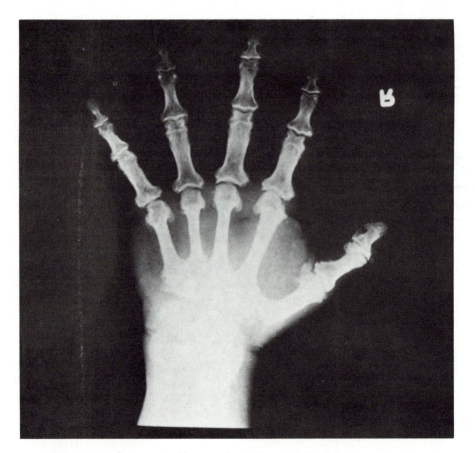

Fig. 17-1. Enlargement of bony and soft tissues of the hand in acromegaly.

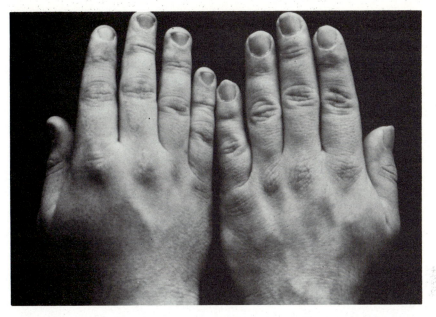

Fig. 17-2. Soft tissue enlargement of the hand secondary to myxedema.

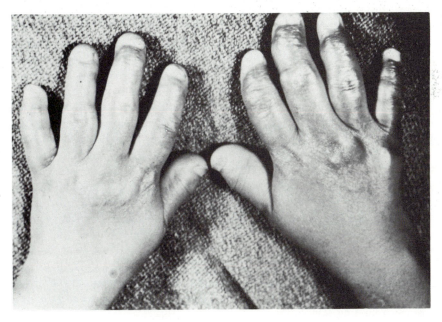

Fig. 17-3. Sarcoid arthropathy.

edema may indicate obstruction of the superior vena cava, especially when associated with cyanosis and edema of the face and neck. Similar patterns of edema may be seen in anasarca from severe congestive heart failure or renal disorders, such as nephrotic syndrome. Unilateral upper extremity edema may result from lymphatic or venous obstruction. Upper extremity stasis secondary to venous thrombosis is infrequent, so other causes, such as malignancy, should be considered.

Muscle mass. Among the normal population, there is considerable variation in muscle mass. Congenital defects, traumatic injuries to one extremity, or neurologic problems, such as hemiplegia, can result in asymmetry of the upper extremity muscle mass. Symmetric loss of upper extremity muscle mass is commonly seen in serious systemic illnesses, such as severe lung disease, malignancy, and intractable congestive heart failure. However, the muscle loss is usually not restricted to the upper extremity, being apparent in other areas.

Vasculature. Normally the veins in the hand and forearms are visibly distended when the upper extremities are in a dependent position. As the hands are elevated above the level of the manubriosternal junction, these veins gradually collapse unless there is a local obstruction of venous return or abnormally elevated venous pressure, as occurs in severe congestive heart failure. Thrombosis of the axillary or subclavian veins can result in marked dilatation of the superficial veins, in addition to swelling and discoloration of the involved extremity. In such cases, the possibility that the obstruction is secondary to neoplasm or to enlarged regional lymph glands should be thoroughly investigated. Thrombophlebitis of the superficial upper extremity veins results in local redness, tenderness, swelling, and heat. The involved vessels are quite prominent, being visibly elevated above the surrounding skin surface.

The examiner should palpate the brachial and arterial pulses in both extremities. More subtle abnormalities can only be detected by carefully comparing the pulses in one upper extremity to those in the other. Diminished or absent pulses in one upper extremity can result from a blockage of the subclavian or axilllary artery. Another cause of abnormal upper extremity arterial pulses is extrinsic compression at the thoracic outlet area as a result of cervical rib or soft tissue impairment. To determine if there might be external compression of the subclavian artery at the thoracic outlet, the patient should be sitting with the forearms supinated and resting on the thighs. Instruct the patient to turn the head toward the side being tested while extending the neck. A diminished or absent radial pulse with inspiration indicates compression of the subclavian artery by the anterior scalene muscle.

The extremities should be palpated for skin temperature and texture. In Raynaud's phenomenon or arteriosclerotic vessel disease, the fingers may be cold. Again, it is important to carefully compare one extremity to the contralateral side, thereby permitting the detection of subtle, localized arterial insufficiency.

Skin, hair, and nails. Although the superficial lymphatics normally are not visible, infections of the lymphatic ducts may be seen as red streaks *(lymphangitis)*.

In hyperthyroidism, the palms are usually moist and warm, with the skin being soft in texture. Moist, but definitely cooler hands occur in nervous patients and occasionally in patients with rheumatoid arthritis. Typically, the skin of the hands is coarse and dry in myxedema. Scleroderma can also result in very dry skin and marked sclerosis, particularly involving the skin overlying the digits *(sclerodactylia)* (Fig. 17-4). Inspection of the hands may reveal features suggestive of certain other diseases. Erythema over the thenar and hypothenar em-

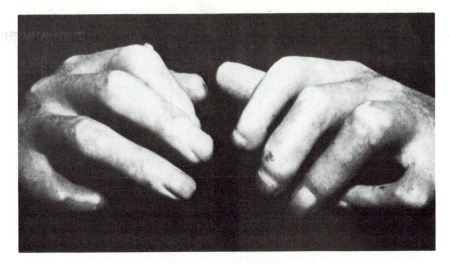

Fig. 17-4. Sclerodactylia.

inences of the palm is occasionally observed in chronic liver disease, being referred to commonly as *liver palm*. In xanthomatosis, inspection of the palms may reveal orange nodules. Petechial hemorrhages or vasculitic lesions may be seen on the extremities as well as on the mucous membranes and the conjunctivae. Petechial lesions are small red or purplish spots that are not raised above the surface of the surrounding skin. The lesions do not fade on pressure and can spontaneously disappear within several days. Vasculitic lesions are actually infarctions of the microvasculature secondary to ischemic occlusion (Figs. 17-5 and 17-6). A raised reddish or purplish lesion is very suggestive of a cutaneous vasculitis. Occasionally, certain infections such as gonococcemia can be manifested as skin lesions closely resembling a cutaneous vasculitis (Fig. 17-7).

In the male, a moderate growth of hair is usually present on the arms and dorsal aspects of the hands. In some endocrine disorders and chronic liver disease, hair over the extremities, in the axillae and elsewhere on the body may

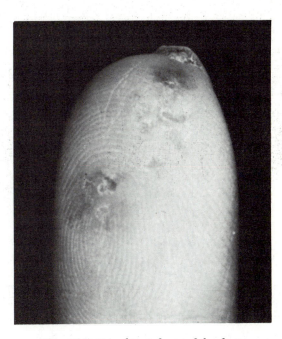

Fig. 17-5. Vasculitic infarcts of the digit.

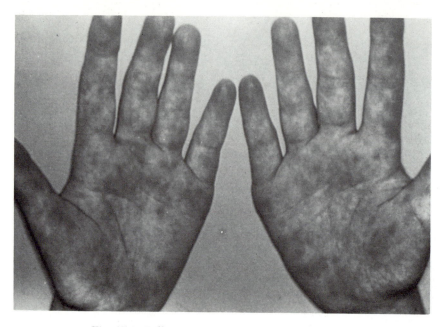

Fig. 17-6. Diffuse cutaneous vasculitis of the hands.

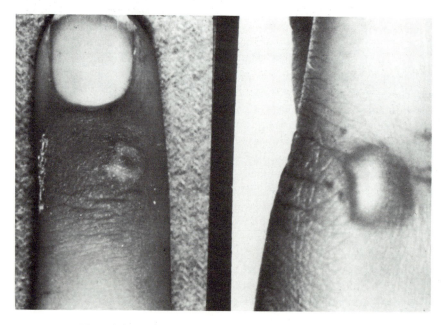

Fig. 17-7. Erythematous papular lesion of gonococcemia.

be sparse or absent. In the female, there is little hair on the arms and dorsal aspects of the hands. Although the growth does vary considerably among normal females, hair patterns more closely resembling males can result from certain endocrine disorders.

Inspection of the nails can be helpful in the diagnosis of certain systemic diseases. In anemia, the nails are pale, as are the mucous membranes and conjunctivae. Cyanotic nail beds may indicate congenital heart disease or severe respiratory insufficiency. The alternate blanching and flushing beneath the nails, termed *capillary pulse*, may be seen in aortic regurgitation. This can best be elicited by exerting slight pressure on the tip of the nail while observing for the blanching and flushing that occur in synchrony with the cardiac cycle. A *paronychia* is a suppurative or infected lesion involving the soft tissues adjacent to the nails. Occasionally, normal individuals may dis-

play a convexity of the nails without associated clubbing. This is usually congenital and may be distinguished from clubbing by the normal angle present between the nail and dorsum of the terminal digit. Fungal infections can involve the nails and without further laboratory tests sometimes are difficult to distinguish from psoriasis.

Congenital defects are extremely variable in their manifestations. Occasionally persons are born without arms or with a part of one extremity missing. Supernumerary digits, the absence of a hand, and webbing of the fingers are among the many possible congenital abnormalities.

In hyperthyroidism there may be a fine tremor involving the hands. This can be demonstrated by having the person extend his hands and by placing a thin sheet of paper on the dorsal aspects of the extended fingers. In parkinsonism there is a pill-rolling movement,

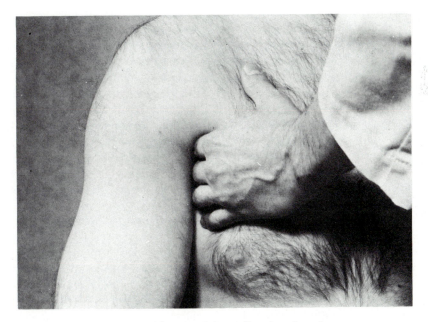

Fig. 17-8. Palpation of the axillary lymph nodes.

in which the thumb rolls over the palmar aspects of the index and second fingers. In this condition the patient also has a rest tremor. When his hands are relaxed, the tremor is present, but it disappears with voluntary movement. In multiple sclerosis just the opposite is seen—an activity tremor. In this condition the tremor is manifested on attempted movement of the extremities but is absent when the limbs are at rest. The liver flap of hepatic coma (asterixis) was discussed previously.

A careful inspection and palpation of the epitrochlear and axillary lymph glands is mandatory whenever the upper extremities are examined. Unfortunately, this is often neglected. If enlarged glands are present, they should be described as to their location, size, consistency, tenderness, state of fixation, and whether they are discrete or matted together.

The axilla, for purposes of examination, should be considered as a pyramid consisting of an apex and four walls: anterior, posterior, lateral, and medial. It is essential to inspect and palpate all dimensions of this anatomic pyramid. The axilla should be examined with the arm first partially adducted and then abducted to palpate adequately for the presence of enlarged lymph glands (Fig. 17-8).

LOWER EXTREMITIES

It should be emphasized that the lower extremities must be completely exposed to detect asymmetry and other more subtle abnormalities. The lower extremities should be examined with the patient in the standing as well as the supine position.

Symmetry. Asymmetry of the lower extremities can be the result of several abnormalities, including unilateral edema, atrophy, trauma, and congenital defects. If there is any suspicion of asymmetry, the examiner should precisely measure both lower extremities at identical levels to quantitate the difference in circumfer-

ence. For the calf, this can be accomplished by making a mark at a prescribed number of centimeters distal to the inferior border of the patella. Measurement of both calves at this specific level permits the valid determination of possible differences. Similarly, the circumference of the thighs can be compared by measuring at specific distances proximal to the superior border of the patella. Such quantitative measurements are not only helpful in initially detecting differences but also are extremely useful in accurately assessing the response to treatment.

One of the most common causes of enlargement of the lower extremities is edema. When edema is present, the tissues will pit (indent) if firm pressure is applied by the examiner. This pitting phenomenon distinguishes edema from synovial thickening, which fails to indent following firm palpation. Edema may be limited to the feet or ankles or may extend to the knees or even to the thighs. Bilateral edema in the lower extremities may result from congestive heart failure, portal cirrhosis, nephritis, and pressure on the inferior vena cava caused by ascites or an intra-abdominal tumor mass. During pregnancy, the pressure of the fetus on the vena cava will often produce bilateral edema in the legs. Unilateral edema in the lower extremities may result from varicose veins, thrombophlebitis (inflammation of veins), lymphangitis, and enlargement of the regional lymph glands compressing the femoral veins. In patients who have a hemiplegia edema of the paralyzed leg often develops as a result of stasis caused by disuse.

The shape of the legs may be altered by rickets, osteitis deformans, syphilis, poorly aligned fractures, and various deformities resulting from tumors and arthritis. Rickets may cause bowlegs or knock-knees. In osteitis deformans (Paget's disease) the legs are bowed, and the anterior tibial aspects are markedly convex. In syphilitic periostitis caused by congenital syphilis tibial surfaces also are bowed anteriorly (saber shins).

The patient's muscular status is usually well demonstrated in the legs. Muscle atrophy may be unilateral or bilateral. Atrophy usually follows lower motor neuron paralysis but may be caused by disuse resulting from previous injury or disease.

Vasculature. Diseases of the veins and arteries are more common in the lower than the upper extremities. Tortuous, dilated, and elongated superficial veins are commonly encountered in adult patients, especially women. They are referred to as *varicose veins* and may be accompanied by varicose ulcers and a bronze pigmentation, termed *stasis dermatitis*. In superficial thrombophlebitis the involved veins are red, swollen, and tender. The surrounding tissue may be edematous. The regional femoral lymph glands may also be en-larged and tender. Embolic complications are rare in superficial thrombophlebitis.

When varicose veins are present to a significant degree, it is important to determine the competency of valves in the saphenous and communicating veins and also to determine the presence of an obstruction in the deep venous circulation. Although a number of tests have been devised to investigate these possibilities, one of the simplest and most informative is that known as Perthes' test. In this procedure a tourniquet is applied to the thigh tightly enough to compress the long saphenous vein and prevent the flow of blood in the superficial circulation past this constriction. The patient then is instructed to walk briskly, and the prominence of the varicose veins is noted. This test depends on the fact that the blood flow in the venous system of the leg is definitely aided by muscular action and normally goes from the superficial to the deep system. If the varices

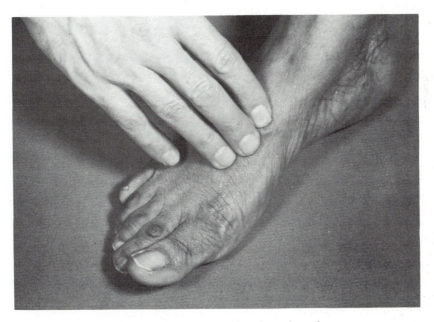

Fig. 17-9. Palpation of the dorsalis pedis pulses.

disappear rather rapidly when the patient walks, the test is interpreted as indicating that the valves in both the saphenous and communicating veins are incompetent. If the varices become more prominent when the patient walks and if he expresses actual discomfort, the test is interpreted as indicating that there is obstruction in the deep veins and that the valves of the communicating veins are incompetent.

Thrombus formation (phlebothrombosis) frequently occurs in the deep veins of the calf following surgery, in patients with congestive heart failure, after childbirth, in carcinomatosis, and in chronic debilitating diseases. As a rule, this process causes relatively little reaction in the vein wall, with the consequence that the thrombus is prone to dislodge and be carried into the pulmonary vascular system, resulting in pulmonary embolization. This constitutes a very serious complication that may and often does prove fatal. Generally, phlebothrombosis is accompanied by pain and tenderness in the calf of the leg. At times the leg may be visibly swollen, and the superficial veins may be slightly distended. On occasion tenderness on pressure and pain in the calf on dorsiflexion of the foot may be the only positive signs. There may be increased warmth in the leg, and in the very early stage, arterial pulsations on the affected side may be decreased temporarily. Finally, there is a measurable increase in the circumference of the involved leg, which may not be visible on inspection.

A routine examination of the legs should include palpation of the femoral, popliteal, posterior tibial, and dorsalis pedis pulses. The femoral pulse is palpated in the femoral triangle, and the popliteal pulse is palpated in the popliteal fossa. The popliteal pulse is best detected with the patient lying on his abdomen with his knees flexed about 45 degrees. The posterior tibial artery lies posterior to the internal malleolus. The dorsalis pedis artery can usually be palpated between the first and second metatarsal bones (Fig. 17-9). It is important to bear in mind that, as the result of anomalies in approximately 8% to 10% of normal people, either or both dorsalis pedis arteries are absent or so anomalously located that they are not palpable. Thus, the absence of dorsalis pedis pulsations alone does not verify a diagnosis of occlusive arterial disease.

In advanced arteriosclerosis it is often impossible to detect either the dorsalis pedis or posterior tibial pulses. The distal portions of the

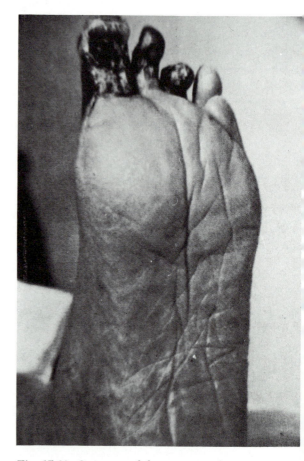

Fig. 17-10. Gangrene of the toes secondary to arteriosclerotic insufficiency.

extremities are usually cold to palpation, they blanch (pallor) when the leg is elevated, and they become red or reddish purple (rubor) when the extremity is in a dependent position. If the pallor in an elevated ischemic extremity does not disappear within 15 seconds after the position has been changed from elevation to dependency, one may conclude that the degree of ischemia is moderate to severe. Ulceration or gangrene of the toes may follow mild trauma to an arteriosclerotic limb (Fig. 17-10).

Arteriosclerosis of the peripheral vessels at

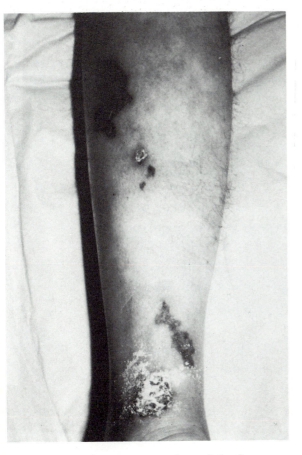

Fig. 17-11. Cutaneous vasculitis of the lower extremities.

times produces significant narrowing (stenosis) of the iliac, femoral, and more distal arteries in the lower extremities. Significant obstruction within these vessels is often accompanied by a bruit. By lightly placing the diaphragm of the stethoscope over the femoral artery in the femoral triangle, one may detect a bruit when this vessel is narrowed or obstructed. Similar bruits may be heard over the lower midabdomen when the abdominal aorta is obstructed.

In obstruction of the femoral artery, the popliteal and all distal pulses on the involved side cannot be palpated. If the obstruction involves the common or external iliac artery, the femoral and all distal pulses on the ipsilateral side cannot be palpated. By careful attention to the color and temperature changes and by systematic palpation of the femoral, popliteal, posterior tibial, and dorsalis pedis pulses, the physician has an excellent opportunity to determine the approximate level of the arterial obstruction. This is of extreme importance in light of the ever-increasing advances in peripheral vascular surgery.

Raynaud's phenomenon is occasionally seen in the lower extremities but is rarely as severe as in the hands.

Thromboangitis obliterans *(Buerger's disease)* most frequently involves the lower extremities and occurs more commonly in men than in women. It is an inflammatory process, not arteriosclerosis, that involves the arteries, veins, and often the accompanying nerve fibers.

Skin, hair, and nails. Cutaneous ulcerations are often observed on the lower extremities. These are usually caused by compromised blood supply in association with arteriosclerotic vessel disease or vasculitis (Fig. 17-11). The lesions of erythema nodosum frequently occur over the pretibial areas (Fig. 17-12). These raised, painful, erythematous lesions are often observed in conjunction with severe edema of

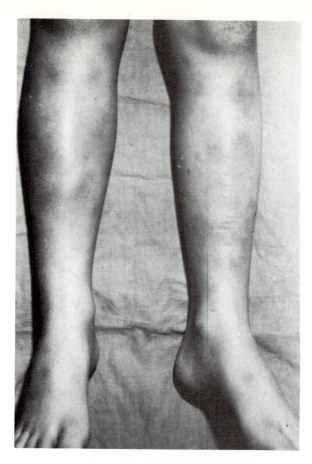

Fig. 17-12. Tender, raised erythematous pretibial lesions of erythema nodosum.

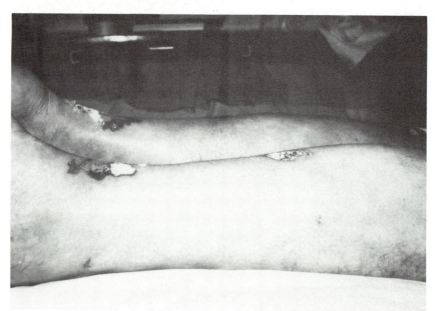

Fig. 17-13. Deep necrotic ulcers secondary to systemic vasculitis.

can be involved with keratoderma blennorrhagia of Reiter's disease, which often is indistinguishable from the pustular form of psoriasis (Fig. 17-14). Onychomycosis and less severe psoriasis can be limited to the toenails.

Feet. Supernumerary digits and webbing of the toes are among the numerous defects involving the feet. Several varieties of talipes, or clubfoot, are also seen.

Unusual movements of the lower extremities are in most instances manifested by disturbances of gait. These are discussed in Chapters 7 and 18.

Lymph glands. Examination of the lower extremities should include a careful inspection and palpation of the inguinal regions for hernia and enlargement of the inguinal and femoral lymph glands. The procedure for detecting inguinal and femoral hernias is discussed in Chapter 15.

Two groups of lymph glands are present in the groin:

1. *Inguinal* glands, located in the region of the inguinal ligament, drain the genitalia, perineum, lower abdomen, buttocks, and parts of the thighs.

2. *Femoral* glands, located in the femoral triangle, drain the thighs, legs, and feet.

The inguinal lymph glands may be enlarged as the result of acute infections in any of the areas mentioned, systemic diseases (such as lymphomas), and metastasis from malignant processes along the course of the lymph channels draining these areas.

The femoral lymph glands are usually enlarged and tender in the presence of inflammatory disease involving the thighs, legs, and feet. They also may become enlarged in various systemic diseases or as the result of metastasis from tumors in the legs and feet.

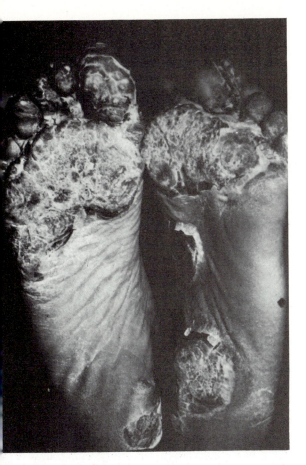

Fig. 17-14. Keratoderma blennorrhagica of Reiter's syndrome.

the adjacent uninvolved tissues. Other vasculitic lesions occur in the lower extremities and, when severe, result in deep necrotic ulcerations with a slightly raised erythematous border next to the uninvolved tissue (Fig. 17-13).

Other signs of nutritional changes resulting from arterial ischemia can include trophic changes of the nails and loss of hair over the pretibial area and dorsum of the feet. The feet

CHAPTER 18

NERVOUS SYSTEM

It is essential that the neurologic examination be adapted to the problem of the individual patient. A complete neurologic examination may occupy many hours, but it is not necessary to perform detailed evaluations of all aspects of neurologic function on every patient when these are irrelevant to the problem under consideration. The nature of the complaint and the history yield the most important clues in planning the examination. For instance, in the case of a middle-aged businessman complaining of forgetfulness, it is essential that a thorough mental status examination be accomplished. In an individual complaining of progressive weakness in his legs, a thorough evaluation of muscle strength and motor system is required. When no neurologic disorder has been indicated on the history, a satisfactory screening examination to detect any unexpected abnormalities can be accomplished within 15 or 20 minutes. If, however, a neurologic deficit is revealed, then the examiner must be prepared to extend his examination appropriately in order to elucidate the problem.

The experienced physician can obtain important neurologic information during the period of history-taking. Evidence of abnormalities in speech, language function, memory, emotional status, and judgment can be detected. With history completed and patient undressed and draped, it is generally convenient to observe gait and stance. After that, the fundi and cranial nerves I through XII are examined. Motor examination proceeds through neck muscles, arms, trunk, and legs; tendon and superficial reflexes are elicited in the same order. Sensory examination is then completed. Examination of relevant skeletal functions, arteries, and autonomic functions, and auscultation of the neck and head are then carried out. Many examiners prefer to defer formal testing of orientation, intellectual functioning, language, and speech until the end of the examination.

MENTAL STATUS

The examination of the mental state from the neurologic point of view places major emphasis on the detection and analysis of disorders in higher function resulting from organic disease. It is especially important to relate disturbances in mental function to anatomic structures, both in order to aid in anatomic localization of disease processes and also to obtain clues as to etiology. Accordingly, the present system of examination is designed to evaluate functions in the three phylogenetic divisions of the human brain, the central and midline systems, the limbic system, and the neocortex (Fig. 18-1 and Table 18-1). With respect to the neocortex, functions having a general relationship to the structure will be described, followed by more localized functions related to the dominant and nondominant hemispheres.

Central and midline system

It is appropriate to group within the central and midline category the ascending reticular projections, diffuse projections from the thalamus, midline nuclei of the brain stem, and the hippocampi. The reticular and diffuse thalamic pathways relate to general arousal of the brain, and the midline brain stem nuclei to sleep mechanisms. The hippocampus plays a major role in the consolidation of memory recordings. Lesions that destroy the reticular nuclei of midbrain and pons bilaterally or that completely interrupt their projections result in *coma*. In examining a patient with impaired consciousness it is important to record specific functional levels, such as the following: drowsy but can be aroused to respond appropriately, stuporous with eyes closed but will wince or

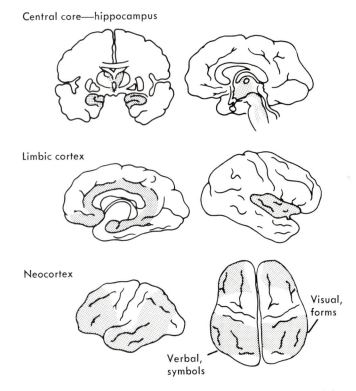

Fig. 18-1. Distributions of three major cerebral systems related to mental functions. (After Dr. P. I. Yakovlev. From Allen, N., and Burkholder, J.: Degenerative diseases of the nervous system. In Farmer, T. W.: Practice of medicine, Hagerstown, Md., 1972, Harper & Row, Publishers, Inc.)

Table 18-1. Outline of the neurologic mental examination

Structures	Observations
Central and medial systems	
Reticular alerting system	State of consciousness
Hippocampus	Orientation in time
	Ten-minute recall of test objects, address
Limbic system	Sociability, affection, aggression, sexuality, emotional expression
Neocortex	
General	Serial sevens, similarities, proverbs and metaphors, emotional control, previous knowledge
Dominant	Language tests, calculations, digit span, right-left discrimination, apraxia tests
Nondominant	Awareness of opposite limbs, awareness of neurologic deficit, facial recognition, orientation in space, dressing ability, ability to construct simple forms

withdraw a limb to strong stimulus, comatose with no evidence of cerebral responsivity. It is important for the examiner to recognize two other states of disturbed consciousness. One is *akinetic mutism* (vigilant coma), which is a state of immobility and speechlessness in which the subject makes no effect to communicate. The eyes often remain open and may occasionally turn toward large objects or the examiner. The patient is incontinent of bowel and bladder and displays no emotional response to pain. He can swallow but has to be fed. The condition has been associated particularly with lesions in the posterior part of the thalami and anteromedial surface of the frontal lobe. Another condition is the *"locked in"* syndrome (de-efferented state). This condition results from destruction of the ventral portion of the pons, resulting in complete paralysis of the limbs and the lower cranial nerves. Because the pontine tegmentum and the midbrain are spared, the patient may be conscious. He can hear and may communicate with the examiner by a system of eye blinks. *Delirium* is a state of disturbed awareness that is accompanied by excitation, confusion, and hallucinations. It usually results from toxic, metabolic, or inflammatory processes acting on brain stem pathways or the cerebrum in a diffuse fashion.

Destructive processes of the hippocampi or the medial thalamic structures may produce a severe disorder in the consolidation of new memory traces. This results in disorientation in time and inability to recall test material, such as three or four common objects or a test name and address (see memory testing following).

Limbic system

The limbic cortex and its subcortical nuclei relate to the emotional life of the individual and to innate behavior specific to the species, including sexual activity, defensive and attack responses, and expressions of inner feeling states, such as laughter or anger. The system may be conveniently divided into two major portions. The anterior and medial portion comprises the cingulate gyrus, the orbital frontal gyri, and the septal nucleus. These structures appear to function primarily with respect to affectionate feelings and responses, sexuality, and ability to relate to other members of society. A lateral and inferior portion contains the pyriform lobe, parahippocampus, uncus, and underlying amygdala. Its function includes aggressive behavior and responses related to self-preservation. A major lesion in one system bilaterally may allow for distorted or exaggerated functions of the remaining division. Thus, tumors or traumatic lesions affecting the medial and inferior portion of the frontal lobes and the septal area can result in extraordinary states of aggression with shouting, biting, and attack behavior precipitated by trivial or inappropriate stimuli. On the contrary, bilateral lesions of the lateral and inferior division can result in pathologic docility and excessive or abnormal sexuality.

The examination of the limbic system requires nonverbal direct observations and indirect accounts of behavior. In the history the physician seeks evidence from informants of alteration in personality that could include carelessness, indifference, inability to sense the emotions in others, loss of sympathetic reactions, loss of libido and sexual activity, excessive irritability or rage reactions, or unusual docility. The examiner himself must interpret the patient's language or gestures, which may be distorted. Facial expressions may be defective in emotional content or bizarre and uninterpretable, often producing a vague sense of discomfiture in the observer (Fig. 18-2).

Neocortex

Most of the higher integrated activities of the human brain are functions of the neocortex. From practical clinical needs several groups of functions can be emphasized. These include language and the use of arithmetic and other symbols. There are the processes of orientation of the patient to his own body shape and to the discrimination of the right and left sides. Perception of extrapersonal space and forms relates to orientation to rooms and environment, to abstract space represented by maps, and to

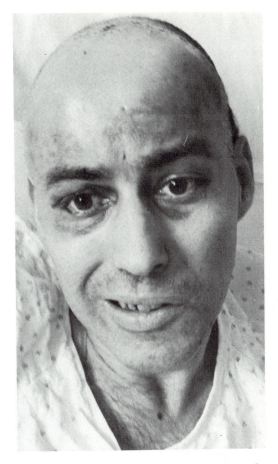

Fig. 18-2. Patient with a presenile cerebral atrophic disorder affecting frontal limbic areas. Emotional expressions are impaired and replaced by quizzical or unusual expressions.

the construction of geometric forms. Other important functions include reasoning, the ability to perform abstractions, the ability to project into the future and plan for it, and the achievement of remote or complex goals.

The neocortex can be examined in terms of specific properties of the hemispheres and of major lobes as well as more general properties that are disturbed by diffuse or multifocal disease. Tests relevant to general properties include serial sevens, similarities, proverb and metaphor interpretation, and reasoning. If there is no specific impairment of ability to perform simple calculations from localized dominant parietotemporal disease, the serial sevens test is a good general index of neocortical performance. The patient is asked to subtract seven from 100 and then to continue the process of serial subtraction. An average patient may make one or two minor errors, but a cortically damaged individual may make numerous errors, may lose track of the process, or may be unable to maintain attention for serial operations. The test is rather sensitive and may be impaired in severe depression or anxiety. Similarities testing requires the recognition of a general or abstract characteristic common to specific objects. Thus, the patient is asked to state what is similar about or what there is in common between an apple and an orange, a table and a sofa, an automobile and a motorcycle. The expected responses would be: "They are both fruit, articles of furniture, motor vehicles." Some abnormal responses could be "one is red and one is orange," "they go together," or "they both have wheels." Interpretation of proverbs and metaphors also deals with the ability of a patient to abstract a generalization from concrete examples. An abstraction deals with the essential or universal properties of a class or group of objects. A concrete observation is concerned with the particular aspects of a specific object detected by the senses. The patient can be given a proverb or common fable and asked for its meaning. An example would be, "A rolling stone gathers no moss." The normal person will interpret this in terms of the inability of an habitual wanderer to acquire material possessions. The person with cerebral disease will speak of the failure of moss to stick to a stone. The fund of general knowledge and vocabulary usually reflects educational background and level of cerebral function in early life. Except in the case of gross social deprivation, it is reasonable to expect a patient of average intellect to be able to name five large cities, major rivers, several countries, commonly known geographic distances, or recent presidents of the United States. Loss of common information and vocabulary, after it is once acquired, takes place only in advanced dementias or in acute confusional states.

Another property of the neocortex is the modulation or control of emotional behavior. In diffuse brain disease one may observe emotional lability with an unstable shifting of mood from extremes of sadness and weeping to jocularity and laughter. Bilateral or unilateral lesions of the frontal lobes are often associated with characteristic defects, including euphoria and inability to maintain sustained efforts. Euphoria is a superficial elevation of mood and a state of relative unconcern in the face of serious events or threatening symptoms. It often coexists with flippancy, loss of social inhibitions, and crude attempts at humor.

Dominant neocortical functions

Language is one of the most important functions of the dominant hemisphere. The left side of the brain is dominant in most right-handed individuals and also in about half of left-handed individuals; therefore, the left hemisphere is dominant in approximately 95% of the general population. Language is not represented in a highly localized fashion, as in the case of the primary sensory projection areas or the motor cortex; rather, it may be thought of as concentrated in a cortical field, including the superior and lateral temporal lobe, the temporoparietooccipital junction, and the lower or opercular region of the frontal lobe. First, the recognition of spoken language requires the perception of sound in the superior temporal cortex. The immediate retention of these sound perceptions and the automatic probability calculation that they represent words is the function of the surrounding temporal cortex. Similarly, recognition of visualized forms corresponding to letters and words requires the occipital cortex surrounding the primary visual projection area. The memory of the names of objects appears to require participation of the lateral temporal lobe. The interpretation of perceived words in terms of meanings and the formulation of a reply with new meanings and new words is a poorly localized function that may be a property of the entire language field. The function of processing language being thought into language to be spoken or written requires the integrity of the frontal operculum. The arcuate bundle connects the temporal cortex and the operculum.

Aphasia. Impairment of the understanding or the use of language is termed *aphasia*. The classification will generally follow that of Geschwind (Table 18-2). Aphasia is usually a combination of several types; however, in some cases relatively pure forms may be found and are of localizing value. It is important to distinguish between aphasias with reduced output or very slowly spoken words and aphasias with well-preserved or fluent output but abnormal word content.

Those with reduced output can be produced by isolated lesions above the Sylvian fissure. *Broca's* or motor aphasia is characterized by very slow speech, poor articulation, and a curious tendency to delete pronouns, prepositions, and other small words (telegraphic speech). The patient is generally aware of a defect and displays evident frustration and impatience. Ability to write may also be impaired, and the written material may be characterized by small deletions. The understanding of written or spoken words is preserved. Broca's aphasia is commonly accompanied by a partial or complete hemiparesis involving the right face and arm. *Aphemia*, or mutism, is a rather uncommon disorder in which there may be gross inability to use the muscles of articulation to form words. The patient may also be unable to perform specific movements of the lips or tongue on request, even in the absence of hemiparesis.

Aphasias with preserved or fluent output may be caused by lesions below the Sylvian fissure. *Wernicke's*, or auditory receptive, aphasia appears with lesions of the posterior superior temporal cortex. Comprehension of spoken words is defective, and the patient may be unable to repeat test phrases. Despite this, abundant speech with appropriate melody and expressiveness is present, although many incorrect words are used (paraphasia). In severe

Table 18-2. Classification of aphasias

Type	Site of lesion
Reduced output	
Motor (Broca's) aphasia	Frontal operculum
Aphemia or mutism	Frontal subcortical white
Preserved or fluent output	
Auditory receptive (Wernicke's) aphasia	Posterior superior temporal
Nominal aphasia	Posterior temporal parietal
Conduction aphasia	Inferior parietal
Dyslexia	Occipital
Global aphasia	Frontotemporoparietal

cases there is a jargon speech—a multitude of sounds having no word meanings. This may be interspersed with some correctly uttered, commonly used words or phrases. An example is the following transcription from a taped record: "Now then, mer dee whan no is from shey sahl. I don't know palla came to plewba and well." In contrast to reduced output aphasias, patients with this type of aphasia often are unaware of their incorrect utterances. The condition is commonly associated with a right homonymous hemianopia or superior quadrantanopia. *Nominal aphasia* is commonly associated with other types, but may occasionally exist alone. It is characterized by inability to name common objects, although recognition is preserved. The patient comprehends spoken language and is able to repeat test phrases and sentences. Spontaneous speech is characterized by deletion of unusual nouns and circumlocutions. It is often accompanied by elements of the parietal temporal syndrome. *Conduction aphasia* appears to occur with the lesions in the lower parietal cortex and has been attributed to involvement of the arcuate bundle. It is characterized by fluent speech with paraphasic errors. There is good comprehension of spoken words but poor ability to repeat test phrases, particularly involving small words. *Dyslexia* consists of the reduced comprehension of written or printed language. It may be accompanied by other aspects of the parietotemporal syndrome and by visual field defects. Abnormalities in writing with incorrect spelling or repetition of words or letters is commonly seen in all of the forms of fluent aphasia. *Global aphasia* consists of almost total loss of all language functions. It is produced by a massive lesion in the language field and is commonly associated with hemiplegia, hemisensory loss, and hemianopia.

In examining for aphasia one first listens to the conversation. In some patients there may be a gross and obvious disorder in language, but in others there may be subtle defects detectable only by careful listening. One first determines whether the spontaneous speech is fluent and voluble or reduced in quantity with hesitancy and slow utterances. With the reduced output types the examiner usually can establish good rapport with the patient and can request him to make some spontaneous statements or to read aloud. Observations are made for imperfect pronunciation, markedly slow speech, and deletions of prepositions and pronouns. In the abundant output types the examiner observes for the comprehension of his own spoken words. It is well to start with simple, slowly spoken commands and work up to larger more complex assertions. The patient is asked to repeat language samples, again starting with simple words or phrases and progressing to more complex phrases. Single words should be used first, such as "cat" or "window." Phrases are then tried, such as "under the table." Next simple sentences can be used, such as "The sky is clear," "The book is on the table," "The dog chased the cat through the garden." In the case of nominal aphasia one listens for hesitancy in the use of nouns or verbs during spontaneous speech; substitutions or circumlocutions may be observed. The patient is then asked to name common objects, such as comb, key, wristwatch, watchband, second hand, pencil, handkerchief; he is asked to read, again starting with simple printed words, such as "cat" or "door," followed by sentences or paragraphs; and he is requested to write spontaneously and also in response to dictation. Common to all forms of aphasia is *perseveration*, in which the word expressed in response to a question is given repeatedly to new and different questions.

Apraxia. The apraxias are defined as disorders in the execution of skilled or learned motor acts that cannot be accounted for simply by paralysis or lack of comprehension (Geschwind, 1975). Implicit in this definition is the concept of the dominant neocortex as the principal brain area acting not only in acquisition of learned movements but also in primary control of muscles of face (perioral area), hand, and foot and in the use of these body parts in the utilization of external objects, such as instruments or tools. Examples of such actions would be drinking from a cup, brushing the teeth, combing the hair, blowing out a match, or operating a foot pedal. The premotor area of the left frontal cortex appears to serve as a processing zone for activation of the motor cortex both of the left and right hemispheres. Information from this center is transmitted by way of the anterior corpus callosum to the comparable area of the nondominant frontal lobe. The defects appearing after destructive lesions of these systems are most pronounced in the case of commands given as verbal or written instructions. Presentation of an actual object to a patient with this disorder often results in improved motor action because of direct visual and tactile influences from older parts of the cortex. Preserved are movements having an older phylogenetic basis and that involve actions of the body on the body or with the use

of a body part as a tool. Also preserved are a variety of skilled movements involving axial parts of the body, such as walking, standing up, sitting, or even dancing. Thus, a patient with apraxia may be unable to respond adequately to commands such as: "Show me how you would drink from a cup," "Pretend to comb your hair," or "Pretend to use a hammer to drive a nail." He may form his hand into a cup and then pretend to drink from it or may use his fingers in a claw fashion to run through his hair, or may make a fist and pound it against the imaginary nail; yet, if he is given a real cup, comb, or hammer his performance may be much improved or quite accurate.

Lesions likely to produce apraxia are listed in Table 18-3. Destruction of the anterior corpus callosum may prevent transmission of information from the dominant to the right frontal lobe. In this case the patient will carry out normal skilled acts on command with his right hand or foot but cannot execute these with his left hand or foot. When the movement is shown him by the examiner or when a concrete object is presented to him, then the right hemisphere is able to coordinate the activity on the basis of visualized information, and the movement is completed. Skilled acts involving

Table 18-3. Apraxias and disorders of innate movements

Type	Site
Apraxias	
1. Left limb deficits in skilled acts on command, corrected by imitation	Corpus callosum
2. Bilateral face and limb deficits in skilled acts on command, improved on imitation	Left frontal premotor
3. Similar to 2, usually milder	Left inferior parietal
Disorders of innate movements	
1. Reflex grasp and suck responses	Opposite superior medial frontal
2. Reflex avoiding responses	Opposite parietal
3. Gait disorder and backward falling	Medial frontal and parietal cortex
4. Midline face movement (close eyes, stick out tongue)	Nondominant or bilateral parietal

the face are generally spared, since the lower motor cortex on the left has some degree of control over facial muscles bilaterally. A lesion in the left frontal premotor area can prevent activation either of the right or left motor cortex for skilled acts. Consequently, there will be a bilateral apraxia involving face and limbs. Lesions in the left inferior parietal area have also been associated with apraxia. This has been at-tributed to interruption of pathways extending from temporal and parietal areas to the frontal premotor cortex.

Parietotemporal syndomes. Disorders commonly seen in lesions affecting the dominant parietal and temporal cortex also include calculation difficulties, right-left disorientation, defects in construction of geometric forms, and defective finger identification. Calculations are

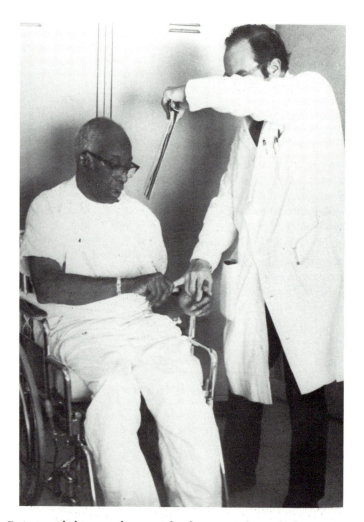

Fig. 18-3. Patient with large, right parietal infarction. When asked to find his left index finger with vision occluded, patient misidentified examiner's finger for his own.

tested by problems in simple mental arithmetic. The average patient may be expected to perform addition such as 25 + 13, multiplication such 3 × 15 or 3 × 1½. Right and left orientation is tested by asking the patient to identify his own right or left limb as well as those of the examiner. Geometric constructions are tested by asking the patient to draw forms, such as a triangle, a square, a cube, or a five-pointed star. With left parietal lesions major errors may be made that are improved by observing a model of the desired figure. In major dominant parietal lesions a patient may have difficulty in discriminating the fingers of his own hand.

Visual agnosia. Visual agnosia (impairment of the ability to recognize objects observed visually) has been associated with bilateral lesions of the occipital cortex bordering primary projection areas. Common objects, such as a paper clip or book of matches are presented. The patient cannot identify these by sight but can detect them by palpation.

Nondominant cortical disorders

The nondominant hemisphere is particularly important in visual recognition and orientation in space. Lesions of the nondominant parietal lobe produce a characteristic series of effects with distortions of concepts of space and form and marked loss of awareness of the left side of the body. Such a patient directs little attention to any stimulus approaching from the left side and literally may neglect the left side of the body. He may fail to recognize his own left hand when placed in front of his eyes. When asked to use his right hand to find and identify his left index finger, he may very well grasp the examiner's finger and declare it to be his own (Fig. 18-3). If he is hemiplegic on the left side he may steadfastly deny any disability. The patient with a right parietal lesion has dif-

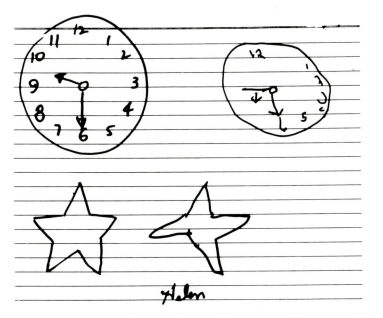

Fig. 18-4. Drawings of patient with parietal cortex lesions caused by trauma. The patient deletes elements on the left sides of the clock face and star.

ficulty in dressing himself, often leaving the left side unclothed. Defects in construction of geometric forms can be revealed by drawing simple figures. In attempting to reproduce the face of a clock, the patient may omit the numerals on the left (Fig. 18-4). Another sensitive indicator is the simple bedside test of matchstick constructions. Designs, such as a simple house or a five-pointed star, are made by the examiner, removed, and the patient asked to reproduce them. He may again neglect the left side of the figure or make gross errors in assembling the matches. These errors are usually not corrected by the presence of a model before him. Patients with relatively minor parietal lobe damage may tend to lose their way in familiar environments and have difficulty in identifying and drawing relationships of their hospital room and ward. Other defects associated with nondominant posterior hemisphere lesions include loss of ability to recognize familiar faces and impairment of musical ability.

Memory testing

Forms of memory or alteration of behavior by experience are common to many parts of the nervous system. In fact, classical conditioning can occur at subcortical levels. For practical clinical purposes, however, the neurologic examiner is mainly concerned with three forms of memory. The first is immediate memory, or recall, that consists of the brief retention of a spoken sentence, written material, or visualized object for a matter of seconds. This process is subserved by the cortex near the primary projection areas (temporal, postcentral, or occipital) and is lost only in localized disease of these regions or of the cerebral cortex in general. The process appears to require local cortical circuits and decays in a very brief period unless memory consolidation is activated. A good test for immediate memory is the digit span. Numerals are spoken at intervals of about 1 second, starting with a series of three digits and

increasing in length until the patient fails to repeat the series correctly. An average person can repeat a series of seven digits forward and five digits backward.

A second form of memory is recent memory in which the process of consolidation takes place. Testing of this function requires persistence of the perceived material for longer periods and involves the function of the hippocampus and its connections. To test this aspect of memory, the patient is presented with three or four common objects and is asked to remember them. He is then given verbal memoranda, such as an address (John Warner, 54 North Broadway, Springfield, Illinois). He is required to repeat it until he can immediately give it correctly. Ten minutes later he is requested to recall all of the items. Recent memory can also be evaluated by orientation to time. It is important to test for this function with tact and consideration. For example, the patient may be asked, "Have you been able to keep up with dates since you've been in the hospital?" He is then requested to give the day of the week, date of the month, and the year. Early in the course of presenile dementia, the patient may appear as a person of proper demeanor and social graces, but on direct questioning may show a surprising lack of orientation in time.

The third process relates to established permanent or remote memories. During this process, there is an element of abstraction of the meaning of remembered material with completion of the consolidation process. The function cannot be well localized but appears to require large areas of the cerebral cortex. It is tested in terms of recollections of verifiable past events and basic knowledge. This function is usually not lost except in rather profound diffuse disease or destruction of large areas of brain.

CRANIAL NERVES

Cranial nerve I (olfactory nerve). In testing olfactory sense, one nostril is occluded while the patient sniffs an unknown substance. Readily available and nonpungent materials, such as soap, tobacco, and coffee are used. Care has to be taken that the patient's air passages are patent. In many elderly people or after years of chronic rhinitis, sense of smell may be lost. Unilateral loss is significant because it may indicate olfactory groove meningioma or laceration of the olfactory nerve from trauma to the head.

Cranial nerve II (optic nerve). Visual acuity can be measured at the bedside with a reading card. To eliminate the influence of refractory errors, the patient should use his reading glasses. Loss of visual acuity with central scotoma is characteristic of retrobulbar neuritis. Initially, papilledema caused by acutely increased intracranial pressure produces little visual loss, but may cause increase of the blind spot and constriction of peripheral fields.

Visual field testing in the office or at the bedside may be performed by confrontation, as described in Chapter 10. In uncooperative patients a rough estimate of the visual field can be achieved by observing the turning of the patients's head and eyes toward an object intro-

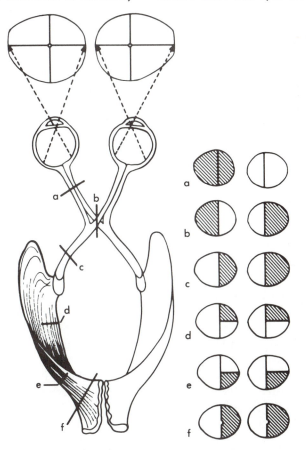

Fig. 18-5. Diagram of major lesions of optic pathways with field defects. *a*, Left optic nerve; *b*, optic chiasm; *c*, left optic tract; *d*, left temporal lobe; *e*, left parietal lobe; *f*, left occipital lobe.

duced into the visual fields. Some classical defects of the visual fields are depicted in Fig. 18-5. A pituitary tumor compressing the optic chiasm produces a bitemporal hemianopia or loss of vision in the temporal halves of each eye field. Temporal lobe lesions may involve the lower portions of the optic radiations and result in a superior quadrantanopia in the opposite visual field. Parietal lesions produce an inferior quadrantanopia. Involvement of the occipital lobe commonly results in contralateral homonymous hemianopia, sparing central vision. Visual extinction may be observed in the field of vision opposite to a posterior parietal lesion. With a right parietal lesion, for example, a single object can be detected throughout the left field. If, however, two objects are introduced simultaneously, one in the left field and one in the right, the object on the left is not perceived.

Cranial nerves III, IV, and VI (oculomotor, trochlear, and abducens nerves). The oculomotor nerve III supplies the superior rectus, inferior rectus, medial rectus, inferior oblique, and the levator palpebrae, as well as the muscles of the iris and ciliary body. The superior oblique is supplied by the trochlear nerve IV, and the lateral rectus by the abducens nerve VI. Eye movements are tested by having the patient keep his head stationary while his eyes follow the finger of the examiner. Fig. 10-16 and Table 10-1 summarize the cardinal directions of gaze of extraocular muscles.

Subtle degrees of extraocular muscle weakness can be detected by observing for diplopia (double vision) on eye movement. Since patients quickly learn to suppress false images, the use of a red glass in front of the eye facilitates the test. The patient will then see superimposed red and white images when a flashlight is held before the eyes, and will be able to report any separation of the two images. Maximal separation occurs when the eyes are moved into the direction toward which the par-

alyzed muscle would normally pull the eye. The more distant image can always be attributed to the eye with the weakened muscle. For example, in a right lateral rectus paresis the images remain fused in the primary position or on looking to the left. On right conjugate deviation the patient will note horizontal diplopia. If the red glass is placed over the right eye, then the red image will be seen to the right of the white one.

Retinal nerve fibers subserving the pupillary light reflex course posteriorly in the optic nerve and both optic tracts. As they leave the tract, they enter the pretectal area and innervate the Edinger-Westphal nucleus of either side. Consequently, the illumination of one retina induces constriction of each pupil (see Chapter 10). In unilateral loss of the pupillary light reflex, the consensual reactions are of diagnostic importance. If the disorder is caused by unilateral atrophy of the right optic nerve, a light directed into the right eye will evoke neither a direct nor a consensual response, whereas a light into the left eye will result in bilateral constriction. This effect is well shown by the swinging flashlight test. A light shone into the right eye produces little reaction, but as it is swung over, into the left eye, the pupil constricts. On swinging back to the right eye, the constricted right pupil dilates. If the unilateral loss of the pupillary light reflex has resulted from destruction of the pupillomotor fibers of the right third nerve, then a consensual reaction results from illuminating the right eye, but only a direct response results from illuminating the left.

If an object is held about 4 inches away, there will normally be convergence of the eyes on the object, accommodation, and pupillary constriction. The Argyll Robertson pupil, which may occur in tertiary syphilis, is typically small and irregular; the response to convergence is preserved, but the reaction to light is lost.

Pupillary dilatation is brought about by stimulation of sympathetic nerve fibers that innervate the radially oriented dilator pupillae muscles. These fibers originate in the hypothalamus, course laterally through the brain stem, leave the spinal cord at first and second thoracic segments, synapse in the superior cervical ganglia, and reach the iris by accompanying the internal carotid and ophthalmic arteries. In a complete third nerve lesion with loss of parasympathetic pupillomotor fibers, pupillary dilatation results from unopposed action of the

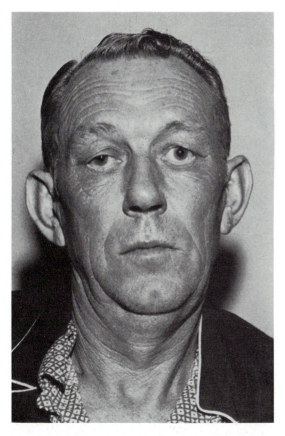

Fig. 18-6. Horner's syndrome, right side. Notice drooping of upper lid, enophthalmos, and smaller pupil.

sympathetic nerves. With interruption of the sympathetic pathways to the eye, there is found a constricted pupil, enophthalmos, and a narrowed palpebral fissure (lowering of the upper eyelid and raising of the lower eyelid). If these signs are accompanied by loss of sweating on the same side of the face, the combination is called *Horner's syndrome* (Fig. 18-6).

So far, impairment of individual muscles or nerves has been considered. Perfectly conjugate movements of both eyes are necessary to assure that a given image always falls on homologous areas of both retinas. This is achieved by several centers for conjugate eye movement. The field for volitional conjugate movements is in the frontal lobe, and that for following moving objects is in the occipital lobe. The pathway determining voluntary horizontal conjugate gaze to the right begins in the left frontal lobe (Fig. 18-7). Fibers descend in the internal capsule and cross in the midbrain to reach a pontine conjugate gaze center in the vicinity of the right sixth nerve nucleus. Some of the fibers end in this nucleus, while others, after synapsing, cross the midline to ascend in the left medial longitudinal fasciculus, terminating on that portion of the left oculomotor nucleus supplying the medial rectus. The system thereby induces contraction of the right lateral rectus and the left medial rectus. The conjugate gaze center is also activated from below by vestibular influences and by passive rotation of the head. Consequently, in paralysis of right lateral gaze caused by a left frontal lesion (Fig. 18-7, *a*), brisk rotation of the head to the left or irrigation of the right ear canal with cold water will still cause reflex deviation of the eyes to the right side. On the other hand, with destruction of the right pontine gaze center (Fig. 18-7, *c*), the eyes remain deviated to the left of the midline, and neither volitional nor reflex influences can induce deviation to the right.

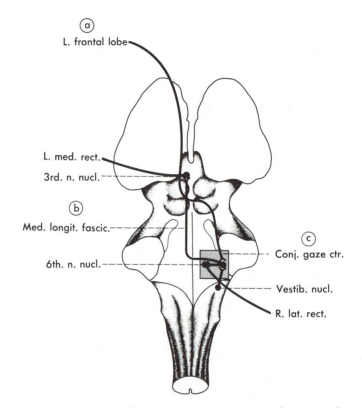

L. frontal lobe

L. med. rect.

3rd. n. nucl.

Med. longit. fascic.

6th. n. nucl.

Conj. gaze ctr.

Vestib. nucl.

R. lat. rect.

Fig. 18-7. Supranuclear control of horizontal conjugate gaze, showing pathways involved with turning of both eyes to the right. Lesion at site *a* results in paralysis of voluntary gaze to the right with preservation of reflex eye movements. Lesion at site *b* produces an internuclear ophthalmoplegia. At site *c* both voluntary and reflex movements are lost.

Lesions of the medial longitudinal fasciculus produce an important and common sign called *internuclear ophthalmoplegia,* in which the medial rectus component of horizontal gaze is defective (Fig. 18-8). With a lesion of the left medial longitudinal fasciculus (Fig. 18-7, *b*), attempted gaze to the right is characterized by failure of the left eye to adduct. The right eye abducts satisfactorily but shows a coarse monocular nystagmus. The act of convergence utilizes a different pathway, and this response is quite normal. Bilateral involvement of the fasciculi is most commonly found with multiple sclerosis.

The paths for vertical gaze follow a different course. From the cortex, fibers enter the dorsal portion of the midbrain tegmentum, ending in nuclei of the third and fourth nerves. Injury to this region of the midbrain by infarction or tumor usually prevents upward gaze and may be accompanied by paralysis of convergence and loss of light reflex.

Nystagmus is a rhythmic involuntary movement of the eyes and is of two main types. *Pendular* nystagmus is hereditary or associated with defective vision of early onset in life. It is present in the primary position as well as on lateral gaze, and it shows oscillations about the

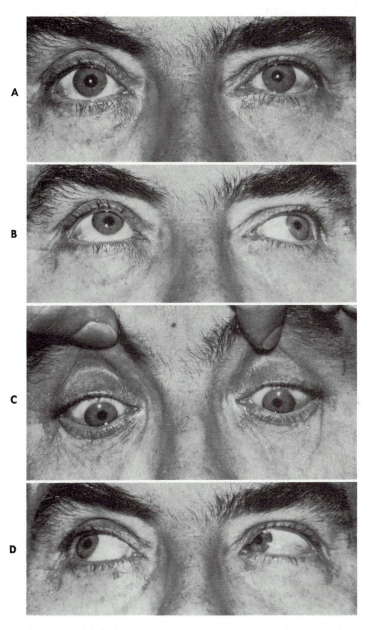

Fig. 18-8. Internuclear ophthalmoplegia, right side. In the primary position, **A,** the eyes are directed straight ahead. On attempted gaze to the left, **B,** the right eye fails to adduct, and the abducting left eye shows a coarse nystagmus. Convergence, **C,** and conjugate deviation of the eyes to right, **D,** are normal.

fixation point. *Jerk* nystagmus consists of a slow drift away from the point of fixation, with a rapid correcting movement. This may be horizontal, vertical, or rotatory. In acute labyrinthine destruction, there is found a nystagmus with slow component toward the side of the lesion, together with vertigo, nausea, and falling to the same side. In medullary and pontine lesions, nystagmus is usually more prominent in one direction and may be horizontal or rotatory. It commonly persists in the absence of vertigo or nausea. Vertical nystagmus is seen in lower medullary compressions. Nystagmus of cerebellar origin is. most pronounced on looking to the side of the lesion and is associated with ipsilateral cerebellar motor signs. In toxic nystagmus caused by diphenytoin or sedatives,

abnormal movements frequently appear in all directions of gaze.

Cranial nerve V (trigeminal). Motor fibers of the fifth nerve innervate the masseter, temporalis, and pterygoid muscles. Masseter and temporalis muscles are tested by having the patient close his jaw against resistance of the examiner's hand placed against the chin. At the same time, the muscles are palpated, and asymmetry of contraction is noted. The pterygoid muscles move the jaw forward and to the contralateral side. In testing these muscles, the patient moves his jaw to the contralateral side and resists the examiner's attempt to push it to the opposite side. In pterygoid weakness, the opened jaw tends to deviate to the side of the weak muscles.

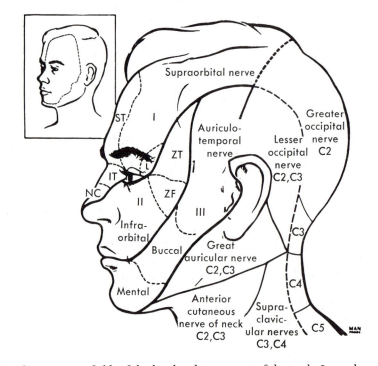

Fig. 18-9. The cutaneous fields of the head and upper part of the neck. Inset shows the area of sensory loss in the face following resection of the trigeminal nerve. (From Haymaker, W., and Woodhall, B.: Peripheral nerve injuries, ed. 2, Philadelphia, 1959, W. B. Saunders Co.)

The three sensory divisions of the trigeminal nerve are the ophthalmic, maxillary, and mandibular, whose superficial boundaries are outlined in Fig. 18-9 as areas I, II, and III, respectively. The corneal reflex, which is mediated through the ophthalmic division, is tested by touching the cornea lightly with cotton twisted into a point. The cotton should be introduced away from the direction of gaze to minimize blinking. Prompt partial or complete closure of the eyelids bilaterally is the normal response. Patients with unilateral facial weakness and inability to close the eyelids on that side will close the contralateral eye. Aside from the examiner observing the reflex eyelid closure, the patient is also asked to report difference in sensation from the stimulus. Cerebellopontine angle tumors frequently reduce the corneal reflex on the same side.

In addition to superficial sensation, the maxillary division supplies sensation for the upper teeth and jaw, mucosal surfaces of the uvula, hard palate, nasopharynx, and lower part of the nasal cavity. The upper part of the nasal cavity is innervated by the ophthalmic division. The mandibular division also supplies the tongue, lower teeth, gums, floor of the mouth, and buccal surface of the cheek. All these areas may be tested for light touch (cotton), pain (pin), and temperature (Fig. 18-10, *A*).

Cranial nerve VII (facial nerve). The motor portion of the seventh cranial nerve innervates all the facial muscles, the platysma, and the stylohyoid. The sensory portion mediates taste from the anterior two thirds of the tongue, somatic sensation from a portion of the external ear canal, and in addition carries fibers that innervate the lacrimal, submaxillary, and sublingual salivary glands.

During the initial interview, the patient's facial movements are observed, and gross weakness, such as inability to smile or close the eyelids, are apparent. The frontalis muscle is tested by asking the patient to look upward and to wrinkle his forehead. To test the orbicularis oculi, the patient closes his eyes tightly and resists the attempt to pry them open. The lower facial muscles are tested by having the patient show the teeth, purse the lips, and blow the cheeks out. The platysma is seen to contract when the patient makes a vigorous effort to show his teeth. Lesions of the corticobulbar tracts at any point above the facial nucleus will produce contralateral lower facial weakness with sparing of the forehead movement because of bilateral cortical representation of upper facial muscles (Fig. 18-11, *C* and *D*). In nuclear or peripheral seventh nerve lesions, the entire facial musculature on the same side is weak (Figs. 18-10, *A*, and 18-11, *A* and *B*).

The sensation of taste is tested with sodium chloride (salty), sugar (sweet), quinine (bitter), and vinegar (sour). The patient protrudes his tongue, which must be moist, and with a wet applicator one of these substances is gently rubbed on one side of the tongue. The patient is instructed not to withdraw the tongue until he identifies the substance as sweet, sour, bitter, or salty.

Cranial nerve VIII (acoustic nerve). Tests for auditory acuity and for differentiation of conduction and sensorineural deafness are described in Chapter 11. Watch tick and voice discrimination are especially useful in the detection of nerve deafness.

Vestibular function is tested by injecting 5 to 10 ml. of ice water into the external auditory canal, with the patient's head tilted forward 30 degrees while he is in the supine position. This position assures maximal stimulation of the horizontal semicircular canal. The normal response is: (a) sensation of vertigo; (b) nystagmus, with the fast component in the direction contralateral to the stimulated ear; and (c) past pointing. In testing for the latter, the patient's finger is placed on that of the examiner. With eyes closed, the patient elevates his arm and seeks to return his finger to the original position. The finger will drift toward the side of the irrigated ear. The time from the beginning of the irrigation to the onset of nystagmus and the duration are noted and compared with results from the other side.

Cranial nerves IX and X (glossopharyngeal and vagus nerves). The glossopharyngeal nerve supplies tactile and taste fibers to the posterior

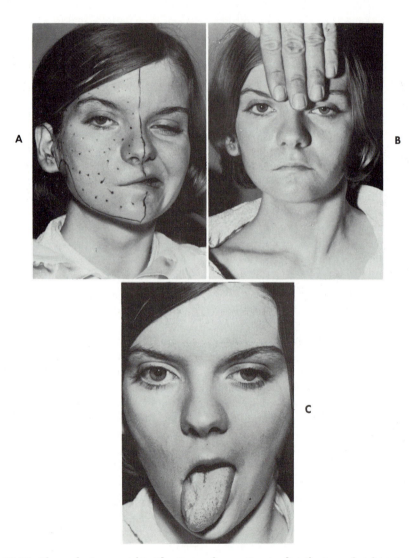

Fig. 18-10. Chemodectoma, right side. Loss of sensation in distribution of right trigeminal nerve with right facial weakness, **A,** atrophy of right sternomastoid, **B,** and atrophy of tongue, **C.**

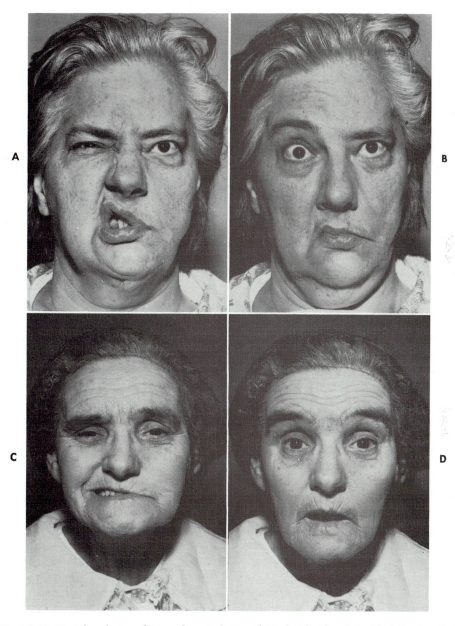

Fig. 18-11. Peripheral, **A** and **B**, and central, **C** and **D**, facial palsy, left-sided. In **A** and **C** the patients attempt to show their teeth. In **B** and **D** the patients attempt to wrinkle their foreheads. Notice left frontalis weakness in patient with peripheral facial palsy, **B.**

third of the tongue, tactile fibers to the naso-pharynx and upper pharynx, and motor fibers to the stylopharyngeal muscle. Because of intermixing of glossopharyngeal and vagal fibers in the pharyngeal plexus, independent clinical testing of the glossopharyngeal nerve is difficult. The afferent arm of the gag reflex is mainly mediated by the glossopharyngeal nerve, and the motor arm by the vagus. The normal response to a tongue blade touching the posterior wall of the pharynx is contraction of pharyngeal muscles and elevation of the palate. The absence of reflex may be unilateral or bilateral and usually indicates impairment of function of glossopharyngeal as well as vagus nerves. Unilateral impairment of motor function of the vagus leads to ipsilateral palatal and vocal cord weakness or paralysis. When the patient is asked to say "ah," the soft palate will deviate to the normal side. Vocal cord paralysis produces a hoarse voice, while a weak palate produces a nasal voice. Bilateral vagal lesions cause severe dysarthria and dysphagia with regurgitation of liquids through the nose.

Cranial nerve XI (accessory nerve). The accessory nerve supplies the sternomastoid (Fig. 18-10, B) and upper portion of the trapezius. Weakness of the sternomastoid is detected by having the patient rotate his head to the contralateral side against resistance. The patient then elevates his shoulders, and the examiner tries to depress them. Since elevation of the shoulders is principally done by the levators scapulae, the upper trapezius should be observed and palpated in order to detect weakness secondary to a lesion of the accessory nerve.

Cranial nerve XII (hypoglossal nerve). The hypoglossal nerve supplies extrinsic and intrinsic muscles of the tongue. Atrophy of one side of the tongue, fasciculations, and deviation of the protruded tongue toward the atrophied side indicate a lesion of the hypoglossal nucleus

or nerve (Fig. 18-10, C). Strength of the tongue is estimated by the amount of force exerted as the tongue is pressed laterally against a wooden blade.

MOTOR FUNCTION

Motor performance is dependent first of all on intact contractile mechanisms of muscle, neuromuscular transmission, and the cranial and spinal motor nuclei with their respective nerves. These in turn are modified and controlled by the gamma system, other proprioceptive pathways, the reticulospinal system, the pyramidal system (motor cortex and corticospinal tracts), the extrapyramidal contributions (extrarolandic motor cortex, basal ganglia, and reticular formation), and the cerebellum. Initial observations of the patient's posture and spontaneous movements prior to formal examination frequently will yield clues to possible abnormality of one or more of these systems. Afflictions of the lower motoneuron, neuromuscular junction, and muscle produce flaccid weakness and atrophy. Involvement of the corticospinal pathway leads to loss of fine digital movements and spasticity, while gross movements are relatively well preserved. Disorders of the extrarolandic motor cortex, basal ganglia, and brain stem reticular motor nuclei are accompanied by abnormalities of posture and by involuntary movements. Disturbances of proprioceptive components of the cerebellum are characterized by *ataxia* (unsteadiness or reeling of movement).

Muscle and anterior horn cell. Generalized wasting of muscle occurs only in nutritional or wasting diseases or in advanced stages of anterior horn cell and muscle disease. More localized wasting or that corresponding to a spinal segmental distribution is encountered in lower motor neuron disease, in which case fasciculations may be observed in the affected muscles. *Fasciculations* are involuntary twitches of small muscle bundles or motor units observed when the muscle is completely relaxed. They are quite coarse in muscles that have large motor units but quite fine and delicate in hand muscles with their small motor units. Fasciculations may be present in normal individuals. These take the form either of occasional twitches of muscles of the thigh or eyelid, or of a myokymia (continuous fasciculation) of calf muscles. The subject is often keenly aware of these benign fasciculations.

The features of lower motoneuron disease include segmental or localized muscle atrophy, weakness in the same distribution, fasciculations, and diminished stretch reflexes in the affected muscles. *Facial myokymia* is an undulating wavelike contraction of facial muscles, which simulates showers of innumerable fasciculations. It occurs with brain stem tumors and multiple sclerosis.

Localized muscle atrophy may occur in primary diseases of muscle in which fasciculations are not present. In patients with myositis, the involved muscles may be tender to palpation. In muscular dystrophy, pseudohypertrophy may be found (Fig. 18-12); the weakened muscle is paradoxically enlarged and feels rubbery to the touch.

Percussion of a muscle normally elicits only a brief contraction at the point struck. In emaciated and myxedematous patients, a local swelling *(myoedema)* lasting several seconds may follow the tap. Myotonia is a prominent local contraction that is sustained for several seconds after percussion. It is best elicited by tapping the thenar muscles with a percussion hammer or the tongue with the edge of a tongue depressor. In tetany, percussion of the facial nerve evokes a twitch of the facial muscles *(Chvostek sign)*, while compression of nerves in the upper arm by a blood pressure cuff inflated above systolic pressure evokes contraction of wrist and finger flexors *(Trousseau's sign)*.

The myasthenic phenomenon is most commonly encountered in the disease *myasthenia gravis* and consists of a steady decrease of muscle strength with sustained or repetitive contractions. It is readily demonstrated in the levator palpebrae muscle by the maintenance of steady upward gaze for 1 minute, after which progressive drooping of the lid develops. In limb muscles, repetitive exercise can demonstrate or increase weakness. In myasthenia gravis, the injection of 10 mg. edrophonium chloride (Tensilon) in small increments intravenously or 1 mg. of prostigmin methylsulfate (Prostigmin) subcutaneously abolishes or lessens the weakness.

Muscle strength. In testing the strength of individual muscles, it is essential to have a thorough knowledge of their origins and insertions, their function, and their innervation (Table 18-4). In the preferred method of testing muscle strength, the patient places a limb in the desired position and resists the examiner's attempt to displace it. With this method almost all patients comprehend easily what is wanted of them, assuring a more reliable examination. Muscle strength depends to some degree on age; therefore, the examiner has to know what strength to expect normally at a given age. Furthermore, what represents normal strength in an untrained individual may represent significant weakness in a highly trained athlete or manual laborer. Proper evaluation of muscle strength requires that all these different factors be taken into account. Only after examining many different patients with and without muscle weakness will the student acquire sufficient experience to become competent. Normal patients will contract their muscles promptly and maximally. When weakness is present, the muscles will lengthen smoothly. In hysterical patients all resistance against the examiner's pressure will abruptly cease, or the contraction will be ratchety. It is desirable to test homolo-

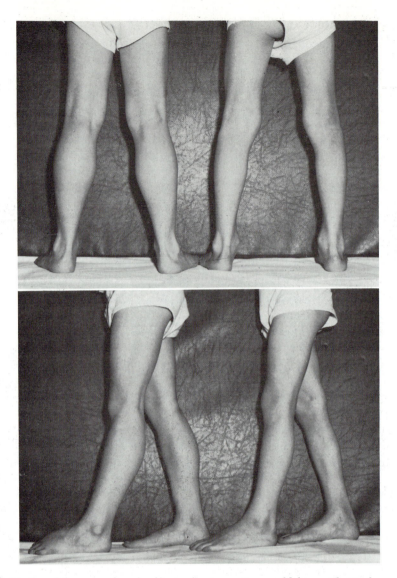

Fig. 18-12. Pseudohypertrophy of calf muscles in an 8-year-old boy with Duchenne type muscular dystrophy on left. Normal 7-year-old sibling on right.

gous muscles simultaneously; this facilitates detection of unilateral weakness.

The strength of the neck flexors is assessed by the resistance encountered with the examiner's fingertips placed against the patient's forehead. Extensors are measured by the palm

of the hand against the occiput. The sternocleidomastoid is assessed by rotation of the head toward the opposite side against the examiner's hand held against the jaw on the side not being examined. The upper part of the trapezius is evaluated by observing the muscle contract on

Table 18-4. Commonly tested muscles and their innervation

Serratus anterior	C5,6,7	Long thoracic nerve
Supraspinatus	C4,5,6	Suprascapular nerve
Infraspinatus	C4,5,6	Suprascapular nerve
Pectoralis major	C5,6,7,8,Tl	Pectoral nerve
Latissimus dorsi	C6,7,8,	Thoracodorsal nerve
Deltoid	C5,6	Axillary nerve
Biceps, brachialis	C5,6	Musculocutaneous nerve
Triceps	C7,8	Radial nerve
Brachioradialis	C5,6	Radial nerve
Supinator	C5,6,7	Radial nerve
Extensor carpi radialis brevis and longus	C6,7,8	Radial nerve
Extensor carpi ulnaris	C7,8	Radial nerve
Extensor digitorum	C7,8	Radial nerve
Flexor carpi radialis	C6,7	Median nerve
Flexor carpi ulnaris	C8,T1	Ulnar nerve
Flexor digitorum sublimis	C8,T1	Median nerve
Flexor digitorum profundus		
Radial portion	C8,T1	Median nerve
Ulnar portion	C8,T1	Ulnar nerve
Abductor pollicis brevis	C8,T1	Median nerve
Opponens pollicis	C8,T1	Median nerve
Interossei	C8,T1	Ulnar nerve
Hypothenar muscles	C8,T1	Ulnar nerve
Iliopsoas	L2,3	Femoral nerve
Thigh adductors	L2,3,4,5	Obturator and sciatic nerves
Thigh abductors	L4,5,S1	Superior gluteal nerve
Gluteus maximus	S1,2	Inferior gluteal nerve
Quadriceps femoris	L3,4	Femoral nerve
Hamstrings	L5,S1	Sciatic nerve
Tibialis anterior	L4,5	Deep peroneal nerve
Extensor digitorium brevis and longus	L5,S1	Deep peroneal nerve
Peroneus longus and brevis	L5,S1	Superificial peroneal nerve
Gastrocnemius-soleus	S1,2	Tibial nerve
Tibialis posterior	L5,S1	Posterior tibial nerve

shrugging the shoulders. The main part of the trapezius must be tested with the patient prone, with arms abducted fully and thumbs pointing upward. The patient is then asked to move his arms in a backward direction.

Finger flexors are estimated by the effort necessary to straighten the flexed fingers of the patient. The patient then extends his fingers and resists attempted flexion. Dorsal interossei and abductors of the thumb and fifth digit are tested as the patient spreads his fingers and resists the examiner's attempt to approximate them. Opponens pollicis strength is assessed by separating the thumb and little finger as the subject brings these two together. Abductor pollicis brevis is tested in a position of abduction of the thumb perpendicular to the plane of the palm. Abduction of the thumb in the plane of the palm is accomplished by the abductor pollicis longus. In compression of the median nerve at the wrist (carpal tunnel syndrome), the opponens pollicis and abductor pollicis brevis may be weak.

The patient is then asked to make fists, bend his elbows to 90 degrees, hold the elbows close to his chest, and resist any movement by the examiner to displace any part of his upper extremities. Strength of pronation is tested by outward rotation of the patient's fist and strength of supination by inward rotation. Supination with the elbow flexed is largely a function of the biceps. Supination by the supinator is tested with the arm extended. Downward pressure on the wrists with the elbow flexed tests the brachioradialis and biceps, while upward pressure tests triceps strength. Attempts to separate the fists evaluates medial rotation of the arm at the shoulder (latissimus dorsi, teres major, subscapularis, deltoid, and pectoralis). Conversely, attempts to bring the fists together checks lateral rotators at the shoulder (infraspinatus, teres minor, and deltoid). Adduction of the arms is a function of the pectoralis and latissimus dorsi and is tested by having the patient resist adduction. Downward pressure on the abducted arms with internal rotation at the shoulder (hand and forearm down) tests supraspinatus strength. With the arm abducted but externally rotated at the shoulder (hand and forearm up), downward pressure evaluates deltoid strength.

Strength of the abdominal muscles and trunk flexors is evaluated as the patient attempts to sit up from the supine positon. Raising the head and shoulders in the prone position estimates strength of back extensors.

Flexion of the thigh at the hip is a function of the iliopsoas and is tested with the patient in a supine position, with one leg raised, by application of downward pressure directed against the knee. The attempt to separate the tightly adducted knees tests thigh adductors, which also function as medial rotators of the thigh. Gluteus medius and minimus abduct the thigh, and their strength is assessed by approximation of the knees against the patient's resistance. Extension of the thigh is accomplished by the gluteus maximus and is best tested by observing the patient ascending a step or rising from a squatting position. The quadriceps extends the leg at the knee, and the hamstrings flex it. Their strengths are estimated by the attempt to overcome extension and flexion of the knee, respectively. The gastrocnemius soleus is a very powerful muscle, and mild weakness can only be detected by application of downward pressure on the shoulder while the patient stands on his toes. The tibialis anterior is tested by downward pressure on the dorsiflexed foot. To test the strength of the peronei, the patient plantar flexes and everts his foot, while resisting inversion of the foot by the examiner. Similarly, to test posterior tibialis function, the foot is plantar flexed and inverted. Toe flexion and extension are tested in a fashion similar to that of finger flexion and extension.

Muscle tonus. Muscle tonus is tested by the passive movement of a limb through its full range of motion. The range of motion for the principal joints of the body is shown in Tables 19-1 and 19-2. Muscle *contracture* is a state of shortening of the muscle and is characterized by a decreased range of motion. In pyramidal *spasticity* resistance to passive movement rapidly increases to a point and then gives way (lengthening reaction or "clasp-knife" phenomenon). Steady plastic resistance throughout the range of movement typifies *parkinsonian rigidity;* the superimposition of parkinsonian tremor adds small regular jerks to the resistance (cogwheel rigidity). Another type of resistance to passive movement is called *dystonia* and is usually seen in extrapyramidal disease. Dystonia may be defined as a persistent abnormal posture. With passive movement, resistance increases progressively as the limb is displaced. On release the limb springs back to its previous posture. Resistance to passive movement throughout the range of motion and somewhat proportional to the amount of force applied is called *paratonia* or "Gegenhalten" and is seen in frontal lobe disease. Resistance to passive movement is also seen in decorticate rigidity, in which the upper limbs are flexed and pronated and the lower limbs are extended. *Decerebrate rigidity* is characterized by extension and pronation of the upper limbs and extension of the lower limbs. It results from functional or structural brain stem transection above the lower third of the pons. This characteristic posture may be evoked or exaggerated by painful stimuli about the face.

Decrease of muscle tonus is also determined by passive movement. The examiner notes increased range of joint motion and looseness of the extremities on shaking them. Overextension or overflexion is frequently seen in *hypotonia*. The hypotonic limb in cerebellar disease lacks the normal braking action. For example, the physician resists the patient's attempt to flex his elbow by pulling on his wrist. On sudden release the hand flies toward the patient's face (rebound phenomenon), and the patient may actually hit his own face.

Coordination. Coordination in skilled acts can be impaired by disorders at any level of motor systems. Incoordination is particularly relevant, however, in respect to cerebellar disease and to hemiplegia caused by corticospinal tract interruption. Some simple tests help to differentiate the causes. The patient is instructed to perform certain rapid rhythmic movements. He pats his knee with his hand alternately using the palm and the back of the

hand; he rapidly pats one hand against the opposite palm; or he rhythmically touches the tip of his thumb to the first crease of the index finger. In cerebellar disease these movements become slowed, nonrhythmic, and occasionally "hung up." In hemiplegia they are simply slowed and stiff. The patient may be instructed to quickly and consecutively touch the tip of his thumb to each of his four fingertips, and then quickly repeat the sequence. In hemiplegia the fingers tend to act in unison, and the oppositional movement of the thumb is impaired. In cerebellar disease the movements are slowed and inaccurate. In parkinsonism the fingers are held together and only tiny but rapid movements are made. In the finger to nose test the patient moves his index finger quickly and smoothly back and forth between his nose and the examiner's finger. In cerebellar ataxia the hand will deviate irregularly away from the axis of movement and may miss the target. In hemiplegic spasticity, jerky clonic movements may be produced in the direction of the movement.

In examination of the lower extremities, the patient is asked to wiggle his toes rapidly up and down. With hemiplegia the rapidity of this motion is grossly reduced. The heel to shin test is performed by placing the heel on the patella and running it quickly down the tibial surface in a straight line. Cerebellar disease results in irregular deviations of the heel to either side.

Involuntary movements. Rhythmic involuntary movements are called *tremors*. *Parkinsonian tremor* has a regular rhythm of four to six cycles per second, is best seen in moderate relaxation, disappears during sleep and complete relaxation and lessens with voluntary movement. It is often called a "rest" tremor and is distributed in the distal joints of the limbs and about the mouth. The most characteristic feature is the pattern of tremor occurring in the hand in which the thumb beats rhythmically against the flexing fingers. *Familial* and *senile* *tremor* is characterized by rhythmic oscillations of the head (titubation) and of the fingers of the outstretched hands. The tremor is rapid and is accentuated in amplitude by action and emotional stress (action tremor). *Cerebellar tremors* are characteristically action tremors, with an oscillation perpendicular to the line of movement and increasing in amplitude as the target is approached.

Sporadic loss of tonus in muscles under steady contraction results in brief lapses of posture, with an irregular flapping tremor *(asterixis)*. This is best demonstrated with arms outstretched and wrists extended and occurs in hepatic encephalopathy as well as in many other metabolic encephalopathies. The adult form of hepatolenticular degeneration *(Wilson's disease)* is frequently associated with a coarse flapping or wing-beating of the wrists and shoulders, increasing in violence and amplitude as the outstretched posture of the arm is maintained. Sudden, irregular, and asymmetric jerks of individual muscles or limbs are called *myoclonus*. The jerks are usually stimulus sensitive and may be evoked by light flashes, loud noise, or manipulations of the limbs. The disorder occurs with diffuse neuronal diseases and with lesions of the cerebellum and its outflow paths. *Athetosis* is a rather slow writhing movement of the arms and foot that may be accompanied by a twisting of the neck and retraction of the lips. The hands tend to swing alternately but irregularly between two extremes of posture—one consists of extension at the elbow with supination of wrist and hyperextension of fingers; the other consists of elbow flexion with pronation and finger flexion. Athetosis is associated predominantly with lesions in the putamen. *Choreic* movements appear with bilateral disease of the caudate nuclei. These movements are quick and erratic, without an easily discernible pattern. They affect individual digits, wrists, proximal parts of limbs, and the trunk. Twisting or lurching movements of trunk may appear on walking. Smacking and sucking movements of the lips and darting motions of the tongue are common. Destruction of the subthalamic nucleus is attended by wild uncontrollable flinging movements of the contralateral arm, with coarse rotatory motions at shoulder and hip *(hemiballism)*.

Stance and gait. Standing and walking are largely automatic, but are really very complex activities depending on adequate muscle strength, coordination, proprioception, vestibular function, and vision. In observing stance, the patient is asked to stand with his feet close together, first with his eyes open and then with his eyes closed. Patients with impairment of proprioception—as in tabes dorsalis, subacute combined degeneration, or sensory neuropathy—show increased swaying and unsteadiness with their eyes closed. In cerebellar disease normal stance is difficult to maintain even with the eyes open, and the patient separates his feet widely in order to stand on a broader, and therefore steadier, base. In acute unilateral impairment of vestibular function, the patient has a tendency to fall to the ipsilateral side.

Gait is usually observed by asking the patient to step out freely. Many normal patients have a tendency to walk slowly and deliberately when observed by an examiner. A gait abnormality may be exaggerated and more easily observed by asking the patient to walk a straight line and to touch his big toe with his heel. Decrease of associated movement, such as arm swing, occurs in hemiplegia or rigidity. It is characteristically seen in patients with Parkinson's disease. Further, patients with this disorder walk with slow short steps, stoop forward as if chasing the center of gravity, turn clumsily in one block, and have difficulty in stopping abruptly. *Gait apraxia* is a disorder of stance and gait, which may occur in the absence of weakness, hemiplegia, or other motor disorders. It is characterized in some patients by diminutive steps in place without any effective movement and flexion of toes against the floor. In others there is instability and a consistent tendency to fall backward, either when standing or sitting. These disorders are associated with destructive processes in the medial aspects of frontal and parietal lobes, usually bilateral. The patient with cerebellar disease walks with a wide base and staggers or reels laterally. In the hemiplegic gait the leg is circumducted, the knee is held stiffly, and the ankle is extended. Bilateral spastic paresis of the legs produces scissoring of the knees while the legs are moved forward in a jerky manner. This is often accompanied by extreme compensatory movements of the trunk. When weakness of dorsiflexion of the ankles is present, the legs are lifted excessively high in the manner of a high-stepping horse and the feet flop onto the ground, producing a characteristic sound (steppage gait). The hysterical gait is characteristically bizarre; close observation will usually show rather delicate balancing movements that cause the patient to walk in a bizarre fashion.

REFLEXES

Stretch reflexes. To test muscle stretch reflexes, the muscle is briefly stretched by a tap on the tendon. Stretch receptors in the muscle (muscle spindles) send impulses via afferent fibers in peripheral nerves and dorsal roots to anterior horn cells. These are excited and send efferent impulses via anterior roots and motor nerve to the same muscle, leading to a brief contraction. This is a simple monosynaptic reflex that may be diminished or lost with interruption of afferent (sensory) fibers. It is also diminished with extensive destruction of efferent (motor) fibers and anterior horn cells. Release of this monosynaptic reflex from the influence of suprasegmental fibers (pyramidal tract) pro-

duces hyperreflexia that, when extreme, leads to clonus. *Clonus* is a rapid repetitive contraction of muscles and is elicited by stretching a muscle briskly and maintaining a certain degree of stretch.

Adequate relaxation of the patient is necessary to elicit a muscle stretch reflex, but to elicit the stretch reflex, some tension of the particular muscle being tested is at times helpful. To achieve this the patient is instructed to contract the muscles slightly. For example, the patient is asked to push gently with his shin against the examiner's finger while he taps the quadriceps tendon just below the knee. It is advisable to place one finger on the tendon and tap the finger with the reflex hammer. In this fashion the tension of the muscle tested, the strength of the tap with the hammer, and the vigor of the muscle contraction can all be assessed. The response is evaluated as to its briskness and ease of elicitation and is compared with that of the homologous muscle on the other side. Slow relaxation after muscle contraction is observed in myxedema. If the leg is allowed to swing freely when testing the quadriceps reflex, it quickly returns to complete rest. In hypotonia caused by cerebellar disease, the leg continues to swing back and forth four or five times after a single contraction of the muscle (*pendular reflex*). Differences between sides are best detected by eliciting a muscle stretch reflex first on one side and then immediately in the homologous muscle on the other side. If a reflex cannot be elicited or if asymmetries are found, the reflex should be tested in several different positions to verify its absence or diminution. Reflexes may be brought out by a reinforcement maneuver (pulling against the interlocked fingers or clenching the fist).

All muscles can be made to contract reflexly, but only a few are tested clinically (Table 18-5). The jaw jerk is elicited by having the pa-

Table 18-5. Reflexes and their innervation

Biceps reflex	C5,6	Musculocutaneous nerve
Brachioradialis reflex	C5,6	Radial nerve
Triceps reflex	C7,8	Radial nerve
Superficial abdominal reflexes		
Upper abdomen	T8,9,10	
Lower abdomen	T11,12	
Cremasteric reflex	L1,2	
Anal reflex	S3,4	
Quadriceps reflex	L3,4	Femoral nerve
Hamstrings reflexes		
Medial hamstring	L5	Sciatic nerve
Lateral hamstring	S1	Sciatic nerve
Gastrocnemius-soleus reflex	S1,2	Tibial nerve

tient let his jaw sag open, placing one finger on the chin, and tapping it with the hammer. In the normal person no response or only a faint contraction may be felt. With hyperactivity of the reflex in upper motor neuron lesions, the jaw closes briskly, and the teeth click audibly. The brachioradialis reflex is tested by striking the distal radius (Fig. 18-13, *C*). In the supine position the patient puts his hand on his abdomen with his arms flexed, or in a seated position the examiner supports one or both hands. A commonly used position to elicit the biceps reflex is to support the patient's elbow with the hand, place the thumb over the tendon, and have the patient's hand rest on the examiner's forearm. Muscles, if percussed directly, will have a brief contraction; this direct contraction is to be disregarded. When eliciting the triceps reflex, which is performed best with the patient's arms folded across his chest or with the patient's arm supported by the examiner and the forearm swinging freely (Fig. 18-13, *B*), care is taken to strike the triceps aponeurosis rather than the muscle. The triceps reflex is frequently diminished or absent with compression of cervical root 7 because of herniation of a cervical nucleus pulposus. The pectoralis re-

flex is evoked by striking a finger placed under the tendon in the axilla while the arm remains in a relaxed position at the side. The finger flexor reflex may be tested by a tap against the examiner's fingers, which are held lightly beneath the slightly flexed fingers of the patient. Flicking the patient's fingernail has the same effect and provides a sudden stretch, which is followed by quick flexion of the fingers. Normally this contraction is minimal. With hyperreflexia, finger flexion is more pronounced; the thumb also flexes (*Hoffmann's sign*).

The abdominal muscles can be made to contract reflexly by tapping a finger placed just below the costal margin.

The quadriceps reflex is easily elicited by striking the tendon just below the patella while the patient sits at the edge of the bed with his legs dangling (Fig. 18-14, *A*). In the recumbent position it may be advantageous to place a finger just above the patella and tap it with the hammer. Adequate relaxation of the gastrocnemius-soleus muscle is accomplished by having the patient kneel on a chair (Fig. 18-14, *C*). Hamstring reflexes are elicited with the patient in the prone position. The patient flexes his leg, the foot rests on the physician's arm, and

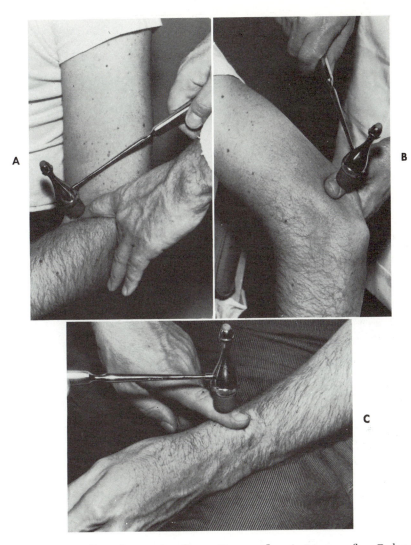

Fig. 18-13. Testing of muscle stretch reflexes. Biceps reflex, **A,** triceps reflex, **B,** brachiora-dialis reflex, **C.**

the examiner's finger is placed directly on the medial or lateral hamstring tendon just above the insertion. The adductor reflex is evoked by tapping the medial aspect of the knee. In upper motoneuron lesions the contralateral adductors may contract simultaneously (crossed adductor response).

Superficial reflexes. The reflexes just described are simple monosynaptic reflexes, and the appropriate stimulus is muscle stretch. Other reflexes are considerably more complex and may be elicited by cutaneous sensory stimulation. Many of these reflexes are facilitated by the cerebral motor cortex and are abolished

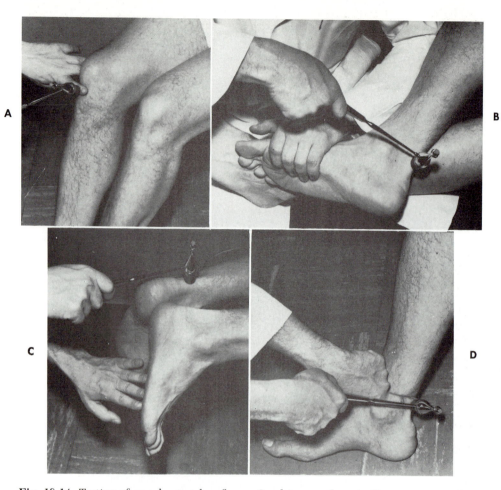

Fig. 18-14. Testing of muscle stretch reflexes. Quadriceps reflex, **A.** Gastrocnemius-soleus reflex in different positions: patient supine, **B,** patient kneeling on chair, **C,** and patient sitting, **D.**

or modified by lesions of the corticospinal tract. *Abdominal* reflexes are elicited by briskly stroking the abdomen with an applicator stick moved toward the umbilicus; the normal response is a brief movement of the umbilicus toward the side of stimulation. This reflex should be tested in the upper and lower quadrants of the abdomen. It is abolished on the side of a hemiplegia and is frequently absent bilaterally in multiple sclerosis. The *cremasteric* reflex is evoked by stroking the inner aspect of the thigh and consists of a quick elevation of the ipsilateral testis. In patients with low back pain or suspected lesions of the cauda equina or sacral nerve roots, it is essential to test the *anal* reflex. With the patient on his side, the buttocks are spread and the perianal area is scratched or pricked. The normal response is an obvious quick contraction of the external anal sphincter, which also may be felt when the gloved finger is inserted into the rectum.

Stimulation of the sole of the foot produces

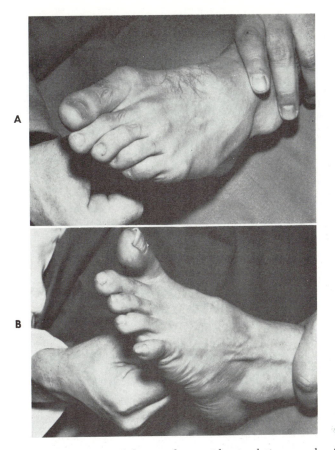

Fig. 18-15. Plantar reflexes. Normal flexion of toes with stimulation on sole of foot, **A.** Dorsiflexion of big toe, fanning of other toes (Babinski sign), **B.**

flexion of the toes (flexor plantar response, Fig. 18-15, *A*). In 1896 Babinski first drew attention to dorsiflexion or extension of the toes upon pricking the sole of the foot in patients with upper motoneuron lesions. The "Babinski sign" now refers to the pathologic reflex of toe extension. The *plantar reflex* is tested in a relaxed recumbent patient who has his legs extended. Firm pressure with the tip of the thumb or a blunt instrument is exerted against the sole of the foot on its lateral aspect, and the finger or instrument is moved slowly upward toward the little toe and then across the sole toward the big toe. Dorsiflexion of the big toe and fanning

of the other toes constitutes the pathologic reflex (extensor plantar response, Fig. 18-15, *B*). A times this response is accompanied by flexion of the thigh at the hip, knee flexion, and dorsiflexion of the foot. In severe upper motoneuron lesions the response may be elicited by stimulation of other parts of the leg as high as the thigh. It is well to remember that dorsiflexion of the big toe is seen normally in infants up to approximately 8 to 10 months of age.

Pathologic reflexes. A number of reflexes are present in infancy but are suppressed early in life. However, they may be released in later life by acquired disease of the cerebrum.

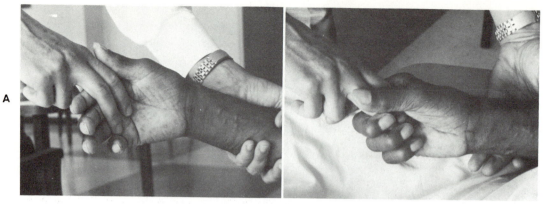

Fig. 18-16. In **A**, the examiner's fingers move across the palm and base of fingers, followed by reflex closure of patient's fingers, **B.**

A group of pathologic reflexes may appear that cannot be ascribed to lesions in any specific location of the brain, but are caused by cerebral cortical atrophy and other diffuse disorders of the cerebral hemispheres. The *snout* reflex consists of a quick pursing or pouting expression of the lips; it is elicited by a light tap beneath the nose. The *palmomental* response involves the contraction of mentalis muscle on one side after stroking the palm on the same side with a sharp object. Traces of this are present in about a third of normal individuals, but a brisk response is pathologic. The *blink* reflex consists of forced closure of the eyes when they are quickly approached by the examiner's hand or by a flashlight or when a light tap is delivered against the glabella.

Another group of reflexes is directly attributable to destruction of the medial premotor portions of the frontal lobe. The reflexes are released on the side opposite the lesion. The *sucking* reflex is elicited by gently stroking the lips with a tongue blade, moving from the center laterally. In mild form the lips contract reflexly on the blade. With more severe release, the tongue moves toward the blade, and the lips and head follow it as if to take hold of the object. The *grasp* reflex of the hand is elicited by stroking the patient's palm with one's fingers (Fig. 18-16). The patient's fingers are flexed, and the thumb opposes, serving to entrap the examiner's fingers in a persistent grasp. The reflex may be released by stroking the dorsum of the hand. In more extensive frontal lobe lesions there may appear the "instinctive grasp response." Under these circumstances the mere touching of any part of the hand with an object or even the introduction of the object into the visual field may result in a following of the object in an effort to grasp it. A grasp reflex of the foot occasionally may be found and is elicited by stroking the sole toward the base of the toes. Although all of these reflexes can be found in discrete frontal lobe lesions, they may also be found in diffuse cerebral diseases as well as in metabolic encephalopathies (hepatic or uremic coma).

In large lesions of the parietal lobe a different set of responses may be noted on the opposite side of the body. A stroke on the patient's palm may evoke extension of the fingers and wrist (Fig. 18-17). If the arms are held outstretched in front of the patient, the affected arm may slowly rise (*levitation* phenom-

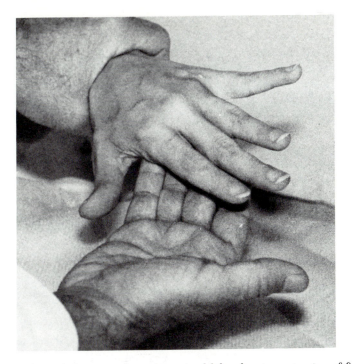

Fig. 18-17. Patient with lesion in the right parietal lobe showing extension of fingers in an avoidance reflex on stimulation of the palm.

enon). Stroking of the lips may elicit a retraction of the mouth and turning of the head away from the stimulus.

COMMON MOTOR AND REFLEX PATTERNS IN NEUROLOGIC DISEASE

Hemiplegia. Hemiplegia appears with interruption of the corticospinal tract and shows a fundamentally similar pattern wherever the interruption is located (from motor cortex to lateral column of spinal cord). Certain topographic features, however, may impart modifications of the pattern that are of localizing value. Since the body's representation is distributed over a considerable length in the motor cortex, lesions at the cortical level seldom produce complete hemiplegia. Instead, one finds a combination of face and arm involve-

ment or involvement of the leg alone. Small lesions in the posterior limb of the internal capsule (lacunar infarcts) commonly produce complete hemiplegias affecting face, arm, and leg. Lesions affecting both capsule and basal ganglia (hypertensive hemorrhages) also produce dense hemiplegias in which spasticity and rigidity are quite prominent. Interruption of corticospinal tract in the cervical spinal cord involves only the arm and leg.

In any acute lesion the hemiplegia is initially flaccid, and only later do spasticity and abnormal reflexes appear, at which time the posture is characteristic. The arm is adducted at the shoulder, flexed at the elbow, and pronated at the wrist, while the leg is extended. Weakness in the face is restricted to the lower group of muscles. In the upper extremity rapid individual digital movements are markedly impaired. The distribution of maximal weakness is characteristic and includes the extensors of wrist and fingers, extensor of the elbow, and abductor of the shoulder. Maximal spasticity is found in exactly the opposite group of muscles; namely, elbow flexors and finger flexors. In the lower extremity weakness is most marked in the dorsiflexors of the ankle, flexors of the knee, and flexors of the hip, whereas maximal spasticity is noted in extensors of the knee and plantar flexors of the ankle. All stretch reflexes are increased on the involved side, and Hoffmann's sign is present. There is loss of corneal, abdominal, and cremasteric reflexes. The Babinski reflex is present and ankle clonus may be elicited.

It is often important for the physician to detect minimal signs of corticospinal tract disease before the appearance of overt hemiplegia. For early detection several tests may be performed. The serial touching of thumb to fingertips is reduced in speed. The *coin test* is a sensitive index of impairment. Several coins are placed on a smooth surface, and the patient is asked to pick up the coins one at a time, placing each one in his palm before going to the next. With early corticospinal tract disease the patient cannot maintain the coins in his grasp while independently moving thumb and index finger. In the *pronator* sign, the patient extends his arms before him with his palms up and his eyes closed (Fig. 18-18). On the affected side, the wrist gradually moves into a pronated position. In the lower extremity rapidity of toe wiggling is decreased. If the patient is placed prone and his knees are bent at right angles, the affected leg will gradually drift downward (Barré's sign, Fig. 18-19).

Pseudobulbar paralysis. With the exception of the lower facial muscles, most muscles innervated by cranial nerves are represented bilaterally. Profound upper motor neuron disorders of these muscles are seen only with bilat-eral disease of corticobulbar tracts or bilateral putaminal lesions. There is slowness and weakness of attempted voluntary movement of the facial muscles, muscles of mastication, tongue, and the palate. Speech is slow and harsh. Reflexes are increased, with exaggeration of the jaw jerk and persistence of the gag reflex. The control of emotional facial expression requires a different motor pathway; namely, from the hypothalamus to the brain stem motor nuclei. In pseudobulbar paralysis this is preserved and excessively active, producing the phenomenon of pathologic laughing and crying. A relatively minor or inappropriate stimulus may set off an exaggerated and prolonged expression of either laughter or weeping.

Paraplegias caused by spinal cord injury. With severe injury or complete transection of the spinal cord, there is an initial phase of spinal shock in which all movement and reflex activity is abolished below the lesion. Gradually the stretch reflexes reappear and become increased. Subsequently, flexor spasms of the legs appear; finally, extensor spasms of the legs develop and prevailing extensor tonus ensues. With very chronic compressive injuries of the cervical spinal cord, the prevailing pattern is one of marked spasticity and increased stretch reflexes. There is slowing of voluntary movement but remarkably little weakness.

Paralysis agitans (parkinsonism). The patient with parkinsonism tends to remain immobile for long periods, with diminished eye blinking and reduction of normal "fidgets." His facial expression is flat and apparently emotionless. His posture is stooped with little flexion of the upper extremities (Fig. 18-20, *A*). He walks and turns in a block. His equilibrium is impaired (Fig. 18-20, *B*), and he is easily pushed off balance or may shift off his center of gravity in walking. The typical parkinsonian tremor is present. Plastic or cogwheel rigidity is noted on passive movement.

Cerebellar disorders. With destruction of a

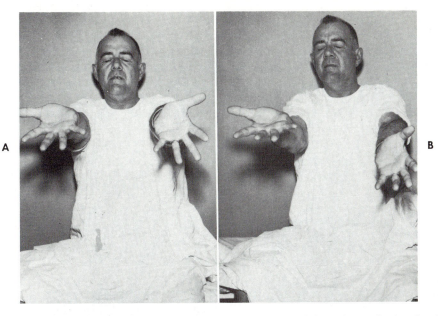

Fig. 18-18. Pronator sign. The patient suffered from an infarct of the right cerebral peduncle. When asked to maintain the position of both arms and hands, **A,** the left arm drifts downward and the hand pronates slightly, **B.**

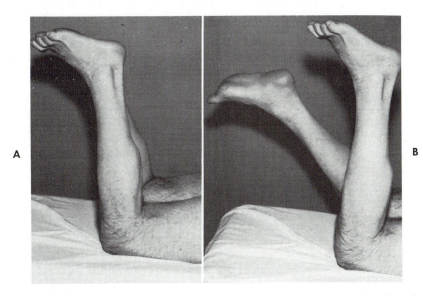

Fig. 18-19. Barré's sign. The patient had an infarct of the right cerebral peduncle. After the lower legs are positioned at right angles to the thighs, **A,** the patient is unable to maintain the position of the affected left leg, **B.**

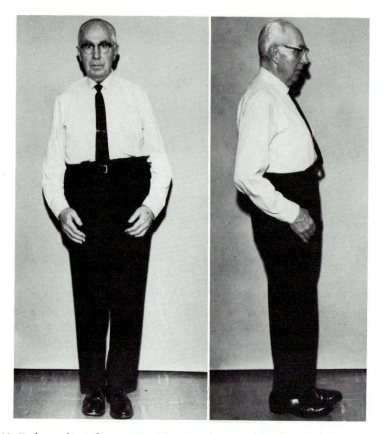

Fig. 18-20. Parkinson's syndrome. Fixed facial expression, adduction and flexion of arms and fingers, and slightly retroverted position.

cerebellar hemisphere motor abnormalities appear on the ipsilateral side. There is ataxia of the upper extremity on active movement, and an irregular lurching or falling toward the affected side on walking. Rapid alternating movements become slow and arrhythmic. Ataxia and tremor appear on the finger to nose and heel to shin tests. Rebound phenomenon is present as well as pendular knee jerks. Coarse nystagmus is noted on gaze to the side of the lesion.

With involvement of the midline portions of the cerebellum, tremor and ataxia of the arms and legs may not be noted. The principal find-

ing is a gross distrubance of equilibrium and an obvious ataxia on walking, both of which may be overlooked if the patient is examined only in bed.

SENSATION

Sensory examination. Ideally a patient should be intelligent, alert, cooperative, and not suggestible when undertaking a sensory examination. Only rarely are all of these attributes present in an individual patient at a given time. In order to yield optimal and reliable information, each sensory examination has to be adjusted according to the patient's particular abilities. A fatigued patient may perform poorly and may superficially give the impression of sensory loss, which disappears when the patient is retested after rest. Whenever the patient or the examiner becomes fatigued, it is better to reexamine at a later time. In a totally uncooperative or obtunded patient the only sensory modality that can be examined may be pain. The patient's face is observed for grimacing in response to a painful stimulus. Even though this is a very crude sensory examination, it may still provide important information.

Without the patient's knowing exactly how to respond, the results of a sensory examination will be confusing, and the examiner may become frustated. Therefore, it is essential to explain to the patient what will be done and how he is expected to respond. A brief practice demonstration before the actual testing will quickly elucidate any misunderstanding.

It is certainly not practical or necessary to examine every square inch of skin surface for every sensory modality in every patient. However, the face, trunk, arms, and legs should be routinely tested for light touch and pain sensation. In addition, position sense and vibratory perception in the fingers and toes should be examined in every patient. The equipment needed for a sensory examination is simple and consists of a cotton wad, a sharp pin, test tubes for cold and warm water, a tuning fork, and a compass with dull tips.

Loss of sensation is usually relative in degree. It is not sufficient to determine whether or not a patient perceives a painful stimulus as pain. The intensity of the stimulus should be minimal at first and then gradually increased. In areas of sensory impairment a higher threshold is found more frequently than total loss of sensation. Vibratory perception in the feet and legs is normally decreased past the age of 60 years; a difference between left and right may indicate a significant neurologic deficit. In ad-

dition to comparing left and right it is important to determine whether there is gradual or abrupt transition from an abnormal to a normal area. In peripheral neuropathies involving the legs, the most severe deficits are usually found in the feet and are gradually reduced as the stimulus is moved up the leg. On the other hand, an isolated nerve or root lesion will show a clear oval or bandlike zone or loss corresponding to its dermatome.

Examination of individual sensory modalities. Light touch is tested by gently touching the skin with a wisp of cotton; the patient responds with "yes" or "now" whenever he feels the stimulus. The testing should be done at irregular intervals, because the patient may begin to respond repetitively whether or not he feels the stimulus if it is applied at regular intervals. If the patient does not feel the lightest touch, the pressure of the stimulus or the area of stimulation is increased until a response is elicited. If an area of decreased touch perception is found, the stimulus is then moved from the point of maximal impairment into several normal areas to delineate the exact boundaries of the deficit. It is well to repeat this procedure several times until the same boundaries are determined repeatedly. Different areas of the skin normally have different thresholds for touch. The back, buttocks, and thickened parts of the skin require more pressure than do the face or fingertips. With damage to the sensory cortex, there may be impairment in tactile localization even though the appreciation of light touch is retained. To detect this disturbance, parts of the limbs are touched with cotton. After each contact the patient, with his eyes closed, tries to place his index finger on the site of touch.

Pain perception is usually tested next. Since it is important to apply stimuli of about equal intensity, it has been found helpful to attach a sharp pin to an applicator stick. With this simple instrument it is easier to apply a uniform stimulus. Again the threshold is determined, and areas of loss are mapped out. The skin is usually touched in an irregular fashion either with the sharp end of the pin or the dull head, and the patient responds with "sharp" or "dull." In some patients with peripheral neuritis or tabes dorsalis the initial response to a painful stimulus may be "dull," only to be corrected within 1 to 3 seconds by the response "sharp." This delayed pain appreciation may be overlooked unless the patient is instructed to watch for this phenomenon. Poorly localized or deep pain is mediated by a different pathway system from sharp pin-prick sensation. It is elicited by application of heavy periosteal or testicular pressure.

For temperature testing, one test tube is filled with cold water and another with warm water. The temperature of the water from the faucet is usually quite adequate. The patient responds with either "cold" or "warm." In some areas of sensory loss neither warmth nor coldness is felt. Under these circumstances the test tube should be rolled on the skin from the involved to uninvolved areas, and the patient is asked to respond when he first feels a cold or warm sensation, depending on which tube is used. The areas of sensory loss for temperature usually overlap with those for pain but are slightly smaller.

Vibratory sensibility is not a separate sense, nor is it bone sensibility. Superficial and deep pressure receptors are involved, and a temporal pattern of pressures is perceived as vibration. Placing a tuning fork over bone mechanically intensifies the stimulus. The greatest sensibility is between 200 to 400 cycles per second; therefore, a tuning fork within this frequency range should be used. It is advantageous to use a large tuning fork, since its tensile strength is of longer duration. Usually the vibrating fork is placed over the sternum, elbows, fingers, iliac crest, knees, ankles, and toes. Threshold is determined by having the patient respond when he no longer feels the vibration. The tuning fork is then quickly placed on other parts of the body to determine if vibration is still perceived there. The patient's threshold may be compared with that of the examiner. Normal persons past the age of 60 years usually have some decrease of vibratory perception in the feet and legs.

The patient's ability to detect small passive movements is tested by holding a finger or toe between the examiner's fingers. The digit should be held by its lateral surfaces. The patient's muscles should be completely relaxed in order to test joint receptors rather than muscle stretch receptors. The digit is moved up or down irregularly and the patient responds with "up," "down," or "I don't know." The patient should clearly understand that "up" or "down" refers to the last position of the digit and not to the midposition. To avoid any misunderstanding, the patient should look at a few movements first; if he responds properly, he is then asked to close his eyes. A normal person can easily detect movements of a few millimeters. Should the patient be unable to detect finger movements, motion of the hand is then tested. If a patient's responses are consistently opposite to the actual movements, this usually indicates hysteria. It is just as difficult to call a movement consistently wrong as it is to call it properly.

A pair of calipers or a compass with dull points is used to test two-point discrimination. The two points have to be applied simultaneously; otherwise, the patient perceives two stimuli because they are separated in time. Two-point discrimination varies considerably over different areas. In the fingertips, points separated by 2 or 3 mm. may be identified as "two," whereas on the back they have to be separated by at least 3 to 4 cm. before they are felt as "two." The minimal distance between points at which the patient consistently feels two stimuli is noted and then comparable areas on the other side of the body are tested. Because objective measurements are made, this test lends itself readily to the detection of minimal abnormalities as well as to serial evaluations of a patient's progress.

High-level sensory discrimination can be tested by tracing numbers on the fingertips, palms, and soles. The size of the number should be smaller on the fingertips than elsewhere. In addition, the patient is asked to feel and identify common objects placed in his hand, such as a pencil, a key, a book of matches, or a ring. *Finger finding* is a valuable test of the patient's ability to locate his limb in space, a function of the parietal cortex. With the patient's eyes closed, his hand is placed and held in a fixed position while he uses the opposite hand to locate and grasp his index finger. When the test is positive, the patient has difficulty in locating or identifying the index finger on the side opposite the lesion.

COMMON PATTERNS OF SENSORY LOSS

While taking the history in many patients, it will become apparent which structures of the nervous system are most likely to be involved. During the sensory examination major emphasis will be placed on those areas that are reasonably expected to show impairment, whereas others are checked in a briefer fashion. Some knowledge of peripheral and central sensory pathways is indispensable.

Peripheral neuropathies. In peripheral neuropathies caused by nutritional deficiencies and metabolic diseases, distal portions of the body are more severely involved than proximal ones; consequently, the feet and legs are usually more severely involved than the hands and arms. Usually all sensory modalities are decreased, and the degree of loss decreases as the stimulus is moved proximally (glove-and-stocking type of sensory loss). Because peripheral nerves are more vulnerable in these conditions, a nerve may be damaged at points nor-

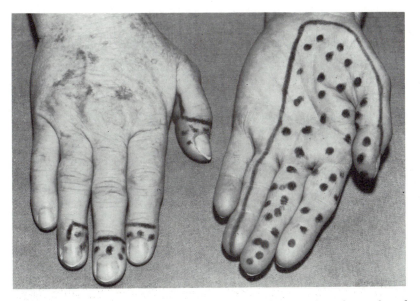

Fig. 18-21. Bilateral compression of the median nerve at the wrist (carpal tunnel syndrome). Atrophy of thenar eminence, sensory loss in distribution of median nerve.

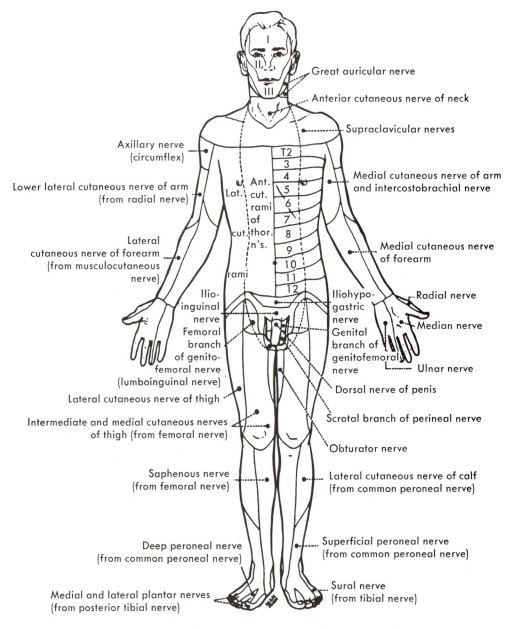

Fig. 18-22. The cutaneous fields of peripheral nerves from the anterior and posterior aspects. (From Haymaker, W., and Woodhall, B.: Peripheral nerve injuries, ed. 2, Philadelphia, 1959, W. B. Saunders Co.)

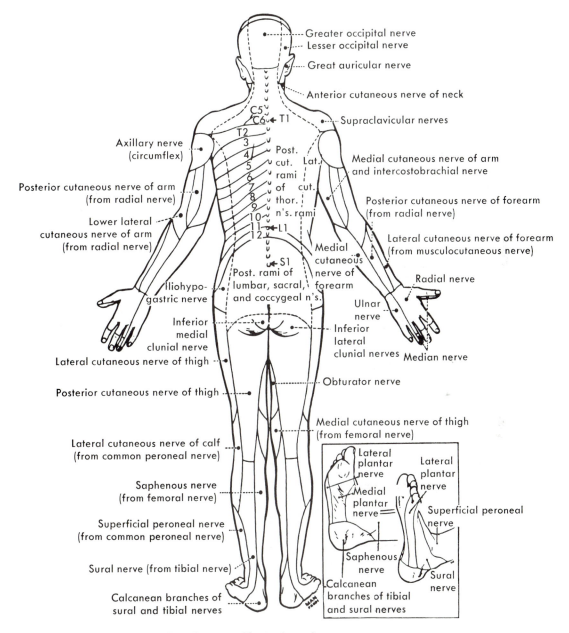

Greater occipital nerve
Lesser occipital nerve
Great auricular nerve
Anterior cutaneous nerve of neck
Supraclavicular nerves

C5
C6 ← T1
T2
3
4
5
6
7
8
9
10
11
12 ← L1
← S1

Post. cut. rami of thor. n's. rami

Lat. cut.

Axillary nerve
(circumflex)

Medial cutaneous nerve of arm
and intercostobrachial nerve

Posterior cutaneous nerve of arm
(from radial nerve)

Posterior cutaneous nerve of forearm
(from radial nerve)

Lower lateral
cutaneous nerve of arm
(from radial nerve)

Lateral cutaneous nerve of forearm
(from musculocutaneous nerve)

Medial
cutaneous
nerve of
forearm

Radial nerve

Iliohypo-
gastric nerve

Post. rami of
lumbar, sacral,
and coccygeal n's.

Ulnar
nerve

Inferior
medial
clunial nerve

Inferior
lateral
clunial nerves

Median nerve

Lateral cutaneous nerve of thigh

Posterior cutaneous nerve of thigh

Obturator nerve

Medial cutaneous nerve of thigh
(from femoral nerve)

Lateral cutaneous nerve of calf
(from common peroneal nerve)

Lateral
plantar
nerve

Lateral
plantar
nerve

Saphenous nerve
(from femoral nerve)

Medial
plantar
nerve

Superficial peroneal
nerve

Superficial peroneal nerve
(from common peroneal nerve)

Sural nerve (from tibial nerve)

Saphenous
nerve

Sural
nerve

Calcanean branches of
sural and tibial nerves

Calcanean
branches of tibial
and sural nerves

Fig. 18-22, cont'd. For legend see opposite page.

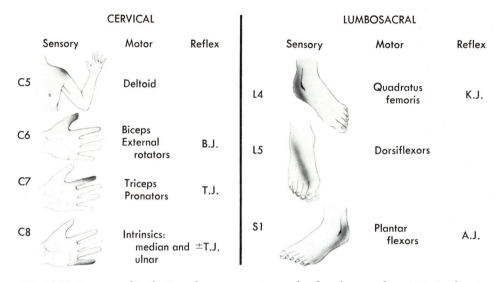

Fig. 18-23. Common distribution of sensory, motor, and reflex changes characteristic of root compression. (From Hunt, W. E., and Paul, S.: Herniated cervical and lumbar discs, Ohio State Med. J. **65:**583-587, 1969.)

mally subjected to repeated trauma, such as the ulnar nerve at the elbow, the median nerve in the carpal tunnel (Fig. 18-21), or the peroneal nerve at the head of the fibula. The resulting sensory loss in the distribution of the particular nerve affected will then be superimposed on the more diffuse peripheral sensory loss.

Individual nerves and roots. A decrease or loss of all sensory modalities is seen also in peripheral nerve lesions (Figs. 18-22 and 18-23) caused by trauma or vascular occlusion. The area of sensory loss depends on the exact site of the nerve injury. For example, compression of the peroneal nerve at the head of the fibula usually spares the lateral cutaneous nerve of the leg and the superficial peroneal nerve, both of which are branches of the common peroneal nerve, while the deep peroneal branch is damaged. The resulting sensory loss consists of a small triangular area on the dorsum of the base of the first and second toes extending a short distance proximally onto the dorsum of the

foot. Involvement of a few or many peripheral nerves or their branches is called *mononeuritis multiplex* and is frequently seen in periarteritis nodosa. If many nerves are involved, the picture may resemble a peripheral neuropathy, but it will be clear from the history that individual nerves or their branches were involved one after the other.

At times it is difficult to distinguish between a nerve and a nerve root lesion. In each the sensory impairment involves all modalities, and only careful testing and comparison of the findings with sensory charts will solve this problem (Figs. 18-22 and 18-24). The common distribution of sensory, motor, and reflex changes characteristic of root compression in disc disease is shown in Fig. 18-23.

Spinal cord. Lesions of the spinal cord produce sensory deficits unlike those of peripheral neuropathy or isolated nerve or nerve root lesions. For example, hemisection of the spinal cord produces loss of pain and temperature perception on the contralateral side, beginning

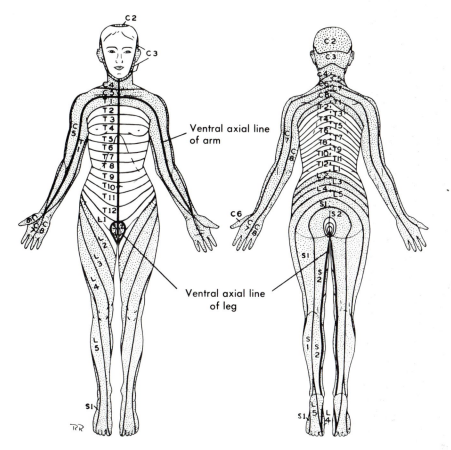

Fig. 18-24. Distribution of spinal dermatomes. (From Keegan, J. J., and Garrett, F. D.: Anat. Rec. **102:**411, 1948.)

at a level one to two segments below the lesion. Vibratory perception, position sense, and two-point discrimination are lost below the level of the lesion on the ipsilateral side. This pattern is explained by the decussation of fibers subserving pain and temperature sensation that cross to the contralateral side via the anterior white commissure within one or two segments of the level of entry into the spinal cord. Nerve fibers required for vibratory perception, position sense, and two-point discrimination ascend in the spinal cord on the ipsilateral side until they reach lower medullary levels. In addition,

there may be ataxia on the ipsilateral side below the lesion as a result of involvement of the ipsilateral dorsal spinocerebellar tract.

Pain fibers, after crossing to the contralateral side, are layered in an orderly fashion. Fibers of caudal origin will be most dorsal and lateral, while those of leg, trunk, and arm will be successively placed in ventromedial positions. When the anterior spinal artery that supplies the anterior two thirds of the spinal cord is occluded, the most caudal fibers of the spinothalamic tract may be spared. If the occlusion occurred at the level of the seventh thoracic segment, there would be loss of pain and temperature perception bilaterally below the lesion on the trunk and in both feet and legs, but sparing the perineal area that is supplied by sacral segments. Proprioception would also be spared because proprioceptive stimuli are transmitted via fibers in the dorsal columns.

Brain stem. In the lower medulla a laterally located lesion, such as an infarct, will produce a distinctive sensory loss that results from the involvement of the lateral spinothalamic and the descending tract of the trigeminal nerve. There will be loss of pain and temperature sensation on the contralateral arm, trunk, and leg. Pain and temperature sensation will be lost on the ipsilateral side of the face, since fibers serving this zone are located in the descending tract of the trigeminal nerve and are not crossed at the medullary level.

Thalamus. Destructive lesions in the posterior ventral nucleus of the thalamus produce a sensory loss involving all modalities on the contralateral side of the body. Small unmyelinated pain fibers synapse widely in the brain stem and diffuse thalamic nuclei; as a consequence, the deep, poorly localized pain mediated by them may be preserved.

Cortex. Since perception of pain, vibration, and crude touch is managed at the thalamic level, there will be little loss of these modalities in lesions of the post-central cortex. In such lesions discriminatory sensation is impaired or lost on the contralateral side of the body. Position sense and two-point discrimination are abolished. Furthermore, the patient is unable to identify traced figures, identify objects by feeling, judge different textures, or estimate different weights. Finger finding will be inaccurate.

AUTONOMIC NERVOUS SYSTEM

Pupillary responses were discussed previously. In idiopathic orthostatic hypotension the iris atrophies, and reactions to light and accommodation are usually decreased. In addition to the pupillary abnormalities, sweating may be lost over the entire body. Ipsilateral absence of sweating on one side of the face is often seen in lateral medullary lesions, lateral cervical cord lesions, or interruption of sympathetic fibers along their path to the superior cervical ganglion. In patients with hypothalamic lesions that destroy the heat loss center, sweating in response to high temperature is lost. Otherwise, discrete central nervous system lesions rarely abolish sweating on the body or extremities because of bilateral sympathetic innervation of sweat glands.

The urinary bladder receives extensive autonomic as well as somatic innervation. Lesions at all levels of the neuraxis from cortex to peripheral nerves produce abnormalities of micturition. Bilateral damage to the medial aspect of cerebral hemispheres near and posterior to the motor area can cause loss of bladder inhibition with incontinence. Bilateral lesions of the lateral columns of the spinal cord are associated with a spastic bladder, with micturition reflex set off at lower-than-normal urinary volume, leading to frequency, urgency, and incontinence. With involvement of sacral cord segments or sacral roots, the micturition reflex may fail, with difficulty in voiding and bladder distention.

COVERINGS (SKULL, SPINE, MENINGES)

Inspection of the skull will readily reveal abnormalities of size and shape. In order to verify the impression of an abnormally large or small head, the circumference should be measured. This is of particular importance in infants and children, since head circumference is the most reliable parameter of physical growth. Bony defects or bony overgrowth can be detected by palpation. The points at which the three branches of the trigeminal nerve and the occipital nerves leave their bony canals should be palpated to detect unusual tenderness. The skull is percussed with a finger. Occasionally the percussion sound may be less resonant over the side of a subdural hematoma, and the patient may wince from pain.

When the spine is inspected, abnormal curvatures, loss of normal cervical or lumbar lordosis, impairment of mobility, and unusual shortness of some segments should be looked for. For example, in basilar impression, the cervical spine looks short, and the head appears to sit on the shoulders. Palpation and percussion will reveal tenderness of spinous processes and paraspinal muscles, as well as unusual degrees of paraspinal muscle contractions. These signs will frequently be found over areas of root compression. In radiculopathies, flexion, extension, lateral rotation, and lateral

flexion of the cervical and lumbosacral spine may produce pain and may be limited in one or more directions. At times a moderate pull on the head will relieve the pain of cervical root compression. In compression of a lumbar or sacral root the examiner can frequently reproduce or aggravate the patient's pain by raising the extended leg in the supine position (straight-leg–raising test). The angle of elevation at which the patient feels pain should be noted. Dorsiflexion of the foot will aggravate the pain by stretching the nerve even more. Raising of the contralateral leg or flexion of the neck also may reproduce the patient's pain.

Meningeal irritation causes a stiff neck. In the recumbent position little resistance is met when moving the head gently from side to side

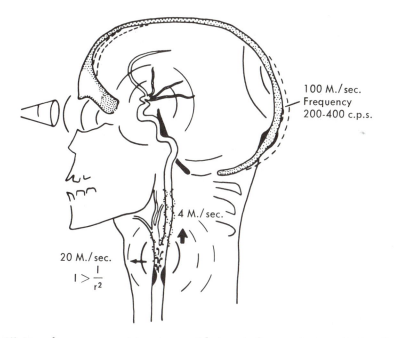

100 M./sec.
Frequency
200-400 c.p.s.

4 M./sec.

20 M./sec.
$I > \frac{1}{r^2}$

Fig. 18-25. Vascular murmurs arising at a carotid stenosis decrease in intensity in soft tissues with the square of the distance. The murmur is propagated with little decrement along the vessel. On entering the cranial cavity it may be transmitted through the orbit. Loud murmurs or those involving intracranial arteriovenous fistulae may be transmitted widely over the skull. (From Allen, N.: Geriatrics **20:**525, 1965; reprinted from Geriatrics © 1965 by The New York Times Media Company, Inc.)

but marked resistance is encountered with any attempt to flex the head. At times neck extensor contractions are so powerful that the back is arched (*opisthotonus*), and the patient can be lifted by his head like a board. With meningeal irritation from any cause, attempts to completely extend the legs at the knees with the thighs flexed at a right angle cause neck and head pain and meet definite resistance to extension (*Kernig's sign*).

Auscultation of the head and neck is of value in the diagnosis of cerebral vascular diseases. Murmurs generated by a carotid stenosis are propagated distally with little decrement and on reaching the intracranial cavity may be transmitted through the orbit (Fig. 18-25). Murmurs of arteriovenous fistulae are often continuous and may be heard over cranium and orbit. The examiner should auscult the great vessels of the neck with the stethoscope bell, taking care to avoid compression of the vessel. For orbital auscultation, the patient is asked to close his eyes while the bell is placed gently but snugly over the eyelids. He is then asked to open his other eye and relax.

NEUROLOGIC EXAMINATION OF THE COMATOSE PATIENT

Coma is a condition commonly encountered by every physician. Often the cause is readily apparent. In those patients in whom the cause is not obvious, a systematic neurologic examination will frequently lead to the correct diagnosis.

Mechanisms of coma. Consciousness is impaired by two different mechanisms: (1) Function of both cerebral hemispheres is directly and widely depressed by toxic-metabolic derangement. (2) Hypothalamic, diencephalic, mesencephalic, or pontine activating mechanisms are depressed or destroyed. The former condition is usually encountered in toxic-metabolic diseases, anoxia, or widespread destructive lesions. The latter is seen with lesions in-

volving the brain stem, either directly by a tumor or infarct or indirectly by a supratentorial tumor or edematous brain that herniates downward. In general, toxic-metabolic disturbances do not alter brain stem functions until late in their development.

Different states of impaired consciousness (drowsiness, obtundation, stupor, and coma) were previously described. Their recognition is not only useful in diagnosis but also serves as a valuable guide in following the patient's progress.

Examination. Immediate general observations should include adequacy of ventilation, blood pressure, evidence of head trauma, skin color (cyanosis, pallor, jaundice), signs of dehydration, and breath odor (alcohol, ketones, uremia).

Measures to provide adequate circulation and oxygenation are instituted prior to a detailed examination. In doubtful situations, intravenous glucose is given after first drawing blood for glucose determination. These measures protect brain function and may prevent serious brain damage.

Neurologic examination of the comatose patient should proceed in the following sequence: state of consciousness, pattern of respiration, size and reactivity of pupils, eye movements, and motor responses. Table 18-6 serves as a guide in the examination of a comatose patient.

Respirations. Several common abnormal patterns of respiration are recognized. *Periodic respiration* was described in Chapter 9. Metabolic brain dysfunction or bilateral lesions in the vicinity of the internal capsule give rise to this respiratory abnormality. In *central neurogenic hyperventilation*, respiration is rapid, deep, and regular. This pattern evolves with impairment of function of the midbrain and pons. *Cluster* breathing characterized by irregular clusters of respiratory movements is indicative of lower pontine or upper medullary disturbances. Respiration completely irregular in

Table 18-6. Neurologic examination of the comatose patient

Function or structure	Observation and appropriate test
Mental status	Definition of level of consciousness
Optic nerve	Light reflex, funduscopy
Oculomotor, trochlear, and abducens nerves	Pupillary responses, reflex eye movements
Trigeminal nerve	Corneal reflex
Facial nerve	Cheek puffing, sucking reflex, responses to painful stimulation
Vestibular nerve	Caloric responses
Glossopharyngeal and vagus nerves	Gag reflex
Motor	Spontaneous movements, muscle tonus with passive manipulation, movements in response to painful stimulation
Reflexes	All reflexes
Sensory	Response to painful stimulation, superficial reflexes
Autonomic	Respiratory pattern, pupillary responses
Coverings (skull, spine, meninges)	Stiff neck, Kernig's sign, wince to head pressure, evidence of external injury

depth and frequency is called *ataxic* (meningitic) respiration. This pattern is seen with destructive lesions of dorsomedial medullary areas. Since apnea may occur in this condition during sleep or light sedation, it is extremely important to anticipate this complication and provide respiratory assistance. Progressive rostral to caudal impairment of brain stem function is accompanied by respiratory abnormalities changing from periodic respiration to ataxic breathing in the sequence given.

Pupils. Normal pupillary responses indicate intact optic pathways and sympathetic and parasympathetic structures governing pupillary activity. In general, pupillary abnormalities are not seen in toxic-metabolic conditions until terminal stages. (A few exceptions are mentioned later.) Cerebral or hypothalamic lesions have variable and diagnostically unreliable effects on the pupil. Midbrain tectal or pretectal lesions interrupt the light pathway; the pupil is in midposition or slightly large and will not react to light. Third nerve involvement, such as in compression of the nerve against the tentorium, leads to wide pupillary dilatation. Bilateral pinpoint pupils commonly indicate pontine hemorrhage. Lateral medullary or lateral cervical cord lesions cause ipsilateral ptosis and pupillary constriction, but the light reflex is preserved. In opiate intoxication the pupils are pinpoint, but with a strong light a light reflex can be elicited. Widely dilated and fixed pupils are seen in atropine intoxication and anoxia. Glutethimide (Doriden) intoxication characteristically produces midposition unequal pupils that may not respond to light stimulation for several hours.

Eye movements. Eye movements can be elicited by quickly turning the head from side to side and up and down (Fig. 18-26). In the comatose patient, the eyes will move in a direction opposite to the head movement (*oculocephalic reflex*). When head position is maintained, the eyes rapidly return to their resting position. Further information about reflex eye movements can be obtained by caloric stimu-

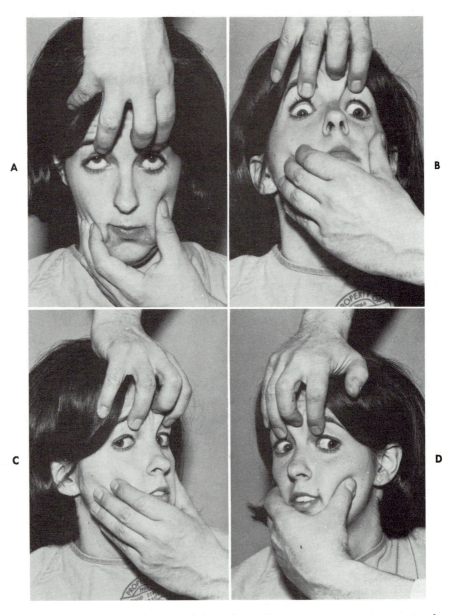

Fig. 18-26. Demonstration of oculocephalic reflexes. Eye movements are in opposite direction of head movement.

lation. In the unconscious patient ice water stimulation is followed by tonic deviation of both eyes toward the irrigated side, provided brain stem function is normal (oculovestibular reflex). Ice water irrigation of both ears simultaneously with the head elevated 30 degrees produces tonic downward deviation of both eyes, while tonic upward deviation is seen with the head 60 degrees below the horizontal.

Conjugate gaze disorders in comatose patients result from destructive lesions. Because of unopposed contralateral innervation, in hemispheric lesions the eyes are deviated toward the side of the lesion and away from an associated hemiparesis. With brisk turning of the head the eyes will briefly turn past the midline to the other side, indicating an intact brain stem. Deviation of the eyes away from a hemispheral abnormality is seen in irritative lesions but rarely persists longer than a few hours. Unilateral pontine lesions involving supranuclear oculomotor fibers below their decussation produce deviation of the eyes away from the lesion. If the patient has an associated hemiparesis, the eyes look toward the paralyzed side. Head turning or caloric stimulation will not modify this condition. Paralysis of upward gaze usually results from compression or destruction of the pretectal area. Persistent downward deviation of the eyes frequently results from compression of the midbrain tectum. Intermittent, brisk, conjugate downward movements of the eyes (*ocular bobbing*) occur with severe destructive caudal pontine lesions. When the head is turned quickly from side to side, failure of *adduction* of one eye suggests involvement of the medial longitudinal fasciculus on the same side, while failure of *abduction* is indicative of a lesion of the abducens nerve. Bilateral destruction of the vestibular nuclei or labyrinth abolishes caloric responses, while eye movements in response to head turning (oculocephalic reflex) remain intact.

Motor responses. All motor responses to painful stimulation may be lost in deep coma. In light coma failure to elicit movement of ipsilateral and contralateral muscles with painful stimulation suggests sensory impairment on the ipsilateral side. If the stimulated extremity does not move but a response is seen in contralateral muscles, weakness of the ipsilateral extremity is probably present. Decorticate or decerebrate posturing may be elicited by painful stimulation of the head or may occur spontaneously. Spasticity, rigidity, dystonia, or paratonia can be detected by moving the patient's extremities. Manipulation of the head will reveal stiffness of the neck.

Tentorial herniations. Central or transtentorial herniation and uncal herniation may all eventually lead to coma. The herniation is usually the result of mass lesions such as tumor, intracerebral hemorrhage, subdural hematoma, or edema secondary to tumor and infarct. Since the resulting coma is frequently irreversible, it is imperative to recognize these conditions before the patient lapses into coma.

Central or *transtentorial herniation* is the result of downward displacement of the hemispheres and basal ganglia compressing and displacing the diencephalon and mesencephalon caudally through the tentorial notch. Superiorly placed cerebral or extracerebral lesions usually lead to such a shift. Clinically, the development of this condition is characterized by the following sequence of events. The first manifestation is usually a change in alertness, accompanied by deep sighs or yawning. As the patient becomes somnolent, periodic respiration develops. At a slightly more advanced stage, paratonic resistance, grasp reflex, and Babinski sign emerge on the side contralateral to a preexisting hemiplegia. Without such a hemiplegia, these signs develop bilaterally. Decorticate posturing eventually appears that initially may be seen only in response to noxious stimulation. If the herniation progresses beyond this diencephalic stage, midbrain failure ensues. Central neurogenic hyperventilation replaces periodic respiration. Pupils dilate moderately, the ciliospinal reflex disappears, and oculovestibular responses become progressively more difficult to elicit. Decorticate posturing changes to decerebrate rigidity. Midbrain damage after tentorial herniation is caused by secondary ischemia, and most patients either die or remain in coma for many months. When further progression of rostrocaudal brain stem dysfunction occurs, the pupils become fixed in midposition, oculovestibular responses are unobtainable, and Babinski signs remain, but the limbs become flaccid. In the last or medullary stage, which occurs terminally, respiration becomes ataxic, the pulse is irregularly slow or fast, and the blood pressure drops.

When breathing finally stops, the pupils dilate widely. At this stage blood pressure and respiration can be maintained artificially, but death is inevitable.

Expanding lesions in the *lateral middle fossa* frequently shift the medial uncus and hippocampal gyrus over the free edge of the tentorium. The most consistent, early, and at times the only, sign is ipsilateral pupillary dilatation caused by pressure on the third nerve. Impaired consciousness or respiratory changes ordinarily are not early signs of uncal herniation because the diencephalon is not the first structure encroached on. Once the pupil is fully dilated, external oculomotor paralysis occurs. As the contralateral cerebral peduncle is pushed against the tentorial edge, ipsilateral hemiplegia develops. When external ophthalmoplegia appears, the patient usually lapses into coma. From this point progression is indistinguishable from that of central herniation. A striking feature of uncal herniation is early midbrain involvement and rapid progression. Uncal herniation requires prompt emergency treatment, since any delay inevitably results in irreversible damage.

SELECTED READINGS

Allen, N., and Burkholder, J.: Practice of medicine, vol. 10, New York, 1972, Harper & Row, Publishers.

Allen, N., and Mustian, V.: Origin and significance of vascular murmurs of the head and neck, Medicine **41**:227, 1962.

DeJong, R. M.: The neurologic examination, ed. 4, New York, 1979, Harper & Row, Publishers.

DeMyer, W.: Technique of the neurologic examination: a programmed text, ed. 3, New York, 1980, McGraw-Hill Book Co.

Denny-Brown, D.: Handbook of neurological examination and case recording, Cambridge, 1960, Harvard University Press.

Geshwind, N.: Current concepts—aphasia, N. Engl. J. Med. **284**:654, 1971.

Geshwind, N.: The apraxias: Neural mechanisms of disorders of learned movement, Am. Sci. **63**:188, 1975.

Medical Research Council War Memorandum No. 7: Aids to the investigation of peripheral nerve injuries, ed. 2, London, 1962, Her Majesty's Stationery Office.

Paulson, G. W., and Gottlieb, G.: Developmental reflexes: the reappearance of fetal and neoplastic reflexes in aged patients, Brain **91**:37, 1968.

Plum, F., and Posner, J. B.: Diagnosis of stupor and coma, ed. 2, Philadelphia, 1972, F. A. Davis Co.

Rucker, C. W.: The interpretation of visual fields, ed. 3, Omaha, 1957, American Academy of Ophthalmology and Otolaryngology.

CHAPTER 19

MUSCULOSKELETAL SYSTEM

A carefully conducted examination of the musculoskeletal system is required to diagnose specific types of arthritis and bursitis. In addition, distinct abnormalities of the musculoskeletal system are frequently indicative of systemic diseases such as acromegaly, hemochromatosis, inflammatory bowel disease, and sickle cell anemia.

The accurate physical examination of the peripheral joints and spine can be accomplished only after a detailed history is taken. Since inspection and palpation are the primary means of evaluating the musculoskeletal system, it is mandatory that the patient be disrobed and wear an examination gown.

The primary purpose of this chapter is to present a systematic routine for examining the musculoskeletal system. Although abnormal findings are occasionally presented as illustrative examples, the reader is directed to the selected references at the end of this chapter for detailed descriptions of pathologic states.

EXAMINATION OF THE PERIPHERAL JOINTS

Effective evaluation of the peripheral joints is best accomplished in a systematic routine that permits the detection of subtle physical abnormalities. Although the particular approach may vary among different examiners, the following procedure is commonly utilized by most rheumatologists.

Hand

First, inspect the hand for deformities and carefully examine the nails for evidence of clubbing, psoriasis, subungual microinfarcts, and anemia. In certain cardiopulmonary diseases and malignant disease states, the fingers may exhibit *clubbing* with a marked exaggeration of the normal curvature of the nails and loss of the angle between the nail and the terminal digit (Fig. 19-1). *Dupuytren's contracture* is caused by thickening and tightening of the palmar fascia, first usually involving the little finger and ring finger. Inability to fully extend the fingers is an early sign of this disorder, and careful palpation of the palmar aspect of the hand is required to reveal thickening and nodularity of the fascia (Fig. 19-2). Psoriasis involving the nails is typically evidenced by pitting and severe destruction of the normal nail architecture (Fig. 19-3). If advanced, psoriatic

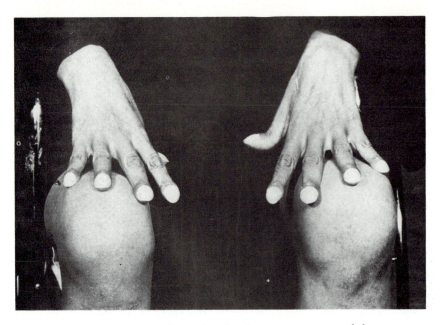

Fig. 19-1. Clubbing of nails and peripheral arthritis in a patient with lung cancer.

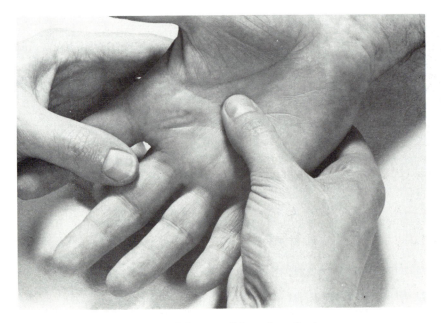

Fig. 19-2. Palpation of the palmar fascia.

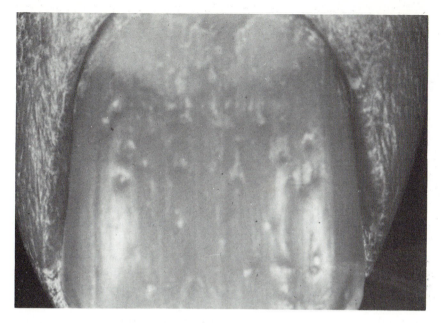

Fig. 19-3. Nail pitting secondary to psoriasis.

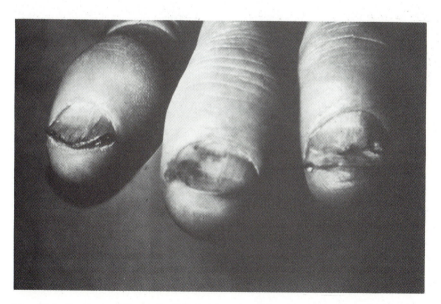

Fig. 19-4. Psoriasis of the nails with destruction of the distal interphalangeal joints.

involvement of the nails can result in a severe destructive arthritis of the small joints of the hand, especially the distal interphalangeal joints (Fig. 19-4). *Sclerodactylia* refers to the hand changes observed in progressive systemic sclerosis. Depending on the severity, the skin overlying the digits and hand is thickened and demonstrates a loss of normal elasticity. In more aggressive and advanced forms of sclerodactylia, flexion contractures rapidly develop, and the fingers become tapered with a loss of the distal tufts (Fig. 19-5). Small hemorrhages under the nails and about the subungual regions are commonly referred to as *splinter hemorrhages*, or *microinfarcts* (Fig. 19-6). These can be seen in bacterial endocarditis and other illnesses that result in occlusion of the small arteries. For example, vascular occlusion secondary to a systemic vasculitis may be observed in lupus erythematosus, idiopathic small vessel vasculitis, or rheumatoid arthritis. In rheumatoid arthritis, digital vasculitis can be

extremely aggressive, resulting in ischemia, gangrene, and autoamputation (Fig. 19-7). Other causes of distal digit and nail abnormalities include *paronychias*, which are suppurative lesions of the soft tissues. Fungal infections of the nails are referred to as *onychomycosis*.

Next, one should inspect and carefully palpate the distal interphalangeal, proximal interphalangeal (Fig. 19-8), and metacarpophalangeal joints (Fig. 19-9). Heberden's and Bouchard's nodes are seen in osteoarthritis involving the distal and proximal interphalangeal joints respectively. These present as firm, bony protuberances secondary to the hypertrophic bone formation in osteoarthritis (Fig. 19-10). Occasionally, considerable inflammation can occur in osteoarthritis of the hands that is commonly referred to as "inflammatory osteoarthritis" (Fig. 19-11). Cyst formation is sometimes associated with Heberden's nodes and may be mistaken for a septic joint (Fig. 19-12). Evidence of synovial thickening is not prominent

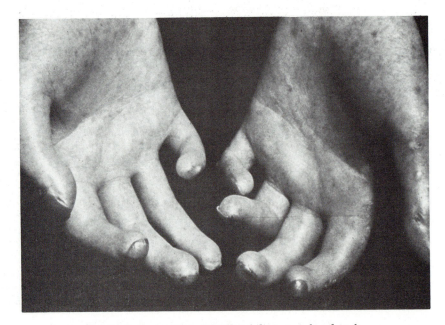

Fig. 19-5. Resorption of the distal digits in sclerodactylia.

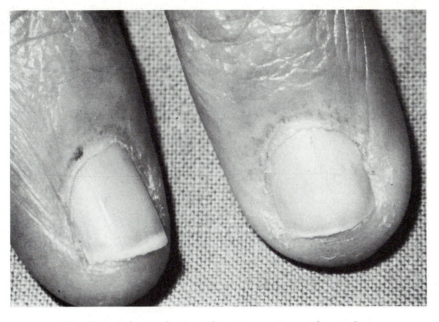

Fig. 19-6. Subungual microinfarcts in a patient with vasculitis.

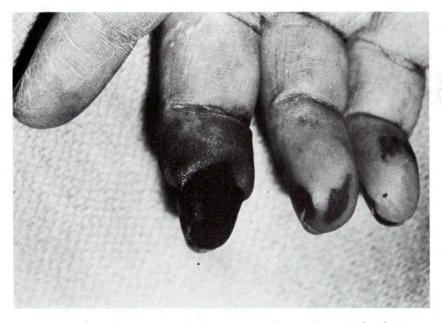

Fig. 19-7. Digital vasculitis and infarction secondary to rheumatoid arthritis.

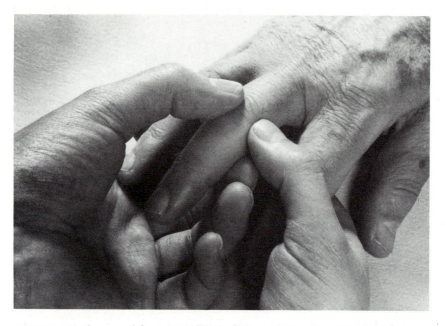

Fig. 19-8. Evaluation of the proximal interphalangeal joint for synovial thickening.

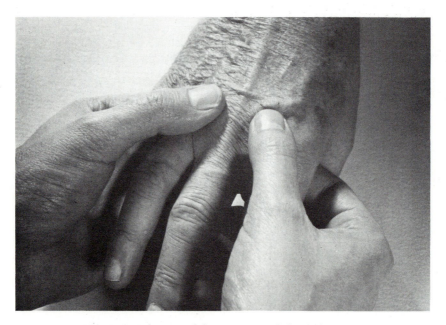

Fig. 19-9. Palpation of the metacarpophalangeal joints.

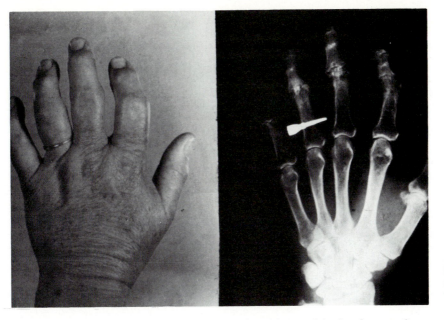

Fig. 19-10. Heberden's and Bouchard's nodes in osteoarthritis of the hands. Spur formation and destruction of the distal and proximal interphalangeal joints are evident in x-rays of the hand.

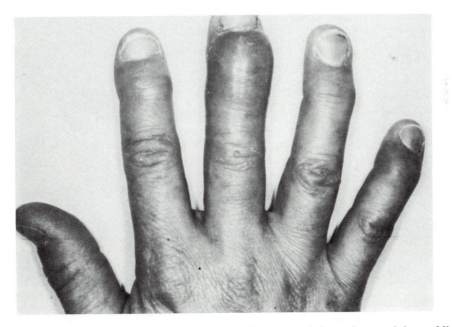

Fig. 19-11. Intense inflammatory synovitis of the distal interphalangeal joint of the middle finger in osteoarthritis.

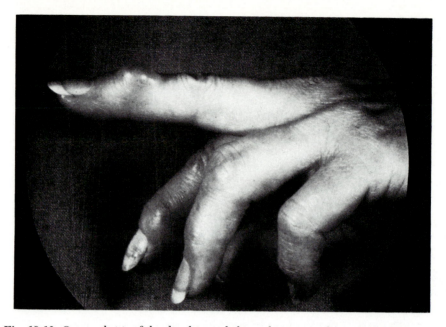

Fig. 19-12. Osteoarthritis of the distal interphalangeal joint, resulting in cyst formation.

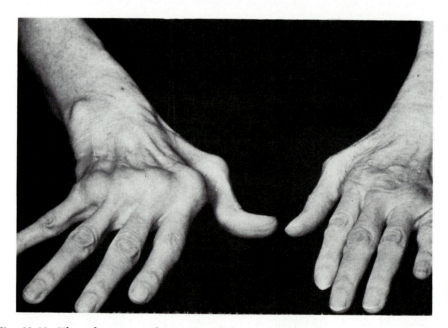

Fig. 19-13. Ulnar deviation and synovitis of the metacarpophalangeal joints secondary to rheumatoid arthritis and mainly involving the dominant (right) hand. Note that the nondominant hand is relatively unaffected.

in osteoarthritis, rather the bony protuberances are the most striking abnormality. In contrast, joint involvement secondary to rheumatoid arthritis is mainly characterized by synovial thickening. In rheumatoid arthritis one finds fusiform swelling of the joints usually with a fairly symmetric involvement of the proximal interphalangeal and metacarpophalangeal joints bilaterally. On palpation, synovial thickening is best described as a sensation of "bogginess." Appreciation of subtle synovial thickening requires considerable experience in examining normal joints, thereby permitting comparison with peripheral joints involved with rheumatoid arthritis. It should be emphasized that the degree of synovial thickening present in a joint is partially related to the amount of use. Therefore, rheumatoid arthritis can occasionally be somewhat asymmetric with, for example, the joints of the dominant hand displaying more noticeable changes than those of the nondominant (Fig. 19-13). Slight asymmetry is not un-

common during the very early phases of rheumatoid arthritis and if not recognized can be a source of confusion.

In the more active and long-standing forms of rheumatoid arthritis, ulnar deviaton of the fingers is observed as a result of synovitis of the metacarpal joints, with subsequent laxity of the capsule. Although erythema is occasionally mentioned as a sign of the synovitis secondary to rheumatoid arthritis, this is an uncommon finding. Indeed, significant joint erythema and tenderness occurring during the course of rheumatoid arthritis are suggestive of either an acutely infected joint or an acute crystal-induced synovitis, such as gout or pseudogout. Slight warmth is usually present over joints with active rheumatoid arthritis.

Pallor of the digits, associated with coldness, is indicative of Raynaud's phenomenon (Fig. 19-14) or other processes compromising the distal circulation, such as peripheral embolization. Patients with Raynaud's phenomenon

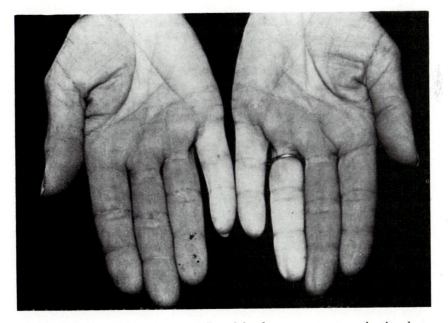

Fig. 19-14. Raynaud's phenomenon. Pallor of the digits in a patient with scleroderma.

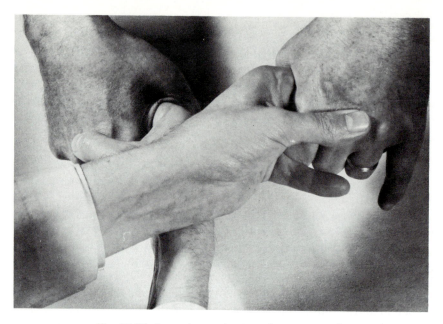

Fig. 19-15. Screening evaluation of grasp strength.

usually experience digital pallor on exposure to cold. This is followed by a phase of cyanosis and then by erythema on rewarming. In the individual patient there may be considerable variation in the severity of these triphasic changes, with some patients not experiencing certain changes. Raynaud's phenomenon can occur in association with scleroderma, rheumatoid arthritis, or other connective tissue diseases.

Test active and passive ranges of motion of the fingers to detect joint contractures, muscular weakness, peripheral neuropathies, or tendon ruptures. For example, extensor tendon rupture secondary to rheumatoid synovitis of the wrists results in the inability to actively extend the digits, while the passive range of motion is relatively normal. Similarly, a palpable nodule within the flexor tendon, associated with a clicking sensation as the finger is extended or flexed is indicative of a "trigger" or "snapping" finger. Again, the patient experi-

ences difficulty in performing full, active range of motion, but the passive range of motion is preserved. The ability to grasp can be estimated by having the patient squeeze the examiner's digits (Fig. 19-15). More quantitative assessment of grip can be obtained by having the patient squeeze a folded blood pressure cuff. Serial recordings on the sphygmomanometer can be helpful in evaluating the clinical course.

Wrist

Inspect the contour of the wrist and particularly note any fullness about the soft tissues adjacent to the styloid process of the ulna. Occasionally, rheumatoid synovitis can result in quite marked changes about the ulnar styloid. Also, carefully observe for abnormal angulation of the wrist, as can occur in aggressive synovitis, leading to destruction of the carpal bones.

Next, palpate the bony and soft tissues of the wrists. Again, the synovial thickening of rheu-

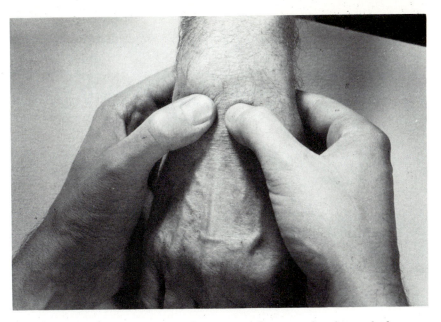

Fig. 19-16. Palpation of the wrist and synovium adjacent to the ulnar styloid process.

matoid arthritis results in a boggy sensation while the examiner is gently palpating the soft tissues (Fig. 19-16). It is extremely important to palpate the flexor aspect of the wrists, because inflammation and swelling of the soft tissues within the carpal tunnel can sometimes be detected as a tense tautness of the transverse carpal ligament. *Tinel's sign* is localized tenderness on percussing over the transverse carpal ligament and often is associated with pain and paresthesias radiating distally along the median nerve distribution (Fig. 19-17). This is suggestive, but not diagnostic, of median nerve compression secondary to carpal tunnel syndrome. *Phalen's sign* is generally less helpful in diagnosing median nerve compression at the wrist. This is elicited by forcibly flexing the wrist, with pain and paresthesias occurring in the distribution of the median nerve when positive (Fig. 19-18). In addition to pain and paresthesias, patients with carpal tunnel syndrome may experience a loss of normal sensation in-

volving the flexor aspect of the thumb, the index and middle fingers, and part of the ring finger. With more severe or long-standing median nerve compression, there may be weakness and even atrophy localized to the muscles of the thumb innervated by the median nerve (Fig. 19-19).

The two common causes of pain along the radial aspect of the wrist and the first carpometacarpal joint include stenosing tenosynovitis and osteoarthritis.

Stenosing tenosynovitis is often referred to as *de Quervain's disease*. On examination, there is tenderness to palpation over the tendon sheaths of the extensor pollicus brevis and abductor pollicus longus along the distal radius (Fig. 19-20). When severely inflamed, a tender nodule is occasionally present within the tendinous structures, and pain may be referred distally to the anatomic snuffbox. In more aggressive forms of stenosing tenosynovitis, it is sometimes possible to elicit a positive Finkel-

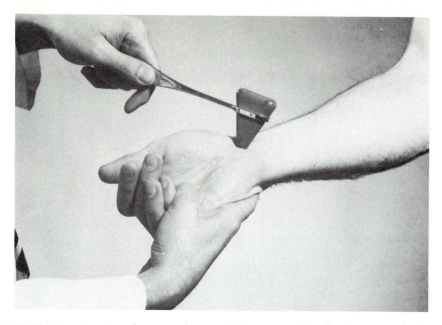

Fig. 19-17. Percussion over the transverse carpal ligament to elicit Tinel's sign, indicative of median nerve compression.

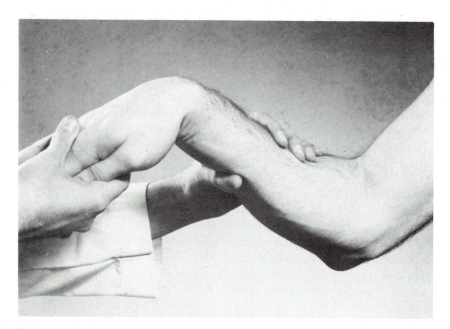

Fig. 19-18. Forced flexion of the wrist to evaluate the Phalen's sign sometimes observed in the presence of median nerve compression.

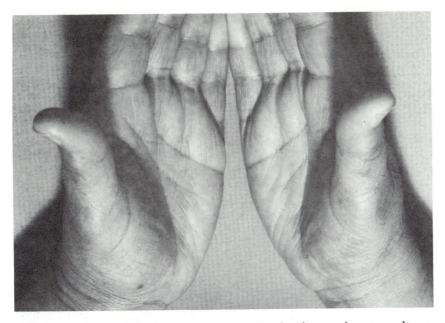

Fig. 19-19. Asymmetry of the musculature about the thumb secondary to median nerve compression.

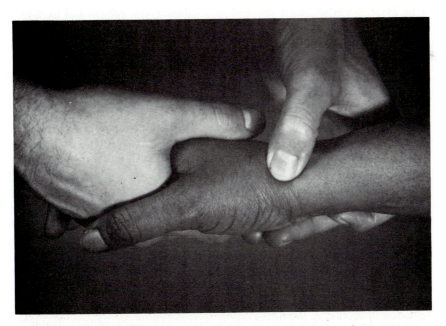

Fig. 19-20. Examination of the radial aspect of the wrist to detect tenderness present with stenosing tenosynovitis (de Quervain's disease).

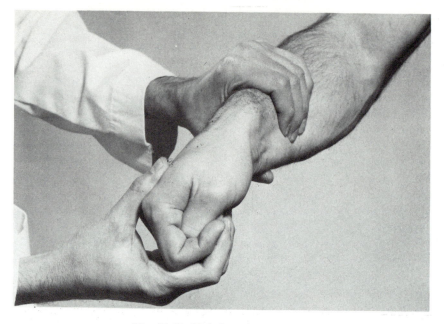

Fig. 19-21. Finkelstein's maneuver.

stein's test. This is performed by rapidly moving the wrist in ulnar deviation, with the patient flexing the thumb in the palm (Fig. 19-21). When positive, sudden pain is experienced over the distal radius often radiating into the first carpometacarpal joint and the thumb.

Osteoarthritis involving the first carpometacarpal joint is fairly frequent and can result in considerable disability. Although the pain is usually localized to the joint, rather diffuse radiation can sometimes occur, and the patient may experience difficulty in precise localization. On physical examination, the most helpful sign is bony protuberances representing the hypertrophic changes. The range of motion is usually fairly well preserved unless far-advanced osteoarthritis is present.

Finally, examine carefully the passive and active range of motion of the wrist. Especially in those patients on therapy, the careful recording of the range of motion is important in evaluating the future treatment response.

Elbow

Inspect the elbow and in particular determine if the patient can fully extend the elbow. Inability to fully extend the elbow may be seen in rheumatoid arthritis, trauma, or osteoarthritis and is one of the earliest signs of abnormality. Only with far-advanced, aggressive forms of arthritis does one detect significant functional defects in flexion or supination-pronation.

The detection of thickened synovium about the elbow is very important in assessing the extent of peripheral joint involvement by inflammatory synovitis. However, accurate evaluation requires considerable practice in carefully palpating the exposed synovium between the olecranon process and epicondyle (Fig. 19-22). After acquiring sufficient expertise, the examiner can determine the degree of synovitis present within the elbow.

Tenderness lateral to the proximal radial head is usually indicative of *lateral epicondyli-*

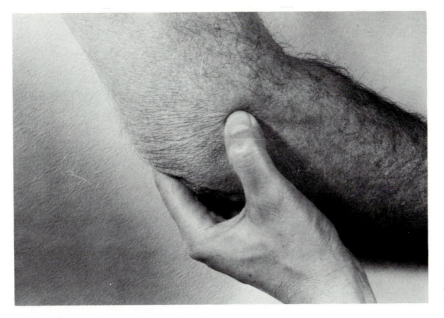

Fig. 19-22. Palpation of the exposed elbow synovium for evidence of synovitis.

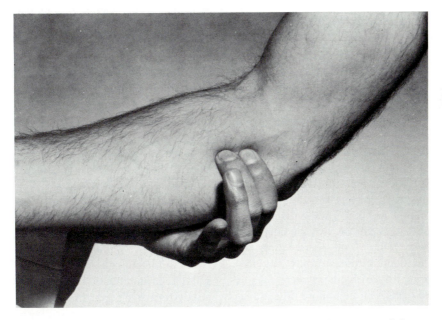

Fig. 19-23. Palpation of the ulnar nerve for tenderness along the posterior medial aspect of the forearm.

tis, which is often termed *"tennis elbow."* The area of tenderness is over the bony surface of the lateral epicondyle, and the pain may be better appreciated by having the patient extend the wrist and pronate the forearm against resistance.

Pain and paresthesias of the hand and forearm in the distribution of the ulnar nerve may be the result of local trauma or compression of the ulnar nerve. Palpation of the ulnar nerve should begin at the groove posterior to the medial condyle of the humerus. This is followed by palpation of the ulnar nerve as it transverses the cubital tunnel along the medial aspect of the forearm (Fig. 19-23). Localized tenderness or pain radiating into the ring and little fingers should alert the examiner to either localized trauma or compression. If far advanced, there may be weakness of the adductor pollicis, the interossei, and the third and fourth lumbrical muscles.

Shoulder

Similar to evaluation of the elbow, physical examination of the shoulder requires knowledge of normal function to identify subtle abnormalities.

Before any attempt is made to palpate the shoulders, it is imperative that the examiner carefully inspect the shoulders anteriorly and posteriorly, especially noting any displacement or asymmetry. Comparison of the musculature and contour is important in diagnosing unilateral disorders. Thus, a systematic inspection can detect visible atrophy of the deltoid muscle, such as might occur following disuse secondary to traumatic arthritis, axillary nerve injury, or severe rotator cuff tears. Bilateral, symmetric shoulder girdle atrophy, as frequently occurs with involvement secondary to rheumatoid arthritis, can be a more difficult diagnostic problem; however, history can often be quite helpful.

A systematic inspection of the bony contour of the shoulders may detect abnormalities such as prominence at the distal portion of the clavicle, possibly suggesting a dislocation of the acromioclavicular joint. A subcoracoid dislocation of the humeral head can sometimes be seen as a flattening over the lateral portion of the shoulder. Swelling of the shoulder joint is often difficult to detect but, if present, is usually most apparent over the anterior aspect.

The structures about the shoulder should be palpated for areas of localized tenderness. This is best performed with the upper extremity thoroughly relaxed and not resisting gravity. The examiner should determine if there is any tenderness about the rotator cuff that would indicate either a tear, inflammatory synovitis, or active periarthritis. Anteriorly, the long head of the biceps tendon passing through the bicipital groove of the humerus at the shoulder should be palpated for tenderness (Fig. 19-24). Localized tenderness is indicative of *bicipital tendinitis,* and the diagnosis is further supported by aggravation of the pain when the forearm is flexed and supinated against resistance.

Particular attention should be devoted to palpating the rotator cuff area underlying the deltoid muscle (Fig. 19-25). Frequently, shoulder pain can result from bursitis in this region, and localized tenderness is detected by deep palpation.

Next, determine the active and passive motion of the shoulder while comparing with the opposite side. With long-standing bursitis or tendinitis, it is not uncommon to observe diminished motion of the shoulders. Subtly impaired rotation and hyperextension of the shoulder are common features of early, relatively milder bursitis or tendinitis. The end results of chronic bursitis and tendinitis are commonly termed "periarthritis," "adhesive capsulitis," or "calcific tendinitis," because the predominant finding is decreased range of motion with pain being less prominent or even absent.

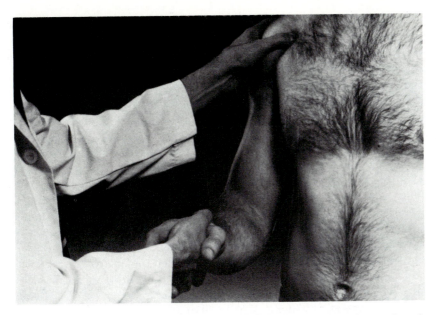

Fig. 19-24. Palpating over the bicipital groove with the thumb to detect bicipital tendinitis.

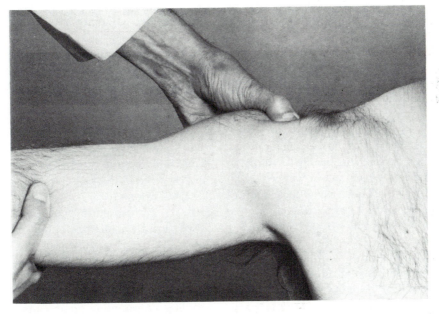

Fig. 19-25. Examining the shoulder for evidence of subdeltoid tenderness indicative of bursitis.

Considerable valuable information regarding the nature of shoulder disability can be gained by comparing active and passive range of motion. For example, marked impairments of active motion and intact passive range of motion are highly suggestive of proximal muscle weakness, such as exists in various types of muscular dystrophies, neurologic disorders, or polymyositis. Equivalently diminished active and passive motions are more indicative of shoulder disease and disuse atrophy, such as occurs with active rheumatoid arthritis. Movement of both the glenohumeral and scapulothoracic components contribute to the shoulder motions. To determine abduction, move the shoulder away from the body with the elbow in 90-degree flexion. Upward forearm rotation measures external rotation, while rotating the forearm downward indicates internal rotation. Normally, external and internal rotation of the shoulders should be approximately 80 to 90 degrees. The degree of flexion is determined by bringing the arm forward. Extension is the ability to swing the arm backward. Adduction is evaluated by bringing the arm anteriorly over the chest toward the contralateral side. Evidence of synovial thickening is usually observed in patients with severe rheumatoid arthritis involving the shoulders.

Foot

Obvious deformities of the foot include tilting of the heel toward the midline, which is termed a *varus deformity* and is frequently associated with clubfoot and cavus foot. Deviation of the heel away from the midline is known as a *valgus deformity* and commonly occurs with pes planus. A frequent abnormality, resulting in considerable disability, is a *bunion*. When present, bunions are usually quite prominent swellings over the medial aspect of the metatarsophalangeal joint of the great toe and are noted in association with lateral deviation of the great toe, which is termed *hallux valgus*.

Next, the foot should be palpated for points of tenderness over joints or bursa. Tenderness over the calcaneus is occasionally observed in the various spondyloarthropathies, particularly *Reiter's syndrome* (Fig. 19-26). Other causes of heel pain include calcaneal spurs and plantar fasciitis localized to the calcaneal insertion of the plantar fascia. In the foot, evidence of rheumatoid arthritis is usually localized to the metatarsal phalangeal joints, which should be individually palpated to detect synovial thickening (Fig. 19-27). By exerting pressure on the lateral and medial aspects of the forefoot, one can elicit subjective tenderness, which is another sign of metatarsal synovitis (Fig. 19-28). Untreated rheumatoid arthritis can significantly deform the foot, resulting in hallux valgus deformity of the great toe (Fig. 19-29) and subluxation of the metatarsal heads (Fig. 19-30).

Acute inflammation of the joints of the foot usually represents either gout or septic arthritis. Gout commonly involves the great toe (Fig. 19-31) and can be indistinguishable from an acutely infected joint. Often the history and joint fluid examination are helpful in establishing the diagnosis. Although not frequent, tenderness between the metatarsal heads may result from an interdigital neuroma (Morton's neuroma). *Metatarsalgia* is a purely descriptive term and does not imply a particular etiology nor connote a known disease process.

By moving the heel medially and laterally while holding the tibia stationary, inversion and eversion of the foot can be assessed. Flexion and extension of the toes in conjunction with the appropriate movements against resistance permit evaluation of range of motion and individual muscle strength.

Ankle

Inspect the ankle for gross deformity and swelling. Attempting to distinguish between synovitis and ankle edema at times can be somewhat difficult. As mentioned previously, however, synovial thickening has a boggy con-

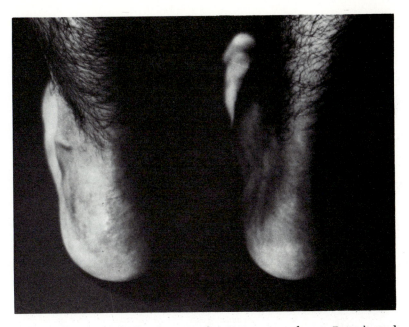

Fig. 19-26. Swelling of the heel and surrounding tissues secondary to Reiter's syndrome.

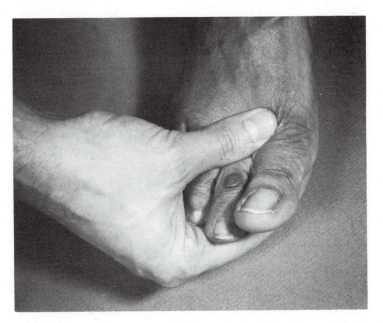

Fig. 19-27. Palpating the metatarsal phalangeal joints for evidence of thickening.

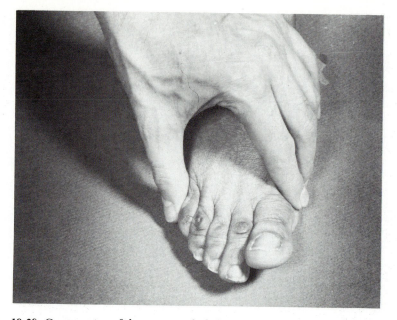

Fig. 19-28. Compression of the metatarsal phalangeal joints to evaluate tenderness.

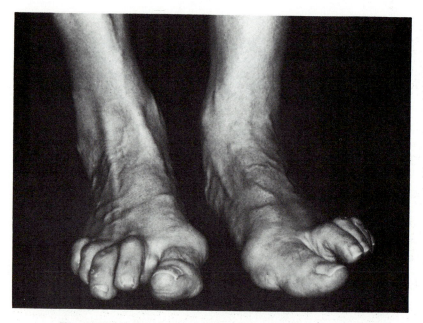

Fig. 19-29. Hallux valgus deformity in rheumatoid arthritis.

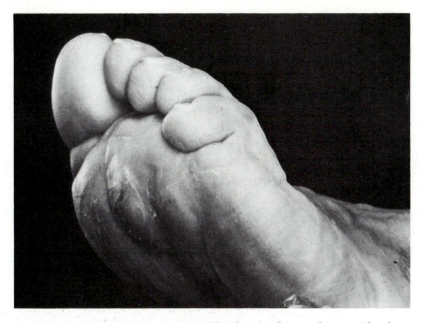

Fig. 19-30. Subluxation of the metatarsal heads secondary to rheumatoid arthritis.

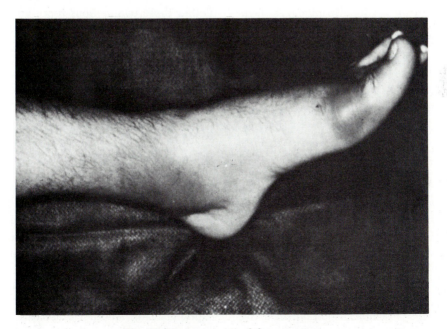

Fig. 19-31. Acute gout of the great toe.

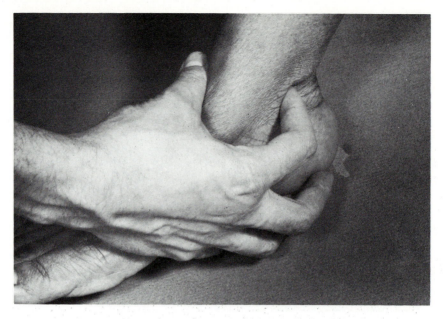

Fig. 19-32. Examining for tenderness posterior to the medial malleolus.

sistency and does not indent as observed in pitting edema. In some patients, edema and synovitis can occur together, but the history can be helpful in determining if the edema is secondary to arthritis involving the ankle. Tenderness is usually not a prominent finding of ankle synovitis and when present should alert the examiner to either tendon sheath inflammation or ligamentous strain. Thus, tenderness posterior to the medial malleolus over the posterior tibial tendon is a fairly common cause of ankle pain. Similar inflammation of the peroneal tendon sheaths results in tenderness to palpation posterior to the lateral malleolus. Careful palpation of these areas is required to elicit localized tenderness (Fig. 19-32). Another cause of ankle pain is inflammation adjacent to the insertion of the Achilles tendon, which most likely is a result of an inflamed bursa.

Normally, the ankle should demonstrate at least 25 degrees of plantar flexion during active and passive range-of-motion testing. Dorsiflex-ion is usually approximately 15 degrees, and together these two motions represent the majority of normal ankle functions. Stability is determined by inversion and eversion against resistance.

Muscle strength can easily be tested by having the patient bear weight on the heels, followed by weight-bearing on the forefeet.

Knee

Considerable information can be obtained by the careful inspection of the knees. First, determine if there is any deformity, swelling, or evidence of asymmetry. Unilateral swelling of the knee can be seen in traumatic arthritis and in various types of internal derangement. Other causes include infectious etiologies such as tuberculosis and fungal diseases. Acute synovitis of the knees manifested by intense erythema, tenderness, and heat is seen in acute septic arthritis. Another cause of acute synovitis of the knees, particularly in the elderly pop-

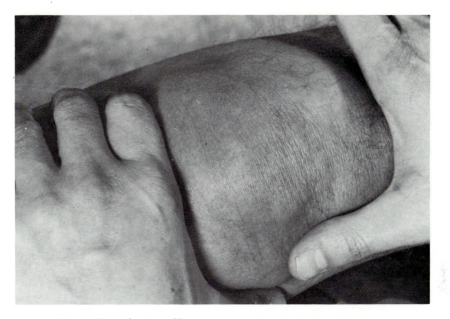

Fig. 19-33. Palpation of knee joint synovium to detect thickening.

ulation, is pseudogout. The presence of chondrocalcinosis helps in the diagnosis of pseudogout, and it is important to exclude associated systemic diseases such as hyperparathyroidism and Wilson's disease.

In rheumatoid arthritis, bilateral knee involvement is usually present, although some asymmetry may be evident, depending on the stage of disease and unilateral stress secondary to gait abnormalities.

Next, the knees should be inspected while the patient is standing. During weight-bearing, one can better assess if there is a significant *genu valgus* (knock-knee) or *genu varus* (bowleg) deformity. Also, significant atrophy of the quadriceps muscle is frequently present with knee dysfunction.

Second, the knee should be palpated to detect the presence of synovial thickening or excess synovial fluid (Fig. 19-33). Boggy, edematous synovium is a sign of an inflammatory synovitis, as can occur in rheumatoid arthritis.

Also, particular attention should be directed to the suprapatellar pouch, since abnormal fullness is indicative of fluid accumulation. Thus, by gently compressing the suprapatellar pouch with one hand, the examiner can more readily detect subtle synovial effusions by brisk ballottement of the patella (Fig. 19-34). When properly performed, one notes the sensation of the patella being buoyed anteriorly by an underlying cushion of fluid.

Even more subtle knee effusions can be detected by effectively eliciting the *"bulge sign."* In attempting to elicit the bulge sign, the examiner should first compress any synovial fluid to one side of the patella by palpating with the hands (Fig. 19-35). Then, this side of the knee is lightly stroked or tapped while the opposite side is carefully observed for a bulge or visible fluid wave (Fig. 19-36). Expertise in examining for the bulge sign is extremely important because this is often the only clue of more subtle knee disorders.

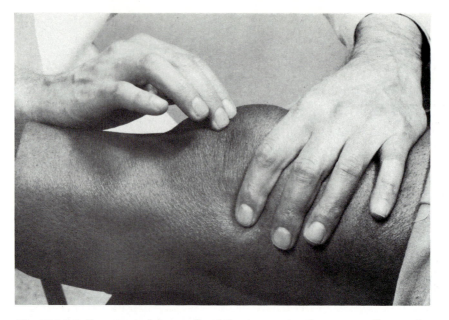

Fig. 19-34. Ballottement of the patella while compressing the suprapatellar pouch.

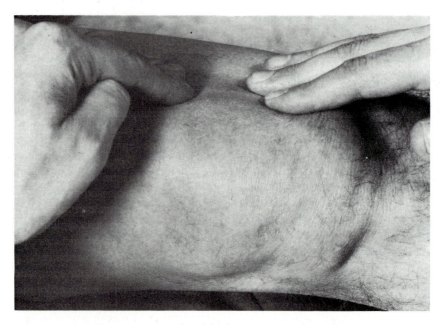

Fig. 19-35. Compressing one side of the knee prior to testing for the bulge sign.

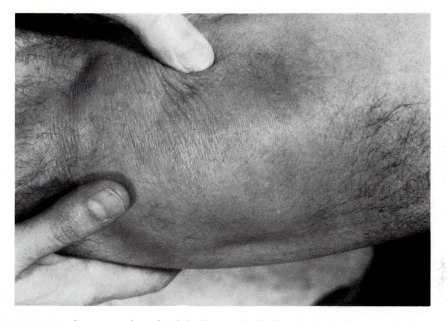

Fig. 19-36. Gently tapping the side of the knee with the thumb while observing the opposite side for a fluid wave or bulge.

Palpable bony protuberances about the knee are present in osteoarthritis, being the result of hypertrophic bone formation and spurs.

It is important to palpate about the joint margins for areas of localized tenderness. Frequently patients experience pain localized to the knee as a result of tenderness localized to the bony insertions of ligaments and tendons. These are usually detected about the circumference of the patella and the lateral aspects of the knees.

An extremely common, but not well emphasized, cause of knee pain is *anserine bursitis*. The anserine bursa is located on the medial posterior aspect of the proximal tibia, approximately 3 cm. distal to the joint line. Tenderness is best evaluated by palpating over this area with the thumb while the index finger is placed along the lateral aspect of the joint line, which serves as a landmark (Fig. 19-37). If anserine bursitis is present, the patient will ex-

perience severe pain on forcible palpation. Not infrequently, anserine bursitis may involve both knees and should be suspected in those patients experiencing knee pain in the absence of either previous trauma or significant abnormalities indicative of arthritis.

Next, the popliteal fossa should be palpated to detect abnormal fullness, which is frequently associated with knee effusions, or the presence of popliteal (Baker's) cyst. Popliteal cysts are actually an outpocketing of the synovial lining secondary to increased intrasynovial pressure and excess synovial fluid. Sometimes these are more evident after having the patient walk, since more intrasynovial fluid is forced into the communicating popliteal cyst (Fig. 19-38).

Third, the knee must be examined for abnormalities during passive and active range of motion. With one hand placed over the patella and the other hand firmly grasping the distal tibia, the examiner evaluates the passive range

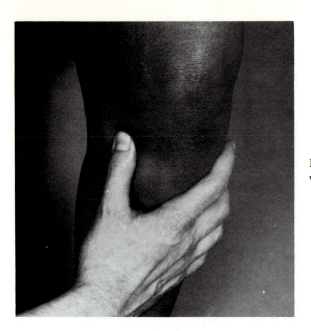

Fig. 19-37. Palpating over the anserine bursa with the thumb.

Fig. 19-38. Calf swelling secondary to a popliteal (Baker's) cyst.

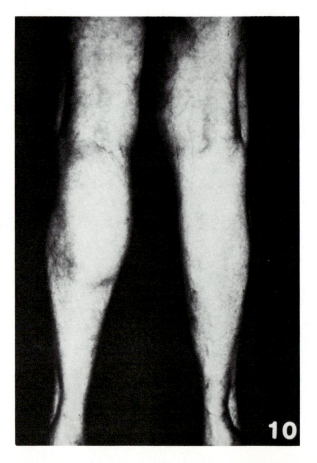

10

of motion. Palpable crepitation of the patella during passive motion is frequently referred to as "patella grating." Though not specific, this is often seen with loss of the normal cartilage surfaces, such as occurs in osteoarthritis, rheumatoid arthritis, or advanced chondromalacia. Sometimes minimal palpable crepitation is observed in normal individuals and, in the absence of other abnormalities, should not be considered evidence of underlying disease.

The patient is then asked to actively flex and extend the knee as far as possible. Patients with rheumatoid arthritis frequently are unable to fully extend the knee against gravity because of quadricep weakness. Also, flexion contractures occasionally develop quite early in the course of rheumatoid arthritis, which prevents full knee extension during both active and passive range of motion.

If locking of the knee is observed during range of motion, then one should suspect either an internal derangement, such as a torn meniscus or the presence of bony fragments.

In certain patients, a torn meniscus may be suggested by a positive *McMurray sign*. To perform this maneuver, the knee is flexed while the patient is lying supine. While palpating the knee with one hand, the examiner slowly extends the internally rotated tibia. The identical maneuver is then performed with the tibia held in external rotation. Acute pain and a palpable snap are very suggestive of a meniscus tear. However, it should be cautioned that the absence of a positive McMurray sign does not exclude the presence of a torn meniscus. Indeed, further diagnostic procedures, such as arthrography or arthroscopy, are frequently warranted if the clinical picture, such as a history of trauma, is compatible with this diagnosis.

The fourth step in examining the knee is evaluation of the integrity of ligamentous and soft tissue supporting structures. Laxity of the medial collateral ligament is determined by attempting to force the knee into a valgus or knock-knee deformity while the knee is fully

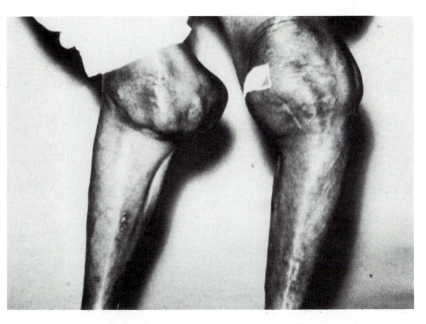

Fig. 19-39. Charcot joints in neuropathic arthropathy.

extended. Normally, movement is barely detectable, being less than 5 degrees deformity. To test the lateral collateral ligament, the examiner again extends the patient's knee and attempts to force the knee into a varus or bowleg deformity. No more than 5 degrees deformity is normally present.

Next, one should determine if there is anterior or posterior subluxation of the knees. The patient should be sitting with the knee flexed 90 degrees. The examiner then firmly grasps the tibia and attempts to displace it forward. If the tibia subluxates anteriorly from under the femur, there is abnormal laxity of the anterior cruciate ligament. The ability to posteriorly dislocate the tibia indicates abnormal laxity of the posterior cruciate ligament.

An accurate evaluation of these supporting structures is especially important in sports medicine, since the knee is particularly prone to injuries. Patients with uncontrolled rheumatoid arthritis frequently display both lateral-medial and anterior-posterior subluxation. This is in part because of cartilage loss in addition to the diminished integrity of supporting structures. The most marked degrees of subluxation

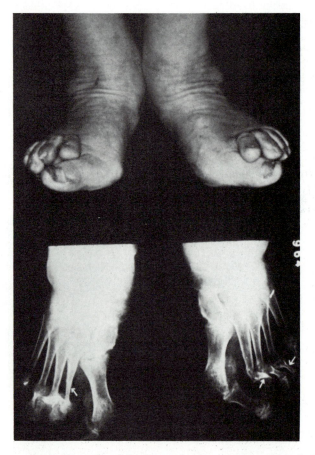

Fig. 19-40. Neuropathic arthropathy of the feet and ankles resulting from diabetes mellitus.

exist in those patients with neuropathic arthritis, commonly referred to as Charcot joints (Fig. 19-39). In the past these resulted from syphilis, but more recently diabetic neuropathy is a common cause of neuropathic joint disease, which particularly involves the ankles and feet (Fig. 19-40).

Hip

Gait abnormalities are frequently seen in those patients with significant hip disease. These abnormalities may range from more subtle changes, such as a slight limp or inability to hyperextend the hip during normal walking to more specific defects occurring in advanced hip disease. Probably the most common abnormality associated with advanced hip disease is referred to as the *"antalgic gait."* Clinically, one observes the patient extending the upper torso laterally over the involved hip so as to minimize the movement and relieve stress placed on the joint. In essence, the patient minimizes the hip pain by assuming a gait in which the diseased hip functions somewhat as a cane. Thus, this gait permits the diseased hip to be relatively fixed while bearing weight.

Although various types of myopathies and neuropathies can result in a *Trendelenburg gait,* this is sometimes observed with intrinsic hip disease. In the Trendelenburg gait, weight-bearing on the diseased hip results in a fall of the pelvis on the opposite side because of abductor muscle weakness about the involved hip. In the normal situation, there is a rise in the pelvis opposite the weight-bearing hip, which facilitates flexion of the lower extremity at the hip.

Another type of gait abnormality occurs in those patients unable to normally rotate the pelvis while walking. Most commonly this is seen in ankylosing spondylitis, and the patient's pelvis appears relatively fixed, with

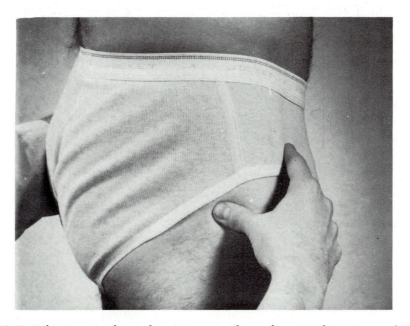

Fig. 19-41. Palpating over the trochanteric process for tenderness indicative to trochanteric bursitis.

more marked flexion of the lower extremity at the hip required to accomplish a normal step.

Other abnormalities include a spastic, erratic gait caused by central nervous system disease, the *foot drop* gait secondary to paralysis of the foot dorsiflexors, and the wide-based *ataxic gait*, which reflects unsteadiness associated with certain neurologic disorders.

With any gait disturbance, the length of the lower extremities should be compared because minimal differences can account for uneven gait. The distance between the anterior-superior iliac spine and the medial malleolus represents the true leg length and is not influenced by scoliosis or abnormal tilting of the pelvis.

While palpating about the hip, special attention should be directed to the trochanteric bursa (Fig. 19-41). Tenderness over the trochanteric process is usually a result of *trochanteric bursitis*, which is a common cause of hip pain.

Hip motions that should be evaluated in addition to internal and external rotation include flexion, extension, abduction, and adduction. To test hip flexion, the patient is instructed to move the flexed knee toward the abdomen. To detect flexion deformities of the hip, attempt to fully extend the hip examined while holding the opposite hip in full flexion to prevent rotation or tilting of the pelvis. Abduction is determined by moving the lower extremity laterally. The ability to adduct is examined by moving the lower extremity across the midline over the contralateral side. External rotation is tested by rotating the lower extremity outward, and internal rotation is evaluated by the ability to roll the lower extremity inward.

EXAMINATION OF THE SPINE

As in examination of the peripheral joints, evaluation of the spine is best performed in a systematic routine that can be incorporated into the physical examination.

Posture. With the patient in a standing position, carefully inspect the spine for any postural abnormalities. Three basic types of abnormalities are generally recognized, and occasionally two or more types may coexist in the patient. *Kyphosis* is the term used to describe forward curvature of the spine. *Lordosis* refers to a backward curvature of the spine. A lateral curvature of the spine is known as *scoliosis*. An abnormal forward and lateral curvature of the spine occurring together is called *kyphoscoliosis*.

Cervical spine

The cervical spine should be thoroughly examined for abnormalities in range of motion. These include forward flexion, hyperextension, and rotation. In addition, assessment of lateral flexion or bending can be performed by asking the patient to attempt to touch the shoulder with the the lateral aspect of the head (Fig. 19-42). Abnormalities of lateral flexion are an important clue to relatively milder forms of cervical arthritis. Usually, significant flexion-extension or rotation impairments are indicative of relatively advanced cervical spine disease. It should be emphasized that rheumatoid arthritis involving the cervical spine can result in considerable instability and subluxation. Maneuvers to elicit signs of subluxation are particularly well described for the atlantoaxial (C1-C2) articulation; however, these are of rather limited value. In addition, such maneuvers can result in high cervical cord compression or even transection. Thus, patients suspected of having cervical spine subluxation secondary to rheumatoid arthritis are more appropriately evaluated by *passive* flexion-extension x-rays of the cervical spine. Often confusing to the less-experienced examiner is the more prominent protuberance of spinous process of the eighth cervical vertebrae. This is a normal finding and should not be mistaken for localized angulations or subluxed vertebrae.

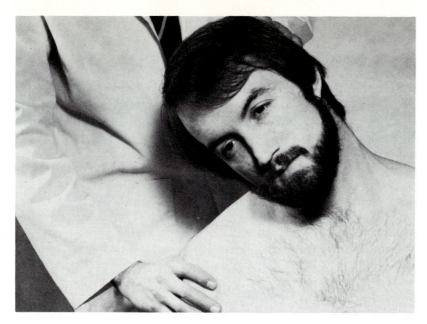

Fig. 19-42. Lateral flexion of the cervical spine.

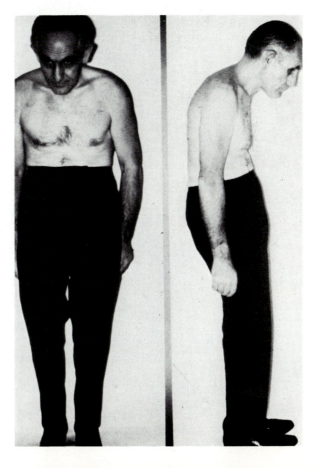

Fig. 19-43. Loss of lumbar lordosis and increased thoracic kyphosis in a patient with far-advanced ankylosing spondylitis.

Complete the examination of the cervical spine by palpating the cervical muscles for points of tenderness. Often, arthritic changes and cervical disc disease are accompanied by spasm and tenderness of the trapezius, scalene, or posterior paraspinal muscle groups, or a combination of them. Also, carefully palpate the bony insertion areas of these muscle groups since location of exquisite tenderness is helpful in planning appropriate local physiotherapy.

The thoracic spine is frequently involved in ankylosing spondylitis, osteoarthritis, and compression fractures of the vertebral bodies. In general these result in abnormal dorsal ky-phosis (Fig. 19-43) and diminished range of motion. In the patient with ankylosing spondylitis, the measurement of chest expansion is important not only to detect thoracic involvement but also to permit future evaluation of possible disease progression.

Lumbar spine

While the patient is standing, inspect the contour of the lumbar spine. Normally, a lumbar lordosis is evident. An absence is indicative of either lumbar paraspinal muscle spasm or significant arthritis. Low back pain and decreased range of motion of the lumbar spine

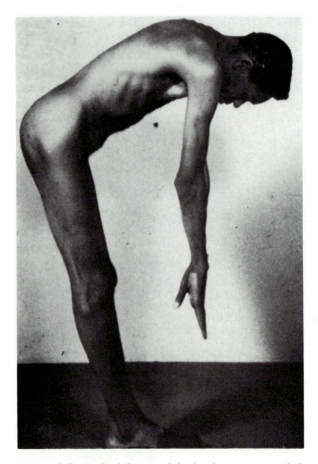

Fig. 19-44. Flattening and diminished flexion of the lumbar spine in ankylosing spondylitis.

can be a result of numerous disorders. Probably the most common cause of low back pain is spasm of the paraspinal musculature. This pain syndrome is best termed mechanical low back pain. Although frequently associated with arthritis of the lumbar spine, mechanical low back pain can occur as an isolated finding.

On physical examination, mechanical low back pain is evidenced by decreased range of motion and firmness of the paraspinal muscle to palpation. If unilateral, the spasm can result in asymmetry of the paraspinal musculature, and a slight lumbar scoliosis may be present. Mild flattening or loss of lumbar lordosis can occur in association with mechanical low back pain. More severe loss of lordosis and range of motion are usually present in ankylosing spondylitis or advanced osteoarthritis of the lumbar spine (Fig. 19-44).

There are two generally accepted methods for evaluating range of motion of the lumbar spine. Both have inherent advantages and dis-

advantages; therefore, it is not possible to recommend one over the other.

One method is to have the examiner seated behind the patient with the knees firmly placed lateral to those of the patient. The patient's pelvic girdle is stabilized by the examiner firmly grasping the lateral aspects of the pelvis. The patient is first instructed to attempt to touch the toes with the fingertips (Fig. 19-45). Normally, most individuals are capable of touching the toes or lack not more than approximately 2 inches. While in flexion, the lumbar spine is inspected for increased lordosis or flattening in addition to any asymmetry of the paraspinal musculature. Next, the patient is instructed to hyperextend the lumbar spine by bending backwards as far as possible toward the examiner. By firmly grasping the pelvis and by exerting lateral pressure on the patient's knees, it is possible to accurately assess the hyperextension mobility. Proper stabilization is extremely important, because the normal tendency is to

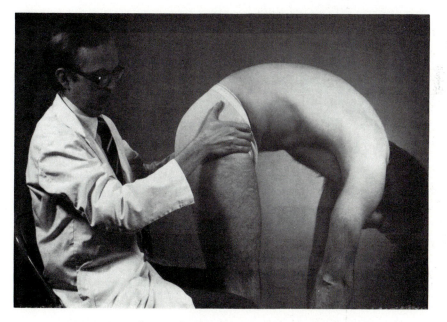

Fig. 19-45. Evaluating flexion of the lumbar and thoracic spine.

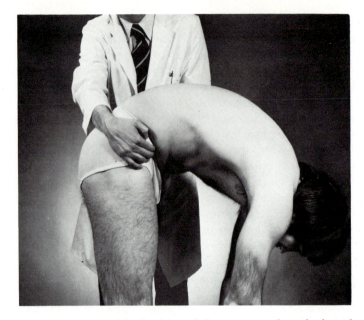

Fig. 19-46. Testing flexion of the lumbar and thoracic spine from the lateral position.

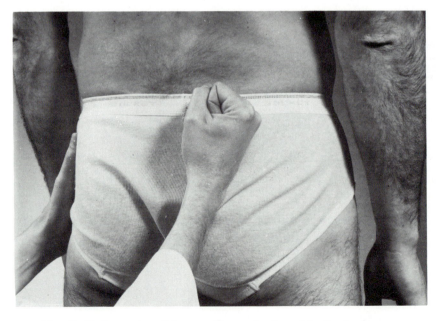

Fig. 19-47. Percussion of the sacroiliac region for subjective tenderness.

rock the pelvis posteriorly or to flex the knees, resulting in the spurious appearance of normal hyperextension. Lateral flexion or lateral bending of the lumbar and thoracic spines should be assessed to complete evaluation of the range of motion. Again, the patient's pelvis must be adequately stabilized by the examiner to accurately evaluate spinal motion.

In the second method commonly utilized to evaluate motion of the lumbar and thoracic spines, the examiner is lateral to the patient while firmly grasping the patient's pelvis (Fig. 19-46). During flexion the examiner can accurately assess the curvature of the spine from the side. However, since the patient's knees are not stabilized, care must be taken to prevent knee flexion, especially during evaluation of hyperextension.

Examination of the spine is not complete without a thorough examination of the sacroiliac joints, especially in those patients suspected of having spondylitis. Tenderness over the sacroiliac joints is one of the earliest signs of sacroiliitis and the presence of spondylitis. Two examinations are helpful in the detection of tenderness associated with sacroiliitis. First, deep palpation is accomplished by firmly pressing the posterior aspects of the sacroiliac joint with the thumb. In normal individuals little subjective tenderness is elicited by this maneuver, but often patients with sacroiliitis experience localized pain. Second, more subtle tenderness can be detected by percussing over the sacroiliac joints with the fist (Fig. 19-47). Again, little tenderness is noted in the absence of disease. A relatively less helpful sign, but one that may be present in patients with severe, active sacroiliitis, is pain localized to the sacroiliac joints with lateral compression of the pelvis. However, this is negative in the majority of patients with less active sacroiliitis.

SELECTED READINGS

McCarty, D. J.: Arthritis and allied conditions, ed. 9, Philadelphia, 1979, Lea & Febiger.

Moskowitz, R. W.: Clinical rheumatology, Philadelphia, 1975, Lea & Febiger.

CHAPTER 20

PEDIATRIC EXAMINATION

In this chapter the unique characteristics of children are emphasized. It is important to recognize these differences, to know how long these differences normally last, and to know when their persistence represents a delay in growth and development. The term growth and development describes a continuing and orderly process through which the child matures physically, psychologically, and socially into an adult. The key ages in this aging process are: the newborn; infancy and early childhood; the school-aged child; and the adolescent. The examination procedure for each of these four stages has some unique features and specialized goals. There are many physical differences that an examiner accustomed to adults might consider abnormal but that are normal in a child. Also, there are variations among children in the same age group that should alert the examiner to the wide spectrum in normal growth and development. Normality in children includes the many variations around the age of the child with consideration of the child's background. A 2-month-old infant weighing 7 pounds, 8 ounces and measuring 20 inches in length is quite normal in physical growth when it is known that this infant was born at 32 weeks' gestation weighing 3 pounds,

8 ounces and measuring 19 inches in length. Thus, his physical growth is understandably different and is related to his conceptual age. However, by 2 years of age this prematurely born infant should be within the average range for weight and height if he is to be considered normal.

APPROACH TO PATIENT AND PARENTS

The child and his parent usually come to the physician as a package. Thus, the physician must establish rapport with two people simultaneously. Both the child and parent should be spoken to, with more interest directed to the parent at the onset of the interview. With toddlers and preschoolers it is often helpful to offer the child a toy or pencil and paper with which to amuse himself during the history-taking. This provides the examiner with the opportunity to observe the child's spontaneous behavior and also gently separates him from his parents. Infants under 6 months separate freely, and adolescents prefer to have most of the history and examination performed with the parent in a separate room. Generally, 6- to 12-year-old children prefer a parent in the room for either verbal or nonverbal moral support. It is quite acceptable for a parent to help

in the examination of a preschooler by holding the child's hand or by simply standing next to the examining table. Encourage the child to be as independent as he can, but allow the parent to be your assistant to whatever degree is necessary.

EXAMINATION OF THE NEWBORN

The newborn examination is performed in two steps. The first examination is brief and is performed at 1 and 5 minutes of age by a physician or nurse in the delivery room. Called the Apgar evaluation, this examination assesses five characteristics of the baby: heart rate, respiratory effort, muscle tone, reflex irritability, and color. The purpose of this examination is to determine if the infant has asphyxia and needs resuscitation. Table 20-1 describes the Apgar scoring method. A score of zero is given for each of the following: no heart beat, no respiratory effort, no muscle tone, no reflex response to a slap on the soles of the feet, and a blue or pale color. A score of one each is given for: slow heart beat, slow or irregular respiratory effort, some flexion of the extremities, a grimace or cry in response to a slap on the soles, and a pink body with blue extremities. Finally, a score of two each is given for: heart rate over 100, good respiratory effort accompanied by crying, active voluntary movements, a cry in response to a slap on the feet, and a completely pink color. The total score is a sum of the individual numbers assigned to each of the five characteristics. The majority of infants are vigorous, with a total score of eight to ten. A score of two or less indicates severe asphyxia; three to five, moderate asphyxia; and six to seven, mild asphyxia. Low 5-minute Apgar scores are correlated with high infant mortality or neurologic injury, especially at lower gestational ages.

The second stage of the newborn examination should be performed in the nursery, preferably during the first 6 hours of life. The purpose of this examination is to detect the presence or absence of congenital anomalies. The mother's prenatal and delivery record should be reviewed, paying particular attention to her age, blood type, expected date of confinement (EDC), and the presence or absence of any acute maternal illnesses during pregnancy and chronic illnesses. The infant should be kept warm during the examination, and a bottle of water should be available to quiet him. If the patient is quiet at the onset of the examination, listen to the heart and lungs first and then palpate the abdomen. Thereafter, proceed systematically from the head downward. A small tube should be passed through the nose and down to the stomach to rule out posterior choanal atresia and esophageal atresia. The position of the tube in the stomach should be checked by auscultation over the stomach area while blowing a small amount of air through the tube. Aspirate the gastric contents and estimate the quantity of fluid removed. Excessive

Table 20-1. Apgar evaluation method

Sign	0	1	2
Heart rate	Absent	Slow (below 100)	Over 100
Respiratory effort	Absent	Slow, irregular	Good, crying
Muscle tone	Flaccid	Some extremity flexion	Active motion
Reflex irritability	No response	Cry	Vigorous cry
Color	Blue, pale	Body pink, extremities blue	Completely pink

amounts of gastric fluid are found in infants born by cesarean section and those with high intestinal obstructions. The tip of the catheter can then be gently inserted in the rectum to check for patency.

Assessment of the baby's gestational age is a practical clinical component in the newborn examination. With gestational assessment the neonate's maturity is evaluated and is labeled as small for gestational age (SGA), appropriate for gestational age (AGA), or large for gestational age (LGA). The clinical course of each group and problems encountered by each group are quite different. For example, hypoglycemia and congenital malformations are more common in SGA babies, while idiopathic respiratory distress syndrome and hyperbiliru-

binemia are more common in prematurely born but AGA neonates. The weight, length, and head circumference of all newborn infants should be compared to a set of normal standards, for in this way SGA and LGA infants can be recognized in a simple and reliable way. Fig. 20-1 depicts the most commonly used normal vaues as compiled by Lubchenco, which are valid data for singleton, white births at both high altitude and sea level. The curves were constructed so that the lowest 10% of values in each week of gestation represents the tenth percentile. A newborn whose birth weight is on or below the tenth percentile curve is considered SGA, while an LGA baby has a birth weight on or above the ninetieth percentile curve.

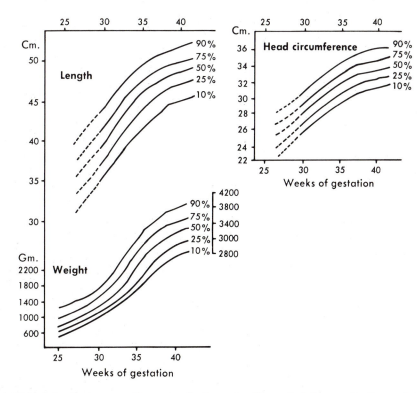

Fig. 20-1. Intrauterine growth curves, both sexes. (From Lubchenco, L. O., and others: Pediatrics **37**[3]:403, 1966.)

Dubowitz devised a scoring system combining neurologic findings with physical characteristics to assess gestational age. This method, when carefully performed, is reliable during the first week. Although mother's dates are also useful, they are sometimes misleading because of bleeding in the first trimetster or a history of irregular menstrual periods. Thus Dubowitz' procedure provides the examiner with a method of determining the physical and neurologic maturity of the infant independent of the mother's history.

EXAMINATION OF INFANTS AND YOUNG CHILDREN

Infancy and early childhood (1 month to 6 years) provide the examiner with the opportunity of observing dramatic and rapid changes in the physical and neurologic status of the child. During each examination of a child in this age group, questions should be asked about the child's eating, sleeping, and elimination. In addition the child's motor and sensory development should be determined by history-taking and direct examination. Accurate assessment of the child's development is best performed by obtaining serial determinations and by recording the child's progress. The concept of developmental testing is based on the assumption that mature behavior is achieved through the progressive unfolding of increasingly complex behavior. Furthermore, it is believed that age norms can be established for the stages in the process against which an individual child can be compared at a given age so that a judgment can be made about the child's current rate of development. Developmental testing should be a part of each well-child examination from birth to age 6. This type of examination emphasizes several aspects of child behavior. The Denver Developmental Screening Test (DDST) is a frequently used developmental test that assesses gross motor, language, fine motor, adaptive, and personal social skills. It has been well constructed and evaluated and provides an excellent method for assessing a child's development. A child evaluated by means of this screening device is found to be either normal, abnormal, or questionable. The DDST is not an intelligence test; it is intended as a screening instrument to determine whether the development of a particular child is within the normal range. When used for this purpose, the DDST is a valuable component in examining infants and preschool children.

Developmental assessment is best done prior to performing the physical examination because it allows the child to play some games with the examiner, which encourages the development of cooperation. Gaining the cooperation of a 1- or 2-year-old child is often a challenge. However, if the youngster is fighting and struggling, the value of the examination is markedly reduced; therefore, it is worth spending a little time developing rapport. Many preschoolers can be partially examined with the child on the parent's lap, standing next to the parent, or in the physician's lap. It is mandatory that the child be completely undressed except for underpants, but it is wise to remove the diaper only briefly while the abdomen and genitalia are checked. From age 1 year on, be sure to show the child the instruments before they are used and allow him to listen with your "telephone" and "blow out" your otoscope. It is best to tell a child what you will do in a firm, but friendly, voice rather than to ask him if you may check his tummy. Many preschoolers will tell you no when and if you give them a chance. The order of the examination should take into consideration the child's developmental level and the amount of discomfort that is associated with each portion of the examination. Generally, the chest, heart, lungs, and extremities can be examined before the child is told to lie down on the table. Sometimes the supine position provokes anxiety and resistance on the part of the child, but gently and slowly laying the child down may avert that type of storm. If the child resists the examination, the examiner must remain free of anger and calmly assure the parent that this type of behavior is not surprising.

EXAMINATION OF SCHOOL-AGED CHILDREN

The ages from 6 to 12 years are often described as the golden or halcyon years. Cooperation, conversation, and coordination are the hallmarks of school-aged children. They can answer questions and describe their problems without assistance. Care should be taken to avoid "talking down" to them, for they quickly respond to verbal and nonverbal behavior. History-taking at this age should include information about peer relationships, school performance, and the assumption of chores and other responsibilities. Generally, children 6 years and older are modest and should be provided with gowns. If siblings of the opposite sex are to be examined at the same visit, it is better to separate them for the actual undressing and physical examination. Vision and hearing screening should be performed as part of the complete examination, with the order of examination the same as is used for adults.

EXAMINATION OF ADOLESCENTS

Adolescents mature at different ages and at different rates and are far from being a homogeneous group. They no sooner become used to one change than they must contend with another. Regional, ethnic, cultural, and economic influences result in many different kinds of adolescent behavior; however, the inner drive for freedom and independence is essentially the same for all adolescents, even if their abilities to achieve and to handle frustrations vary.

It is helpful to make a semantic distinction between puberty and adolescence. Puberty is the purely biologic state of sexual development at which it is first possible to bear or beget children, and adolescence is the period when so-

cial, psychologic, and cognitive maturation take place. Prior to adolescence, about the eighth year, boys and girls are quite similar, although body composition and reproductive organs differ. After adolescence, the two sexes are markedly different in terms of anthropometric measurements and body composition. A rapid rise in height and weight characterizes the adolescent growth spurt, although growth increments are smaller in girls than in boys and occur approximately 2 years earlier.

The physician should establish certain basic ground rules during the initial interview of an adolescent. The physician is the teenager's personal physician; and he is the patient's advocate with whom any subjects may be discussed and any questions may be asked. The physician should tell his patient that all information will be handled in a confidential manner; however, if the teenager reveals plans that could be seriously harmful to himself, the physician will inform his parents. No information should be discussed with his parents without the adolescent's full knowledge.

The physical examination of a teenager should be performed with the parents out of the room. Girls, when examined by a male physician, should have a female attendant present. Height and weight, blood pressure, and hearing and vision screening should be performed and discussed with the patient. The order of the examination should be as is used for adults.

Because of the varying ages at which puberty begins, chronologic age is a poor indicator of the teenager's physiologic growth and development. Physicians caring for adolescents frequently utilize the pubertal classification developed by Tanner (Table 20-2). Using this scale, a rating on a 1 to 5 scale is given for pubic hair. A second rating is given for genital development in boys and for breast development in girls. Stage 1 is preadolescent and Stage 5 is adult.

Table 20-2. Tanner pubertal stages

Boys: Genital development

Stage 1   Preadolescent: Testes, scrotum, and penis are about the same size and proportion as in early childhood.

Stage 2   Scrotum and testes are enlarged. Skin of scrotum reddened and changed in texture. Little or no enlargement of penis is present at this stage.

Stage 3   Penis is slightly enlarged, which occurs at first mainly in length. Testes and scrotum are further enlarged.

Stage 4   Increased size of penis with growth in breadth and development of glans. Testes and scrotum larger; scrotal skin darker than in earlier stages.

Stage 5   Genitalia adult in size and shape.

Girls: Breast development

Stage 1   Preadolescent: Elevation of papilla only.

Stage 2   Breast bud stage: Elevation of breast and papilla as small mound. Enlargment of areola diameter.

Stage 3   Further enlargement and elevation of breast and areola with no separation of their contours.

Stage 4   Projection of areola and papilla to form a secondary mound above the level of the breast.

Stage 5   Mature stage: Projection of papilla only, due to recession of the areola to the general contour of the breast.

Both sexes: Pubic hair

Stage 1   Preadolescent: The vellus over the pubes is not further developed than that over the abdominal wall; i.e., no pubic hair.

Stage 2   Sparse growth of long, slightly pigmented downy hair, straight or curled, chiefly at the base of the penis or along labia.

Stage 3   Considerably darker, coarser, and more curled. The hair spreads sparsely over the junction of the pubes.

Stage 4   Hair now adult in type, but area covered is still considerably smaller than in the adult. No spread to the medial surface of the thighs.

Stage 5   Adult in quantity and type with distribution of the horizontal (or classically feminine) pattern. Spread to medial surface of thighs but not up linea or elsewhere above the base of the inverse triangle.

Stage 6   Spread up linea alba

From Tanner, J. M.: Growth and endocrinology of the adolescent. In Gardner, L. I., editor: Endocrine and genetic diseases of childhood, Philadelphia, 1969, W. B. Saunders Co.; cited in The approach to the adolescent patient, Pediatr. Clin. North Am. **20**(4):785, 1973.

The maturation of the sex organs is important. In girls, breast budding occurs almost concurrently with the appearance of pubic hair. The average development of both these secondary sex characteristics is completed in 3 years. Menstruation may occur at any time after the growth spurt, from 9 to 17 years. If a girl has not reached menarche by 13½ years, she can be considered as significantly delayed for the onset of puberty. Ninety-five percent of boys begin pubertal development between 9½ and 15½ years, with adult stages of genital development reached within 3 to 5 years.

Peak growth velocity in height occurs 2 years later in boys than in girls, with maximum rate of growth in boys achieved by 14.1 years. In contrast to girls, who achieve their maximal height early in genital development, boys usually reach their maximal height when genitalia are quite well developed. Voice change in boys is a gradual process and cannot be used as an index of any one particular stage of puberty.

OUTLINE OF PEDIATRIC HISTORY

Just as in taking the medical history of the adult (Chapter 3), a systematic approach is essential to a well-organized and accurate pediatric history.

Informant. The interviewer should identify the informant and evaluate the reliability of his observations. Information obtained from the child should be so indicated.

Chief complaint. State the main reason or reasons for the visit to the physician. Whenever possible, use the informant's own terms. It is worth noting that an interview is often most productive if the initial focus is on the parent's and the child's impressions of the problem and, hence, the reason for being there. This simple step—of inviting the parent, and the child as well, to explain why they came to see the physician—can avoid false starts, confirm the physician's interest in and respect for his patient, and reassure the family about the physician's competence as he directs himself quickly to the problem they perceive as critical (even though other problems may later prove to be of much greater significance).

Present illness. To begin with, a statement should be made: "This 7-year-old child was well until . . .," defining as accurately as possible the precise onset of the present illness. It is important to emphasize the last time the child was well and free from symptoms.

Symptoms should be described in chronologic order, with appropriate paragraphing and underlining for emphasis, so that others may obtain maximum information in a minimum of reading time. All symptoms should be ampli-

fied; for example, cough (onset, course, character, severity, time of occurrence, frequency, associated symptoms, exacerbations, and remissions).

The examiner should list absent pertinent symptoms that would help to exclude other diseases capable of producing similar complaints; for example, "There have been no nosebleeds, abdominal pain, or growing pains" in an attempt to assess the likelihood of rheumatic fever in a patient complaining of a sore knee and fever.

The following brief report of a present illness illustrates how symptoms may be emphasized, amplified, and arranged for usefulness.

PRESENT ILLNESS
Informant: Mother (reliability—good)

This 3-year-old Negro boy was entirely well until 4 days ago (June 20)* when he seemed to have a "head cold," runny nose, sneezing, and a slight dry cough. He ate and played normally, but was restless in his sleep.

Two days ago (June 22) he suddenly came in from play and lay down. He felt warm and appeared sick. That evening he had cramping abdominal pains, severe enough to make him cry out, occurring every 2 to 3 hours and lasting 10 to 15 minutes. He ate little and slept poorly.

One day ago (June 23) he seemed more feverish, "talked out of his head,"† and vomited several times during the morning, following the intake of food and fluids. During the evening he seemed slightly better but began to pass large, watery, foul stools, which were at first brown and later green in color. This morning (June 24) he has had no stools, seems less feverish, but his cough has been much more frequent, harsh, and "tight."

---

*Avoid using days of the week unless definitely related to the present illness; for example, headache only on Sunday morning or rash every Monday morning.
†The informant's own words, although nonmedical, are often more enlightening than technical medical terms. Denote informant's phrases by quotations.

There have been no convulsions, blood in the stools, grunting or rapid respirations, pain on coughing, earache, or any instance of illness similar to that of the patient among his siblings and playmates.*

Family history. Family history should include the health and age of the mother, father, and siblings who are living. In the case of deceased members of the family, the cause of death and age should be recorded. Also, make note of abortions, and whether they were spontaneous or induced.

One should inquire about history of familial disease, making clear he is talking about the larger family, not just parents and siblings. The physician should use terms familiar to the parents, not technical language. Questions may be answered incorrectly if they are not understood by the informant. The list should include infections such as tuberculosis, syphilis; mental illness, retardation, cerebral palsy; allergies, eczema, hay fever, asthma, migraine, hives, vomiting; intestinal problems such as ulcers, colitis, hernias; congenital deformities; heart and lung disease; and growth problems.

Environmental and emotional conditions in the home may be of considerable importance in assessing a child's illness.

Past history. The past history of infants and young children should include the following points.

1. *Mother's health and prenatal care.* Any history of venereal disease and its treatment. (Specific questions referable to weight gain, swelling, vaginal bleeding or "spotting," nausea or vomiting, high blood pressure, and proteinuria or pyuria may be helpful.)

2. *Birth.* Length of gestation, duration and nature of labor, type of delivery, need for resuscitation and condition at birth. (It is relevant to ask where the child was born and who delivered the child.)

3. *Postnatal adjustment.* Cyanosis, convulsions, hemorrhage, bruising, jaundice, appetite, time of regaining birth weight, use of incubator or oxygen, other special treatment.

4. *Feeding (breast).* Interval, regularity, length of nursing, ability to nurse, cause and age of weaning.

5. *Feeding (artificial).* Kind of food at present and in sequence since starting artificial feeding, proportions, amount, and interval; cause of change; reaction to food and rate of growth and gain; age at which solid foods were added and reactions to each addition; quantity of and reaction to various vitamins, orange juice, and so on. (It is important during late childhood and early adolescence to know specifically what a child eats at various meals and the amounts of carbohydrates, protein, and fat.)

6. *Development.* Age of smiling, sitting alone, crawling, walking, saying first words, and talking in sentences; weight progress; comparison with sibling's development; quality of schoolwork; and psychologic and emotional progress.

7. *Diseases.* Age at which they occurred; severity; complications following measles, mumps, pertussis, diphtheria, chickenpox, sore throat, rheumatic fever, chorea, skin eruptions, upper respiratory infections, and other infectious conditions.

8. *Immunizations,* including booster injections, with dates. Diphtheria, pertussis, tetanus (DPT); poliomyelitis; measles, mumps, and rubella.

---

*In looking over the history at this point, several diagnoses suggest themselves, such as severe acute upper respiratory infection, dysentery, and pneumonia. Thus, a statement is inserted showing that some of the more common accompanying symptoms of these diseases have not occurred.

9. *Skin tests.* Tuberculin and histoplasmin
10. *Injuries and operations.*
11. *Recent contact with contagious diseases.*

In obtaining the past history of adolescent patients one does not ordinarily seek detailed information about the mother's prenatal health and medical care or specific information concerning early infancy unless there appears to be a relationship between the current health problem and conditions in early life. However, in caring for teenage patients, the interview should include inquiries about pubertal development, relationships with family members and peers, school achievement and feelings about school, dating, jobs, and plans for future career.

System review. The system review in the child is similar to that of the adult, with a few exceptions. As an example, in the review of the genitourinary system the examiner asks about enuresis (bed-wetting). It may be necessary to ask the parents if the child has had specific diseases. After each affirmative answer it will be essential to characterize fully the symptoms that led to this diagnosis.

PHYSICAL EXAMINATION

Begin the examination with careful observation of the child's state of activity, mood, nutrition, hydration, and presence or absence of distress. The child may be examined in a crib, on a table, or, initially, on the parent's lap. With preschool children it is ideal to be at eye level with the child rather than towering over him (Fig. 20-2). Routine hand-washing with warm water before and after the examination gives

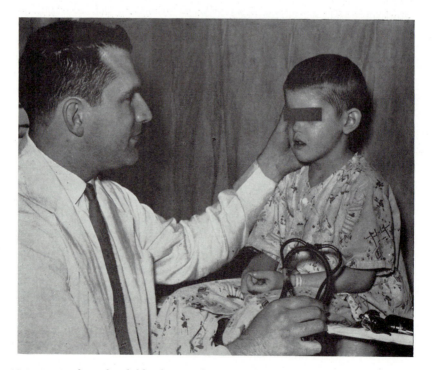

Fig. 20-2. Approaching the child at his own level is indicative of an attitude of mutual respect between physician and patient.

you clean and warm hands that are appreciated by both the child and the parents. Approach the child slowly, gently, and kindly. Your sensitivity to the child and his feelings is as important as the facility with which you use your instruments.

Measurement

Measurements of body length, weight, and head circumference of infants are fundamental components of good medical supervision. The physician is interested not only in comparing an individual's measurements to a norm but also in relating them to the range of values. The norm indicates the approximate midpoint (but nothing else) of the range of values established from measurements of a large number of infants and children. It should be remembered that there are wide variations in patterns of growth and that it is erroneous to expect each

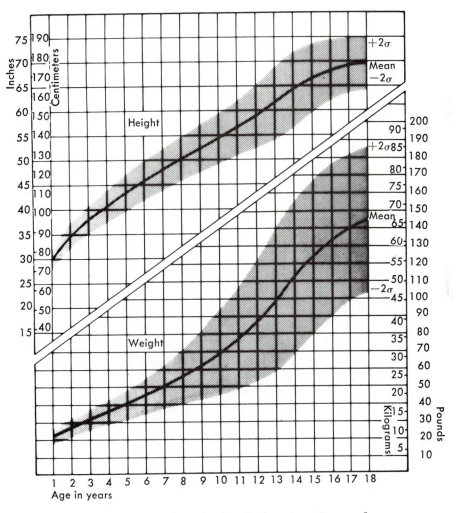

Fig. 20-3. Height and weight chart for boys 1 to 18 years of age.

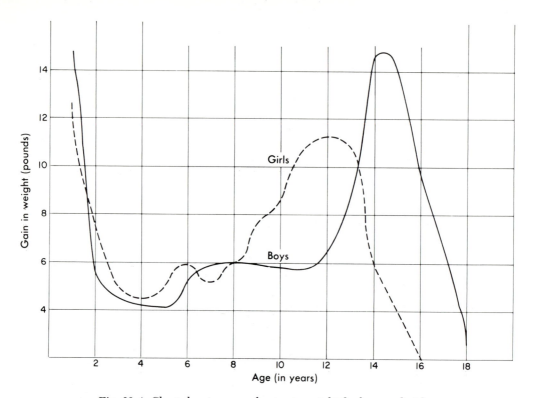

Fig. 20-4. Chart showing annual gains in weight for boys and girls.

infant or young child to follow some specified growth channel.

The growth chart ordinarily used by the physician to record height and weight measurements is a plot of distance (Fig. 20-3 for boys 1 to 18 years). If one plots the average annual gains in weight (or in height), a very different curve is evident (Fig. 20-4); this reveals more clearly the dynamic character of growth of children. Determination of rate of growth and reference to incremental growth data are potentially useful to the physician at any interval from infancy through adolescence but particularly during infancy and adolescence, when growth is progressing very rapidly.

It is difficult to accurately measure an infant's length. However, once a child is able to stand alone, satisfactory measurements of height can be made. Growth retardation, particularly in weight, is among the earliest indicators of illness or of improper nutrition in the infant. As the physician charts weight measurements of his patient during routine health supervision, he will be alerted to possible early malfunction by deviations from usual or expected growth achievements.

Skin

The newborn infant is covered with *vernix caseosa*. When the vernix is removed, the smooth red skin of the infant is seen. Postmature infants have dry, wrinkled skin with little or no vernix. Anemic infants have pale skin, conjunctivae, and palmar creases. The jaundice of *erythroblastosis fetalis* stains the skin, sclerae, and mucous membranes a reddish yellow color, while obstructive jaundice tends to have a distinct green hue. In the newborn, jaundice is best detected by pressing on the tip of the nose briefly, removing the finger, and observing the color before the red hue given by the baby's high hemoglobin returns. Jaundice is best appreciated in natural daylight, because fluorescent lighting significantly changes visual perception of the color.

Milia which may appear on the cheeks and forehead during the neonatal period, are pinpoint-sized white spots that represent retention of sebum in the ostia of the sebaceous glands. *Seborrhea capitis (cradle cap)* is a greasy exudate on the scalp, eyebrows, and cheeks and may be confused with atopic eczema. *Intertrigo* (chafing) occurs in the folds of the axilla, neck, ears, and inguinal areas. *Diaper rash* appears as red, raw areas or as discrete, punchedout ulcers in the diaper area as the result of ammonia released from breakdown of urea. *Miliaria* (heat rash) is a fine, papular eruption resulting from warmth and moisture of the neck, arms, and chest. Another form of miliaria may occur on the forehead or at the hairline as small, superficial vesicles resembling beads of sweat.

Many infants have a pink or red *capillary nevus* at the nape of the neck. About 10% of infants have similar lesions in the central portion of the face, most commonly on the forehead and eyelids. These disappear spontaneously in time. *Strawberry nevi (capillary hemangiomas)* are well circumscribed, slightly elevated, bright red to deep purple vascular tumors that incompletely blanch with pressure. Most strawberry nevi will eventually disappear; at least 75% will have disappeared by the seventh year. In contrast to the capillary and strawberry nevus, the *port wine stain* is permanent and may be cosmetically disfiguring. It may occur on one side of the face and may correspond to the distribution of the trigeminal nerve. These flat, purple lesions are present at birth and may be accompanied by central nervous system involvement. *"Café au lait"* spots are flat, brown spots that may be seen with hyperparathyroidism. During adolescence, *acne vulgaris*, an inflammatory disease of the pilosebaceous glands, appears on the face, neck, and back.

In newborn infants of dark or Mediterranean races the lower lumbar and buttock region may contain blackish-blue areas known as *Mongolian spots*. These are caused by large stellate pigmented cells in the deeper layers of the skin and may be mistaken for bruises or hemangiomas. They are of no clinical significance.

Head

The fronto-occipital circumference of the head of a newborn infant approximates that of the chest and abdomen; it measures a fourth of the body length. Depending on the infant's posture in utero and duration of labor and character of delivery, he may have a molded head immediately after birth. The skull molds easily because the bones are relatively soft, with pliable fibrous attachments between them. Therefore, the head molds quite like artist's clay but assumes a normal shape within the first few days of life. Less molding occurs in infants born to multiparous mothers. Overriding of one cranial bone by another is a frequent occurrence as a result of a difficult labor; it may persist for a few days following birth.

In the newborn, trauma to the skull during parturition may be manifested by *caput succedaneum* or by *cephalohematoma*. The former is an edematous swelling in the superficial tissues of the scalp of infants born head first. It is usually generalized, not bounded by the sutures, and pits on pressure. It is caused by venous obstruction of the scalp as the fetus traverses the birth passage. A cephalohematoma (Fig. 20-5) results from extravasation of blood between the periosteum and underlying skull. The trauma of birth causes separation of the

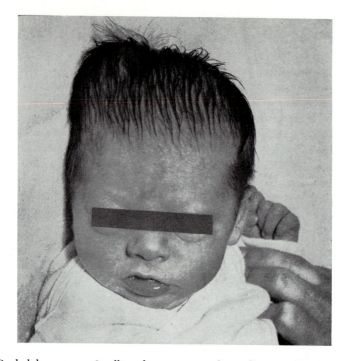

Fig. 20-5. Cephalohematoma. Swelling does not cross the midline as in caput succedaneum.

periosteum from the bone with escape of blood between the two. In contrast to caput succedaneum, the swelling never extends across sutures. It is usually detected in the first 24 hours of life and may even increase in size for a few days. The cephalohematoma may persist for weeks or months but will eventually disappear. At first the mass is soft, but with time it may become calcified. Neither the caput nor the cephalohematoma is cause for concern.

The suture lines of the skull are easily palpated as ridges until 6 months of age. The sutures are open at two areas to form the anterior and posterior fontanelles, or "soft spots." The anterior fontanelle, situated in the midline between the parietal and frontal bones at the intersection of the sagittal and coronal sutures, measures about 4 to 6 cm. in diameter at birth and slowly decreases in size until closure at about 18 months of age. The posterior fonta-

nelle is smaller than the anterior, measuring 1 to 2 cm. in diameter, and may be overlooked on physical examination. It usually closes at about 2 months of age. Delayed closure of the fontanelles may be seen in rickets, hypothyroidism, increased intracranial pressure, and certain bone disorders.

The anterior fontanelle may normally pulsate because of pulsations of the cerebral arteries. If the pulsation is marked, it may reflect intracranial disease, such as increased pressure, venous obstruction, and hydrocephalus. Tenseness of the fontanelle is most commonly seen in the crying, coughing, vomiting, or straining infant; it is abnormal if the child is quiet and in the sitting position. This observation is of great importance, since it may indicate meningitis or encephalitis, benign intracranial hypertension, and various encephalopathies, including that caused by lead intoxication. On the other hand,

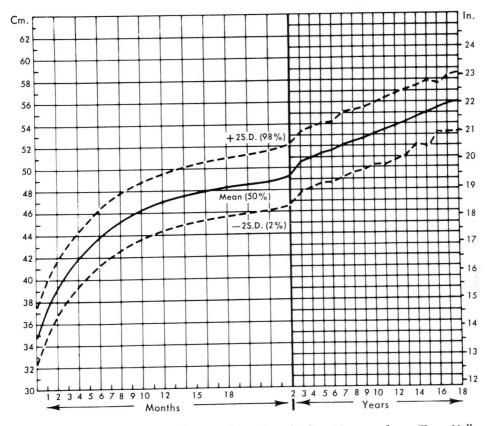

Fig. 20-6. Chart for head circumference of boys from birth to 18 years of age. (From Nell-haus, G.: Pediatrics 41:106-114, 1968.)

a depressed fontanelle usually indicates dehydration.

The newborn's scalp hair is often useful in estimating gestational age. A full-term baby will have fine silky hair, whereas an infant born at 36 weeks' gestation will have fuzzy and woolly hair.

Craniotabes are thin, parchmentlike areas in the flat bones of the skull in the neonate. Pressure over these regions elicits a crackling sound similar to that of a compressed ping pong ball and represents a softening of the outer table of the skull. This condition may be associated with several disorders, including hydrocephalus, syphilis, rickets, osteogenesis imperfecta,

and hypervitaminosis A; it may occasionally be present in normal children.

Asymmetry of the skull is usually found in children with irregular closure of the sutures. For example, a baby might have a tower skull (*turricephaly*) caused by premature closure of the coronal sutures during intrauterine life; this may be associated with cerebral agenesis, atrophy, and precocious bone growth. A long and narrow skull, often seen in premature infants, is known as *dolichocephaly*, or *scaphocephaly*; a broad cranial vault is labeled *brachycephaly*. Flattening of one side of the head may occur in an infant who lies in only one position or has unusual softening of the bones, such as occurs in rickets. *"Bossing,"* or bulging, of the frontal areas results in a square or blocky appearance of the head that may be present in prematurity, rickets, or congenital syphilis.

Inadequate or excessive growth of the head terminates in either *microcephaly* or *macrocephaly*, respectively, each with different underlying causes. Both may be recognized at birth or shortly thereafter. It is important that head circumference be measured and values recorded serially during the first 18 months (Fig. 20-6).

Auscultation of the skull to detect a bruit is of little clinical significance until late childhood because a systolic or continuous bruit may be heard over the temporal areas in normal children until early school age. Bruits heard in nonanemic older children are suggestive of an intracranial arteriovenous shunt or aneurysm or increased intracranial pressure.

Ears

The external ears should be inspected for asymmetry in size, shape, and location. The position or set of the ears is determined by drawing an imaginary line straight back from the inner and outer canthus of the eye to where the ear joins the scalp. When an ear is in the normal position, the line touches the auricle; in low-set ears, the line passes above the auricle. A small skin tag, cleft, or pit may be found just anterior to the tragus. This is a common malformation and is a remnant of the first branchial cleft.

The external canal may be absent or partially occluded by infection, malformation, or cerumen. In the examination of the newborn infant it is important to visualize the tympanic membrane. In infancy the auditory canal proceeds upward from the inside. Thus, the pinna should be pulled down gently for the best view of the tympanic membrane. In early childhood the external auditory canal is directed downward and forward from the inside. Thus, the

pinna should be gently pulled up and backward.

Use the largest speculum possible for the size of the canal in order to completely visualize the tympanic membrane of a child. The mobility of the membrane can be tested by blowing through the otoscope. A large speculum with a small segment of rubber tubing slipped over the tip will assure an airtight fit in the canal.

Hearing should be screened at various ages. At 1 month of age an infant responds to a bell rung one foot away. The common visible responses are eye blink, startle, or cessation of activity. Some babies turn their eyes in an attempt to localize the sound. By 28 weeks of age, an infant should turn his head 90 degrees to search for a quietly spoken voice. Failure to do so requires detailed evaluation of hearing and development. Formal audiometric testing can be performed with infants and older children when delays or defects in speech are noted.

Eyes

Examination of the eyes of the newborn is the most difficult portion of the entire examination because the baby's lids are usually tightly closed, especially in a lighted room. Thus, a dimly lighted room should be used. First, hold the baby upright with your hands under his axilla, supporting his head posteriorly. Rotate the baby slowly in one direction. When the baby is rotated and his head is held in the midline, his eyes will look toward the direction being moved. When the movement stops, the eyes will turn in the opposite direction following a few unsustained nystagmoid movements. This maneuver will provide the examiner with a view of the sclerae, pupils, irides and extraocular movements. Small subconjunctival and scleral hemorrhages are commonly seen in the newborn. Intermittent alternating convergent strabismus is seen frequently during the first 6 months of life. Persistence of this finding after 6 months, or divergent strabismus at any time, deserves evaluation by an ophthalmologist. Pupillary response to light during the first 3 months of life is best tested by obtaining the optical blink reflex. First, cover one eye and then uncover it. The infant will blink his eyes and dorsiflex his head in response to the bright light, demonstrating light perception. Inspect the iris for coloboma and for Brushfield's spots.

When silver nitrate drops are placed in the eyes after birth as prophylaxis against gonococcus, a chemical conjunctivitis usually occurs. This conjunctivitis is characterized by edema of the lids and purulent drainage with an inflamed conjunctiva.

Funduscopic examination should be accomplished during the first few days of life. Place the baby on his back and use a nipple if necessary to quiet him. The examiner may need to retract the lids with his thumb and first finger. The fundus can usually be seen at "0" diopters. Start by obtaining a red reflex. Normally a red or orange color is seen; a partial red reflex or a white reflex is seen with cataracts and other abnormalities of the lens and retina. The disc is paler in the newborn than in older infants and children. The funduscopic examination should be performed as in the adult.

Measured visual acuity changes with the age of the patient. During the first week of life, measured visual acuity is approximately 20/600. Visual acuity can be tested by obtaining an eye blink to bright light and by an object moved quickly toward the eye. Opticokinetic nystagmus is demonstrated by the rapid movement of a cloth with vertical black lines across the visual fields. By 1 year of age the measured visual acuity is 20/200, 20/30 at 3 years, and 20/20 at 5. Thus vision, as it can be measured, seems to improve up to about 5 years of age when most normal children have a measured acuity of 20/20.

In the preschool-aged child checking for amblyopia is the most important part of the routine eye examination because it has a high frequency rate, and early detection and treatment provide for the best prognosis. Both visual acuity and muscle weakness (strabismus) must be tested as described in Chapter 10.

Nose

The nose does not usually grow as rapidly as does the rest of the face. Therefore, a small nose in infancy probably will remain small until adolescence. The saddle nose of syphilis, acrocephaly, or cretinism is easily recognized.

During delivery the septal cartilage may be displaced, producing nasal obstruction. If recognized within the first week, it can be easily replaced. Patency of the posterior choanae of a newborn infant should be ascertained by passing a small rubber catheter through the nose into the pharynx. Also, patency can be determined by holding the baby's mouth closed and alternately occluding each naris. A normal baby can breath comfortably through the unoccluded or patent naris. With choanal atresia or other conditions that block the passage of air through the nose, the infant is visibly distressed during this maneuver.

Flaring movements of the nares should be looked for since they are found in all types of respiratory distress. Next, the color of the mucosa of the nose should be observed. A red, inflamed mucosa indicates infection; and a boggy, blue mucosa may indicate allergy. Note the color and character of the nasal secretions. If unilateral purulent secretions are seen in a preschooler, look for a foreign body!

Mouth breathing may be caused by enlarged adenoids. The presence of enlarged vessels over the anterior part of the septum in Kiesselbach's triangle, if accompanied by dryness of the mucosa, can result in repeated attacks of epistaxis. Cleft palate and cleft lip will produce distinct asymmetry of the corresponding nasal orifice. Mongolism is accompanied by lack of development of the nasal bones; during the first few months of life, a roentgenogram of the skull shows this characteristic lack of development.

Mouth

In the newborn the movement of the mouth and lips with crying should be observed carefully as evidence of facial paralysis. The lower jaw may be poorly developed (Andy Gump type) or may be grossly underdeveloped as in micrognathia (Fig. 20-7). In the newborn infant micrognathia usually requires some corrective or supportive apparatus to prevent suffocation.

Next, open the mouth with a small tongue blade laid on the tongue just off the midline. The hard and soft palates should be complete

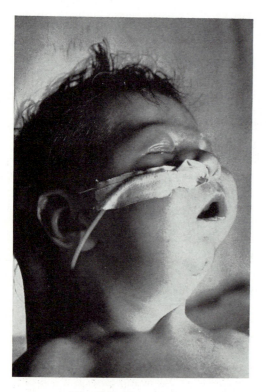

Fig. 20-7. Micrognathia.

in the midline, and the uvula should be single. Small, white pinhead-sized cysts, called Epstein's pearls, frequently are seen along the midline of the hard palate, and are collections of retained secretions, which spontaneously disappear in infancy.

Observe the buccal mucosa for thrush. These white plaques cover the oral mucosa, do not wipe off, and are a common type of monilial infection acquired from mothers with vaginal moniliasis. Next examine the tongue and the frenulum. As long as the tongue can touch the alveolar ridge there will be no impairment with feeding or with speech.

In older children the mouth examination should be performed as in adults. However, special emphasis should be directed toward the teeth and tonsils.

The teeth are inspected for number, order of dentition, caries, alveolar abscesses, and the state of occlusion ("overshot" upper jaw, "undershot" lower jaw, or "rocking bite"). Malocclusion should be carefully observed, since it may impair speech and breathing and lead to frequent upper respiratory infections. Teeth may be notched, peglike, or spotted with yellow or brown deposits. The frenum of the upper lip may be attached low between the two upper central incisors, producing varying degrees of separation. This condition can be corrected by orthodontia.

After inspection of the mouth, the pharynx should be examined. The tonsils should be inspected for size, crypts, abscesses, and infection. The tonsils, being part of the lymphatic system, are proportionately larger in the growing child than in the adult. Tonsillar enlargement may affect swallowing and eating, and at times may be so great that there is interference with proper oral breathing. An adenoid mass that is located on the posterior nasopharynx above the level of the soft palate may occasionally be visualized to a slight extent when the oropharynx is exposed. Excessive mouth breathing is nearly always indicative of adenoid hypertrophy and is associated frequently with serous otitis media. Nasal quality of the voice is another clue to hypertrophied adenoids.

Larynx

When there are voice changes or stridor, the larynx should be observed directly for evidence of paralysis, inflammation, and obstruction. Stridor is fairly common in the young infant and is usually caused by lack of maturation of the cartilages of the epiglottis, the larynx, and at times the tracheal rings. Stridor is loudest when the infant is at rest and disappears during crying or straining, when the immature structures are supported firmly by muscle contraction. If associated with hoarseness, stridor usually is caused by vocal cord paralysis, inflammation, edema, or tumor in the glottic area.

Attention should always be given to the voice. Is it nasal, muffled, mushy, highpitched, or low pitched? In the young infant the quality of the cry may be quite significant. Hoarseness is an indication of disease of the larynx.

Neck

The neck should be inspected for symmetry, masses, and abnormal structures. Shortening of one sternomastoid muscle may result from inflammation, pain, or masses, with resulting temporary or permanent *torticollis*. A hematoma of the sternomastoid muscle, first seen at 2 to 8 days of life and usually complicating a breech delivery, may become fibromatous. Surgical treatment may be necessary within the first few months to prevent a permanent wryneck.

Deep cervical lymphadenitis associated with a lateral or retropharyngeal abscess may produce little superficial swelling, but may cause much pain and limitation of motion with the head held in a fixed position. Superficial adenitis, which may occur in any group of the cervical lymph glands, usually appears rapidly and resolves slowly. In mumps *(epidemic parotitis)* the bulk of the swelling is above and in front of a line connecting the angle of the jaw with the tip of the mastoid process, whereas in cervical adenitis the swelling is below this line.

The isthmus of the thyroid gland is occasionally palpable below the larynx, with the lateral lobes felt on either side. The asthenic child with the long neck and a drooping "debutante" posture may thrust the neck forward, producing a false appearance of an enlarged thyroid.

Cysts or sinuses in the neck may be the result of embryonic rests from gill arches or clefts. Branchiogenic sinuses or cysts are located at the anterior border of the sternomastoid muscle; in contrast, thyroglossal duct sinuses or cysts occur in the midline and move when the patient swallows.

Chest

Examination of the chest of infants and young children should be performed early in the general examination, since examination of the head and neck especially may provoke crying and resistance. An apprehensive child may be examined in the mother's lap or when held on her shoulder (Fig. 20-8).

Inspection. The newborn infant's thorax is nearly circular and relatively short, in contrast to his abdomen (Fig. 20-9). With age this proportion approaches that of an adult. Abnormality may be present in the form of a flat, barrel-shaped, pigeon-breasted, flaring, or funnel-shaped chest. *Pectus excavatum* (funnel chest) is a congenital depression of the sternum and costal cartilages that is accentuated during inspiration. The deformity may be sufficient to cause significant cardiac or respiratory embarrassment or both, and surgical correction may be indicated. Occasionally the chest may become asymmetric as the result of absence of external musculature, collapse or surgical removal of a lobe or lung, fibrothorax, or cardiac enlargement forcing the ribs outward in the

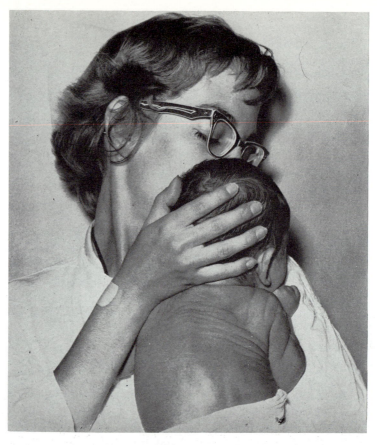

Fig. 20-8. Upright position for examination of the infant's chest.

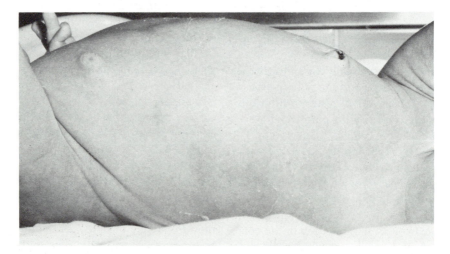

Fig. 20-9. Nearly circular and relatively short thorax in the newborn infant, in contrast to abdomen.

precordial area. The anteroposterior diameter often is increased in chronic obstructive lung disease.

The tip of the xyphoid cartilage may be felt normally as a rather sharp point in the epigastrium of the young infant. The enlargement of the chondrocostal junctions that occurs in rickets, syphilis, and scurvy may be seen. The presence of *dilated* veins over the lower thoracic wall suggests superficial collateral circulation caused by portal hypertension. Nondilated veins are frequently observed on the thorax and abdomen in healthy children.

In the newborn, premature, and young infant, normal respiration is mainly abdominal. Abnormal forms of respiration, such as meningitic, periodic, and paradoxical, should be noted. In addition, the examiner should observe for signs of retraction or bulging of the intercostal, suprasternal, and supraclavicular regions, which are indicative of inspiratory or expiratory obstruction. The respiratory rate should be recorded in the presence of dyspnea or hyperpnea.

The breasts of newborn infants of either sex may be slightly enlarged, and even a small amount of secretion may be present as a result of estrogenic stimulation from the mother. At 8 to 11 years of age, the breasts of girls begin to enlarge, and this enlargement is usually accompanied by some tenderness. Normal breast enlargement may occur as early as 4 to 5 years of age in females who are hypersensitive to small amounts of estrogen. Abnormal precocious development also occurs in adrenocortical imbalance. In early adolescence girls and, not infrequently, boys will show tender hypertrophy of breast tissue. Early breast development is frequently asymmetric.

Palpation. Tenderness, masses, and defects of bony structures may be detected by palpation. The smooth enlargement of chondrocostal junctions seen in rickets (*rachitic rosary*) may be differentiated from the sharp, bayonet type

of enlargement found in *scorbutic rosary*. The examiner should palpate for tactile fremitus and friction rubs, as noted in Chapter 12. The extent and symmetry of lateral movements of the chest should be determined.

Percussion. The chest wall of the infant is substantially more resonant than that of the adult, so percussion should be light to better appreciate the variations of sounds produced. Direct percussion on the chest wall is sometimes a better method to delineate dullness or other changes in the chest of neonates and small children (Fig. 20-10). Any decrease in resonance detected over the lung fields of an infant is of the same importance as dullness or flatness in the adult.

Auscultation. Utmost cooperation is necessary to obtain satisfactory information from this procedure. The young child may be engaged in a game of counting, talking, and "blowing out" the otoscope light in lieu of direct instructions for deep breathing or coughing. When prolonged deep breathing is necessary, it should be alternated with periods of rest. The stethoscope head should be relatively small in order to localize the source of the sounds. The bell type with soft rubber margins is preferable to the diaphragm type, since the latter frequently will not make complete contact with a small curved chest wall. The breath sounds of the infant and young child are relatively louder than those of the adult because the stethoscope is closer to the origin of the sounds. Also, infant breath sounds are normally characterized as being bronchovesicular. There may be alteration of breath sounds with changing positions. Thus, the young infant should be examined in both the upright and supine positions. The grunting respirations of dyspnea and the presence and variation of breath sounds are noted. Vocal resonance may be detected during crying or during conversation with the child.

The stethoscope head may be held in front of the infant's mouth as a means of determining

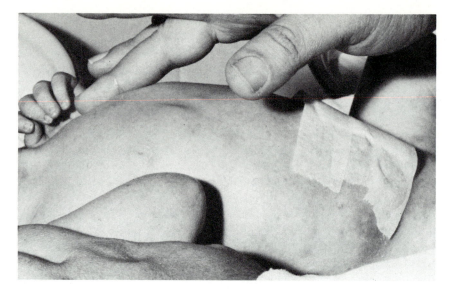

Fig. 20-10. Direct percussion on the chest wall.

relative air exchange and evidence of hyperpnea; rhonchi can also be heard by this technique, but rales cannot.

Pulse

The pulse rate of the healthy neonate is about 120 beats per minute but may vary from 80 to 160 per minute. It gradually falls to 80 to 90 per minute by 7 to 9 years of age. The rate varies greatly with fever, emotional tension, and exercise. Sinus arrhythmia is a normal observation in the infant and child. The palpation of pulses in all extremities should be a routine procedure. Weak pulses in the arms and legs suggest an obstruction to left ventricular blood flow, whereas bounding pulses are typical of a patent ductus arteriosis. Femoral pulses are palpated along the inguinal ligament midway between the iliac crest and the symphysis pubis. Absence of pulsations in the femoral arteries, in the presence of pulses in the brachial arteries connotes coarctation of the aorta.

Blood pressure

Blood pressure reading is an important procedure; the technique varies with the size of the child. The cuff size is essential to the accuracy of the reading. It should be not more than two thirds or less than one half the length of the upper arm. In a facility where many ages of children are seen, standard cuff sizes of $2\frac{1}{2}$ inches, 5 inches, 8 inches, and 12 inches should be available. The child should be sitting, and the arm should be at heart level. Table 20-3 provides a chart of normal blood pressure readings for different ages.

Thigh blood pressures also may be valuable and should be taken in a patient with cardiac disease and when femoral pulses are thought to be abnormal. In a child under 1 year, the systolic thigh pressure should be equal to that in the arms. After that age it may be 10 to 40 mm. Hg higher. The diastolic pressure should always be the same. If it is lower, coarctation should be suspected.

In children under 1 year of age, the blood

Table 20-3. Normal blood pressure for various ages

Ages	Mean systolic ± 2 S.D.	Mean diastolic ± 2 S.D.
Newborn	80 ± 16	46 ± 16
6 months to 1 year	89 ± 29	60 ± 10*
1 year	96 ± 30	66 ± 25*
2 years	99 ± 25	64 ± 25*
3 years	100 ± 25	67 ± 23*
4 years	99 ± 20	65 ± 20*
5 to 6 years	94 ± 14	55 ± 9
6 to 7 years	100 ± 15	56 ± 8
7 to 8 years	102 ± 15	56 ± 8
8 to 9 years	105 ± 16	57 ± 9
9 to 10 years	107 ± 16	57 ± 9
10 to 11 years	111 ± 17	58 ± 10
11 to 12 years	113 ± 18	59 ± 10
12 to 13 years	115 ± 19	59 ± 10
13 to 14 years	118 ± 19	60 ± 10

From Haggerty, R. J., Maroney, M. W., and Nadas, A. S.: Essential hypertension in infancy and childhood, Am. J. Dis. Child. **92**:536, 1956; copyright 1956, American Medical Association.
*In this study the point of muffling was taken as the diastolic pressure.

pressure is best taken by the flush method. Elevate the arm and wrap it in an elastic bandage to drain the blood from it. The blood pressure cuff is then applied and inflated, and the arm is lowered. Gradually deflate the cuff and note the point at which the arm distal to the cuff flushes pink. This point is the median between the systolic and diastolic readings and is called the flush blood pressure.

Heart

The examination of the heart in infants and children is conducted as described in Chapter 14 with a few exceptions. The first exception is the location of the apical impulse (PMI). In normal infants and children the PMI is frequently visible in the fourth intercostal space to the left of the midclavicular line until age 7, when it is then located in the fifth intercostal space to the right of the midclavicular line. In the newborn and infant the heart percusses relatively larger because of its more horizontal position and because of the thymus located at the base of the heart.

Almost all children, particularly teenagers, normally have sinus arrhythmia. Occasional runs of premature ventricular contractions are quite common in childhood and are of no clinical significance.

Recognition of the innocent murmur is another important aspect of the pediatric cardiac examination. Approximately half or more of all children have an innocent murmur during childhood. The innocent murmur is systolic, of short duration, and grade 3 or less in intensity. It is usually loudest in either the second or third intercostal space along the left sternal border. It sounds low pitched, musical, and groaning in quality. It is poorly transmitted and varies in its intensity and presence with position, respiration, and activity. It is an asymptomatic finding and is associated with no other signs of cardiovascular disease.

The final unique feature of this examination is the most difficult for the student to appreciate. The hearts sounds in infants and children are louder because of the thinner chest wall. Furthermore, S_1 is louder than S_2 at the apex. Narrow splitting of S_2 that varies with respiration can be heard in many normal children.

The heart of the newborn infant should be examined repeatedly during the first few months of life, since murmurs may not become apparent until some time after birth. If a murmur is heard at birth, the chances are one in twelve that the infant has congenital heart disease; if it persists until 1 year of age, the chances are three in five that there is a heart defect. The observation of cyanosis, poor weight gain, fatigue, rapid respiration, persistent tachycardia, or stridor indicate that early and complete evaluation of the heart is necessary. Surgical correction of major heart defects is possible even in the newborn period. The generalist physician should be able to differentiate normal from abnormal findings on completion of the pediatric cardiac examination. Precise diagnosis of organic cardiac lesions is best accomplished with the assistance of a pediatric cardiologist.

Abdomen

A friendly approach, warm hands, a comfortable room, and a child relatively free of anxiety, embarrassment, and discomfort will greatly facilitate the abdominal examination. Feeding from a bottle may aid in obtaining the relaxation so essential in the examination of an infant's abdomen.

Inspection. Distention, masses, scaphoid abdomen, weakness or absence of abdominal muscles, dilated veins, and peristaltic activity should be noted. The abdomen of an infant is relatively larger than his chest. Children under 4 years of age may thus appear "pot-bellied," especially following a meal or if their ribs are flaring. True increase in size of the abdomen may be caused by enlargement of solid organs, the presence of a tumor or cyst, ascites, or congenital defects of the abdominal wall. The crying infant and the child with gastrointestinal infection may accumulate large amounts of intraluminal air, causing abdominal distention. A depressed (scaphoid) abdomen may be seen with emaciation or dehydration or with large diaphragmatic hernias. Prominent superficial abdominal veins may be seen in premature and normal small infants. Dilated veins may accompany portal hypertension, ascites, and hepatic or portal vein thrombosis. The peristaltic waves

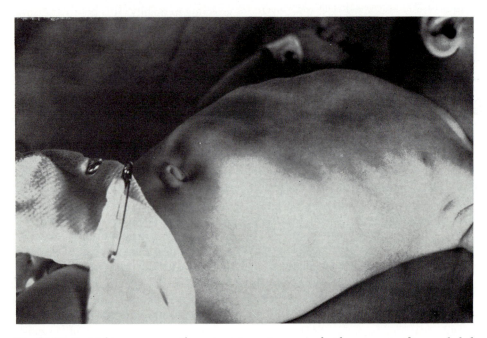

Fig. 20-11. Peristaltic waves over the epigastrium. A wave is clearly seen extending cephalad from the umbilicus.

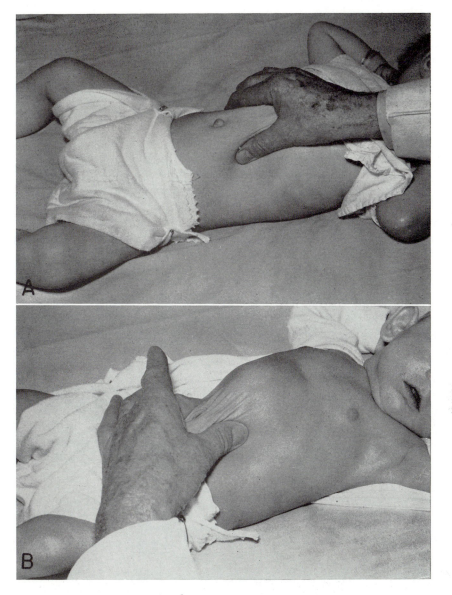

Fig. 20-12. A, Good tissue turgor. **B,** Poor tissue turgor.

of pyloric stenosis or small bowel obstruction are best observed under oblique lighting conditions (Fig. 20-11) and may be elicited by gently stroking the upper abdomen after feeding the infant several ounces of water. Prominent intestinal loops often seen in small premature babies should not cause concern.

The umbilicus of a neonate should be inspected for state of healing, vessels, discharge, granulation tissues, and protrusions. The umbilical cord ordinarily dries up by 5 days of age and sloughs off by the eighth to fourteenth day. If the cord fails to drop off by 2 weeks of age or if the navel is persistently wet or draining, one must consider the possibility of granulation tissue, omphalitis, or urachal remnant.

Defects of the abdominal wall in the midline may present as omphalocele, diastasis recti, exstrophy of the bladder, or umbilical hernia. The latter, best observed in a crying child, may vary in diameter from a few millimeters to 2 or 3 cm. They occur more often in Negro than in Caucasian children; most will disappear during the preschool years. Inguinal hernias may present as a swelling in the groin, although it is more commonly detected as a mass in the scrotum.

Palpation. The technique of laying the infant longitudinally in the lap of the parent with his legs on the examiner's knees may facilitate palpation. Regions suspected of being painful should be examined last.

The condition of the subcutaneous tissue should be determined. Dryness or loss of turgor accompany dehydration (Fig. 20-12). The general resistance of abdominal muscles may reflect overall muscular tonus. In the normal newborn one may, by superficial palpation, feel the sharp edge of the liver 1 to 2 cm. below the right costal margin. The tip of the spleen is

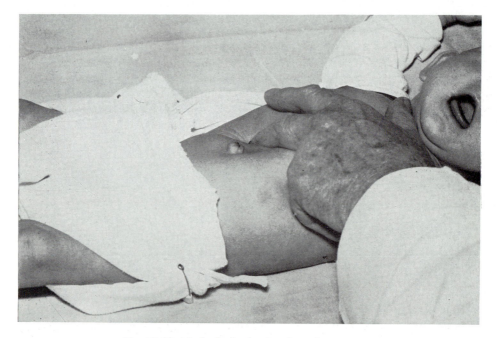

Fig. 20-13. Method of palpation for pyloric tumor.

frequently felt under the left costal margin. To avoid missing the edge of these organs, palpation should begin in the lower quadrants and progress cephalad.

Deeper palpation may reveal masses, which should be described as to size, location, consistency, contour, mobility or fixation, tenderness, and ability to transilluminate. By deep palpation one may normally feel the kidneys, especially in a thin infant. The tumor of pyloric stenosis is best palpated with the fingertips in the angle formed by the lateral margin of the right rectus muscle and the lower margin of the liver (Fig. 20-13) or at the point where visible peristaltic waves disappear. The right upper quadrant is a common, but not constant, location for the sausage-shaped tumor of intussusception. A distended urinary bladder may present as a suprapubic mass.

Percussion, auscultation, and transillumination. Percussion may be used to outline the boundaries of the liver, spleen, and tumors; and it may be helpful in the diagnosis of intestinal obstruction, peritonitis, and ascites. Auscultation of bowel sounds should be carried out prior to palpation, while the child is quiet. Transillumination with a strong light may help differentiate solid from cystic masses.

Anorectal area

The anorectal area is examined routinely in infants and children, but rectal examination is reserved for individuals with diagnostic problems, intra-abdominal complaints, or neurologic disorders.

The infant is placed in the prone position with the legs adducted and extended; fullness and symmetry of the buttocks and gluteal folds are noted (decrease in muscle mass or asymmetry may indicate chronic disease or a dislocated hip, respectively). The buttocks are then separated; the lower back is observed for sacrococcygeal dimple, sinus, and masses; and the anus is observed for fissure, polyps, and prolapse.

The rectal examination of infants, preschool, and school-aged children is best done with the child in the supine position. The feet should be kept together in the midline and the knees should be flexed while the gloved and lubricated index finger is slowly introduced into the rectum. Then the other hand is placed on the abdomen to conduct a bimanual examination. The index finger is preferred for rectal examination, but in some infants the fifth finger must be used.

Imperforate anus or stenosis is immediately evident. Sphincter tone is noted. A shelflike protuberance 2 to 3 cm. above the anus may be felt in megacolon. Masses, tenderness, the pea-sized prostate, the cervix, and the character of stool are noted. Imperforate anus in the female is always accompanied by a genitovesical fistula.

Genitalia

The foreskin of the newborn male is adherent to the glans penis and almost completely covers it. The foreskin does not retract over the glans until the infant is several months of age and then only if it has been retracted on a regular basis. The distal urethral opening should always be observed as part of the newborn examination and before circumcision is performed. If the urethral opening is not centrally located on the tip of the glans, the ventral and dorsal surfaces of the glans and the shaft of the penis should be examined for hypospadias and epispadias. The foreskin is incompletely formed in these congenital malformations. The testes are normally located in the scrotum or can be easily milked down from the inguinal canal into the scrotum. If the testes are not palpable or cannot be moved down out of the canal, the boy should sit in a crosslegged, tailor's position. The inguinal canal and scrotum should then be re-examined for the testes. If the testes are still not in the scrotum, undescended testes are diagnosed. Hydroceles are common in boys under 2 years of age and are often associated with an inguinal hernia. If the mass (except the testes) transilluminates when a light is shown through it and is irreducible, this is a hydrocele. A hydrocele is asymptomatic and nontender. Next, the examination for the presence of an inguinal hernia is performed in the same manner as in an adult.

In the newborn female the labia minora are prominent, and the labia majora are small; thus, the clitoris appears prominent. The labia minora quickly recede in size and are almost nonexistent until puberty. A mucoid or sanguineous vaginal discharge usually is present in the first week of life. The physician should observe the urethral and vaginal orifices (hymenal skin tags are normal). Adhesions or fusion of the labia minora may be seen during the first 2 or 3 years with ventral displacement of the posterior fourchette, which covers the vaginal or urethral openings or both. Profuse vaginal discharge may be caused by a foreign body, infection, or tumor. Vaginal examination is not performed routinely in childhood or during adolescence. Until a girl has reached puberty the vagina may be visualized easily when the patient is in the knee-chest position.

Musculoskeletal

At birth, the full-term newborn normally assumes a position of flexion with some limitation of extension of the major joints of the extremities. This results from the intrauterine position and subsides spontaneously in the early weeks of life. Frequently the feet appear malformed when they retain their intrauterine positioning. However, when the malposition is only temporary, the foot and ankle can be easily rotated into a normal or neutral position. With a true clubfoot, the foot cannot be rotated into any other position. All newborns have some bowing of their legs for the first weeks of life because of the intrauterine position. There may be further apparent bowing at 6 to 8 months of age, as a result of the development of the peroneal muscle. When the child begins to walk, bowing is often quite visible because the toddler stands with his toes turned in, his knees and thighs slightly flexed, and his gastrocnemius muscles turned out. The bowlegged growth pattern begins to disappear at 18 months of age when a transition from bowlegs to knock-knees occurs. This appearance lasts until adolescence, when the legs tend to straighten out.

All infants under 1 year of age are apparently flatfooted as a result of the fat pad in the longitudinal arch. This condition disappears at about 18 to 30 months of age.

The hips should be examined carefully for evidence of congenital dislocation. The baby is placed on his back with his legs pointing toward the examiner. The legs are flexed at the knee to form a right angle and then both legs are abducted until the lateral aspect of each knee touches the table. When a congenital dislocation exists, the femoral head lies posterior to the acetabulum, and this maneuver will cause the head to "click" as it rotates in and out of the acetabulum. This procedure is called Ortolani's test, and the "click" is Ortolani's sign. After the newborn period, as muscle strength about the hip increases, the "click" may be difficult to elicit but decreased abduction of one or both legs will be present when a congenital dislocation exists. Leg symmetry should also be noted and may be easily checked by placing the child on a flat surface with his legs and thighs flexed and his heels close to his buttocks. Asymmetry in the relative height of the knees is indicative of a short leg.

In school-aged children the presence of musculoskeletal problems can often be detected by careful observation of the child walking, stooping to recover an object from the floor, and rising from the supine position on the floor. When rising from the floor is observed, the examiner should note the manner in which the child reaches the sitting position and then the standing position. Muscular weakness can be detected in this manner.

In adolescence, especially in adolescent girls, the position of the spine should be carefully noted. A lateral curvature of the spine (scoliosis) can be detected in its earliest stages by having the child bend forward while the examiner marks a vertical line with a felt tipped pen along the spinous processes. With this visible line a straight or a curved spine will be apparent. Some adolescents may have a "fatigue," or drooping, posture as a result of an anterior curvature (kyphosis).

Neurologic system

The neurologic examination of infants and children begins when the examiner has his initial contact with the child. For example, a 2-year-old child is unable to follow the commands for some portions of a formal neurologic examination, but watching this same child as he spies a small piece of paper on the floor about 3 feet away, runs over, picks it up with a neat pincer grasp, and turning to his parent clearly says, "Mommy, see paper?" provides a great deal of information about the child's neurologic system. From age 1 month to 6 years a developmental test, such as the Denver Developmental Screening Test, should always be used in conjunction with a formal neurologic examination since they are complementary. When both are used, a more complete and accurate picture of the developing child is obtained. While older children and adolescents can be examined in the same manner as adults, the newborn, infant, and toddler are best tested by observing characteristic posture, spontaneous activity, and play activity that are then compared to standardized norms of development.

The newborn neurologic examination is unique because the central nervous system is incompletely developed and operates at subcortical levels. Cortical function develops slowly after birth and is better tested in early childhood. Thus, the newborn neurologic examination reflects brain stem and spinal cord activity.

The newborn's reflex behavior is the basis for the examination. The startle or Moro reflex is elicited by any stimulus that suddenly moves the head in relation to the spine or is perceived by the newborn as being noxious or frightening (Fig. 20-14). The reflex may be elicited by holding the baby in the supine position supporting head, back, and legs then suddenly lowering the baby 2 feet and stopping abruptly, by jarring the bed, or by making a loud sound. The reflex disappears between 4 and 6 months of age, and its persistence is an abnormal neurologic sign. In addition this reflex provides the examiner with a good view of how the baby moves his arms, since with a brachial plexus injury or fractured clavicle the response is asymmetric.

The *tonic neck* reflex is elicited by turning the infant's head sharply to one side, which causes the ipsilateral arm and leg to extend and the contralateral arm and leg to flex. This reflex may be absent at birth, but will appear by 2 months only to disappear again between 4 and 6 months if normal maturation of the central nervous system is occurring.

To elicit the *palmar grasp* reflex the examiner's index fingers are placed from the ulnar side into the baby's hands and pressed against the palmar surfaces. A positive response is flexion of all of the fingers with equal strength in both hands. This grasp reflex disappears by 3 to 4 months; persistence after 4 months suggests cerebral dysfunction, as does persistence of the fisted hand in an infant after 2 months. Extension of the thumb and fingers second, third, and fourth is elicited by stroking the ul-

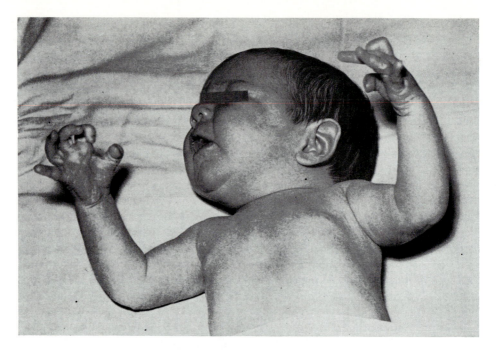

Fig. 20-14. Moro or startle reflex.

nar side of the hand and the fifth finger. The deep tendon reflexes are variable, and their presence or absence is of little significance.

The *rooting* reflex is demonstrated by placing the infant's head in the midline with his hands held against his anterior chest. The examiner then strokes the perioral skin at the corners of the mouth and the midline of upper and lower lips. When the corner is stroked, the infant's mouth opens and turns toward the stroked side. When the upper lip is stroked, the head retroflexes and when the lower lip is stimulated, the jaw drops. This reflex disappears at 3 or 4 months of age.

The neurologic examination of the newborn should include observation of the infant's spontaneous and induced movements and performance of rooting, grasp, Moro, and tonic neck reflexes. Also the physician should listen to the infant's cry. If abnormalities exist in the results

of any of these procedures, a full assessment of the infant's neurologic system should follow.

The absence of nuchal rigidity is of little diagnostic value in infants under 12 to 15 months of age. At this age lethargy, vomiting, convulsions, and bulging of the fontanelle are much more significant and indicate examination of the spinal fluid and central nervous system.

Older children. If the child's mental development and nervous system maturation are normal, he will present the reflex pattern of the adult with comparable interpretations. Gait should be considered a reflex. The infant beginning to walk independently at 12 to 15 months of age normally has a broadly based gait. Persistence or reappearance of this type of gait is indicative of gross central nervous system disease. The "scissors" gait of the spastic child is easily detected. Occasionally, normal small children run on their toes, but this is most likely to be observed in children with spasticity, mental retardation, or in association with the clumsiness of poor nutritional states.

SELECTED READINGS

Barness, L. A.: Manual of pediatric physical diagnosis, Chicago, 1966, Year Book Medical Publishers, Inc.

Barnett, H. L.: Holt's pediatrics, ed. 14, New York, 1968, Appleton-Century-Crofts.

Dubowitz, L. M. S., Dubowitz, V., and Goldberg, C.: Clinical assessment of gestational age in the newborn infant. J. Pediatr. **77**:1, 1970.

Frankenburg, W. K.: The Denver developmental screening test, Dev. Med. Child Neurol. **11**:260-262, 1969.

Haggerty, R. J., Maroney, M. W., and Nadas, A. S.: Essential hypertension in infancy and childhood, Am. J. Dis. Child. **92**:536, 1956.

Hammer, S. L.: The approach to the adolescent patient, Pediatr. Clin. North Am. **20**(4):779-788, 1973.

Heald, Felix P.: Growth and development in adolescence. In Wallace, Gold, and Lis., editors: Maternal and child health practice, Springfield, Ill., 1973, Charles C Thomas, Publisher, pp. 827-829.

Hoekelman, R. A.: Section on pediatric physical diagnosis. In B. A. Bates, ed.: A guide to physical examination, Philadelphia, 1974, J. B. Lippincott Co., p. 375.

Holt, L. B.: Pediatric ophthalmology, Philadelphia, 1964, Lea & Febiger.

Lubchenco, L. O., and others: Intrauterine growth in length and head circumference as estimated from live births at gestational ages from 26 to 42 weeks, Pediatrics **37**:403, 1966.

Nelson, W. E., Vaughan, V. C., and McKay, R. J.: Textbook of pediatrics, ed. 9, Philadelphia, 1969, W. B. Saunders Co.

Smith, D. W., and Bierman, E. L.: The biologic ages of man from conception through old age, Philadelphia, 1973, W. B. Saunders Co.

Tanner, J. M.: Growth at adolescence, ed. 2, Oxford, England, 1962, Blackwell Scientific Publications Ltd.

Tanner, J. M.: The approach to the adolescent patient, Pediatr. Clin. North Am. **20**(4):785, 1973.

CHAPTER 21

REASSURANCE

One of the most important ingredients of the therapy program that a physician renders to his patient is intangible—it cannot be seen, touched, or weighed. It is not medication to be written on a prescription pad nor a stroke of the surgeon's scalpel, and it is independent of our present-day sophisticated electronic equipment. However, its effects are frequently beneficial, at times even miraculously so. This remarkable component is the art of medicine. Often this important factor is played down in deference to the modern, more sophisticated scientific approach to the practice of medicine. Certainly it is true that the charlatan has little to offer his patient except the art of medicine. However, it must be accepted that this same charlatan frequently has a profoundly reassuring influence on his patient. Consequently by combining the art and science of medicine, an ethical, well-educated physician certainly should have an even greater influence on his patients.

We are all familiar with stories about the medicine men of the Indian tribes, grandmother's herb cure for warts (often accompanied by mystical incantations), numerous worthless but highly ballyhooed cancer cures, the notorious shrines of religious healing, and

most recently, acupuncture. While it is generally acknowledged that there is no scientific basis underlying any of these forms of therapy, they all have one common force—a strong, metaphysical form of reassurance. When human beings are sick, they are fearful of their unknown illnesses, afraid of death, concerned for their economic security and the welfare of their families, annoyed with the frustrations of illness, isolated in the strange environment of a hospital, and alone as they try to deal with their illnesses (even though family and friends are all about). In fact all of their usual fears, concerns, anxieties, and apprehensions become greatly exaggerated on a relatively basic and primitive level. All human beings desire and need to be comforted, loved, supported, and reassured. These needs become greatly magnified when people become ill.

For centuries it has been recognized that patients suffering from even the most serious illnesses often recover in spite of and at times irrespective of the various therapeutic regimens to which they are subjected. The human body possesses remarkable recuperative powers, even under the most critical conditions. In some instances recovery can be attributed to sound native defense mechanisms, in others the exact reasons for recovery are not known, Faith and courage may even be factors. As physicians, we may be inclined to credit medication for the patient's recovery when actually it may have had little or no effect.

The effectiveness of reassurance may be demonstrated by a brief discussion of a medical practice that is still employed—placebo therapy. Medical students as well as practicing physicians are well aware of the term *placebo*, which means any therapy that has no known value in the treatment of a given medical condition. For example, if the physician treats the common cold (a virus infection) with sugar pills or with penicillin, both are placebos; yet many patients are firmly convinced that penicillin is of definite benefit in curing their colds. On the other hand if the physician similarly treats streptococcus infection, the sugar pill is a placebo, whereas penicillin has definite medical value.

It is frequently observed that patients suffering from any one of many diseases are cured or greatly improved after using a placebo. The response to a placebo is not a property of the medication but instead is a function of the personality of the patient and of the effectiveness of the power of suggestion employed by his physician. The composition and quantity of the placebo are irrelevant, so long as it is not detected by the patient as being a placebo. It is the positive attitude of the physician that results in the beneficial response to a placebo. Thus, the placebo is not necessarily worthless since it may be profoundly reassuring to the patient—in fact, it may be one of the more potent forms of therapy available to the physician. At the same time it never is a substitute for accurate diagnosis and appropriate treatment skillfully applied.

The preceding serves to stress the important role of reassurance in the practice of medicine. Every patient requires reassurance to a lesser or greater degree, but for some patients reassurance may be the only treatment required in the management of their symptoms.

Reassurance begins when the physician enters the hospital or examining room. This is the physician's first introduction to the patient whose impressions depend on the physician's appearance, attitude, concern, and skill in taking the history. Patients are reassured by a physician who is neat, clean, and well-dressed, pleasant, optimistic, and courteous; who manifests an interest in and understanding of the patient's problem; and who displays an attitude of professional competence. The history is the major portion of the verbal communication between physician and patient and often is laden with significant emotional content. Consequently, it is of great importance in developing the patient's relationship with his physician. The patient readily perceives when his physician is genuinely interested in him and his health, understands his feelings, and is on his side in the battle to regain his health and with it to return to all the important roles that he must daily play in his family, business, community, and circle of friends. In this kind of physician he can have confidence and faith. On the other hand, the patient promptly senses when the physician is hurried, abrupt, and disinterested in him and his welfare.

When the physical examination is performed with confidence, obvious skill, and a sense of orderliness, it becomes a form of communication between physician and patient and clearly enhances the confidence of the patient in his physician, which is most essential to his reassurance.

Reassurance therapy involves six steps that frequently overlap:

Step 1: *Recording the standard medical history*. This is a definite indication of interest and concern for the patient's problem and for him as a person.

Step 2: *Evaluation of affect*. While taking the history the physician should be evaluating the emotional and intellectual status of the patient, observing his mannerisms and his tone of voice. The patient's affect indicates to the physician the emotional significance of his symptoms and also suggests how much reassurance will be necessary and how it may be most effectively provided. Patients are not alike and must be evaluated and managed individually.

Step 3: *Examination of the affected part.* The gentleness, thoroughness, and confidence displayed during the physical examination has a reassuring effect on the patient's estimation of the physician's ability.

Step 4: *Medical diagnosis.* As noted before, diagnosis involves an accurate assessment of the patient's problem, which in turn determines the definitive medical care to be rendered to the patient and the probable nature of his response. Arrival at a specific conclusion is definitely reassuring because for many patients living with uncertainty is even worse than dealing with the diagnosis of a fatal illness.

Step 5: *Explanation.* Although it is generally recognized that a full understandable explanation of the patient's problem is necessary for the development of confidence, it is also basic to the legal doctrine of informed consent. The patient does not need to thoroughly understand the physician's explanation in order to be reassured, but it is essential that the patient believe that the physician understands his problem, is not uncertain about the management of his case, and is sympathetic toward his cause.

Step 6: *Reassurance.* Only too frequently physicians are overheard saying to the patient, "Don't worry, you're going to be alright." To the average patient who is ill, anxious, and concerned for his welfare these are empty words with little or no impact. To convincingly reassure the patient the physician must be able to establish an accurate diagnosis, outline the treatment, and predict the prognosis as specifically as possible. The physician should stress the positive aspects of the patient's therapy, be sensitive to his fears and superstitions, and attempt to bolster the patient's morale by being as optimistic as possible.

In conclusion we do not in any sense want to deprecate or minimize the necessity of delivering the best and most modern scientific medical care possible. However, to practice complete medicine the physician must combine high-quality medical care with reassurance, with the result that the patients feel gratitude and in many instances make a more rapid recovery and have an earlier return to normal activities.

INDEX